COLPOSCOPY
Principles and Practice

An Integrated Textbook and Atlas

COLPOSCOPY
Principles and Practice

An Integrated Textbook and Atlas

2nd Edition

Barbara S. Apgar MD, MS

Professor
Department of Family Medicine
University of Michigan Medical Center
Ann Arbor, Michigan

Gregory L. Brotzman MD

Professor
Department of Family and Community
Medicine
Medical College of Wisconsin
Milwaukee, Wisconsin

Mark Spitzer MD

Professor of Clinical Obstetrics and
Gynecology
Weill Medical College of Cornell University
Chairman, Department of Obstetrics and
Gynecology
Brookdale University Hospital and Medical
Center
Brooklyn, New York

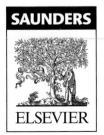

SAUNDERS

ELSEVIER

SAUNDERS
ELSEVIER

1600 John F. Kennedy Blvd.
Ste 1800
Philadelphia, PA 19103-2899

COLPOSCOPY: PRINCIPLES AND PRACTICE SECOND EDITION   ISBN: 978-1-4160-3405-6

Notice

Knowledge and best practice in this field are constantly changing. As new research and experience broaden our knowledge, changes in practice, treatment and drug therapy may become necessary or appropriate. Readers are advised to check the most current information provided (i) on procedures featured or (ii) by the manufacturer of each product to be administered, to verify the recommended dose or formula, the method and duration of administration, and contraindications. It is the responsibility of the practitioner, relying on their own experience and knowledge of the patient, to make diagnoses, to determine dosages and the best treatment for each individual patient, and to take all appropriate safety precautions. To the fullest extent of the law, neither the Publisher nor the Editors assumes any liability for any injury and/or damage to persons or property arising out of or related to any use of the material contained in this book.

The Publisher

Library of Congress Cataloging-in-Publication Data

Colposcopy, principles and practice / [edited by] Barbara S. Apgar, Gregory L. Brotzman, Mark Spitzer. – 2nd ed.
  p. ; cm.
  Includes index.
  ISBN 978-1-4160-3405-6
  1. Colposcopy–Atlases. I. Apgar, Barbara S. II. Brotzman, Gregory L.
III. Spitzer, Mark. IV. Title: Colposcopy, principles and practice.
  [DNLM: 1. Colposcopy–methods. 2. Colposcopy–Atlases. WP 250 C721 2008]

RG107.5.C6C65 2008
618.1'40754–dc22

2007030086

Acquisitions Editor: Druanne Martin
Developmental Editor: Lucia Gunzel
Project Manager: Bryan Hayward
Design Direction: Gene Harris

Working together to grow
libraries in developing countries

www.elsevier.com | www.bookaid.org | www.sabre.org

ELSEVIER   BOOK AID International   Sabre Foundation

Printed in China
Last digit is the print number: 9 8 7 6 5 4 3 2 1

To my beloved teachers, Virginia and Gloria, whose spirits continue to enrich my life; to Larisa for teaching me about rainbows; and to my caring and energetic residents, who have given me a wealth of fond memories over the years.

B.A.

To my mother Mary Brotzman, whose love and support helped me along the way as I pursued a career in medicine. To my children, Ethan, Isaac, Elyse, Isaiah and Eliana, who continue to love and support me and bring me joy; and most of all, to my wife Cindy, my love and my friend.

G.B.

To my beloved parents, Sam and Miriam Spitzer, of blessed memory, who sacrificed everything for their children's happiness and success; to my wonderful daughters, Gila, Ayelet, and Elkie; and, most of all, to my beloved wife and partner through life, Peri, without whose love and understanding this book could not have happened twice.

M.S.

Contents

Preface

It has been a pleasure and honor to complete the second edition of this colposcopy textbook and atlas. Since the first edition, knowledge about human papillomavirus (HPV) continues to emerge, especially in special populations. Although colposcopy has been practiced for more than 50 years and its place in the management of women with cytological abnormalities is well established, recent studies have shed new light on our understanding of this procedure and its role in the care of our patients. Cytology, HPV DNA testing, colposcopy and surgical excision have each evolved and now both compete with and complement each other. The Consensus Guidelines for the management of cervical cytological and histological abnormalities sought to find a clinical balance between these modalities and were revised in 2006 by the American Society for Colposcopy and Cervical Pathology (ASCCP). Colposcopic principles and practice are evolving. Practitioners from various disciplines are training in colposcopy and including it in their practice. This integrated textbook and atlas provides a modern framework for all students and practitioners of the art and science of colposcopy. This second edition is written to put these advances within easy reach for all our colleagues.

A comprehensive textbook and atlas is not possible, especially a second edition, without the help of countless individuals. In our search for authors for this edition, we looked not just for experts in the field, but rather to those national and international thought leaders whose research and clinical practice initiatives have defined and shaped the field.

One of the stumbling blocks in writing a colposcopy textbook is the large number of high-quality images needed to illustrate each clinical condition. Without the awesome and superb assistance of Mr. Fred Kostecki, president of National Testing Laboratories (NTL), we would not have been able to publish the first or second edition. Fred spent innumerable hours selecting the best Cervigrams from NTL's extensive collection. His extraordinary generosity enabled Dr. Brotzman to successfully digitalize and format the exceptional images in our books.

In addition to Mr. Kostecki, we want to gratefully thank our colleagues, Federico M. di Paola, MD, and Vesna Kesic,

MD, PhD, for allowing us to use their Cervigrams. They provided invaluable assistance. Mr. John R. Voelz, Audiovisual Specialist at Columbia—St. Mary's Hospital, Milwaukee, Wisconsin, helped in obtaining images of procedures and photofinishing pathology sections.

Two pathologists provided immeasurable help in selecting and labeling cytologic and histologic images. We would like to thank Edward J. Wilkinson, MD, Professor of Pathology and Laboratory Medicine at the University of Florida, Gainesville, Florida, and Joseph Novak, MD, Staff Pathologist, North Shore Pathologists, Milwaukee, Wisconsin, who selected appropriate pathology material for the book.

Our goal with the second edition is to provide an updated comprehensive and practical guide to colposcopic practice. We are deeply appreciative of all those who helped make the first and second edition a reality.

I would like to especially thank the individuals who taught and mentored me in my colposcopic practice. Thanks to my chairman, Thomas L. Schwenk, MD, who has supported me during the writing of both books. Most of all, I want to acknowledge the extraordinary efforts of my coeditors, Greg and Mark. Special and heartfelt thanks go to Greg for his uncanny and masterful ability to process the images and to Mark for his precise and brilliant editing and always sage advice. B.A.

A special thanks to my colleagues at the Medical College of Wisconsin—Columbia St. Marys Family Practice Residency Program, who helped and supported me through this project, and to my editorial partners, Barbara and Mark, who helped make this book a reality. G.B.

In life, the difference between success and failure is often the presence of others who assist or enable an individual to reach his/her goals. I would like to thank Burton A. Krumholz, MD, who has been my colposcopy mentor, and Vicki L. Seltzer, MD, who has been enormously supportive and enabled me to achieve my career goals. Finally, I would like to thank Barbara and Greg for allowing me to join them in this wonderful endeavor. M.S.

Barbara S. Apgar, MD, MS
Gregory L. Brotzman, MD
Mark Spitzer, MD

List of Contributors

Barbara S. Apgar, MD, MS
Professor, Department of Family Medicine, University of Michigan Medical Center, Ann Arbor, Michigan
Principles & Technique of the Colposcopic Exam; Abnormal Transformation Zone; Vagina: Normal, Premalignant, and Malignant; Practical Therapeutic Options for Treatment of Cervical Intraepithelial Neoplasia

Dorothy Barbo, MD
Professor of Obstetrics and Gynecology, Director of the Center for Women's Health at the University of New Mexico, Albuquerque
Colposcopic Assessment Systems: Rubin and Barbo Colposcopic Assessment System

J. Michael Berry, MD
Asst. Clinical Professor, Department of Medicine (Hematology/Oncology), University of California, San Francisco, San Francisco, California
Anal Disease

Gregory L. Brotzman, MD
Professor, Department of Family and Community Medicine, Medical College of Wisconsin, Milwaukee, Wisconsin
Principles & Technique of the Colposcopic Exam; Abnormal Transformation Zone; Vagina: Normal, Premalignant, and Malignant; Psychosocial Aspects of Colposcopy; Practical Therapeutic Options for Treatment of Cervical Intraepithelial Neoplasia

Darron R. Brown, MD
Professor of Medicine, Microbiology, and Immunology, Indiana University School of Medicine, Indianapolis, Indiana
Human Papillomaviruses and Mechanisms Of Oncogenesis

Dennis J. Butler, PhD
Professor of Family Medicine, Medical College of Wisconsin, Milwaukee, Wisconsin; Clinical Assistant Professor, University of Wisconsin Medical School, Madison, Wisconsin
Psychosocial Aspects of Colposcopy

Teresa M. Darragh, MD
Professor of Clinical Pathology, Departments of Pathology and Ob/Gyn, Mt. Zion Medical Center, University of California, San Francisco, San Francisco, California
Anal Disease

Diane Davis Davey, MD, FCAP
Professor of Pathology and Assistant Dean, University of Central Florida, Orlando, Florida
Terminology in Cervical Cytology: The Bethesda System

Peter A. Drew, MD, FCAP
Department of Pathology, Immunology and Laboratory Medicine, University of Florida College of Medicine, Gainesville, Florida
Conventional Cytology

Juan Felix, MD
Professor of Pathology and Obstetrics and Gynecology, USC Keck School of Medicine, Los Angeles, California
Thin-layer, Liquid-Based Cytology

Alex Ferenczy, MD
Professor of Pathology and Obstetrics and Gynecology, McGill University and the Sir Mortimer B. Davis-Jewish General Hospital, Montreal, Quebec, Canada
Vulvar Intraepithelial Neoplasia; External Genital Condyloma

Stanley A. Gall, MD
Professor of Obstetrics, Gynecology & Women's Health, Department of Obstetrics, Gynecology & Women's Health, Professor of Public Health and Information Science, University of Louisville, Louisville, Kentucky
Human Papillomavirus Vaccine

Naomi Jay, RN, NP, MSN
Dysplasia Clinic, University of California, San Francisco, San Francisco
Anal Disease

Jose Jeronimo, MD
Associate Director I, Program for Appropriate Technology in Health (PATH), Seattle, Washington
Epidemiology Applied to Colposcopy

Raymond H. Kaufman, MD
Professor Emeritus, Dept of OB/GYN Baylor College of Medicine, Professor, Dept of OB/GYN, Houston, Texas; Weill Medical College of Cornell University, New York, New York; The Methodist Hospital, Houston, Texas
Lower Genital Tract Changes Associated with In-Utero Exposure to Diethylstilbestrol

Neal M. Lonky, MD, MPH
Department of OB/GYN, Kaiser Anaheim, Anaheim, California; Director, Southern California Permanente Medical Group, Anaheim, California; Clinical Professor, UC Irvine School of Medicine, Irvine, California
Cervical Screening with in Vivo and in Vitro Modalities: Speculoscopy Combined with Cytology

Attila T. Lorincz, PhD
Professor of Molecular Epidemiology, Cancer Research UK Centre of Epidemiology, Mathematics and Statistics, Wolfson Institute of Preventive Medicine, Barts and The London School of Medicine, London, United Kingdom
Human Papillomavirus Testing

Lynette J. Margesson, MD, FRCPC
Assistant Professor of Medicine (Dermatology) and Obstetrics and Gynecology, Dartmouth Medical School, Hanover, New Hampshire
Non-Neoplastic Epithelial Lesions of the Vulva

L. Stuart Massad, MD
Professor of Obstetrics and Gynecology, Division of Gynecologic Oncology, Washington University School of Medicine, St. Louis, MO
High-Grade Squamous Intraepithelial Lesions

Anna-Barbara Moscicki, MD
Professor of Pediatrics, Associate Director, Division of Adolescent Medicine, University of California, San Francisco, California
Human Papillomavirus Infections in Adolescents

Dennis M. O'Connor, MD, FACOG, FCAP
CPA Lab, Louisville, Kentucky; Clinical Associate Professor, Departments of Obstetrics and Gynecology, and Pathology, University of Louisville School of Medicine, Louisville, Kentucky
Normal Transformation Zone

Joel M. Palefsky, M.D.
Associate Dean for Clinical and Translational Research; Professor, Laboratory Medicine and Medicine; Member, Biomedical Sciences Graduate Program and Program in Biological and Medical Informatics (BMI); Co-Leader, Cancer and Immunity Program, UCSF Helen Diller Family Comprehensive Cancer Center, University of California San Francisco, San Francisco, California
Anal Disease

John L. Pfenninger, MD, FAAFP
Senior Consultant, The National Procedures Institute, Medical Director, The Medical Procedures Center P.C., Midland, Michigan; Clinical Professor of Family Medicine, Michigan State College of Human Medicine, East Lansing, MI; Private Practice, Midland, Michigan
Androscopy: Examination of the Male Partner

Richard I. Reid, MD
Consultant Gynaecologist, Hunter New England Health System, Inverell, Australia
Colposcopic Assessment Systems: Reid's Colposcopic Index

R. Kevin Reynolds, MD, FACOG, FACS
The George W. Morley Professor and Chief, Division of Gynecologic Oncology, University of Michigan Hospitals, Ann Arbor, Michigan
Squamous Cervical Cancer

Ann Roman, PhD
Chancellor's Professor and Associate Chairperson Department of Microbiology and Immunology, and Walther Oncology Center, Indiana University School of Medicine and Walther Cancer Institute Indianapolis, Indiana,
Human Papillomaviruses and Mechanisms Of Oncogenesis

Mary M. Rubin, RNC, Ph.D, CRNP
Associate Clinical Professor School of Nursing, Clinical Research Coordinator Gyn Oncology/ Dysplasia, University of California San Francisco, San Francisco, California
Principles and Technique of the Colposcopic Exam; Colposcopic Assessment Systems: Rubin and Barbo Colposcopic Assessment System

Mark Schiffman, MD, MPH
Deputy Chief, Hormonal and Reproductive Epidemiology Branch, National Cancer Institute, Bethesda, Maryland
Epidemiology Applied to Colposcopy

Helena Spartz, PhD
Department of Microbiology and Immunology Indiana University School of Medicine Indianapolis, Indiana
Human Papillomaviruses and Mechanisms Of Oncogenesis

Mark Spitzer, MD
Clinical Professor, Weill Medical College of Cornell University, New York, New York; Chairman, Obstetrics and Gynecology, Brookdale University Hospital and Medical Center, Brooklyn, New York
Practical Therapeutic Options for Treatment of Cervical Intraepithelial Neoplasia; Colposcopy: Pitfalls and Tricks of the Trade

Adolf Stafl, MD, PhD
Professor of Obstetrics and Gynecology (Retired), Charles University, Prague, Czech Republic
Angiogenesis of Cervical Neoplasia

Alan G. Waxman, MD, MPH, FACOG
Professor, Dept. of Obstetrics and Gynecology, Director, Women's Health Center, University of New Mexico School of Medicine, Albuquerque, New Mexico
Low-Grade Squamous Intraepithelial Lesions

David G. Weismiller, MD, ScM
Associate Professor, Department of Family Medicine,
The Brody School of Medicine at East Carolina University;
Assistant Provost, East Carolina University, Greenville,
North Carolina
Colposcopy in Pregnancy

Edward J. Wilkinson, MD, FCAP, FACOG
Department of Pathology, Immunology and Laboratory
Medicine, University of Florida College of Medicine,
University of Florida, Gainesville, Florida
Conventional Cytology

Thomas C. Wright, Jr., M.D.
Professor of Pathology, Columbia University, New York,
New York, Director, Division of Gynecologic and Obstetrical
Pathology, Columbia University, New York, New York
Atypical Squamous Cells

V. Cecil Wright, MD, FRCS(C), FACOG, FSOGC
Professor Emeritus, Department of Obstetrics and
Gynaecology, Schulich School of Medicine and Dentistry,
University of Western Ontario, London, Ontario, Canada
*Cervical Glandular Disease: Adenocarcinoma In Situ and
Adenocarcinoma*

CHAPTER 1

Epidemiology Applied to Colposcopy

Mark Schifman • Jose Jeronimo

Most clinicians perform epidemiologic evaluations more often than they realize. Epidemiology is defined as the scientific study of factors affecting health and disease in populations. When managing women with lower genital tract disorders, clinicians deal with individual patients but frequently think and act epidemiologically. "This is an unusual diagnosis" is a statement of incidence or prevalence. The question, "Should I treat this woman based on what I see?" draws on an understanding of absolute risk and relative risk posed by the colposcopic appearance. The question, "Would my colleague agree with my colposcopic impression?" relates to interobserver agreement and diagnostic reproducibility. Similarly, trends of disease are implicit when a clinician asks, "Why am I seeing so many cases of this type of tumor?" Finally, questions such as "Does human papillomavirus (HPV) cause vulvodynia?" relate to etiology of disease and can be addressed by clinicians performing epidemiologic evaluations or working with epidemiologists.

The main goal of this chapter is to introduce frequently used epidemiologic concepts to colposcopists interested in research or involved in public health work. Most of the examples explained in this chapter come from the authors' experiences in colposcopic practice or cervical cancer epidemiologic research. It is not our intention to write this chapter as a reference for formal epidemiologic training. Clinicians are our intended audience. To encourage readability, terms will be described informally, leaving details to epidemiologic textbooks.[1-4]

COMMON EPIDEMIOLOGIC TERMS AND CONCEPTS

The Many Kinds of Risk

The *frequency* of a disease is very important for clinical evaluation as well as for epidemiologic analysis. Clinicians perform differential diagnosis starting with the more frequent entities because "rare diseases occur rarely." *For epidemiologists, the most reliable way to exclude chance is to have a moderate-to-large number of case subjects when comparing patterns of occurrence among different populations; thus*

KEY POINTS

- Epidemiology is the scientific study of factors affecting health and disease in populations.
- *Prevalence of disease* is the number of subjects who *have* a disease during a given period of time.
- *Incidence of disease* is the number of subjects who *acquire* a disease during a given period of time.
- In highly lethal diseases and those of very short duration, the values of prevalence and incidence are very similar.
- *Mortality rates* measure the rate of death from a disease.
- Patterns of disease occurrence may vary over time within a given area, or they can be very different among two or more geographic regions.
- A prospective or cohort study measures the exposure in a group of subjects and follows them over time.
- *Absolute risk* compares incidence rates of disease in two groups of people: one exposed to the risk factor and the other unexposed.
- *Relative risk* (RR) is the ratio of a rate of a specific disease in the exposed subjects versus nonexposed ones.
- Prospective studies are the best for determining the relationship between exposure to a risk factor and occurrence of disease.
- *Screening* is the action of actively searching for a disease in an asymptomatic population.
- The sensitivity and specificity of a screening technique theoretically do not change regardless of whether the test is applied in a high-risk setting or in the general population.
- *Systematic error*, called *bias*, has a direct impact on the accuracy of the measurement; a study conclusion based on biased measurements will be wrong no matter how large the study is.
- The *chi-square test* is meant to determine whether the disease categories and the exposure categories are associated or independent.
- A *true-positive* screening result occurs when the subject has the disease and tested positive.
- A *false-negative* screening result occurs when the subject has the disease but tested negative.
- The *sensitivity* of a test is the percentage of diseased subjects who test positive.
- The *specificity* of a test is the percentage of subjects without the disease who test negative.
- The key to defining the proper size of the study is to agree on the hypothesis and the range of expected results. Sample size calculations are very assumption dependent and usually demand information not available until the study is completed.

frequency of disease occurrence is very important when planning or analyzing a study.

Because disease frequency is so important, epidemiologists study it several ways. Prevalence of disease *is the number of subjects who have a disease during a given period of time.* For example, 12% of women evaluated in our clinic tested positive for oncogenic HPV types. It is important to note that prevalence is related to a specific point in time, leading to the notion of *point prevalence.* Therefore we can find statements such as "Last year, 5% of women screened with conventional cytology had an abnormal result."

Incidence of disease *is the number of subjects who acquire a disease during a given period of time.* The difference between incidence and prevalence is that prevalence considers all cases in the population, new and chronic, that are found on examination, whereas incidence only counts new cases. The values of prevalence and incidence are very similar if the disease is highly lethal or has a very short duration. We can assume that the yearly prevalence of stillbirths is close to the yearly incidence because the duration is short and it is unlikely that a woman would have more than one occurrence per year. Meanwhile, the prevalence of a long-duration entity such as chronic hypertension largely exceeds the incidence for any time period. As a practical example of the value of studying the incidence and prevalence of a disease, approximately 15 years ago it was noted that the point prevalence and yearly incidence of HPV infection follow the same pattern, with an age peak. This predicted correctly that most HPV infections are transient rather than persistent and accumulating.

Incidence and prevalence *are usually defined as a yearly rate.* Incidence and prevalence rates of cancer are expressed as a fraction in which the numerator is the number of occurrences observed per 100,000 subjects (denominator). For example we know that ≈10,000 incident cases of invasive cervical cancer were diagnosed in the United States in 2006, for a rate of ≈9 per 100,000 women for that year. However, incidence can be also determined for other time periods. A very useful term is *lifetime cumulative incidence,* which shows the estimated risk of suffering a disease over the lifetime. Thus we estimate that ≈13% of women born today in the United States will develop breast cancer during their life. Therefore the chance that these women will never have breast cancer is ≈87%. For neoplastic diseases, recurrence (return of a previously diagnosed and treated incident disease), is related to prevalence. *For acute, self-limited, or curable conditions such as gonorrhea, incidence must be defined over a narrow range of time appropriate to the duration of the illness.*

Mortality rates *measure the rate of death from a disease. Incidence* rate and mortality rate are very similar if the disease is highly lethal *(case:fatality ratio),* but the higher the cure rate, the lower the fatality rate. For example, we know that the incidence of cervical cancer is 17 per 100,000 in women aged 65 or older, but the mortality rate for cervical cancer is 9 per 100,000 in the same group of women.

In summary, *incidence, prevalence, and mortality rates of a disease are basic information when starting the study of a disease.* These rates can be explored or studied for any population, such as a medical office, a hospital, a city, a country, or the entire world. National incidence and mortality rates are very valuable data when evaluating the medical conditions and problems of a country and when planning studies or interventions. Incidence and mortality rates are also good indicators of the health conditions of a country or region and can be used to evaluate the improvement or decline of health care of a population over time.

In the United States, many sources of information about incidence and mortality rates of cancers are available. The *National Cancer Institute's Surveillance, Epidemiology, and End Results* (SEER) Program collects information about incidence rates of cancer for a sample of ≈10% of the U.S. population *(www.seer.cancer.gov).* The most accessible source of SEER cancer incidence and survival data (as well as national cancer mortality data) is *CA-A Cancer Journal for Clinicians,* published annually by the American Cancer Society and mailed free on request.[5] Worldwide information on cancer incidence and mortality can be obtained in the publication *Cancer in Five Continents* from the International Agency for Research on Cancer (IARC).[6,7]

Geographic Differences and Time Trends in Disease Occurrence

Patterns of disease occurrence may vary over time within the same area, or they can be very different among two or more geographic regions. Figure 1-1 shows the incidence of cervical cancer by country in the world.[8] *Almost all the developed countries have a very low incidence rate, whereas developing countries have a high burden of disease. This difference of rates is mainly due to insufficient screening because developing countries do not have the resources to maintain population-based cervical cancer control programs, so undetected and untreated pre-cancer lesions can develop into invasive cancer.* Epidemiologists study geographic and temporal correlations with disease to help find the etiology and to understand the pathogenesis of disease. However, we need to be very cautious to avoid the influence of chance when analyzing the data. In the past, there have been several examples of erroneous epidemiologic evaluations showing differences in the pattern of disease occurrence that were later shown to be due to temporary fluctuations that did not persist over time.

In order to differentiate differences due to chance from true differences, researchers have to rely on statistical tests. First, we need to know the magnitudes of differences likely to be produced by chance. This is critical because *incorrect interpretation of chance differences is one of the most common errors made by inexpert epidemiologists.* For example, periodically we can find news about cancer "outbreaks" that really are no more than clusterings of cases produced by chance. This may be manifest in a group of women who have known each other for many years in a neighborhood and who each develop breast cancer. They suspect an environmental cause but are actually noticing that breast cancers are common among postmenopausal women. Therefore true differences in trends of disease require a long-lasting, unexpected change in the rate of occurrence.

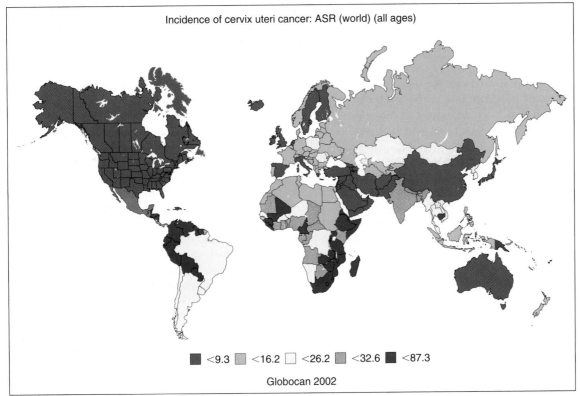

Incidence of cervix uteri cancer: ASR (world) (all ages)

■ <9.3 ▨ <16.2 □ <26.2 ▨ <32.6 ■ <87.3

Globocan 2002

Figure 1-1 Incidence of Cervix Uteri Cancer. *ASR*, (Adapted from International Agency for Research on Cancer [IARC] data.)

When comparing trends, several questions need to be answered, as follows:

- Are the rates comparable? It is important to know exactly how data were collected in two different regions or times. We cannot compare a mandatory population-based registry with an institutional report. *Data should be equally collected in order to be comparable.*
- *Were the same diagnostic criteria used in either places or times?* This is particularly important when evaluating a disease that has had several modifications in the diagnostic criteria or when diagnostic or screening tests have improved dramatically over time. A clear example is related to the diagnosis of HPV-related changes of the cervix because understanding and recognition of subtle changes have evolved during the past decade. Even the diagnosis provided by the same pathologist might have changed over the past years.
- *Do the different populations share similar characteristics such as sex, age, or behavior?* For example, rates of HPV infection vary considerably with age; therefore we need to consider this confounding factor when comparing HPV infection rates between two geographic areas. Similarly, we cannot compare the prevalence of cervical intraepithelial neoplasia (CIN) among women with abnormal cytology who attend a gynecologic referral practice versus the prevalence of CIN among women from the general population who attend a screening clinic. Epidemiologists have some statistical tools to correct and adjust data to

avoid the bias produced by confounding factors such as age or number of sexual partners.

Intraobserver or Interobserver Agreement

Clinicians are concerned with the reliability of their diagnosis. This is particularly important for colposcopists because of several recent reports questioning the validity of the current colposcopic criteria. At the same time, epidemiologists are concerned with uniform case definition in their studies. Colposcopists and epidemiologists can partner for studies on intraobserver and interobserver agreement among colposcopists. Most clinicians tend to agree more in public than in independent (masked) evaluations; therefore an epidemiologist can play the role of organizer and mediator to ensure independence of the reviews and mask colposcopists to the diagnoses of the other evaluators until after the data are complete. *Unmasked evaluations in which evaluators can access the diagnosis of the other experts have very limited scientific value. Usually, the dominant personality rules.*

EPIDEMIOLOGY AND DISEASE ETIOLOGY

One of the main goals of epidemiology is to help determine the causes of disease through the evaluation of risk factors *(exposures)*. These epidemiologic studies, called *analytical studies,* differ from *descriptive studies* that yield rates of disease without directly addressing its etiology.

The following is a brief description of some types of analytical studies. *A prospective or cohort study measures the exposure in a group subjects and follows them over time.* Then the investigators compare incidence rates or *absolute risks* of disease in the group of people exposed to the risk factor and in the unexposed group. If we divide the incidence rate in exposed subjects by the incidence rate in the unexposed subjects, we obtain the *incidence rate ratio.* Similarly, we can calculate the rate ratio for any type of rates such as prevalence, mortality, and others. Frequently such ratios are known as the *relative risk* (RR) of exposed subjects versus nonexposed ones.

Prospective studies attempt to determine the relation between exposure to a risk factor and occurrence of disease. For example, we might have a question such as "If a woman (30 years or older) is infected with an oncogenic HPV type, how much more likely is she to develop CIN 3 within the next 10 years, compared with a similar uninfected woman?" Current data collected during prospective epidemiologic studies permit us to answer for these questions. As shown in Figure 1-2, women infected with the most oncogenic HPV type (HPV 16) have an absolute risk of CIN 3 and cancer of approximately 20% over the next 10 years (despite participation in a prepaid health plan that offers yearly cytology screening). The comparable risk for uninfected women is 1%. Therefore the RR associated with a single HPV test revealing HPV 16 infection is 20 for the subsequent 10-year period.[9]

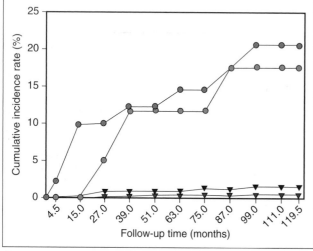

Figure 1-2 Cumulative incidence of cervical intraepithelial neoplasia grade 3 and cancer (CIN 3) over a 10-year period in 12,976 women 30 years old and older with negative cytology at enrollment, according to oncogenic human papillomavirus (HPV) status at enrollment. HPV status is defined hierarchically as: positive for HPV 16 *(blue circles)*, else positive for HPV 18 *(orange circles)*, else positive for the non–HPV 16/18 oncogenic types in Hybrid Capture 2 *(purple triangles)*, else oncogenic HPV negative *(blue triangles)*. (Adapted from Khan MJ, Castle PE, Lorincz AT, et al. The elevated 10-year risk of cervical precancer and cancer in women with human papillomavirus [HPV] type 16 or 18 and the possible utility of type-specific HPV testing in clinical practice. J Natl Cancer Inst. 2005;97:1072–1079.)

Unfortunately, prospective studies of cancer are expensive, may take several years, and require enrolling a high number of subjects to ensure enough observations (cases) for direct calculation of relative risk. In order to avoid great expenses of money and time, epidemiologists have alternative study designs to estimate the relative risk. One option is the *case-control* study, in which cases (women diagnosed with a given disease) are compared with adequately selected controls (women without that disease). Even though the risk factor (exposure) under evaluation is not determined for all cases and controls, we can estimate the RR for developing disease by calculating the ratio of the odds of exposure in random samples of both groups of subjects. This *odds ratio* (OR) is one of the most widely used and important statistical concepts for epidemiologists. However, the validity of an odds ratio depends on a very careful selection of incident cases and, more importantly, selection of adequate controls. *The most common mistake committed by inexpert epidemiologists is the incorrect selection of a control group.* Controls must be at risk of developing the disease being evaluated at the time the incident case was diagnosed; otherwise the estimation of the relative risk is biased and therefore erroneous. The result is considered biased because of nonrandom or systematic error.

It is very difficult to select an unbiased sample of the general population to match and compare with the cases recruited in one hospital or clinic. For example, smoking causes or worsens so many types of illness that it is very difficult to use hospitalized controls to estimate whether a disease is associated with smoking. The exposure to smoking in the hospitalized controls is elevated compared with the general at-risk population, so the odds ratio obtained in a naively conducted hospital-based study of cases tends to provide results that make smoking look less risky than it really is (both the cases and controls smoke more than usual.)

Another common epidemiologic design is the *cross-sectional* study. *In a cross-sectional study, measurements are done at a specific point in time or during a short time period.* Additionally, the risk factor and disease status are ascertained concurrently for a study population. For example, a colposcopist evaluates two simultaneously performed screening methods for cervical cancer (an HPV deoxyribonucleic acid [DNA] test and conventional cervical cytology) in women attending a community clinic. Cross-sectional and case-control studies are alike because they both collect the data at once and are analyzed in a similar manner. They differ mainly in that a cross-sectional study includes all patients seen, including incident and prevalent cases, in whatever ratio to controls they happen to occur within the study group, whereas case-control studies carefully select the number and type of controls. If the disease is rare, a cross-sectional design might not yield enough cases for a reliable study.

Beyond proper choice of controls, the *other critical component of good case-control studies is the adequate measurement of exposure and careful classification of the disease.* Clinicians play a very important role in analytical studies of diseases whose definitions rely on adequate clinical evaluation and diagnosis. Inadequate classification of presence or absence of a given disease can invalidate a study because it can reduce or increase the strength of the association between disease and exposure. A very poor definition of disease does not permit a researcher to find any risk factors even if they exist.[10] Careful exposure assessment with accurate measurements is more important than fancy statistical analyses.

The combination of errors can completely invalidate the results of a study. Early studies attempting to correlate HPV and CIN provide a clear example: they found HPV DNA in fewer than 50% of cases. Also, those studies failed to demonstrate the relation between HPV infection and sexual activity, an already known risk factor for CIN. The development of new more sensitive HPV tests and careful evaluation of pathologic specimens showed that almost 100% of cases of CIN contain HPV DNA and proved that HPV is a sexually transmitted agent, explaining the association of sexual activity and cervical cancer. There is a clear need to have teams of epidemiologists and clinical evaluators in all epidemiologic studies in which a careful definition of disease is required.

Follow-Up Studies of Patients

Clinicians, colposcopists, and epidemiologists are all interested in learning what happens to patients diagnosed with a given disease. For a possibly fatal disease, survival rates are critical, whereas for other chronic diseases progression rates are often estimated. It is often of interest to divide the patients into groups to determine whether subtypes of disease follow different courses or whether different treatments influence outcome. For example, when we face a patient diagnosed with cancer, it is important to know the possibility of survival for that given cancer at a given stage (survival rates), the possibility of cure with a given treatment (cure rate), and the recurrence of the disease in subsequent years (recurrence rate). *The randomized clinical trial* (see later discussion) *is a specialized version of such a follow-up study, in which subjects are randomly assigned to various treatment groups to maximize the comparability of the groups.* The hope is that the randomization will minimize differences in both known and unknown confounding variables that could bias the comparison.

Follow-up studies almost invariably involve the concept of time to an event. In other words, it is important when *incidence, progression, or death occur, not just* whether *they occur.* Let us discuss this issue in the context of studies of disease outcome (as opposed to disease incidence). Clearly, all participants in any follow-up study or clinical trial eventually die; the question is *when* (and *why*). An effective treatment prolongs time to death, whereas a particularly aggressive type of disease shortens it. Because of the critical notion of *time to event* in epidemiologic follow-up studies, such studies depend heavily on actuarial (insurance) methods such as survival curves and life-table analyses when comparing exposed with unexposed patients or treated with untreated patients. This allows us to compare the efficacy of treatments based on the survival (patients alive with or without evidence of disease), survival free of disease (patients alive and without evidence of disease), and rate of severe complications, among other factors.

The central statistical concept in such studies is a kind of rate called a *hazard*, which refers to the risk of an outcome occurring per unit of follow-up time. A hazard is computed as the number of events (e.g., death, cure, progression) divided by the amount of person-time of follow-up. Person-time is computed individually for each participant as the observation time between her entry into the study and her exit. The total person-time for a study group is the sum of all the individual observation periods. For example, 10,000 women followed for 1 year or 100 women followed for 10 years both yield 1000 person-years of follow-up time. Twenty deaths arising during that follow-up would yield an estimated hazard of 20 deaths per 1000 person-years in both situations.

Figure 1-3 is an example of hazard evaluation used by Plummer et al. to measure the risk of persistent HPV infection among several thousand infected women during a 2-year follow-up period.[11] The rapid clearance (the opposite of persistence) was plainly visible.

A hazard is a special kind of rate because it is considered the rate of an outcome (e.g., disease incidence, progression, mortality) at a single moment in time, as the mathematical *limit* of the rate as time *goes to zero*. Accordingly, *the hazard of disease can change from moment to moment as conditions change.* An HPV-infected woman smokes a cigarette, and her hazard for progression to invasive cervical cancer probably increases. She quits smoking the next day, and her hazard is thought to decrease.

Moreover, the computation of the denominator of hazards, person-time of follow-up, requires some training and thought. For each successive time interval during

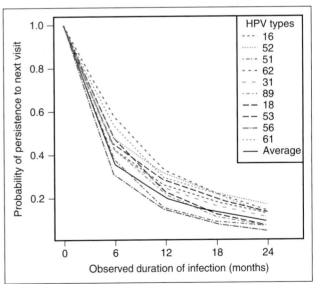

Figure 1-3 Individual human papillomavirus *(HPV)* types typically clear rapidly within 1 to 2 years of first detection. (Adapted from Plummer M, Schiffman M, Castle P, Maucort-Boulch D, Wheeler CM. A 2-year prospective study of human papillomavirus persistence among women with a cytological diagnosis of atypical squamous cells of undetermined significance or low-grade squamous intraepithelial lesion. J Infect Dis. 2007 Jun 1;195(11):1582–9.

follow-up, the denominator of women at risk for an event changes. For example, women are lost to follow-up as they drop out of the study, or they die for other reasons, or they experience the event itself (because one can only progress for the first time or die once). Thus *computing the proper amount of person-time during which the events occurred requires some knowledge of censoring* (the proper deletion of irrelevant follow-up time during which the subject was not truly at risk of the outcome).

In summary, it is relatively straightforward to compute the hazard of conditions such as death, which happen once and do not reverse. Life-table methods are more confusing when a condition can come and go. For example, imagine we want to study "HPV infection" without defining specific types. However, using the term "HPV infection" is similar to using the term "a cold." The presence of multiple HPV types can present a confusing picture of clearance and recurrence. Proper counting of events and censoring of person-time are very difficult in this context, making simpler analyses more appealing, such as the computation of cumulative incidence rate ratios (ever infected versus not infected over the course of study).

Usually, researchers are not content to describe the simple survival or progression curve of a disease after diagnosis. They wish to determine which factors affect the hazard; in other words, what is the relative or proportional hazard of death for women in different groups (defined by pathologic differences or treatment types). The proportional hazard is almost identical to the incident rate ratio already discussed, but the denominator is person-time of observed follow-up, not simply time. Proportional hazard analyses are too complex to be described here, and colposcopists performing follow-up studies might consider consulting an epidemiologist or biostatistician early in the design phase of such projects. Data collection must be organized carefully to permit a correct determination of person-time.

Randomized Clinical Trials

Randomized clinical trials are conceptually simple prospective analyses, with eligible women divided by random draw into treatment arms. Randomization serves to balance known and unknown biases in each arm. A placebo or standard treatment arm is compared with one or more new treatment arms. *Randomized clinical trials are very appealing as a court of judgment regarding best medical practice when we do not know which practice is best.* Such trials are highly influential. However, they are surprisingly difficult and should not be undertaken as quickly as observational studies. The maxim "Do no harm" is applicable because the participants' fates are influenced by the randomization. Clinician judgment as to the individual's optimal treatment must explicitly be set aside. The stakes are always high when a trial is underway. We want a result quickly and definitively, but the two objectives are in conflict. The time-honored rules used to ensure fairness can seem bureaucratic and rigid. *Clinical trialists* are statisticians, epidemiologists, and others who specialize in randomization, data monitoring,

intermediate analyses (*data peeks* before the scheduled end of follow-up), and stopping rules (in case the intermediate analyses reveal an especially good or bad outcome). Clinicians contribute expert review of entry diagnoses and outcomes. Often the burden of clinical review is large, reproducibility is paramount, and the review process is highly controlled by central administration. Of all collaborations with epidemiologists, colposcopists should be most wary of clinical trials because of the inevitable attendant requirements. Still, the rewards are vital.

Screening for Gynecologic Malignancies

Screening is the action of actively searching for a disease in an asymptomatic population. A disease should fulfill some requirements before it is considered as candidate for screening. First, we need a clear understanding of the natural history and progression of the disease; the screening test should be reliable and reproducible; the disease should have a detectable preinvasive or early invasive stage; and once the disease is detected, effective treatment should be available. However, probably the main requirement is that the disease should be important for the community.

Screening is inherently epidemiologic; thus the clinician involved in screening programs (e.g., cervical cytologic screening or transvaginal ultrasound and CA125) needs to understand the interrelated concepts of sensitivity, specificity, and predictive value. The basics are outlined later in a statistical section on screening.

A common mistake in evaluating the results of a screening trial is to ignore the clinical setting. *Although dogma states that the sensitivity of a screening technique* (percentage of diseased women who test positive) *and its specificity* (percentage of disease-free women who test negative) *do not change when the test is taken out of a high-risk hospital clinic to be applied to the general population, this dogma is not true.* It is easy to show[11] that a test may have very different specificity for CIN 3 when it is used in different settings. Figure 1-4 shows what is called a *receiver-operating characteristic (ROC) curve* (see section on Receiver-Operating Characteristic Curve (page 16) for details) that plots the sensitivity versus (1 − specificity) for the importance of individual HPV types in detection of CIN 3. Two curves are shown, one using data from a screening study and another in triage. Twenty HPV types were added in order of best sensitivity for CIN 3 (when the impact of sensitivity was the same, the choices of the next type to add were based on minimum decrease in specificity). It is obvious that the specificity of HPV testing for a given level of sensitivity is much lower in a triage setting, in which HPV infections associated with ASC and LSIL are quite common.

Rather than sensitivity and specificity, most clinicians are more interested in the positive predictive valve and negative predictive value, two statistics that are highly dependent on the clinical setting. *The positive predictive value is the percentage of women testing positive who truly have disease. The negative predictive value is the reassurance that disease does not exist given a negative test result.* **The positive predictive value decreases sharply as the prevalence of the disease decreases.**

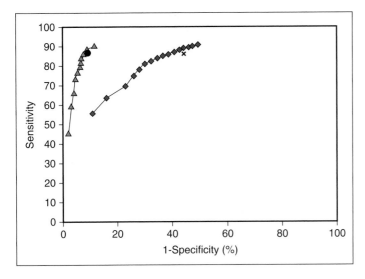

Figure 1-4 Receiver operating characteristic (ROC) curve for human papillomavirus (HPV) types in a screening and triage setting. Sensitivities of detection of cervical intraepithelial neoplasia grade 3 (CIN 3) and cervical cancer were plotted versus (100%–specificity) for increasingly sensitive combinations of HPV types. The results for screening in the Proyecto Epidemiológico Guanacaste (PEG) are plotted with **orange triangles**, and the results for triage of equivocal cytology in the ASC-US-LSIL Triage Study (ALTS) are plotted with **blue diamonds**. As described in the text, up to 20 HPV types were added in order of maximum impact on sensitivity and, when the impact on sensitivity was the same, in order of minimum decrement in specificity. For PEG, HPV types were added in the following order: HPV16, 58, 18, 31, 56, 51, 11, 68, 52, 35, 45, 66, 71, 67, 74, 59, 40, 32, 55, and 89. For ALTS, HPV types were added in the following order: HPV16, 31, 52, 58, 33, 35, 45, 18, 42, 66, 51, 73, 82, 54, 39, 84, 53, 57, 11, and 26. The last several HPV types added in each study did not increase sensitivity, and their corresponding points are indistinguishable on the plots. For each study, we show as a separate point (**solid circle** for PEG, **cross** for ALTS) the estimate performance of a probe set containing the 13 HPV types in the currently FDA-approved HPV DNA test. (Adapted from Schiffman M, Khan MJ, Solomon D, et al. A study of the impact of adding HPV types to cervical cancer screening and triage tests. J Natl Cancer Inst. 2005;97:147–150.)

True positives can be swamped by false positives once the test is applied to a screening population that consists mainly of normal women. Therefore the same screening test that looks promising because of high sensitivity in a high-risk clinic treating many diseased women will often perform poorly in the general population, producing so many false positives compared with the disease yield that the costs outweigh the benefits. As a general rule, specificity is surprisingly important as a requirement for a screening test. A screening test such as a tumor marker must be highly specific (negative in virtually all nondiseased women, certainly 90%) to be cost effective for general population screening.

BASIC STATISTICAL CONCEPTS USED IN EPIDEMIOLOGIC STUDIES OF COLPOSCOPY

It is hoped that the preceding discussion has firmly established the relevance of epidemiology to clinical research and even daily practice. Epidemiology requires an understanding of biostatistics. In fact, it is somewhat artificial to divide the two disciplines. This section presents the bare basics of what the authors believe colposcopists might wish to know about biostatistical methods when collaborating in epidemiologic research. Introductory biostatistics texts are available and easy to read for colposcopists who wish to work independently or want computational formulae for chi-square or other commonly used tests.

Variability as a Fundamental Principle

Virtually all measurements that one could make about a human population are variable. Height, weight, fine points of anatomy, metabolic patterns, serum levels of hormones, and nutrients are all variable. The same variability is seen among colposcopists observing the position of the squamous–columnar junction of the cervix, acetowhiteness of the epithelium, and presence of cervicitis, among others. Even the intricate, multiple-step molecular pathways to

cancer demonstrate substantial variability among individuals who develop the same type of malignancy.

Variability in data may be described as either *categorical or discrete* or as *continuous* (the province of the mean and median, and standard deviation). Variability in colposcopy is mainly described by *categorical or discrete data* and statistics. More attention is paid to the borderlines and overlaps of the categories, rather than subtler differences within the categories (unless splitting into finer categories is being considered). Categorical data analysis relies on *contingency tables*, which are discussed in the section "Measures of Risk: Absolute, Relative, and Attributable Risks" on page 10. Contingency tables such as the common *2 × 2 table* are frequently counts of categorical data; an example is the number (percent) of HPV 16–infected women who demonstrated acetowhite lesions compared with HPV 18–infected women.

The variability in categorical data such as colposcopy categories shows up in *diagnostic error* (the misassignment of a patient to the wrong category). In general, error cannot be avoided. To the epidemiologist, categorization of variable biological continua virtually dictates that there will be error. If two categories blend into each other with regard to a characteristic (even one as complex and general as colposcopic appearance), they cannot be perfectly separated based on that characteristic. Thus colposcopists search for additional characteristics to discriminate difficult-to-distinguish indeterminate cases, such as Lugol's staining, but these ancillary measurements also have error and overlap. In a field of statistics called *discriminant analysis*, the goal is to determine how many characteristics must be measured to maximize correct assignment to overlapping categories. This complicated set of statistical methods underlies one approach to the development of computer-assisted cytology screening.

Error versus Bias

Error is inevitable, but epidemiologists hope that it is mainly random, not systematically pushing the data in one way or the other. Random error *reduces the reliability and precision of repeated measurements, affecting their precision, and it reduces the perceived strength of correlations, but the average measured value still becomes accurate as the study size increases. Systematic error, called* bias, *affects the accuracy of the measurement directly; a study based on biased measurements will be wrong no matter how large it is.* Thus epidemiologists struggle to reduce random measurement error, but they have an even stronger aversion to biased measurements. If the exact direction and magnitude of a fixed bias were known, the data could be adjusted (similar to a scale that always reads 3 lb too heavy), but adjustments for bias are not usually possible.

Epidemiologists combat error and bias in a few standard ways. To quantify and reduce random error, reliability is measured by repeating data collection, which may involve reasking a question, rerunning an assay, or submitting a pathology slide for rereview.

For continuous variables, statistics of reliability begin with the variance. *Variance* is the sum of the squared deviations of measurements from their arithmetic average or mean, divided by the number of data points minus one. The *standard deviation* is the square root of the variance and is commonly used to indicate the *spread* of a group of numbers. The standard deviation of a measurement can be computed for individual members of the overall study population or for repeated samplings of a study statistic such as the mean (in which case it is called the *standard error* of the mean). When we compare different populations to see whether they are statistically significantly different regarding the characteristic being studied, standard errors are important in making confidence intervals around the mean.

When epidemiologists assess laboratory assays, they often consider the *coefficient of variation* (CV), which is the ratio of the standard deviation to the mean. Although they do not ensure accuracy, low CVs (under 10% is excellent) indicate high assay reproducibility. Remember that a reproducible assay can still be biased. For categorical variables such as colposcopy interpretations, statistics of reliability include the simple percentage of agreement as well as more complicated statistics mentioned later in the section on measures of interrater agreement. *Ideally, epidemiologists would compare the colposcopy diagnoses with a reference standard of truth, but such reference standards virtually never exist. There is no source of absolute truth in colposcopy; only advancing degrees of expertise that correlate with decreasing amounts of diagnostic error.* Therefore, to reduce bias in colposcopy, researchers are limited to the comparison of different experts. To the extent that truly independent experts (blinded to each other's opinion) agree, the possibility that either one is biased is reduced. To reduce the possibility of bias, epidemiologists try to ensure that all study measurements are made without knowledge of the other study measurements so that one variable cannot bias a decision about another. The difficulties of masking are discussed in a later section. Unfortunately, colposcopy is based on the direct evaluation of the cervix performed dynamically by one or several evaluators. The only information that could be shared with other experts is the pictures or video collected during the evaluation. *The results of the evaluation of that visual data by experts have been very controversial, probably due to the fact that colposcopy is a dynamic, three-dimensional evaluation, whereas the visual data is two-dimensional, is often static, and may be of relatively poor resolution.*

Descriptive Data

The terms used most often to describe and summarize descriptive data, such as *prevalence* and *incidence*, were defined earlier in the section on geographic differences and time trends and will not be repeated here. A few additional statistical concepts critical to the interpretation of descriptive data are discussed, however.

First, there is an important choice of scale in the plotting of descriptive data. In a graphic description of the data, the scale of the vertical axis greatly affects the appearance of the data and must always be noted when examining plotted data. A *log scale* (in which the log or natural log of y-values is plotted) flattens curves and reduces the apparent strength of trends and differences, whereas an *arithmetic scale* does the opposite. *On a log scale, an increasing, straight-line trend implies an exponential, not a linear rate of increase.*

When interpreting descriptive data, a common error in inference is the *ecologic fallacy*, the attribution of causality to an association seen only in descriptive data. For example, the international mortality rates from colon cancer correlate with several other variables. These include the average dietary intake of those countries for fat, meat, and sugar and the average amount of sunlight (the major determinant of vitamin D levels). To assume automatically that all four variables are true risk factors for colon cancer at the level of the individual would be an example of the ecologic fallacy, confusing descriptive data for analytical (individual level) data.

In the interpretation of time trend data, the possibility of a *cohort effect* must be considered. A cohort effect is the variation in disease occurrence that happens in a population over time, as successive birth cohorts (persons of the same age) experience the unique environment that typifies their life course. This effect may be familiar by analogy to anyone who studies the sociology of baby boomers. A manifestation of the cohort effect may be seen in the cross-sectional prevalence data compiled in Portland, Oregon in 1991. The prevalence rates of koilocytotic atypia of the cervix peaked at about 20 to 25 years and then decreased sharply with increasing age. This age trend might represent a biological phenomenon, the result of immunity, with many women becoming infected with HPV with initiation of sexual intercourse, then becoming increasingly immune and having fewer new sexual partners as they age. Or the age trend could also reflect a cohort effect, with changing sexual practices and increasing prevalence of HPV infection over the past decades placing younger women at higher risk for koilocytotic changes compared with their older sisters and mothers.

A graphic example of a probable cohort effect is presented in Figure 1-5 regarding trends of cervical cancer among black and white women in the United States.[13] During 1976 to 1987, the incidence of squamous cervical

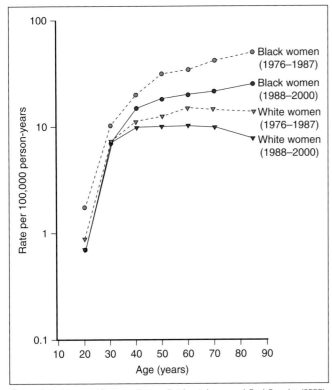

Figure 1-5 Age-specific Surveillance, Epidemiology, and End Results (SEER) incidence rates for cervical squamous cell carcinoma (SCC) in black and white women during 1976 to 1987 and 1988 to 2000. (Modified from Wang SS, Sherman ME, Hildesheim A, et al. Cervical adenocarcinoma and squamous cell carcinoma incidence trends among white women and black women in the United States for 1976–2000. Cancer 2004;100:1035–1044.)

Table 1-1 The Basic Contingency Table

	Disease	**Abnormal**	**Total**
Exposed or test positive	a	b	a + b
Unexposed or test negative	c	d	c + d
Total	a + c	b + d	a + b + c + d = n

(proportions of 100%) that can then be compared, such as "Ninety percent of the group with disease was infected with HPV [a/(a+c)=0.9] compared with 20% of the non-diseased [b/(b+d)=0.2]." These proportions could be compared statistically using the well-known *t-test* or another test of the difference between independent proportions. More often, the *chi-square statistic* is computed, which gives equivalent interpretations.

The chi-square test is meant to determine whether the disease categories and the exposure categories are associated or independent; that is, does being exposed affect the probability of having disease? Chi-square values are derived by comparing the expected counts of *a*, *b*, *c*, and *d* to the values that would be expected if disease and exposure were totally independent. For example, the expected value of *a* is the cross-product of (a+b)(a+c) divided by *n*. The divergence of observed from expected values for all the cells of the table (*a*, *b*, *c*, *d*) are summed to derive the chi-square statistic. The larger the statistic, summarizing how much observed counts differ from the expected, the more likely disease and exposure are associated by more than chance.

The chi-square statistic is compared with the tabled values of the *chi-square distribution* to yield a *p-value*, the probability of observing such a chi-square value if disease and exposure are not related. In other words, this is the probability of concluding that an association exists in error. To falsely accept an association, when the *null assumption* would be correct, is considered a *type 1 error*. This name was perhaps chosen because it is generally considered a more important scientific error than failure to detect a true association (a type 2 error). If the p-value is less than an appropriate cut-point, such as 0.05 or 0.01, then convention dictates that chance is unlikely to explain the degree of association seen in the table, and the association is considered *statistically significant*.

Thanks to many published cautions, most clinicians and researchers know that *a strict dependence on p-values is incorrect because the magnitude of the p-value is dependent on the size of the study*. Smaller studies require stronger associations to achieve the same level of statistical significance; thus a p-value of 0.06 in a small study by no means rules out a true association between exposure and disease, whereas a highly statistically significant difference from a huge study may be so small as to be clinically irrelevant.

cancer was higher for black women at all ages in comparison with white women. During 1988 to 2000, the incidence was the same at young ages (30 years or less), but the racial difference was still evident at older ages. This could indicate that risk and screening had become equivalent in younger cohorts, whereas older black women still suffered from their historically worse risk.

To distinguish cohort effects from simple age trends requires a *cohort analysis*, a type of descriptive graphing in which the age-specific prevalence rates are graphed separately for each birth cohort. These analyses are usually difficult enough to interpret to merit a statistical consultation.

The Basic Contingency Table

Colposcopists are naturally drawn to colposcopic images. The analogous, fundamental tool of epidemiology is the contingency table, the basic form of which is the 2 × 2 table (Table 1-1). Most important epidemiologic findings, relating an exposure to the risk of a disease, have been derived and can be expressed in this simple form. Extension of the table to more rows or columns does not change the concepts, only the statistical complexity.

The most common statistics computed from a contingency table are simple proportions or percentages

Contingency tables larger than 2×2 should be analyzed in a methodic and hierarchic fashion, not restricting the analysis to the most significant-looking internal comparisons. First, the evidence for association in the full table should be assessed and, if none is found, then the analysis should stop or at least proceed cautiously. *A common mistake is to look at a large contingency table, choose the most interesting difference seen, and then test the significance of that extracted comparison. Given a large-enough contingency table, some subtables will yield statistically significant results by chance alone.* Permitting a prescreening of the data before applying a statistical test to the most divergent data points is wrong. If one wishes to define the likely source of the association when the overall contingency table indicates statistical significance, the proper approach is to analyze smaller subtables in a complete and hierarchic manner. A formal description of the proper approach to contingency table analyses can be found in standard biostatistics texts.

When the number of study subjects is very small, (the expected count in any cell is less than about five), then chi-square analyses are unreliable and should be replaced by a test called *Fisher's exact test.* Of course, if the study is too small, no result will be statistically significant.

As one embarks on statistical testing, one other key point about contingency tables to keep in mind is that the two measurements (e.g., disease status and exposure) must be assumed to be independent. Although a significant chi-square statistic indicates that the measurements are not independent, the initial or *null hypothesis* of independence is what the test is designed to reject. Thus standard chi-square analyses should not be performed to test tables where the measurements are explicitly correlated, as in interobserver agreement studies (see later) or comparisons of the efficacy of two sample collection techniques used in the same group of patients. *For these paired-sample comparisons, the McNermar's test is easy to use.* The test ignores the instances of agreement of the two measurements and tests the statistical significance of the amount of divergence.

It would also be wrong to include more than one measurement per subject in a standard contingency table. Measurements from a given person tend to be *autocorrelated;* that is, more alike than random measurements. A difficult and evolving field of epidemiology explicitly considers multiple measurements from subjects. For example, a prospective cohort study to evaluate HPV infection in a group of women, persistence over time, and risk of CIN would need to have multiple HPV tests performed on the same woman. The level of study remains the woman, not the test, and a simple contingency table cannot be used as it would lump together all the interpretations naïvely.

Measures of Risk: Absolute, Relative, and Attributable Risks

The chi-square provides limited information regarding the strength of an association (yes/no). Therefore epidemiologists prefer to compute a more informative statistic, the relative risk (or odds ratio estimate of the relative risk). These key terms were defined earlier in the section on epidemiologic studies of disease etiology. In this section, the terms are defined more formally in the context of the contingency table, with a brief discussion of ancillary topics such as statistical adjustment of confounding variables, interaction, and confidence intervals.

Suppose a prospective study followed two groups of women for disease occurrence: one exposed and one unexposed group. The absolute risk of disease following exposure can be represented as an incidence rate: $a/(a+b)$. The time period for this incidence rate is implicitly the duration of follow-up. The absolute risk of disease in the unexposed group would be the incidence rate: $c/(c+d)$. The ratio of these absolute risks would be the relative risk (specifically, the incidence rate ratio) in exposed versus nonexposed women: $a/(a+b)$ divided by $c/(c+d)$. A relative risk of 1.0 implies the exposure is not related to risk of the disease. A relative risk greater than 1.0 implies an increased risk. For example, a relative risk of 2.0 means that the risk of disease in exposed women is twice that of unexposed women. In contrast, a relative risk between 0.0 and 1.0 indicates a protective association (a relative risk of 0.5 implies a halving of risk associated with the exposure). Prospective studies permit the computational directness and intuitive quality of the relative risk calculation, as well as the ability to decompose the relative risk into the absolute risks among the exposed and unexposed groups.

In contrast, *it is not usually possible to calculate absolute risks in case-control studies* because the true numbers of exposed women $(a + b)$ and unexposed women $(c + d)$ are not known. In fact, in 2×2 tables from case-control studies, the values $a + b$ and $c + d$ are meaningless and should never be computed. The numbers of cases $(a + c)$ and controls $(b + d)$ are chosen first, not in proportion to the true ratio of cases to controls in the population. Cases are almost always sampled in excess; in fact, oversampling cases to overcome the limitation of rarity is the major reason to perform a case-control analysis.

As mentioned earlier, although case-control data do not permit direct calculation of the relative risk, the odds ratio provides a valid estimate of the relative risk if the following assumptions are met: The cases must represent an unbiased sample of all women with disease in the population. The controls must represent an unbiased sample of all women without disease. The disease in question must be rare if prevalent cases are studied; otherwise, the odds ratio will be higher than the relative risk it is meant to estimate. If all the cases are incident, the rare disease assumption is not as important, unless the disease is so common that a non-negligible percentage of the population is developing it at any given time.

To understand these points more intuitively, again consider a prospective study. The odds of disease in exposed women is a/b, very close to the risk of disease $a/(a + b)$ only if a, the occurrence of disease among the exposed, is very infrequent. Similarly, the odds of disease in nonexposed women is c/d, close to the risk of the disease if it is uncommon in the nonexposed women, $c/(c + d)$. With a little algebra, it is easy to see that the relative odds or odds ratio for a rare disease (a/b divided by c/d, often computed as the cross-product ad/bc), is quite close to the relative risk.

The important point is that the cross-product ad/bc can be computed from a case-control study without knowing the total number of exposed and unexposed women. As long as the odds a/c and b/d are unbiased with regard to the entire population, then a/c divided by b/d = ad/bc = the prospective odds ratio of a/b divided by c/d. The key is to select an unbiased sample of cases and controls. Because epidemiologists usually try to recruit all cases occurring in a population, bias among cases is not usually an issue unless participation rates are poor. The place where bias is a major concern is among the controls. Epidemiologists spend most of their intellectual energy attempting to ensure that the ratio b/d in controls (also thought of as the percentage of controls exposed to the risk factor) is unbiased compared with the same ratio in the population that gave rise to the cases. Without the elimination of bias, the odds ratio does not estimate the relative risk, and the case-control design will yield a false result.

Confounding is the type of bias that is of greatest concern to epidemiologists, particularly when they are conducting case-control studies or nonrandomized prospective studies. *Confounding variables* are factors that influence both the risk of disease and the likelihood of exposure to a risk factor under study. The relationship among exposures, confounding variables, and disease outcome is illustrated in Figure 1-6. As shown in the figure, when assessing whether an exposure, such as genital herpes infection, causes cervical cancer, the researcher must consider and adjust for the confounding influence of HPV infection, the sexually transmitted agent that is the central cause of cervical cancer. Women who have more sexual partners are more likely to be both HSV-2 and HPV infected (i.e., the confounding variable [HPV] is linked to the likelihood of the study exposure [herpes]). The apparent influence of HSV-2 on risk of cervical cancer is reduced by statistically adjusting for HPV infection status. In summary of this important point, epidemiologic analyses must adjust statistically for the influence of confounding factors to generate unbiased risk estimates. Note that confounding factors are true risk factors for disease, despite the word *confounding* that suggests confusion; it is

the exposure-disease association and not the confounder-disease association that is under question.

Adjustment for confounding is commonly undertaken by one of three methods: *exclusion*, *stratification*, or *regression modeling*. Exclusion could be exemplified in the foregoing example by restricting the analysis to women known to be infected with HPV. Using stratification, rather than excluding any subjects, the association of sexual behavior with cervical cancer could be examined separately in each of the two strata (HPV–/HPV+), providing two unconfounded estimates akin to those derived by exclusion. The risk estimates could then be pooled to obtain a global estimate for the risk of genital herpes adjusted for HPV. This kind of stratified analysis is commonly performed using a group of procedures called a *Mantel–Haenszel analysis*.

A widely used but more conceptually difficult approach is *logistic regression analysis*, a multivariable regression technique available in the major statistical software packages, such as SAS, STATA, and BMDP. Logistic regression is especially well suited to calculation of the odds ratio as an estimate of the relative risk in case-control studies. This technique permits the simultaneous calculation of the odds ratio for multiple risk factors, adjusted for one another's confounding influences. A discussion of this technique, and its uses and misuses, is beyond the scope of this chapter. The commercially available statistical packages offer multivariable regression packages in a seductively simple format that might inspire some novice epidemiologists to perform complicated analyses. However, to master the art of multivariable regression analysis takes statistical training and apprenticeship. Moreover, the results cannot be *checked* easily. It is wise to both avoid and distrust complicated analyses, especially because the bulk of what can be learned from most data sets can be expressed using simple tables and intuitively approachable statistics. In short, *all modeling should be checked against simple tables for common-sense agreement*.

Adjustment for confounding is often not perfectly achieved, particularly when the confounding variable cannot be measured well or when variables under study are highly correlated. In fact, *it is sometimes virtually impossible using statistical methods to adjust for the confounding influences of correlated variables*. For example, the most conceptually difficult areas of chronic disease epidemiology relate to time. In all data analyses involving time, the correlated effects of age at first exposure, duration of exposure, and latency (time since first exposure) are among the most difficult to determine.

Sometimes the risk of an exposure varies by the level of another exposure. For example, the risk of oral cancer is higher among smokers who also drink alcohol than among those who only smoke. This effect modification is often called *interaction*. Extreme positive-effect modification is sometimes called "synergy," but that term is inexact and probably is worth avoiding. Effect modification is different from confounding, in that no global adjustment is possible to arrive at a single correct risk estimate for the exposure. The risks truly vary by levels of the effect modifier. The

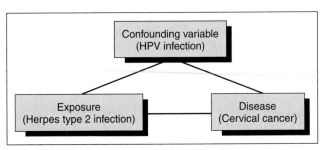

Figure 1-6 Confounding factors. *HPV,* Human papillomavirus.

proper approach is to present the risk estimates for the exposure separately for each level.

It is common to place *confidence intervals* around relative risk estimates to indicate the likely range of the true risk that we are trying to estimate. *Confidence intervals take into account only random error, not bias, and are conceptually similar to p-values, although more informative. Thus a 95% confidence interval and a p-value of 0.05 are both commonly chosen as standard and have analogous interpretations.* For example, if the relative risk of an exposure for a disease is 1.8 with a 95% confidence interval of 1.1 to 3.0, this implies that given random error, the true relative risk has a 95% chance of falling within that range. *If the confidence interval for a relative risk excludes 1.0, the result is conventionally considered statistically significant. A relative risk with confidence intervals including 1.0 indicates no statistically significant association between exposure and disease.* As with p-values, confidence intervals should be used as a guide but not followed absolutely in interpreting data.

Most analytical epidemiologic research centers on estimation of relative risks. Another very useful concept, especially for public health applications of epidemiologic results, is the *attributable risk,* also known as the *attributable proportion* or *etiologic fraction.* These terms subsume several computational forms and subtle differences in meaning, but the general meaning is clear: the percent of the disease (from 0 to 100%) that is due to the exposure and would theoretically disappear if the exposure were eliminated. One useful computational formula for the attributable risk, using the notation in Table 1-1, is: attributable risk $= [(a/a+c) \times (1-1/RR) \times 100\%]$. In words, the fraction of disease attributable to the risk factor is equal to the percentage of cases of the disease that are exposed, adjusted for the strength of the estimated relative risk. Although the formula may appear a bit complicated, it is very easy to use. The adjustment part of the formula $(1-1/RR)$, goes to 0 as the relative risk goes to 1.0 and goes to 1 as the relative risk goes to infinity. Thus even if all cases are exposed, the attributable risk will be 0% if all controls are also exposed because the RR is 1.0 and the adjustment multiplier term is 0.

As a practical example showing the measurements of risk just discussed, our relatively complete understanding of the development of cervical cancer permits the creation of a useful risk table shown in Table 1-2.[14] The table gives the absolute risks of finding CIN 3 post-colposcopy in patients from ASC-US LSIL Triage Study (ALTS) when that first colposcopy found no CIN 2 or worse. The risk of finding subsequent CIN 3 by study exit, despite the initially reassuring colposcopy, was predicted by combinations of cytology, HPV status and the exit colposcopic impression. Knowing the absolute risks permits easy and direct calculation of relative risks and attributable risks.

Causal Intermediates and Surrogate Endpoints

Increasingly, many colposcopy and epidemiology studies of gynecologic neoplasia in the United States do not include invasive tumors. There is a keen interest in the validation of biomarkers and intermediate/surrogate endpoints for screening,

diagnosis, and etiologic research. Cancers arise as multistep processes. An exposure can become a biologically effective internal dose; resultant genetic alteration can lead to a subtle lesion, and the precursor can progress to cancer. For example, most women are exposed and infected with HPV, but almost all of them clear the infection within a relatively short period of time (1–2 years). Only a small percentage become chronically infected and present genetic alterations leading to precancer and cancer. Each step might be reversible and influenced by the genetic susceptibility of the individual. The earliest *intermediate endpoints* (such as HPV infection) are often common and reversible. Later steps (such as progression of a simple HPV infection to CIN 3) are less common and more fixed. *Although molecular biologists may view oncogenesis as a series of* molecular hits, *epidemiologists may discuss* conditional probabilities. For example, "Conditional on a woman being infected with an oncogenic type of HPV, what is the probability of progression to CIN 3?" "Conditional on having CIN 3, what is the probability of invasion?" "If the CIN 3 lasts for 5 years without regression, how does that affect the probability of invasion?" Oncogenesis occurs mechanistically but, lacking all the details, epidemiology presumes that events will happen by useful measurements of *risk.*

The importance of a biomarker or intermediate endpoint can be evaluated using the relative risk of cancer when a biomarker or intermediate endpoint is positive compared to when it is negative. A high relative risk implies importance. A *surrogate endpoint* is a more stringent term. Many studies examining the associations between biomarkers are not necessarily clinically relevant because no association with attributable risk of disease is directly made. If a biomarker is a valid surrogate endpoint, then reducing its occurrence should proportionately reduce the occurrence of the cancer itself. CIN 3 is a good surrogate endpoint for invasive cervical cancer. However, reducing 50% of CIN 1 might not imply reducing 50% of invasive cancer.

The statistical evaluation of possible intermediate endpoints is algebraically linked to the analysis of confounding, but there are important differences of interpretation. When a biomarker or preinvasive lesion is proposed as an intermediate endpoint for a cancer, it should share the general risk factor profile of that cancer. In fact, its consideration by statistical adjustment should *explain* the association of known epidemiologic risk factors for that cancer. If not, the validity of the intermediate endpoint as a surrogate for the cancer is in question. For example, the risk of ovarian cysts detected by transvaginal ultrasound is not reduced by multiparity and oral contraceptive use. These are two very powerful protective factors in the etiology of ovarian cancer, casting doubt on the etiologic relevance of most of the cysts found by ultrasound.[15] On the other hand, HPV infection almost completely explains the strong association of sexual behavior and risk of cervical cancer, as befits a central causal intermediate.[16]

Measures of Intercolposcopist Agreement

Simply put, *there is no universally accepted statistical measure of interrater agreement.* The problem is adjustment for the

Table 1-2 Absolute Risks for Postcolposcopic Two- and Three-Stage Strategies for CIN 3 Outcome

Thin Prep Pap	#CIN 3/Total	Absolute Risk (%)	Hybrid Capture 2 — Negative #CIN 3/Total 19/962	Absolute Risk (%) 2.0	Colposcopy	#CIN 3/Total	Absolute Risk (%)	Hybrid Capture 2 — Positive #CIN 3/Total 103/874	Absolute Risk (%) 11.8	Colposcopy	#CIN 3/Total	Absolute Risk (%)
Normal	36/1157	3.1	9/726	1.2	Normal	1/401	0.2	25/344	7.3	Normal	3/135	2.2
					Low grade	8/308	2.6			Low grade	18/195	9.2
					High grade/CA	0/13	0			High grade/CA	3/9	33.3
ASC-US	37/466	7.9	10/199	5.0	Normal	0/100	0	26/240	10.8	Normal	2/69	2.9
					Low grade	9/94	9.6			Low grade	20/158	12.7
					High grade/CA	1/4	*			High grade/CA	4/11	36.4
LSIL	25/273	9.2	0/25	—	Normal	0/12	0	24/225	10.7	Normal	1/55	1.8
					Low grade	0/13	0			Low grade	19/149	12.7
					High grade/CA	—	—			High grade/CA	4/19	21.0
HSIL	29/69	42.0	0/4	—	Normal	0/1	0	28/62	45.2	Normal	1/1	*
					Low grade	0/3	0			Low grade	15/43	34.9
					High grade/CA	—	—			High grade/CA	12/18	66.7

Reproduced from Walker JL, Wang SS, Schiffman M, Solomon D. Predicting absolute risk of CIN 3 during post-colposcopic follow-up: results from the ASC-US-LSIL Triage Study (ALTS). Am J Obstet Gynecol 2006;195:341–348.

*Denominator < 5.

Cytology predicts CIN 3 absolute risk in second column (bolded). Absolute risks for CIN 3 by HPV-negative and HPV-positive results are presented in the top row (bolded). In the columns below this, the risk by HPV result is further stratified according to the cytology result. Finally, the risk groups defined by HPV and cytology results are further stratified by colposcopy impression. For example, HPV + absolute risk of CIN 3 overall is 11.8% in the last column. HPV+ is then stratified below by cytology result in the values of 7.3 (nL); 10.8 (ASCS); 10.7 (LSIL); and 45.2 (HSIL). Finally, HPV+/cytology results are stratified by colposcopy impression (i.e., HPV+/HSIL with high-grade colposcopy has a CIN 3+ absolute risk of 66.7).

influence of chance agreement, which varies with the numbers of categories and the composition of the study population. All currently available statistical methods have limitations, and therefore it is best, whenever possible, to present the actual data to the reader, in addition to any percentage or statistic.

Consider a study in which two colposcopists are asked to evaluate 100 cases and provide one of two diagnoses: normal or abnormal. As illustrated in Table 1-3, even though evaluators A and B might have good agreement on the number of normal (40% versus 45%) and abnormal cases (55% versus 60%), the real agreement of the evaluators might be mediocre (highlighted boxes). *The Kappa statistic, widely used by epidemiologists, corrects the observed agreement (actual agreement among evaluators) for the expected agreement (what would be expected just by chance).* Using the data in Table 1-3, the observed agreement is calculated with the values in the highlighted boxes (75% = 0.75). The agreement expected by chance is $(45/100) \times (40/100) + (55/100) \times (60/100) = 0.18 + 0.33 = 0.51$. The value of Kappa is calculated as (Observed value − Expected value) / $(1 - \text{Expected value}) = (0.75 - 0.51) / (1 - 0.51) = 0.49$.

A Kappa value close to 1 represents almost perfect agreement. A value close to 0 means that agreement is mainly due to chance. There is no absolute consensus about the meanings of Kappa values between 0 and 1, but in general, values greater than 0.75 represent excellent agreement, values between 0.40 and 0.75 are moderate to good, and values below 0.40 mean poor to mediocre agreement beyond chance.[1]

The Kappa statistic has some limitations.[17] Only tables of identical size can be compared, and the statistic is slightly dependent on the prevalence of disease. An asymmetry chi-square, analogous to a multicategory McNemar's test, is often calculated with the Kappa statistic. The purpose is to test whether one rater is yielding systematically more severe interpretations than the other, or whether disagreements are randomly distributed.

Other factors could influence the evaluation of interobserver agreement. For example, suppose we are evaluating the agreement between two cytotechnicians and select a sample from general screening in which almost 95% of samples are normal. The percentage of agreement would be high. The same could happen if the vast majority of the samples are clearly abnormal. As a general recommendation, better information will be obtained using an adequately balanced sample.

During the last few years, there have been many publications about interobserver agreement in colposcopy showing that it is very difficult to visually distinguish grades of intraepithelial neoplasia. The NIH/ASCCP Research Group (National Institutes of Health/American Society for Colposcopy and Cervical Pathology) recently completed a study with the participation of 20 expert colposcopists that evaluated 939 digitized cervigrams distributed in such a way that each expert was assigned 112 images.[18] After adjusting the results by patient HPV status and age, this study showed that agreement is poor among expert colposcopists evaluating static images, although it was possible to identify groups of evaluators with similar frequency of diagnoses (Table 1-4).

Similar lack of agreement was found among pathologists performing cytologic or even histologic evaluations. HPV DNA testing has proven to be very helpful in distinguishing patients with equivocal cytology at high risk of harboring CIN 3 from those with nonsignificant smears. Based on the rationale explained earlier (Risk Assessment), we forecast a similar role for HPV DNA testing when evaluating colposcopic examinations. For example, women with persistent infection with oncogenic HPV (especially HPV16) would need a more aggressive search for preneoplastic lesions, with multiple biopsies taken possibly even from areas without evident visual alterations.

SCREENING TERMS

Screening is a special area of epidemiology distinct from descriptive or analytic studies. It is rare to find a useful screening test. Finding a strong risk factor for a disease does not imply that we should screen for that risk factor because the factor is often too common in the general population to permit its use as a trigger for clinical action. For example, we do not consider smoking a screening test for lung cancer.

Screening terms have very exact meanings that may vary from other common uses of the same terms. In Table 1-1, the women in cell A have *true-positive* screening tests in that they have the disease and tested positive. The women in cell C have *false-negative* results because they have the disease but tested negative. The *sensitivity* of a test, also called the *true-positive rate*, is the percentage of diseased women who test positive [a/(a+c) in Figure 1-1]. *The screening sensitivity must be clearly distinguished from the analytic sensitivity of a laboratory assay, which has a different meaning. Typically, more analytic sensitivity implies a better laboratory test. However, increasing screening sensitivity often leads to decreasing specificity, as indicated in the following section on ROC curves.*

Table 1-3 Interobserver Agreement

		Evaluator B		
		Normal	**Abnormal**	**Total**
Evaluator A	Normal	30	10	40
	Abnormal	15	45	60
	Total	45	55	100

Table 1-4 Agreement among Expert Colposcopists after Adjusting for Age and HPV DNA Result

Raters	Ratio: High Grade+ to Normal	Normal	Cervicitis/ Metaplasia	Low Grade/ Condyloma	High Grade/ Cancer
Rater 7	0.13	46%	28%	20%	6%
Rater 11	0.43	28%	29%	31%	12%
Rater 20	0.56	25%	28%	33%	14%
Rater 10	0.73	22%	27%	35%	16%
Rater 16	0.73	22%	27%	35%	16%
Rater 6	0.81	21%	26%	36%	17%
Rater 9	0.81	21%	26%	36%	17%
Rater 13	0.95	19%	26%	37%	18%
Rater 8	1.00	19%	25%	37%	19%
Rater 15	1.06	18%	25%	37%	19%
Rater 12	1.11	18%	24%	38%	20%
Rater 14	1.18	17%	24%	38%	20%
Rater 5	1.24	17%	24%	38%	21%
Rater 19	1.79	14%	22%	39%	25%
Rater 18	1.79	14%	22%	40%	25%
Rater 4	2.33	12%	20%	40%	28%
Rater 1	2.73	11%	19%	40%	30%
Rater 2	2.33	12%	20%	40%	28%
Rater 3	3.20	10%	18%	40%	32%
Rater 17	4.00	9%	16%	39%	36%

Adapted from Jeronimo J, Massad LS, Castle PE, Wacholder S, Schiffman M; National Institutes of Health (NIH)-American Society for Colposcopy and Cervical Pathology (ASCCP) Research Group. Interobserver agreement in the evaluation of digitized cervical images. Obstet Gynecol. 2007 Oct;110(4):833–40. p-trend < 0.0005.

The *true-negative* results are in cell D; the *false-positive* results are in cell B. The *specificity*, also called the *true-negative rate*, is the percentage of women without the disease who test negative [d/(b+d)]. The concept of specificity is more important in screening than most realize. *Because the overwhelming majority of women in a population do not have the disease under study, as the specificity percentage falls even slightly, the absolute numbers of false-positive screening tests rise dramatically in comparison to the number of true positives.* Therefore decreased specificity leads to low *positive predictive value*, the percentage of women with a positive test who truly have the disease [a/(a + b)]. For many diseases, positive predictive value is the major screening statistic of interest. Clinicians ask, "If a woman tests positive, what is the likelihood that she will have disease confirmed on referral to the next clinical step (e.g., colposcopically directed biopsy, laparoscopy, more major surgery)?" *Low positive predictive value leads to over-referral and over-treatment.*

For grave diseases in which over-treatment of normal women is less of a concern than not missing any cases, the *negative predictive value* is a very important concept of reassurance. The negative predictive value is the percentage of women who test negative who are truly diseasefree [d/(c + d)]. A clinician may ask accordingly, "If the test is negative, how safe is it for me to defer any further diagnostic workup?" The sensitivity of the test is usually the key determinant of negative predictive value.

When screening is mentioned, there is always an implicit notion of a *reference standard* or *gold standard* of disease. The performance of screening tests is described statistically in relation to this reference standard. *A flawed reference standard screening will lead to flawed statistics. For example, colposcopically directed biopsy with pathologic diagnosis is often taken as the reference standard of CIN, but the colposcopic biopsy may be misdirected or the histopathologic diagnosis may be in error. Thus the true performance of screening tests such as cytology, cervicography, or HPV testing may be misinterpreted when compared with the results of colposcopically directed biopsies.*[19] *For example, the cytology may identify disease that is missed or misinterpreted as negative by the colposcopy or biopsy. The cytology would be considered falsely positive, but the real flaw is that the colposcopy or biopsies are falsely negative.*

Screening tests may detect prevalent disease or predict the future diagnosis of disease, and the two time frames may be confused. If some type of HPV test could truly predict incipient cervical neoplasia, even when biopsies were still negative, it would be misleading to compare the HPV screening result only with prevalent (same-day) disease defined by biopsies.

Another mistake is the following: Researchers who wish to compare the sensitivity of two screening tests might double-test a research population, referring for a definitive diagnostic procedure only those women who are positive for either screening test. If they then compute and report the *sensitivity* of each test, an error of circular reasoning has been made. Because an unknown number of cases of disease could be missed by both screening tests (double false-negatives), the true sensitivity of either test cannot be known without referring all women in the study population for the definitive workup. Sometimes in large studies it suffices to refer a random sample of the women who screen negative on both tests, as a way of correcting (or of verifying, to think optimistically) the estimates of sensitivity.

A particularly tricky error happens when the gold standard has the same limitations of the screening test. For example, there is a conflict at this time of evaluating visual inspection with acetic acid (VIA) using colposcopy and biopsy as the gold standard because patients with CIN missed by VIA could have a *nonvisible* lesion very likely to be also missed by colposcopy.

The point of this discussion is that, when screening terms such as sensitivity or specificity are mentioned, then the reference standard must be explicitly stated and, if necessary, questioned.

Receiver-Operating Characteristic Curve

Some of the current controversy regarding the proper clinical management of inconclusive cervical cytologic smears centers on the competing needs for a good negative predictive value (assurance that we are not missing any high-grade disease) and a good positive predictive value (desire not to over-treat). This problem highlights an inescapable feature of screening (or, more fundamentally, of trying to categorize overlapping distributions): *Increased sensitivity virtually always leads to decreased specificity and, as a corollary, increasingly reassuring negative predictive value can only be obtained at the price of decreased positive predictive value.*

A formal method exists for choosing the proper screening *cut-point* (for example, the viral load threshold of a DNA-based assay meriting colposcopic referral to detect CIN 2,3 or cancer) to achieve an optimal compromise between sensitivity and specificity. The technique is called the ROC curve because the approach was developed to test how well an electronic receiver could distinguish signals from electrical noise. The concepts are useful and well explained in a few key articles that are recommended to anyone wishing to evaluate a screening test.[20,21]

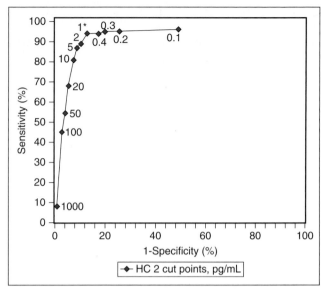

Figure 1-7 Receiver Operating Characteristics Curve for Hybrid Capture II (*HC 2*) test for detection of high-grade cervical lesions and cancer. Asterisk (*) indicates inflection point. (Adapted from Schiffman M, Herrero R, Hildesheim A, et al. HPV DNA testing in cervical cancer screening: results from women in a high-risk province of Costa Rica. J Am Med Assoc. 2000;283:87–93.)

In brief, most test measurements range from 0 to some high value. It is conceivable to set a series of cut-points that define a positive screening test result demanding further attention. Lower cut-points for considering the assay positive detect more cases of disease but refer more women. In a ROC curve, sensitivity for detection of the target disease is plotted against 100% minus specificity. The expression "100% minus specificity" is very close to percent referred if disease is rare. A very good screening test will have very high sensitivity and specificity. In other words, it will detect women with disease but refer few extra women. The quality of screening or diagnostic tests is easy to compare using ROC curves.

As an illustration of their usefulness, ROC curves were used to determine the optimal cut-point for Hybrid Capture II (HC 2). Figure 1-7 shows the ROC curve for detection of CIN 3 and cancer.[20] The plot starts at a viral load of 1000 pg/mL that was very specific for disease but had an extremely poor sensitivity. When the cut-point for viral load was progressively lowered, the sensitivity increased sharply with very small decrease in specificity. This pattern was observed until a viral load of 1 pg/mL. Below that level there was almost no increase in sensitivity but a great decrease in specificity. Based on this and similar ROC curves, a viral load of 1 pg/mL was selected as the clinically useful cut-point to consider a HC 2 result as positive.

PROBLEM AREAS

The major goal of including an introduction to epidemiology in a textbook on colposcopy was to encourage colposcopists to do epidemiologic studies and to work with epidemiologists. Accordingly, it may be worth alerting the colposcopists to recurrent problem areas that exist at the juncture of the two disciplines. This section quite informally catalogs a few practical problems that appear to arise most commonly.

Dividing a Spectrum of Disease into Categories

Unfortunately, some epidemiologists may seek out colposcopists to perform a service function of "making sure the cases are right," without understanding much about colposcopy (just as colposcopists might seek out statisticians to do a rote data analysis or to determine how many cases are needed for statistical significance). Providing rote colposcopy review may prove a difficult collaboration because epidemiologists are prompted by their statistical methods to seek overly simplistic and discrete categorization of disease outcomes. Because the statistical methods for considering a spectrum of disease are difficult to perform and understand, epidemiologists tend to simplify disease measurements into a few (ideally two) reliably distinguished categories, such as *invasive cervical cancer* versus *normal*. However, as the example of cervical neoplasia demonstrates, diseases may exist as a spectrum of changes that are impossible to divide perfectly into a few categories.

If an epidemiologist asks a colposcopist to determine whether a cervigram shows disease (positive) or not (negative), an equivocal or *rule-out* diagnosis is usually not usable because it cannot be forced into a statistical table. Often the epidemiologist must subsequently exclude the uncertain diagnoses from the analyses. It is possible to perform a *malicious analysis* in which the uncertain cases are added to the analysis as cases, then reanalyzed as controls, to see whether the uncertainty in case definition affects the comparisons being made. However, too large a proportion of uncertain diagnoses can make an analytic study unreliable.

The collaborating epidemiologist must be willing to understand diagnostic error as a fact of nature and not a failing of colposcopists. The colposcopist must be willing to sacrifice absolute truth to simplify the statistical data to the point of understanding. The limitations of epidemiology should be recognized. As a great physician-epidemiologist once said, "Epidemiology is a butcher shop; don't try to use a scalpel." In other words, epidemiology can only study strong risk associations because even strong associations are made to appear weak by unavoidable measurement errors and biases. Truly weak associations will probably be missed by all but the largest and luckiest studies. With this in mind, the routine use of diagnostic terms such as "consistent with" and "cannot exclude" should be abandoned for epidemiologic studies, with the recognition that diagnostic errors will exist (the extent of which should be measured by reliability studies and reported).

Need for Masking

Epidemiologists tend to mask all data collection as an automatic part of good research technique in order to avoid the influence of subtle biases that could distort risk estimates. Thus epidemiologists do not routinely tell interviewers the disease status of the subjects to minimize bias in questioning, they do not tell laboratory collaborators the identity of specimens until the results are obtained, and they ask colposcopists to make their diagnoses with a minimum of information regarding the patients. Colposcopists working together (panel reviews) tend to agree more readily than if the independent opinions are compared. The social tendency to promote consensus may be the cause. Epidemiologists are seeking a completely independent decision from colposcopists, without influence from previous diagnoses or clinical tests, which often are being studied as risk factors for the current condition. All common statistical tests assume that the study measurements are completely independent of each other; thus using any piece of data to influence a decision on another piece of data is wrong.

Colposcopists, however, realize that diagnoses are best made in the context of complete information regarding the patient and that asking for a diagnosis out of context, as one would demand a lab result from a machine, risks increased error. Some clinicians incorrectly view the request for masking as a sign of distrust of their intellectual integrity or ability to make an independent decision. The request is actually a sign of the epidemiologist's belief that everyone is biased about every decision unless masked. Epidemiologists practice skepticism as part of their profession, and it eventually characterizes them as a group. As a revealing example, an epidemiologists' beer-tasting group in Maryland drinks from opaque, unlabeled mugs and unmasks the results only after the *data* (opinions) are in. Fortunately, it is usually easy for good collaborators to achieve a balance between automatic demands for complete masking and the kind of complete disclosure of study information that could lead to serious biases.

Standardization of the Scientific Art of Colposcopy

A thornier problem arises when epidemiologists challenge the accuracy and reliability of clinical diagnoses, either as part of a formal colposcopy agreement study or as part of a larger epidemiologic project. This challenge takes the form of calculation and publication of rates of (dis)agreement between experts or between the expert and himself or herself on different days. The epidemiologist is trained to believe that all biological phenomena are variable and that all measurements of biological phenomena are prone to random error. Clinicians have the weighty daily task of being the final arbiter of disease definition, a responsibility that does not mesh well with error.

A colposcopist may feel irritated at the demands for reliability studies from new epidemiologist colleagues. If so, it might help to ask eager-beaver epidemiologists when they had last compared their design or analytic performance in a masked comparison with other epidemiologists. Because such painful comparative exercises are almost never perpetrated by epidemiologists on themselves, mutual humility and curiosity should reign.

Specimen Adequacy versus the Bias of Convenience Samples

Epidemiologists seeking to minimize bias are loath to permit exclusions from a complete series. They suspect that the excluded members of the set will differ from those included in a systematic (biased) rather than a random way. Thus epidemiologists working with colposcopists wish to start their analyses by considering the entire sample available, winnowing out as needed to arrive at usable results, but always with an eye to possible biases of exclusion that could affect the general applicability of the results. Epidemiologists distrust *convenience samples*, groups of specimens that happen to be available for testing or for review. Colposcopists may view the task of defining and retrieving all relevant subjects from their center to be unnecessary. It may be difficult to decide in advance when a convenience sample is sufficient and when a more definitive collection is required. In general, convenience samples are useful for preliminary methodologic work, but such studies cannot be used to reach definitive, generalizable conclusions.[22]

Another example of possible convenience sampling relates to the fact that more frequently, biopsies of CIN 3 come from the 6- and 12-o'clock positions of the cervix. Is CIN really more common at those locations? Or is it due to a bias at sampling because it is much easier for colposcopists to take a biopsy from ratios 6 and 12?

Determining the Size of the Study: Statistical Significance versus Practicality

Bigger is better for the epidemiologist. It is not much more difficult to do a statistical analysis of 1000 patients than 100; in fact, it is methodologically easier because the numbers are clearly sufficient. However, the clinical collaborator may view it differently. The question of study size is almost always negotiable, in that bigger studies permit the detection of smaller differences, but the critical difference that needs to be detected is usually open to discussion.

There are minimum numbers of subjects that permit epidemiologic analyses. It is impossible to generate a statistically significant result with fewer than five subjects, regardless of the strength of an association. Thirty subjects is another breakpoint because a sample of 30 produces common statistics such as arithmetic means that "behave" with reasonable reliability. About 200 cases and 200 controls are needed to find a relative risk of about 2.0 (a doubling of risk), given typical prevalences of common exposures. Case-control studies of more than 1000 subjects are relatively rare. Cohort studies, however, often require thousands or even tens of thousands of subjects to generate enough disease endpoints for analysis. Clinical trials range from small (20 subjects per randomization arm) to large (thousands of subjects) based on the size of the difference being sought. *In general, small studies miss weak associations, do not permit adequate adjustment for confounding, and generate less reliable estimates of risk.* Still, many landmark studies of new topics have been small.

The key to defining the proper size of the study is to agree on the hypothesis and the range of expected results. Sample size calculations are very assumption dependent and usually demand information not available until the study is completed. Most epidemiologists choose a reasonable number based on cost and time available and then compute the statistical power of such a study to detect associations of various strengths. It is standard to require the study to have an 80% or greater chance of finding (as statistically significant) the key disease-exposure association under study, assuming the association truly exists. Epidemiologists therefore commonly accept a 20% chance of making a type 2 error (failing to *observe* a true association), whereas they restrict themselves to approximately a 5% chance of making of a type 1 error (falsely declaring a null association to be significant). As scientific skeptics, epidemiologists stack the deck against themselves to avoid being rash. When they are making multiple comparisons, they often reduce the required level of significance below 1% to even tougher standards of evidence.

For clinicians, boredom and time commitment can be real problems in big epidemiologic collaborations. Quality assurance group members can easily spend many hours a week on review work of fairly monotonous, unchallenging cases. Of course, the friendly epidemiologic collaborator will be monitoring to avoid any drift in diagnostic interpretations over time. The situation requires dedication, trust, and scientific interest. In truth, to answer big questions often takes big studies by a cooperative team.

REFERENCES

1. Fleiss JL, Paik MC, Levin B. Satatistical Methods for Rates and Proportions. 3rd Ed. Hoboken: Wiley, 2003.
2. Gordis L. Epidemiology. 3rd Ed. Philadelphia: Elsevier Saunders, 2004.
3. Last JM, Spasoff RA, Harris SS. A Dictionary of Epidemiology. 4th Ed. New York: Oxford University Press, 2000.
4. Haynes RB, Sacket DL, Guyatt GH. Clinical Epidemiology. How to Do Clinical Practice Research. 3rd Ed. Baltimore: Lippincott, Williams and Wilkins, 2006.
5. Jemal A, Siegel R, Ward E, et al. Cancer statistics, 2006. CA Cancer J Clin 2006;56:106–130.
6. Parkin DM, Bray F, Ferlay J, et al. Global cancer statistics, 2002. CA Cancer J Clin 2005;55:74–108.
7. Parkin DM, Bray F, Ferlay J, et al. Estimating the world cancer burden: Globocan 2000. Int J Cancer 2001;94:153–156.
8. Ferlay J, Bray F, Pisani P, et al. GLOBOCAN 2002. Cancer Incidence, Mortality, and Prevalence Worldwide. IARC CancerBase 5:20. IARC Press, Lyon, France: IARC Press, 2004.
9. Khan MJ, Castle PE, Lorincz AT, et al. The elevated 10-year risk of cervical precancer and cancer in women with human papillomavirus (HPV) type 16 or 18 and the possible utility of type-specific HPV testing in clinical practice. J Natl Cancer Inst 2005;97:1072–1079.

10. Schiffman MH, Schatzkin A. Test reliability is critically important to molecular epidemiology: an example from studies of human papillomavirus infection and cervical neoplasia. Cancer Res 1994;54(7 Suppl):1944s–1947s.

11. Plummer M, Schiffman M, Castle P, et al. A 2-year prospective study of human papillomavirus persistence among women with a cytological diagnosis of atypical squamous cells of undetermined significance or low-grade squamous intraepithelial lesion. J Infect Dis. 2007 Jun 1;195(11):1582–9.

12. Schiffman M, Khan MJ, Solomon D, et al. A study of the impact of adding HPV types to cervical cancer screening and triage tests. J Natl Cancer Inst. 2005;97:147–150.

13. Wang SS, Sherman ME, Hildesheim A, et al. Cervical adenocarcinoma and squamous cell carcinoma incidence trends among white women and black women in the United States for 1976–2000. Cancer 2004;100:1035–1044.

14. Walker JL, Wang SS, Schiffman M, et al. Predicting absolute risk of CIN3 during post-colposcopic follow-up: Results from the ASCUS-LSIL Triage Study (ALTS). Am J Obstet Gynecol 2006;195:341–348.

15. Hartge P, Hayes R, Reding D, et al. Complex ovarian cysts in postmenopausal women are not associated with ovarian cancer risk factors: preliminary data from the prostate, lung, colon, and ovarian cancer screening trial. Am J Obstet Gynecol 2000;183:1232–1237.

16. Schiffman MH, Bauer HM, Hoover RN, et al. Epidemiologic evidence showing that human papillomavirus infection causes most cervical intraepithelial neoplasia. J Natl Cancer Inst 1993;85:958–964.

17. Maclure M, Willett WC. Misinterpretation and misuse of the kappa statistic. Am J Epidemiol 1987;126:161–169.

18. Jeronimo J, Massad LS, Castle PE, Wacholder S, Schiffman M; National Institutes of Health (NIH)-American Society for Colposcopy and Cervical Pathology (ASCCP) Research Group. Interobserver agreement in the evaluation of digitized cervical images. Obstet Gynecol. 2007 Oct;110(4):833–40.

19. Wacholder S, Armstrong B, Hartge P. Validation studies using an alloyed gold standard. Am J Epidemiol 1993;137:1251–1258.

20. Schiffman M, Herrero R, Hildesheim A, et al. HPV DNA testing in cervical cancer screening: Results from women in a high-risk province of Costa Rica. J Am Med Assoc 2000;283:87–93.

21. Zweig MH, Campbell G. Receiver-operating characteristic (ROC) plots: A fundamental evaluation tool in clinical medicine. Clin Chem 1993;39:561–577.

22. Guido RS, Jeronimo J, Schiffman M, Solomon D; ALTS Group. The distribution of neoplasia arising on the cervix: results from the ALTS trial. Am J Obstet Gynecol. 2005 Oct;193(4):1331–7.

CHAPTER 2

Human Papillomaviruses and Mechanisms of Oncogenesis

Ann Roman • Helena Spartz • Darron R. Brown

KEY POINTS

- All papillomaviruses share a similar genomic organization consisting of an early (E) gene region, a late (L) gene region, and a regulatory region. The five "early" proteins (E1, E2, E5, E6, and E7) are required for viral replication and/or cellular transformation. Translation of the "late" structural L1 and L2 transcripts, and of the E1^E4 spliced transcript, are restricted to the differentiating epithelium, where viral assembly occurs.
- Human papillomavirus (HPV) types are assigned numerical designations based on their DNA sequence. A new number is assigned when a sequence has less than 90% sequence identity in the L1, E6, and E7 genes of the virus. An isolate with more than 90% homology to a known HPV type is classified as a subtype.
- All HPV types are epitheliotropic, and fully differentiated squamous epithelium is required for completion of the HPV life cycle. HPV infects keratinocytes, the predominant cell of epithelial surfaces.
- HPV is presumably transmitted by contact with desquamated keratinocytes from an infected individual. This contact may be indirect, as in the case of cutaneous wart viruses, or sexual, in the case of cervical infection. These desquamated keratinocytes contain virus particles that must somehow escape the cell and infect the new host.
- Loss of p53 function by interaction with E6 therefore leads to a failure of growth arrest and to a loss of apoptotic signaling. The failure of cell cycle checkpoint controls in E6-expressing cells results in chromosomal duplication and centrosome abnormalities.
- HPV integration correlates with genomic instability, a poor prognosis, and resistance to treatment. Insertional mutagenesis may provide the cell harboring the integrated HPV with a selective growth advantage.
- Keratinocytes expressing high-risk (HR) HPV E6 and E7 are immortalized; that is, they grow indefinitely in cell culture but do not form tumors in animals. As these cells are passaged in cell culture, they may ultimately become tumorigenic. Therefore additional alterations in the cell must occur in the progression toward malignancy.
- In both precursor lesions such as CIN 3 and invasive cervical carcinomas, alterations of human chromosomes such as centrosome abnormalities and aneuploidy can be observed.
- HR-HPV integration is associated with chromosomal instability and overexpression of the E6 and E7 oncoproteins.

Human papillomavirus (HPV) is an icosahedral, nonenveloped, double-stranded deoxyribonucleic acid (DNA) virus of approximately 55 nm in diameter.[1] The genome of all HPVs consists of an approximately 8-kilobase pair molecule of circular, double-stranded DNA (a map of the HPV 16 genome is shown in Figure 2-1).[2,3] All of the proteins are encoded on one of the two DNA strands. *All papillomaviruses share a similar genomic organization consisting of an early (E) gene region, a late (L) gene region, and a regulatory region. The five "early" proteins (E1, E2, E5, E6, and E7) are required for viral replication and/or cellular transformation. Translation of the "late" structural L1 and L2 transcripts and of the E1^E4 spliced transcript are restricted to the differentiating epithelium, where viral assembly occurs.*[4-7] The 55-kDa L1 protein comprises the majority of the virus shell. The L1 gene is the most highly conserved gene among individual HPV types. The L2 protein of 77 kDa is known as the *minor capsid protein* because it contributes a smaller percentage of the capsid mass than does the L1 protein.

The upstream regulatory region (URR), also called the *long control region* (LCR), is located between the end of L1 and beginning of E6 and does not encode HPV proteins. It contains the "early" promoter (termed p97 for HPV 16, as it begins at the 97th base pair) and enhancer sequences necessary for transcription, as well as the origin of replication.[5,7,8] Keratinocyte-specific enhancers have been described in the URR and are thought to contribute to the tissue-specific tropism of HPVs.[2,3,9] This region has the highest degree of variation in the HPV genome.[3,9]

More than 100 different types of HPV have been identified and fully sequenced, and at least an additional ≈50 to 100 putative types have been partially characterized.[10,11] *HPV types are assigned numeric designations once the DNA sequence has been established and a comparison with previously known types has found less than 90% sequence identity in the L1, E6, and E7 genes of the virus.*[12] An isolate with more than 90% homology to a known HPV type is classified as a subtype.

All HPV types are epitheliotropic, and fully differentiated squamous epithelium is required for completion of the HPV life

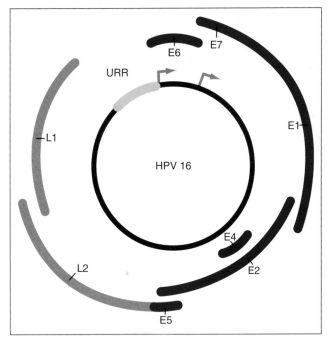

Figure 2-1 Map of the 7905-base pair human papillomavirus (HPV) 16 genome. The *arrows* indicate the positions of the early promoter (upstream of the sequences encoding the E6 protein) and the late promoter (within the E7 gene). The upstream regulatory region (URR) is indicated as a *green band* between the end of the L1 gene and the beginning of the E6 gene.

cycle. HPV infects keratinocytes,[1] the predominant cells of epithelial surfaces. It is believed that only basal or undifferentiated keratinocytes are infected. The viral replication cycle is completed as the keratinocyte undergoes the process of differentiation. Virus is assembled in the nuclei of the most differentiated keratinocytes and can be detected in these cells as desquamation (or shedding of epithelial elements) occurs from the epithelium.[13,14]

HPV is presumably transmitted by contact with desquamated keratinocytes from an infected individual. This contact may be indirect, as in the case of cutaneous wart viruses, or sexual, in the case of cervical infection. These desquamated keratinocytes contain virus particles that must somehow escape the cell and infect the new host. The specific host cell receptor(s) for HPV has not been determined.[15,16]

Approximately 40 HPV types infect the genital tract. HPV infection of the human genitalia causes a range of clinical states including asymptomatic infection, genital warts, cytologic abnormalities of the cervix, and invasive cervical cancer.[17] *The different HPV types can be subdivided into two categories, "high risk" (HR-HPV) and "low risk" (LR-HPV), originally assigned based on whether the HPV type could be found in carcinoma specimens.* The LR-HPV types, such as HPV 6 and HPV 11, are associated with benign, hyperproliferative lesions, commonly referred to as *genital warts* or *condylomata acuminata*, and also cause low-grade cervical dysplastic lesions.[18–20] HR-HPV types, such as HPV 16 and 18, cause low- and high-grade dysplastic lesions of the cervix, including invasive cancer.[21] Other HPV-related genital malignancies include vulvar cancer, particularly the verrucous (warty) form,[22] vaginal cancer, and anal cancer.[23]

Anal cancer is HPV positive in almost all cases.[23] Approximately 45% of cases of penile cancer are associated with HPV.[24] HPV 16 causes more than 50% of these noncervical genital tract cancers.[24]

Six hallmarks of cancer have been identified, which include self-sufficiency in growth signals, insensitivity to antigrowth signals, evading apoptosis, limitless replicative potential, sustained angiogenesis, and tissue invasion and metastasis.[25] HR-HPV gene products, either directly or indirectly, contribute to all of these attributes. In this chapter, we will focus on several key points: the role of specific viral proteins encoded by HPV, the role of viral integration into the host cell genome, angiogenesis induced by HPV, centrosome abnormalities and genetic instability induced by HPV, and nonviral cofactors that help to explain why only some women infected with HR-HPV develop malignancy. We will address the mechanisms shared by LR- and HR-HPV types to induce lesions and why HR-HPV types have the potential to induce malignancy.

ROLE OF SPECIFIC VIRAL ONCOPROTEINS ENCODED BY HIGH-RISK HUMAN PAPILLOMAVIRUS

E6 and E7 are the major HPV oncoproteins, and the expression of the two together optimally immortalizes keratinocytes grown in culture. If expressed at a high level alone in human keratinocytes, E7 can induce immortalization, whereas E6 cannot.[26–28] However, E6 alone does inhibit differentiation.[29] In a transgenic mouse model of cervical carcinogenesis, E7 alone produced microinvasive cancers, whereas E6 alone did not produce neoplasia or cancer.[30] The combined action of both E6 and E7 resulted in large, extensively invasive cancers.[30] *E6 and E7 are the only two HPV proteins whose expression is consistently maintained in cervical carcinomas.*

Expression of the E6 protein allows the infected cell to be insensitive to antigrowth signals and to evade apoptosis (Figure 2-2). The HPV E6 protein binds to a cellular protein, E6-associated protein (E6-AP).[31,32] E6-AP is an E3 ubiquitin-protein ligase.[32] *The E6 and E6-AP complex associates with the cellular tumor suppressor p53, causing rapid ubiquitin-dependent degradation of p53.*[31–33] *The p53 protein normally activates expression of genes involved in cell cycle arrest and/or apoptosis.*[34,35] p53 levels are increased in response to DNA damage or cellular stress, resulting in increased expression of target genes such as the cyclin-dependent kinase inhibitor $p21^{cip1}$. The consequence is cell cycle arrest at the G_1/S interface via inhibition of cyclin-associated kinase activity. Alternatively, if the damage is too extensive, p53 sends a signal for the cells to undergo apoptosis, programmed cell death, through transcriptional activation of proapoptotic genes. Loss of p53 function by interaction with E6 therefore leads to a failure of growth arrest at the G_1/S checkpoint[33] and to a loss of apoptotic signaling. E6 further inhibits apoptosis by interfering with the interaction of cotranscriptional coactivators, CBP/p300, with p53.[36–38] *The failure of cell cycle checkpoint controls in E6-expressing cells results in chromosomal duplication*

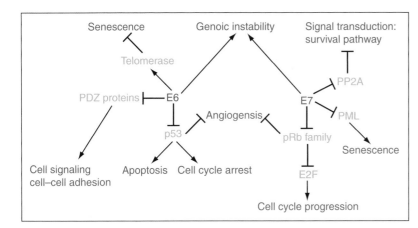

Figure 2-2 A selected set of activities of the E6 and E7 proteins and their potential impact on aspects of the conversion of normal cells to tumor cells. The pathways affected are shown in *red* and the mediators in *green*. E6 has p53-dependent and p53-independent activities that contribute to the development of cervical cancer. A number of the E6 activities are mediated through complex formation with E6-AP, leading to subsequent degradation of the target protein. E7 has pRb-dependent and pRb-independent activities. An *arrow* (→) indicates that an activity is induced or activated; a *bar* (⊣) indicates that the activity is repressed or inactivated. For example, E6 inhibits the ability of p53 to trigger apoptosis or cell cycle arrest; E7 inhibits the ability of pRb to repress E2F. See the appropriate sections of the text for further explanation.

and centrosome abnormalities[39,40] (see later section on Genomic Instability).

HR-HPV E6 proteins also possess transforming activities that are independent of p53 binding. The E6 proteins contain a sequence that mediates interaction with PDZ domain proteins (e.g., hDlg, MAGI, hScrib), which are cellular proteins that play a role in cellular adhesion and/or cellular signal transduction pathways.[41–43] Such interactions might contribute both to self-sufficiency in growth signals and tissue invasion. E6 interaction with PDZ proteins results in their degradation.[44,45] Although E6-dependent degradation of hScrib is mediated by the E6-AP complex, degradation of hDlg and MAGI is not.[45,46] *The importance of the PDZ binding domain to E6 function is well documented. In studies of transgenic mice expressing E6 proteins lacking the PDZ binding domain, epidermal hyperplasias did not develop even when E6 retained the ability to inactivate p53.*[47]

The list of proteins with which E6 interacts continues to grow and includes E6-targeted protein 1 (E6TP1), the focal adhesion protein paxillin and the calcium-binding protein E6-BP (reticulocallin 2). E6TP1 is a GTPase activating enzyme (GAP) that binds and inhibits Rap, a mitogenic signal transducer. Degradation of this protein by the E6:E6AP complex and consequent activation of Rap correlates with the oncogenic potential of E6.[48] Although the biological relevance of the other E6 binding partners is not yet known, it is likely that further research will prove that E6-mediated associations with these cellular factors contributes to one or more of the hallmarks of cancer.

Expression of the E7 protein of oncogenic HPV types leads to insensitivity to antigrowth signals and the immortalization of keratinocytes.[49] This effect is mediated by interactions with the retinoblastoma tumor suppressor protein (pRb), as well as the related pocket proteins p107 and p130 (see Figure 2-2).[49] The pRb family members exert their growth-suppressive function by forming a complex with a group of transcription factors, referred to collectively as *E2F*, resulting in the repression of transcription from promoters that contain E2F binding sites.[49] E2F is a transactivator of many genes involved in cell cycle progression. In normal cells, pRb is hypophosphorylated in early G_1 and becomes phosphorylated by cyclin-dependent kinases (cdk) prior to entry into S phase. Growth factor signaling in normal cells

leads to synthesis and activation of cyclin/cdk complexes that phosphorylate pRb, leading to S phase entry.[4] Inhibition of these cyclin/cdk complexes by cyclin-dependent kinase inhibitors renders them unable to phosphorylate pRb, resulting in cell cycle arrest. E7-pRb complex formation disrupts the pRb-E2F complex and releases transcription factor E2F[49,50] in the absence of any growth factor signaling, sending cells into S phase.

As is true for the E6 protein, there is an ever-increasing list of proteins with which E7 interacts, only a few of which will be described here. In addition to interactions with the pRb family, the E7 protein binds to and modifies the activity of other cell cycle regulatory proteins. E7 binds to both cyclin A and cyclin E, retaining the cyclin-dependent kinase 2 (cdk2) activating capability of both cyclins.[50] As noted previously, the cyclin/cdk complexes drive cell cycle progression by phosphorylating pRb family members. It has been speculated that the association of E7 with cyclin/cdk complexes may alter the time when the kinase is active or the substrates it phosporylates[50] and/or may contribute to abnormal centrosome duplication[51] (see section on Genomic Instability). E7 also interacts with p21^{cip1}, a cyclin-dependent kinase inhibitor.[52,53] The interaction of E7 with p21^{cip1} abrogates p21^{cip1}-mediated inhibition of cyclin A- and E-associated kinase activities. E7 thereby overrides p21^{cip1}-regulated inhibition of the cell cycle.[52,53]

Transcription is regulated by histone acetyl transferases (HATs) and histone deacetylases (HDACs). E7 binds to the class I HDACs, and this binding is required for activation of E2F-responsive promoters and for E7-mediated reversal of pRb-mediated cell cycle arrest.[54,55]

Very recent data also suggest that E7 may contribute to cell survival. Signals are often transduced in the cell through a cascade of protein kinases that phosphorylate their targets, thereby activating them. Protein phosphatases dephosphorylate proteins thereby turning off the signal. E7 binds a particular protein phosphatase, PP2A, and inhibits its function.[56] This would, in turn, allow signal transduction to continue. In this particular case, *it allows cells to survive rather than to undergo apoptosis.*

What happens to HPV-positive cervical cancer cell lines if the expression of E6 and E7 is repressed? Such repression has been achieved two independent ways: using short interfering ribonucleic acid (siRNA) to target the viral transcripts and using the viral E2 protein to repress transcription. Selective silencing of mammalian gene expression has recently been achieved using siRNA, which efficiently targets homologous messenger RNA (mRNA) for degradation. *Several reports have indicated that expression of siRNA directed to E6 and/or E7 mRNA sequences in HPV-positive cervical carcinoma cell lines results in restoration of growth control and apoptosis or senescence.*[57–60]

The E2 regulatory protein is involved in both viral replication and in transcriptional regulation of the viral early genes.[2] E2 binds as a dimer to the E2 binding site of the DNA sequence $ACCG(N_4)CGGT$. There are four E2 binding sites in the URR of genital HPV types.[61,62] E2 binding to the site adjacent to the transcription initiation start site of the p97 promoter represses the expression of the E6 and E7 oncogenes by interfering with the binding of cellular transcription factors, such as TFIID and Sp1.[2,61,62]

Loss of E2 expression results in derepression of the p97 early promoter and increased expression of E6 and E7. This derepression of p97 occurs when the HPV genome integrates into the chromosomal DNA (see next section), a process that usually occurs within the E2 gene, causing loss of E2 protein expression. Reintroduction and expression of exogenous E2 in HPV-containing cancer cells resulted in repression of E6 and E7 expression, reactivation of p53 and pRb tumor suppressor pathways and apoptosis,[61,63] or cellular senescence,[60,64,65] the latter of which will be discussed later.

A third HR-HPV protein, the E5 protein, potentially contributes to uncontrolled cellular proliferation. This is the only virally encoded membrane protein. Its expression results in elevated levels of epidermal growth factor receptor (EGFR) activation and thus may contribute to self-sufficiency in growth signals.[66–68] Upon integration (see next section), expression of E5 is often lost, and thus it is not required for maintenance of the oncogenic state.

ROLE OF VIRAL INTEGRATION INTO THE HOST CELL GENOME

HPV infection is extremely common, yet only a small percentage of infections result in cancer, and cancers usually develop many years after HPV infection. Although HPV infection plays a definitive role in cancer, additional genetic alterations of the cell are required for cancer to occur. One such possible alteration is the insertion, or integration, of the HPV genome into the host cell genome.

Early in HPV infection, the HPV genomes exist as circular, extrachromosomal copies. However, after a period of time, the duration of which has not been established, these *viral genomes can become inserted into the DNA of the host cell chromosomes* (Figure 2-3). This process is called *integration* and is a terminal event for the HPV life cycle.

The integration process has been correlated with the transition from low-grade to high-grade lesions.[69–71] *For example, in one study integrated HPV DNA was shown in 8% of low-grade cervical intraepithelial neoplasia (LG-CIN, 67% of high-grade CIN (HG-CIN), and 83% of invasive cervical carcinomas.*[71] *HPV integration correlates with genomic instability,*[69] *a poor prognosis, and resistance to treatment.*[72]

Studies of HPV integration in cervical malignancies indicate that HPV integrates throughout the host cell genome. Integrated HPV has been found in all human chromosomes except the Y chromosome.[73] Integration sites are apparently not randomly distributed, as HPV integrates in common

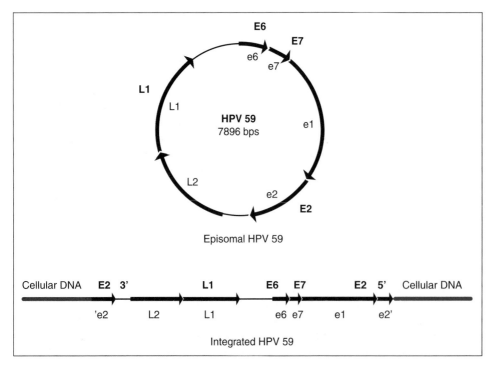

Figure 2-3 Diagram of episomal and integrated viral forms of human papillomavirus *(HPV)* 59, an oncogenic type related to HPV 18. Episomal HPV *(top)* is circular, found inside the nucleus of infected cells, but is separate from host chromosomes. Integrated HPV *(bottom)* is inserted into the host chromosome. Note that the E2 gene has been disrupted, and thus no E2 protein can be made. (Modified from PhD thesis by Helena Spartz.)

fragile sites (CFSs) and near locations of cellular oncogenes. Eighty-seven CFSs are present in the genomes of all individuals and are distributed throughout the genome.[74,75] CFSs are preferential sites for sister chromatid exchange, translocations, deletions, intrachromosomal gene amplification, and also integration of the DNA of tumor-associated viruses.[74,75] Forty to sixty percent of HPV integrations occur in or very near CFSs.[73–76] In addition, HPV integration sites have been observed at or very near the site of translocation breakpoints.[77–79]

Although insertional mutagenesis, the disruption or deregulation of a cellular gene by integration of HPV, has been proposed as a factor in HPV-induced pathogenesis, a review of greater than 190 HPV integration sites showed no evidence for consistently targeted disruption or functional alteration of critical cellular genes by the integration of viral sequences.[80] Repeated integration in the area of a tumor-relevant gene is uncommon. However, repeated integration has occurred in or near a few genes relevant to tumor development. Integration loci described in two or more independent samples from different studies have been described in or close to the MYC locus, FHIT, FANCC, hTERT, and CEACAM5.[73,75,76,81] The important point is that insertional mutagenesis may not be benign and may in some cases provide the cell harboring the integrated HPV with a selective growth advantage.

In addition to the disruption of the human chromosome, other changes such as homologous recombination may occur at the site of HPV integration. In some cases major chromosomal changes occur at the site of integration, including large deletions and complex rearrangements.[72,73] More often, short overlapping sequences one to six nucleotides in length are found at the site of integration. In other cases there is a direct transition from viral to cellular sequences. In still other cases of integration, filler sequences are found at the fusion site derived from neither the viral nor the cellular sequences at the respective locus.

HPV integration has consequences for both the viral and cellular genome.[72] In the case of the virus, integration allows for enhanced expression of E6 and E7 genes.[72,82] The viral oncogenes E6 and E7 are always retained during integration. Three significant changes occur to E6 and E7 transcription upon viral integration. First, the HPV genome is linearized between the E1 and L1 genes. Deletions of viral DNA can occur at the site of linearization. There is a loss, by break or deletion, of the viral E2 gene, which normally functions as a transcriptional regulator of the E6 and E7 genes. Thus, *upon integration, E6 and E7 transcription is no longer down-regulated by the viral E2 gene, and E6/E7 protein levels increase, leading to further alterations in the parameters described earlier in the section on viral oncoproteins.*

Second, the downstream viral DNA sequences normally encoded in E6 and E7 transcripts are often deleted upon integration. Because these viral downstream sequences may interfere with E6 and E7 gene expression,[83] it is possible that their deletion following integration may play a part in up-regulating E6 and E7 gene expression, thereby contributing to cervical oncogenesis.

Third, polyadenylation sites are sequences of DNA signaling the endpoint of a transcript. After integration, the viral polyadenylation signal is no longer available for E6 and E7 gene expression. Viral transcripts are thus made using a cellular polyadenylation signal.[84] It has been demonstrated that viral–cellular fusion transcripts have enhanced stability compared with viral transcripts.[85]

GENOMIC INSTABILITY

It is important to note that keratinocytes expressing HR-HPV E6 and E7 are immortalized; that is, they grow indefinitely in cell culture but do not form tumors in animals. As these cells are passaged in cell culture, they may ultimately become tumorigenic.[86,87] Therefore additional alterations in the cell must occur in the progression toward malignancy, a process that may take many years in humans. One such change is instability of the host cell genome, which is considered to be an early step in the progression to HPV-associated malignancy.[88,89] In both precursor lesions such as CIN 3 and in invasive cervical carcinomas, alterations of human chromosomes such as centrosome abnormalities and aneuploidy can be observed[71,90–92] (Figure 2-4). Centrosomes, the centers for organization of microtubules in interphase and mitotic cells, ensure that chromosomes accurately segregate, thus preventing asymmetry during cell division.[93] Abnormal centrosome numbers are associated with multipolar mitoses and tetraploidy in cervical dysplastic lesions.[94–97] In addition to changes in abnormal chromosome numbers, other mutations accumulate as cervical lesions progress toward malignancy. Losses and gains in specific chromosomes have also been observed in cervical cancers.[72,75,78,98] Also, structural abnormalities of chromosomes such as translocations and rearrangements have been observed in cervical cancers.[78,98]

HR-HPV integration is associated with chromosomal instability[96] and is associated with overexpression of the E6 and E7 oncoproteins as indicated in the previous section. Although HR-HPV integration is associated with chromosomal instability, such changes may occur even before integration occurs. For example, numerous centrosome abnormalities and chromosomal abnormalities were identified in human keratinocytes that contained HPV 16 in the extrachromosomal form.[90]

Expression of the E6 and E7 proteins of HR-HPV types in cell culture systems has been shown to cause abnormalities in chromosomes.[94,99–101] E7 induces abnormal centrosome numbers, multipolar mitotic spindles, chromosomal breaks, and alterations of chromosomal structure.[54] In a mouse model, centrosome aberrations were found in cell lines established from skin tumors of mice expressing either the HPV 16 E6 or E7 oncoproteins, indicating that each oncoprotein was capable of interfering with the centrosome cycle.[102]

HPV AND LIMITLESS REPLICATIVE POTENTIAL: ESCAPE FROM SENESCENCE

Even if HPV-infected cells become self-sufficient regarding growth signals and become resistant to antigrowth signals and apoptosis, they would still not have unlimited replicative

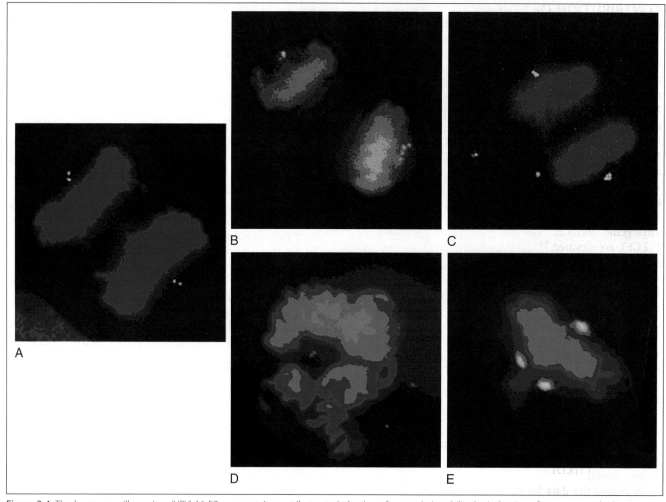

Figure 2-4 The human papillomavirus *(HPV)* 16 E7 oncoprotein contributes to induction of genomic instability by induction of centrosome duplication errors. Examples of different mitotic abnormalities that can be generated by numerical centrosome abnormalities are shown. **A,** Normal bipolar metaphase; each mitotic spindle pole body consists of a single centrosome, which contains 2 centrioles. Individual centrioles are visualized by green fluorescent protein (GFP)-centrin fluorescence. **B,** Abnormal bipolar mitosis due to centrosome aggregation. Individual centrioles are visualized by green fluorescent protein-centrin fluorescence. The mitotic spindle pole on the left contains three centrioles, whereas the one on the right contains four centrioles that may represent two aggregated centrosomes. There is a chance of nonsymmetric chromosome segregation upon completion of cell division. **C,** Abnormal bipolar mitosis in the presence of multiple individual centrosomes. Individual centrioles are visualized by immunofluorescence using a centrin-specific antibody. Although the majority of the chromosomes are segregated in a bipolar fashion, the centrosomes on the left may interfere with symmetric chromosome distribution by apparently capturing some chromosomal material. **D,** Predominantly monopolar mitosis in the presence of multiple centrosomes. Individual centrosomes are visualized by immunofluorescence using a γ tubulin–specific antibody. **E,** Tripolar mitotic figures are hallmarks of high-risk HPV-associated cervical lesions. Individual centrosomes are visualized by GFP-γ-tubulin fluorescence. (Figure and legend courtesy of Karl Munger and reproduced from Ref. 92.[113])

potential. Senescence would occur due to the shortening of telomeres, the repeat DNA sequences (TTAGGG) at the end of chromosomes that have been shown to shorten with age.[103] *Erosion of the chromosomal termini (telomeres) occurs with each round of DNA replication, and shortening of telomeres serves to restrict the proliferative capacity of normal cells.* The cell life span increases when the catalytic subunit of telomerase (hTERT) is expressed.[104–106] Because many human tumor cells express telomerase, it is believed that abnormal telomerase expression may be essential for development of malignancy.[107,108]

The HPV E6 protein contributes to the unlimited replication potential of keratinocytes by activation of hTERT transcription.[109] Transcription of hTERT is regulated by cellular proteins that bind upstream of the hTERT promoter.

Both HPV E6 and the cellular protein c-Myc have been shown to activate transcription of hTERT.[109] Other cellular proteins (USF1/2 and NFX1–91) have been identified that decrease expression of hTERT.[110,111] Interestingly, NFX1-91 is targeted for degradation by the same E6/E6-AP complex that targets p53 for degradation.[110] Thus HR-HPV E6 contributes to escape from senescence by inducing telomerase activity.

Another cellular protein involved in inducing senescence is the promyelocytic leukemia protein (PML), which acts by forming a complex with p53. As noted earlier, E7 also plays a role in blocking senescence because silencing of E7 may also lead to cellular senescence.[60] Although the mechanism is not clear, E7 has been reported to disrupt the PML:p53 complex.[112]

CONTRIBUTION OF HUMAN PAPILLOMAVIRUS TO ANGIOGENESIS

Angiogenesis is the acquisition of a new blood supply from the existing vasculature and is required for tumors to obtain nutrients and oxygen and to remove waste products.[113–115] *Whether endothelial cells are quiescent or are activated to proliferate, migrate, and differentiate is regulated by the ratio of inhibitors of angiogenesis to inducers. The endothelium adjacent to the tumor becomes activated when the level of angiogenic inducers produced by the tumor increases and/or the level of angiogenic inhibitors decreases.*[113] Such changes in angiogenic factors have been reported in biopsies of cervical cancers. For example, the levels of both mRNA and protein of an angiogenic inducer, vascular endothelial growth factor (VEGF), are elevated.[116–119] Transcription of thrombospondin-1 (TSP-1), an angiogenic inhibitor, is decreased in cervical cancer cells.[120] Similarly, cervical carcinoma cell lines have been shown to have increased levels of VEGF and interleukin 8 (IL-8), another angiogenic inducer, and decreased levels of TSP-1.[80]

Angiogenesis is a multistep process initiated in the premalignant stage of disease.[113,120] *There is a progressive change in the ratio of inducers to inhibitors of angiogenesis as the grade of the lesion increases from mild to severe dysplasia and ultimately to invasive carcinoma. This is accompanied by a progressive increase in the number of microvessels as well as their proximity to the epithelium.*[116–118] This progressive alteration is seen in cervical lesions progressing from dysplasia to invasive carcinoma and is recapitulated in the HPV 16 transgenic mouse model.[118,121]

Although the data from HPV-positive human dysplasias and carcinomas and from the transgenic mouse model document changes in expression of VEGF, whether the contribution of HPV proteins to this process is direct or indirect cannot be established in these models because the assessments are conducted long after the initial infection, and other cellular changes have occurred as well (see Genomic Instability, earlier). This same limitation exists for experiments monitoring angiogenic factors in carcinoma cell lines.[80] *However, very recent data indicate that expression of HR-HPV E6 and E7 gene products in their target cell, the human foreskin keratinocyte, is sufficient to cause an angiogenic switch in these cells.*[122] There is an increase in the expression of VEGF and IL-8 and a decrease in the expression of TSP-1 and maspin, another angiogenic inhibitor.

Regulation of angiogenic factors at the transcription level is complex, involving a number of cellular proteins. Identification of some such factors provides a means for understanding how HR-HPV can contribute to the angiogenesis needed for a tumor to thrive. p53 is one of the participants in this regulation. It represses the proangiogenic factor VEGF,[123] and it up-regulates the inhibitor of angiogenesis, TSP-1.[124–126] As noted in an earlier section, the HR-HPV E6 protein targets p53 for degradation. In addition, VEGF is regulated by two other transcription factors, Sp-1 and AP-1. The HR-HPV E6 protein transactivates VEGF transcription through sites that normally bind Sp-1.[127] HR-HPV E7 protein has been reported to enhance activation of transcription of genes containing sites for AP-1 binding.[128,129] The precise mechanism whereby HR-HPV regulates angiogenic factors in vivo has yet to be determined.

An appreciation of the complexity of cells and factors making up the tumor microenvironment has increased over time. In addition to the sprouting of new vessels from the pre-existing vasculature, endothelial progenitor cells can be mobilized from the bone marrow and contribute to the formation of new blood vessels.[130–132] Furthermore, in addition to the tumor itself, different cell lineages within the tumor microenvironment (e.g., stromal fibroblasts) also secrete factors that enhance the recruitment of the blood supply.[133] Thus data indicating that IL-8 is increased in cervical secretions of women with cervical cancer,[134] as opposed to data generated by *in situ* hybridization or immunohistochemistry, add to the total picture of what is occurring in the tumor microenvironment, but not what is happening in individual cells. How HPV-dependent alterations of tumor cells affect communication between these cells and those in the microenvironment remains to be determined.

HUMAN PAPILLOMAVIRUS–MEDIATED ESCAPE FROM INNATE AND ACQUIRED IMMUNE RESPONSE

The immune response plays a critical role in the incidence of cervical cancer because women who are immune compromised are at increased risk (see Nonviral Cofactors, later). However, immunocompetent women also develop disease. Although nonviral factors are described in the next section, it is also clear that HPV gene products play a role in immune evasion. *The innate immune response is the first line of defense against viral infection. This is followed by an acquired immune response.*[135] *HPV has several mechanisms to downregulate both of these aspects of the immune response.* With respect to the innate immune response, HR HPV gene products, for example, inhibit the ability of cellular gene products (IRF-1 and IRF-3) to activate the interferon-β gene and down-regulate transcription of interferon-inducible genes.[136–139] With respect to the acquired immune response, HPV gene products may decrease the presentation of HPV epitopes on the surface of infected cells.[139–141]

NONVIRAL COFACTORS

The majority of women infected with HR-HPV will never develop serious complications of infection. Therefore there must be additional factors that predispose certain women to HPV-related cervical dysplasia. Some of these nonviral cofactors may include cigarette smoking, oral contraceptives, parity, the genetic makeup and immune status of the person infected with HPV, and coinfection with other genital tract pathogens.[11]

Cigarette smoking has long been suspected to be a contributing factor for cervical malignancy.[142-144] Tobacco smoke contains and delivers numerous chemical compounds, many of which are known carcinogens.[145-149] Some of these compounds can be found in the cervical mucous of cigarette smokers, perhaps delivered to the cervix through the bloodstream.[150] A beneficial effect can be shown in randomized studies of smoking cessation among women with low-grade cervical dysplasia.[151]

Oral contraceptives (OCPs) have been studied as a risk factor for cervical cancer. A large series of studies over a number of years have shown inconsistent associations with cervical cancer. It is difficult to separate the influence of the sexual habits of OCP users from the OCP use itself. However, recent literature reviews have suggested that OCP use for more than 5 years is a modest risk factor for cervical cancer.[152-154] Multiparity has also been shown to be a risk factor.[155] Possible mechanisms for this include cervical trauma and maintenance of the transformation zone of the cervix.

A series of early, cross-sectional, case-control studies indicated an association between infection with herpes simplex virus (HSV) and cervical cancer.[156] However several prospective cohort studies failed to confirm that association.[116,157] Infection with *Chlamydia trachomatis* has repeatedly been associated with cervical neoplasia and invasive cancer.[158-162] A history of *C. trachomatis* infection was a significant risk factor for HPV persistence in a large, population-based, cohort study of HPV-positive women.[163]

The genetic makeup and the immune status of the infected host are strong determinants of the clinical manifestations of HPV infection. Genital warts recur more often in immunosuppressed individuals. These individuals also have an increased incidence of cervical cancer, HPV-related squamous cell carcinomas of the face, and a high incidence of anal carcinoma.[164-169] In healthy, non-immunosuppressed individuals, differences in class II HLA haplotypes are suspected to play a role in susceptibility to cervical cancer. DQw3 and DR15/DQ6 are the haplotypes that have shown the most consistent associations.[170,171] DR15/DQ6 has been associated with persistent HPV 16 infections, with cervical dysplasia, and with cervical cancer.[172]

LIMITED ONCOGENIC POTENTIAL OF LOW-RISK HUMAN PAPILLOMAVIRUS

All HPV replicates in the differentiated compartment of the squamous epithelium. Cells in this compartment have normally exited the cell cycle. However, HPV can only replicate its genome and complete its life cycle in cells in S phase. Therefore both LR and HR-HPV need to have the ability to create an S-like environment in the differentiation compartment. Why, then, is the risk of developing cancer following infection with an HR-HPV many times higher than that following infection with a LR-HPV?[173,174]

The reasons for the differences between the oncogenic activity of the HR and LR-HPV are still under investigation.

However, several points are clear. *First, there are quantitative and qualitative differences between the activities of the E7 proteins of HR and LR-HPV types.* HR-HPV E7 proteins bind pRb and its family members, p107 and p130, with higher affinity than LR HPV E7 proteins.[175-177] This could mean that there is less perturbation of the pRb:E2F circuitry with LR-HPV. Perhaps more importantly, pRb degradation occurs with interaction with E7 of oncogenic types only.[178,179] Analysis of specific HPV 16 E7 mutations in the background of the intact genome has shown that binding of HPV 16 E7 to pocket proteins such as pRb is sufficient to induce DNA synthesis in the suprabasal compartment, but that delaying differentiation also requires degradation of these proteins.[180] Because LR-HPV E7 proteins can also induce DNA synthesis in the suprabasal compartment,[181] the more critical activity for both HR- and LR-HPV may be the shared ability to target p130 for degradation.[182] In addition, both HR- and LR-HPV can delay differentiation, perhaps also contributing to the completion of the virus life cycle and this correlates with degradation of p130.[182] Perhaps LR-HPV, by failing to target all pRb family members for degradation also fail to render cells resistant to a sufficient number of antigrowth signals.

Second, there are major differences between the HR- and LR-HPV E6 proteins. *Although HR-HPV E6 proteins target p53 for degradation, LR-HPV E6 proteins do not. They do, however, share the ability of E6 to block activation of p53-mediated transcription.*[37] This may be necessary to subvert p53-mediated apoptosis that might be triggered by p130-mediated alterations in E2F signaling long enough for completion of the virus replication cycle but may not be sufficient for long-term insensitivity to apoptotic signals. In addition, only the HR-HPV E6 proteins bind PDZ-containing proteins and target them for degradation[44] and activate hTERT.[106] Thus the LR-HPV E6 proteins may not protect against senescence.

Finally, as opposed to the HR-HPV E6 and E7 proteins, the LR-HPV E6 and E7 proteins do not induce genomic instability.[99] *Therefore other mutations rendering keratinocytes self sufficient in growth signaling, may be lacking.*

SUMMARY

As an infectious disease, HPV is passed from person to person by sexual contact, and numerous studies indicate the ease and frequency with which this transmission occurs. HPV infection leads to malignancy only in a small percentage of individuals, and although the mechanisms of progression to malignancy have been aggressively studied, there is much that is not understood. The important factors associated with the progression from infection to cancer have been reviewed here, but in the future, it is likely that new factors will be recognized. Similar to other cancers, cancers resulting from HPV infection are composed of cells that have undergone numerous changes. In the case of HPV-mediated carcinogenesis, some of these changes are the direct result of introduction of new genetic information, namely the HPV genome and the ability of HPV gene products, in particular E6 and E7, to subvert the function of a number of cellular proteins. The additional ability of these proteins to induce genomic instability furthers the progression of disease. Prevention and treatment of HPV-related malignancy depends on an understanding of this dynamic process.

REFERENCES

1. Howley P. Papillomavirinae: the viruses and their replication. In Fields B, Knipe D, Howley P (eds). Fields Virology. 3rd ed, 2nd vol. Philadelphia: Lippincott-Raven, 1996, pp 2045–2109.

2. Longworth MS, Laimins LA. Pathogenesis of human papillomaviruses in differentiating epithelia. Microbiol Molecul Biol Rev 2004;68:362–372.

3. zur Hausen H. Papillomaviruses and cancer: from basic studies to clinical application. Nature Rev Cancer 2002;2: 342–350.

4. Brown DR, Bryan JT, Pratt L, et al. Human papillomavirus type 11 E1^E4 and L1 proteins colocalize in the mouse xenograft system at multiple time points. Virology 1995;214: 259–263.

5. Fuchs PG, Pfister H. Transcription of papillomavirus genomes. Intervirology 1994;37:159–167.

6. Stoler MH, Whitbeck A, Wolinsky SM, et al. Infectious cycle of human papillomavirus type 11 in human foreskin xenografts in nude mice. J Virol 1990;64:3310–3318.

7. Turek LP. The Structure, Function, and Regulation of Papillomaviral Genes in Infection and Cervical Cancer. San Diego: Academic Press, 1994.

8. Pfister H, Fuchs PG. Anatomy, taxonomy and evolution of papillomaviruses. Intervirology 1994;37:143–149.

9. Burd EM. Human papillomaviruses and cervical cancer. Clin Microbiol Rev 2003;16:1–17.

10. zur Hausen H. Papillomaviruses causing cancer: evasion from host-cell control in early events in carcinogenesis. J Natl Cancer Inst 2000;92:690–698.

11. zurHausen H. Viruses in human cancers. Eur J Cancer 1999;35:1174–1181.

12. deVilliers EM. Human papillomaviruses—introduction. Semin Cancer Biol 1999;9:377.

13. Bryan JT, Brown DR. Transmission of human papillomavirus type 11 infection by desquamated cornified cells. Virology 2001;281:35–42.

14. Lehr E, Brown D. How do human papillomaviruses escape the infected keratinocyte? Papilloma Rep 2002;13:181–189.

15. Evander M, Frazer IH, Payne E, et al. Identification of the alpha(6) integrin as a candidate receptor for papillomaviruses. J Virol 1997;71:2449–2456.

16. Patterson NA, Smith JL, Ozbun MA. Human papillomavirus type 31b infection of human keratinocytes does not require heparan sulfate. J Virol 2005;79:6838–6847.

17. zurHausen H. Papillomaviruses in human cancers. Proc AAP 1999;111:581–587.

18. Brown DR, Schroeder JM, Bryan JT, et al. Detection of multiple human papillomavirus types in *Condylomata acuminata* lesions from otherwise healthy and immunosuppressed patients. J Clin Microbiol 1999;37:3316–3322.

19. Gissmann L, Wolnik L, Ikenberg H, et al. Human papillomavirus types 6 and 11 DNA sequences in genital and laryngeal papillomas and in some cervical cancers. Proc Natl Acad Sci U S A 1983;80:560–563.

20. Pfister H. Papillomaviruses: general description, taxonomy, and classification. In Salzman NP and Howley PM (eds). The Papillomaviruses. New York: Plenum, 1987.

21. Herrero R, Munoz N. Human papillomavirus and cancer. Cancer Surv 1999;33:75–98.

22. Hildesheim A, Han CL, Brinton LA, et al. Human papillomavirus type 16 and risk of preinvasive and invasive vulvar cancer: results from a seroepidemiological case-control study. Obstet Gynecol 1997;90:748–754.

23. Bosch FX, Schiffman M, Solomon D (eds). Future directions in epidemiologic and preventive research on human papillomaviruses and cancer. J Natl Cancer Inst Mono. 31st vol. Oxford, UK: Oxford University Press, 2003.

24. Dillner J, von Krogh G, Horenblas S, et al. Etiology of squamous cell carcinoma of the penis. Scand J Urol Nephrol Suppl 2000;205:189–193.

25. Hanahan D, Weinberg RA. The hallmarks of cancer. Cell 2000;100:57–70.

26. Halbert CL, Demers GW, Galloway DA. The E7 gene of human papillomavirus type 16 is sufficient for immortalization of human epithelial cells. J Virol 1991;65:473–478.

27. Hawley-Nelson P, Vousden KH, Hubbert NL, et al. HPV16 E6 and E7 proteins cooperate to immortalize human foreskin keratinocytes. EMBO J 1989;8:3905–3910.

28. Munger K, Phelps WC, Bubb V, et al. The E6 and E7 genes of the human papillomavirus type 16 together are necessary and sufficient for transformation of primary human keratinocytes. J Virol 1989;63:4417–4421.

29. Sherman L, Schlegel R. Serum- and calcium-induced differentiation of human keratinocytes is inhibited by the E6 oncoprotein of human papillomavirus type 16. J Virol 1996;70: 3269–3279.

30. Riley RR, Duensing S, Brake T, et al. Dissection of human papillomavirus E6 and E7 function in transgenic mouse models of cervical carcinogenesis. Cancer Res 2003;63:4862–4871.

31. Huibregtse JM, Scheffner M, Howley PM. A cellular protein mediates association of p53 with the E6 oncoprotein of human papillomavirus types 16 or 18. EMBO J 1991;10: 4129–4135.

32. Scheffner M, Huibregtse JM, Vierstra RD, et al. The HPV-16 E6 and E6-AP complex functions as a ubiquitin-protein ligase in the ubiquitination of p53. Cell 1993;75:495–505.

33. Kuhne C, Banks L. Cellular targets of the papillomavirus E6 proteins. Papilloma Rep 1999;10:139–145.

34. Oren M. Decision making by p53: life, death and cancer. Cell Death Differ 2003;10:431–442.

35. Slee EA, O'Connor DJ, Lu X. To die or not to die: how does p53 decide? Oncogene 2004;23:2809–2818.

36. Patel D, Huang SM, Baglia LA, et al. The E6 protein of human papillomavirus type 16 binds to and inhibits co-activation by CBP and p300. Embo J 1999;18:5061–5072.

37. Thomas MC, Chiang CM. E6 oncoprotein represses p53-dependent gene activation via inhibition of protein acetylation independently of inducing p53 degradation. Mol Cell 2005;17:251–264.

38. Zimmermann H, Degenkolbe R, Bernard HU, et al. The human papillomavirus type 16 E6 oncoprotein can down-regulate p53 activity by targeting the transcriptional coactivator CBP/p300. J Virol 1999;73:6209–6219.

39. Duensing S, Munger K. Centrosome abnormalities and genomic instability induced by human papillomavirus oncoproteins. Prog Cell Cycle Res 2003;5:383–391.

40. Duensing S, Munger K. The human papillomavirus type 16 E6 and E7 oncoproteins independently induce numerical and structural chromosome instability. Cancer Research 2002;62:7075–7082.

41. Banks L, Mantovani F. The human papillomavirus E6 protein and its contribution to malignant progression. Oncogene 2001;20:7874–7887.

42. Lee C, Laimins LA. Role of the PDZ domain-binding motif of the oncoprotein E6 in the pathogenesis of human papillomavirus type 31. J Virol 2004;78:12366–12377.

43. Munger K, Scheffner M, Huibregtse JM, et al. Interactions of HPV E6 and E7 oncoproteins with tumour suppressor gene products. Cancer Surv 1992;12:197–217.

44. Gardiol D, Kuhne C, Glaunsinger B, et al. Oncogenic human papillomavirus E6 proteins target the discs large tumour suppressor for proteasome-mediated degradation. Oncogene 1999;18:5487–5496.

45. Nakagawa S, Huibregtse JM. Human scribble (Vartul) is targeted for ubiquitin-mediated degradation by the high-risk papillomavirus E6 proteins and the E6AP ubiquitin-protein ligase. Mol Cell Biol 2000;20:8244–8253.

46. Grm HS, Banks L. Degradation of hDlg and MAGIs by human papillomavirus E6 is E6-AP-independent. J Gen Virol 2004;85:2815–2819.

47. Nguyen ML, Nguyen MM, Lee D, et al. The PDZ ligand domain of the human papillomavirus type 16 E6 protein is required for E6's induction of epithelial hyperplasia in vivo. J Virol 2003;77:6957–6964.

48. Singh L, Gao Q, Kumar A, et al. The high-risk human papillomavirus type 16 E6 counters the GAP function of E6TP1 toward small Rap G proteins. J Virol 2003;77:1614–1620.

49. Munger K, Basile J, Duensing S, et al. Biological activities and molecular targets of the human papillomavirus E7 oncoprotein. Oncogene 2001;20:7888–7898.

50. McIntyre MC, Ruesch MN, Laimins LA. Human papillomavirus E7 oncoproteins bind a single form of cyclin E in a complex with cdk2 and p107. Virology 1996;215:73–82.

51. Duensing S, Munger K. Mechanisms of genomic instability in human cancer: insights from studies with human papillomavirus oncoproteins. Int J Cancer 2004;109:157–162.

52. Funk JO, Waga S, Harry JB, et al. Inhibition of CDK activity and PCNA-dependent DNA replication by p21 is blocked by interaction with the HPV-16 E7 oncoprotein. Genes Develop 1997;11:2090–2100.

53. Jones DL, Alani RM, Munger K. The human papillomavirus E7 oncoprotein can uncouple cellular differentiation and proliferation in human keratinocytes by abrogating p21Cip1-mediated inhibition of cdk2. Genes Develop 1997;11:2101–2111.

54. Brehm A, Nielsen SJ, Miska EA, et al. The E7 oncoprotein associates with Mi2 and histone deacetylase activity to promote cell growth. EMBO J 1999;18:2449–2458.

55. Nguyen D, Westbrook TF, McCance DJ. Human papillomavirus type 16 E7 maintains elevated levels of the cdc25a tyrosine phosphatase during deregulation of cell cycle arrest. J Virol 2002;76:619–632.

56. Pim D, Massimi P, Dilworth SM, et al. Activation of the protein kinase B pathway by the HPV-16 E7 oncoprotein occurs through a mechanism involving interaction with PP2A. Oncogene 2005;24:7830–7838.

57. Butz K, Ristriani T, Hengstermann A, et al. siRNA targeting of the viral E6 oncogene efficiently kills human papillomavirus-positive cancer cells. Oncogene 2003;22:5938–5945.

58. Hall AH, Alexander KA. RNA interference of human papillomavirus type 18 E6 and E7 induces senescence in HeLa cells. J Virol 2003;77:6066–6069.

59. Jiang M, Milner J. Selective silencing of viral gene E6 and E7 expression in HPV-positive human cervical carcinoma cells using small interfering RNAs. Methods Mol Biol 2005;292:401–420.

60. DeFilippis RA, Goodwin EC, Wu L, et al. Endogenous human papillomavirus E6 and E7 proteins differentially regulate proliferation, senescence, and apoptosis in HeLa cervical carcinoma cells. J Virol 2003;77:1551–1563.

61. Demeret C, Desaintes C, Yaniv M, et al. Different mechanisms contribute to the E2-mediated transcriptional repression of human papillomavirus type 18 viral oncogenes. J Virol 1997;71:9343–9349.

62. Steger G, Corbach S. Dose-dependent regulation of the early promoter of human papillomavirus type 18 by the viral E2 protein. J Virol 1997;71:50–58.

63. SanchezPerez AM, Soriano S, Clarke AR, et al. Disruption of the human papillomavirus type 16 E2 gene protects cervical carcinoma cells from E2F-induced apoptosis. J Gen Virol 1997;78:3009–3018.

64. Goodwin EC, DiMaio D. Repression of human papillomavirus oncogenes in HeLa cervical carcinoma cells causes the orderly reactivation of dormant tumor suppressor pathways. Proc Natl Acad Sci U S A 2000;97:12513–12518.

65. Wells SI, Francis DA, Karpova AY, et al. Papillomavirus E2 induces senescence in HPV-positive cells via pRB- and p21 (CIP)-dependent pathways. EMBO J 2000;19:5762–5771.

66. Crusius K, Auvinen E, Steuer B, et al. The human papillomavirus type 16 E5-protein modulates ligand-dependent activation of the EGF receptor family in the human epithelial cell line HaCaT. Exp Cell Res 1998;241:76–83.

67. Gu ZM, Matlashewski G. Effect of human papillomavirus type 16 oncogenes on MAP kinase activity. J Virol 1995;69:8051–8056.

68. Straight SW, Hinkle PM, Jewers RJ, et al. The E5 oncoprotein of human papillomavirus type 16 transforms fibroblasts and effects the downregulation of the epidermal growth factor receptor in keratinocytes. J Virol 1993;67:4521–4532.

69. Hopman AH, Smedts F, Dignef W, et al. Transition of high-grade cervical intraepithelial neoplasia to micro-invasive carcinoma is characterized by integration of HPV 16/18 and numerical chromosome abnormalities. J Pathol 2004;202: 23–33.

70. Nagao S, Yoshinouchi M, Miyagi Y, et al. Rapid and sensitive detection of physical status of human papillomavirus type 16 DNA by quantitative real-time PCR. J Clin Microbiol 2002;40:863–867.

71. Tonon SA, Picconi MA, Bos PD, et al. Physical status of the E2 human papilloma virus 16 viral gene in cervical preneoplastic and neoplastic lesions. J Clin Virol 2001;21:129–134.

72. Lazo PA. The molecular genetics of cervical carcinoma. Br J Cancer 1999;80:2008–2018.

73. Wentzensen N, Vinokurova S, von Knebel Doeberitz M. Systematic review of genomic integration sites of human papillomavirus genomes in epithelial dysplasia and invasive cancer of the female lower genital tract. Cancer Res 2004; 64:3878–3884.

74. Thorland EC, Myers SL, Gostout BS, et al. Common fragile sites are preferential targets for HPV16 integrations in cervical tumors. Oncogene 2003;22:1225–1237.

75. Yu T, Ferber MJ, Cheung TH, et al. The role of viral integration in the development of cervical cancer. Cancer Gen Cytogen 2005;158:27–34.

76. Ragin CC, Reshmi SC, Gollin SM. Mapping and analysis of HPV16 integration sites in a head and neck cancer cell line. Intl J Cancer 2004;110:701–709.

77. Brink AA, Wiegant JC, Szuhai K, et al. Simultaneous mapping of human papillomavirus integration sites and molecular karyotyping in short-term cultures of cervical carcinomas by using 49-color combined binary ratio labeling fluorescence in situ hybridization. Cancer Gen Cytogen 2002;134:145–150.

78. Harris CP, Lu XY, Narayan G, et al. Comprehensive molecular cytogenetic characterization of cervical cancer cell lines. Genes Chromosomes Cancer 2003;36:233–241.

79. Koopman LA, Szuhai K, van Eendenburg JD, et al. Recurrent integration of human papillomaviruses 16, 45, and 67 near translocation breakpoints in new cervical cancer cell lines. Cancer Res 1999;59:5615–5624.

80. Bequet-Romero M, Lopez-Ocejo O. Angiogenesis modulators expression in culture cell lines positives for HPV-16 oncoproteins. Biochem Biophys Res Commun 2000;277:55–61.

81. Durst M, Croce CM, Gissmann L, et al. Papillomavirus sequences integrate near cellular oncogenes in some cervical carcinomas. Proc Natl Acad Sci U S A 1987;84:1070–1074.

82. Jeon S, Allen-Hoffmann BL, Lambert PF. Integration of human papillomavirus type 16 into the human genome correlates with a selective growth advantage of cells. J Virol 1995;69:2989–2997.

83. Vinther J, Rosenstierne MW, Kristiansen K, et al. The 3′ region of human papillomavirus type 16 early mRNAs decrease expression. BMC Infect Dis 2005;5:83.

84. Wentzensen N, Ridder R, Klaes R, et al. Characterization of viral-cellular fusion transcripts in a large series of HPV16 and 18 positive anogenital lesions. Oncogene 2002;21:419–426.

85. Jeon S, Lambert PF. Integration of human papillomavirus type 16 DNA into the human genome leads to increased stability of E6 and E7 mRNAs: implications for cervical carcinogenesis. Proc Natl Acad Sci U S A 1995;92:1654–1658.

86. Hurlin PJ, Kaur P, Smith PP, et al. Progression of human papillomavirus type 18-immortalized human keratinocytes to a malignant phenotype. Proc Natl Acad Sci U S A 1991;88:570–574.

87. Kaur P, McDougall JK, Cone R. HPV-18 immortalization of human keratinocytes. Virology 1989;173:302–310.

88. Hashida T, Yasumoto S. Induction of chromosome abnormalities in mouse and human epidermal keratinocytes by the human papillomavirus type 16 E7 oncogene. J Gen Virol 1991;72:1569–1577.

89. Tlsty TD, White A, Livanos E, et al. Genomic integrity and the genetics of cancer. Cold Spring Harbor Symp Quant Biol 1994;59:265–275.

90. Duensing S, Duensing A, Flores ER, et al. Centrosome abnormalities and genomic instability by episomal expression of human papillomavirus type 16 in raft cultures of human keratinocytes. J Virol 2001;75:7712–7716.

91. Heselmeyer K, duManoir S, Blegen H, et al. A recurrent pattern of chromosomal aberrations and immunophenotypic appearance defines anal squamous cell carcinomas. Br J Cancer 1997;76:1271–1278.

92. Munger K, Baldwin A, Edwards KM, et al. Mechanisms of human papillomavirus-induced oncogenesis. J Virol 2004;78:11451–11460.

93. Urbani L, Stearns T. The centrosome. Curr Biol 1999;9:R315–R317.

94. Duensing S, Munger K. Centrosome abnormalities, genomic instability and carcinogenic progression. Biochim Biophys Acta 2001;1471:M81–M88.

95. Heselmeyer K, Macville M, Schrock E, et al. Advanced-stage cervical carcinomas are defined by a recurrent pattern of chromosomal aberrations revealing high genetic instability and a consistent gain of chromosome arm 3q. Genes Chromosomes Cancer 1997;19:233–240.

96. Pett MR, Alazawi WO, Roberts I, et al. Acquisition of high-level chromosomal instability is associated with integration of human papillomavirus type 16 in cervical keratinocytes. Cancer Res 2004;64:1359–1368.

97. Stanley MA. Personal Communication, 22nd International Papillomavirus Conference, Vancouver, 2005.

98. Cottage A, Dowen S, Roberts I, et al. Early genetic events in HPV immortalised keratinocytes. Genes Chromosomes Cancer 2001;30:72–79.

99. Duensing S, Lee LY, Duensing A, et al. The human papillomavirus type 16 E6 and E7 oncoproteins cooperate to induce mitotic defects and genomic instability by uncoupling centrosome duplication from the cell division cycle. Proc Natl Acad Sci U S A 2000;97:10002–10007.

100. Duensing S, Munger K. Human papillomaviruses and centrosome duplication errors: modeling the origins of genomic instability. Oncogene 2002;21:6241–6248.

101. Thomas JT, Laimins LA. Human papillomavirus oncoproteins E6 and E7 independently abrogate the mitotic spindle checkpoint. J Virol 1998;72:1131–1137.

102. Schaeffer AJ, Nguyen M, Liem A, et al. E6 and E7 oncoproteins induce distinct patterns of chromosomal aneuploidy in skin tumors from transgenic mice. Cancer Res 2004;64:538–546.

103. Meeker AK, De Marzo AM. Recent advances in telomere biology: implications for human cancer. Curr Opin Oncol 2004;16:32–38.

104. Bodnar AG, Kim NW, Effros RB, et al. Mechanism of telomerase induction during T cell activation. Exp Cell Res 1996;228:58–64.

105. Kiyono T, Foster SA, Koop JI, et al. Both Rb/p16INK4a inactivation and telomerase activity are required to immortalize human epithelial cells. Nature 1998;396:84–88.

106. Klingelhutz AJ, Foster SA, McDougall JK. Telomerase activation by the E6 gene product of human papillomavirus type 16. Nature 1996;380:79–82.

107. Blasco MA, Hahn WC. Evolving views of telomerase and cancer. Trends Cell Biol 2003;13:289–294.

108. Hahn WC. Role of telomeres and telomerase in the pathogenesis of human cancer. J Clin Oncol 2003;21:2034–2043.

109. Veldman T, Liu X, Yuan H, et al. Human papillomavirus E6 and Myc proteins associate in vivo and bind to and cooperatively activate the telomerase reverse transcriptase promoter. Proc Natl Acad Sci U S A 2003;100:8211–8216.

110. Gewin L, Myers H, Kiyono T, et al. Identification of a novel telomerase repressor that interacts with the human papillomavirus type-16 E6/E6-AP complex. Genes Dev 2004;18:2269–2282.

111. McMurray HR, McCance DJ. Human papillomavirus type 16 E6 activates TERT gene transcription through induction of c-Myc and release of USF-mediated repression. J Virol 2003;77:9852–9861.

112. Bischof O, Nacerddine K, Dejean A. Human papillomavirus oncoprotein E7 targets the promyelocytic leukemia protein and circumvents cellular senescence via the Rb and p53 tumor suppressor pathways. Mol Cell Biol 2005;25:1013–1024.

113. Bouck N, Stellmach V, Hsu SC. How tumors become angiogenic. Adv Cancer Res 1996;69:135–174.

114. Folkman J. The role of angiogenesis in tumor growth. Semin Cancer Biol 1992;3:65–71.

115. Folkman J. Tumor angiogenesis and tissue factor. Nat Med 1996;2:167–168.

116. Dobbs SP, Hewett PW, Johnson IR, et al. Angiogenesis is associated with vascular endothelial growth factor expression in cervical intraepithelial neoplasia. Br J Cancer 1997;76: 1410–1415.

117. Guidi AJ, Abu-Jawdeh G, Berse B, et al. Vascular permeability factor (vascular endothelial growth factor) expression and angiogenesis in cervical neoplasia. J Natl Cancer Inst 1995;87:1237–1245.

118. Smith-McCune K, Zhu YH, Hanahan D, et al. Cross-species comparison of angiogenesis during the premalignant stages of squamous carcinogenesis in the human cervix and K14-HPV16 transgenic mice. Cancer Res 1997;57:1294–1300.

119. Kodama J, Hashimoto I, Seki N, et al. Thrombospondin-1 and -2 messenger RNA expression in invasive cervical cancer: correlation with angiogenesis and prognosis. Clin Cancer Res 2001;7:2826–2831.

120. Hanahan D, Christofori G, Naik P, et al. Transgenic mouse models of tumour angiogenesis: the angiogenic switch, its molecular controls, and prospects for preclinical therapeutic models. Eur J Cancer 1996;32A:2386–2393.

121. Arbeit JM, Olson DC, Hanahan D. Upregulation of fibroblast growth factors and their receptors during multi-stage epidermal carcinogenesis in K14-HPV16 transgenic mice. Oncogene 1996;13:1847–1857.

122. Toussaint-Smith E, Donner DB, Roman A. Expression of human papillomavirus type 16 E6 and E7 oncoproteins in primary foreskin keratinocytes is sufficient to alter the expression of angiogenic factors. Oncogene 2004;23:2988–2995.

123. Ravi R, Mookerjee B, Bhujwalla ZM, et al. Regulation of tumor angiogenesis by p53-induced degradation of hypoxia-inducible factor 1alpha. Genes Dev 2000;14:34–44.

124. Dawson DW, Volpert OV, Pearce SF, et al. Three distinct D-amino acid substitutions confer potent antiangiogenic activity on an inactive peptide derived from a thrombospondin-1 type 1 repeat. Mol Pharmacol 1999;55:332–338.

125. Kieser A, Weich HA, Brandner G, et al. Mutant p53 potentiates protein kinase C induction of vascular endothelial growth factor expression. Oncogene 1994;9:963–969.

126. Mukhopadhyay D, Tsiokas L, Sukhatme VP. Wild-type p53 and v-Src exert opposing influences on human vascular endothelial growth factor gene expression. Cancer Res 1995;55: 6161–6165.

127. Lopez-Ocejo O, Viloria-Petit A, Bequet-Romero M, et al. Oncogenes and tumor angiogenesis: the HPV-16 E6 oncoprotein activates the vascular endothelial growth factor (VEGF) gene promoter in a p53 independent manner. Oncogene 2000;19:4611–4620.

128. Antinore MJ, Birrer MJ, Patel D, et al. The human papillomavirus type 16 E7 gene product interacts with and transactivates the AP1 family of transcription factors. EMBO J 1996;15:1950–1960.

129. Tischer E, Mitchell R, Hartman T, et al. The human gene for vascular endothelial growth factor. Multiple protein forms are encoded through alternative exon splicing. J Biol Chem 1991;266:11947–11954.

130. Lyden D, Hattori K, Dias S, et al. Impaired recruitment of bone-marrow-derived endothelial and hematopoietic precursor cells blocks tumor angiogenesis and growth. Nat Med 2001;7:1194–1201.

131. Rafii S, Lyden D, Benezra R, et al. Vascular and haematopoietic stem cells: novel targets for anti-angiogenesis therapy? Nat Rev Cancer 2002;2:826–835.

132. Ruzinova MB, Schoer RA, Gerald W, et al. Effect of angiogenesis inhibition by Id loss and the contribution of bone-marrow-derived endothelial cells in spontaneous murine tumors. Cancer Cell 2003;4:277–289.

133. Orimo A, Gupta PB, Sgroi DC, et al. Stromal fibroblasts present in invasive human breast carcinomas promote tumor growth and angiogenesis through elevated SDF-1/CXCL12 secretion. Cell 2005;121:335–348.

134. Tjiong MY, van der Vange N, ten Kate FJ, et al. Increased IL-6 and IL-8 levels in cervicovaginal secretions of patients with cervical cancer. Gynecol Oncol 1999;73:285–291.

135. Stanley M. Immune responses to human papillomavirus. Vaccine 2006;24(Suppl 1):S16–S22.

136. Chang YE, Laimins LA. Microarray analysis identifies interferon-inducible genes and stat-1 as major transcriptional targets of human papillomavirus type 31. J Virol 2004;74: 4174–4182.

137. Nees M, Geoghegan JM, Hyman T, et al. Papillomavirus type 16 oncogenes downregulate expression of interferon-responsive genes and upregulate proliferation-associated and NF-kappaB-responsive genes in cervical keratinocytes. J Virol 2001;75: 4283–4296.

138. Park JS, Kim EJ, Kwon HJ, et al. Inactivation of interferon regulatory factor-1 tumor suppressor protein by HPV E7 oncoprotein. Implication for the E7-mediated immune evasion mechanism in cervical carcinogenesis. J Biol Chem 2000; 275:6764–6769.

139. Ronco LV, Karpova AY, Vidal M, et al. Human papillomavirus 16 E6 oncoprotein binds to interferon regulatory factor-3 and inhibits its transcriptional activity. Genes Dev 1998;12:2061–2072.

140. Ashrafi GH, Haghshenas MR, Marchetti B, et al. E5 protein of human papillomavirus type 16 selectively downregulates surface HLA class I. Int J Cancer 2005;113:276–283.

141. Zhang B, Li P, Wang EZ et al. The E5 protein of human papillomavirus type 16 perturbs MHC class II antigen maturation in human foreskin keratinocytes treated with interferon-gamma. Virology 2003;310:100–108.

142. Winkelstein W. Smoking and cancer of the uterine cervix: hypothesis. Am J Epidemiol 1977;106:257–259.

143. Winkelstein WJr. Smoking and cervical cancer—current status: a review. Am J Epidemiol 1990;131:945–957; discussion 958–960.

144. Winkelstein W Jr. Smoking and cervical cancer: cause or coincidence. J Am Med Assoc 1989;262:1631–1632.

145. Haverkos H, Rohrer M, Pickworth W. The cause of invasive cervical cancer could be multifactorial. Biomed Pharmacother 2000;54:54–59.

146. Haverkos HW. Multifactorial etiology of cervical cancer: a hypothesis. MedGenMed 2005;7:57.

147. Haverkos HW. Viruses, chemicals and co-carcinogenesis. Oncogene 2004;23:6492–6499.

148. Haverkos HW, Soon G, Steckley SL, et al. Cigarette smoking and cervical cancer: part I: a meta-analysis. Biomed Pharmacother 2003;57:67–77.

149. Steckley SL, Pickworth WB, Haverkos HW. Cigarette smoking and cervical cancer: part II: a geographic variability study. Biomed Pharmacother 2003;57:78–83.

150. Prokopczyk B, Cox JE, Hoffmann D, et al. Identification of tobacco-specific carcinogen in the cervical mucus of smokers and nonsmokers. J Natl Cancer Inst 1997;89:868–873.

151. Cuzick J, Szarewski A, Terry G, et al. Human papillomavirus testing in primary cervical screening. Lancet 1995;345: 1533–1536.

152. Castle PE. Beyond human papillomavirus: the cervix, exogenous secondary factors, and the development of cervical precancer and cancer. J Low Genit Tract Dis 2004;8:224–230.

153. Franco EL, Schlecht NF, Saslow D. The epidemiology of cervical cancer. Cancer J 2003;9:348–359.

154. Smith J, Green J, Berrington de Gonzalez A, et al. Cervical cancer and use of hormonal contraceptives: a systematic review. Lancet 2003;361:1159–1167.

155. Schiffman M, Brinton L. The epidemiology of cervical carcinogenesis. Cancer 1995;76:1888–1901.

156. Aurelian L. Herpes simplex virus type 2 and cervical cancer. Clin Dermatol 1984;2:90–99.

157. Vonka V, Kanka J, Hirsch I, et al. Prospective study on the relationship between cervical neoplasia and herpes simplex type-2 virus. II. Herpes simplex type-2 antibody presence in sera taken at enrollment. Int J Cancer 1984;33:61–66.

158. Anttila T, Saikku P, Koskela P, et al. Serotypes of *Chlamydia trachomatis* and risk for development of cervical squamous cell carcinoma. J Am Med Assoc 2001;285:47–51.

159. Ghaderi M, Wallin K, Wiklund F, et al. Risk of invasive cervical cancer associated with polymorphic HLA DR/DQ haplotypes. Int J Cancer 2002;100:698–701.

160. Hakama M, Lehtinen M, Knekt P, et al. Serum antibodies and subsequent cervical neoplasms: a prospective study with 12 years of follow-up. Am J Epidemiol 1993;137:166–170.

161. Koskela P, Anttila T, Bjorge T, et al. *Chlamydia trachomatis* infection as a risk factor for invasive cervical cancer. Int J Cancer 2000;85:35–39.

162. Schachter J. Sexually transmitted infections and cervical atypia. Sex Transm Dis 1981;8:353–356.

163. Dillner J, Silins I, Ryd W, et al. History of *Chlamydia trachomatis* infection is a determinant of HPV DNA persistence. A population-based cohort study. Abstract for HPV conference 2002.

164. Barba A, Tessari G, Boschiero L, et al. Renal transplantation and skin diseases: review of the literature and results of a 5-year follow-up of 285 patients. Nephron 1996;73:131–136.

165. Boccalon M, Tirelli U, Sopracordevole F, et al. Intra-epithelial and invasive cervical neoplasia during HIV infection. Eur J Cancer 1996;32A:2212–2217.

166. Jay N, Moscicki AB. Human papillomavirus infections in women with HIV disease: prevalence, risk, and management. AIDS Read 2000;10:659–668.

167. Orozco Topete R, Archer Dubon C, Valadez Huerta N, et al. 1996. Cutaneous neoplasms and human papillomavirus in renal transplant patients: experience of one center in Mexico. Transplant Proc 1996;28:3314–3316.

168. Palefsky JM, Holly EA, Ralston ML, et al. Prevalence and risk factors for human papillomavirus infection of the anal canal in human immunodeficiency virus (HIV)-positive and HIV-negative homosexual men. J Infect Disease 1998;177:361–367.

169. ter Haar-van Eck SA, Rischen-Vos J, Chadha-Ajwani S, et al. The incidence of cervical intraepithelial neoplasia among women with renal transplant in relation to cyclosporine. Br J Obstet Gyn 1995;102:58–61.

170. Daling JR, Madeleine MM, Schwartz SM, et al. A population-based study of squamous cell vaginal cancer: HPV and cofactors. Gynecol Oncol 2002;84:263–270.

171. Konya J, Dillner J. Immunity to oncogenic human papillomaviruses. Adv Cancer Res 2001;82:205–238.

172. Beskow A, Josefsson A, Gyllensten U. HLA class II alleles associated with infection by HPV16 in cervical cancer in situ. Int J Cancer 2001;93:817–822.

173. Moscicki AB, Schiffman M, Kjaer S, et al. Chapter 5: updating the natural history of HPV and anogenital cancer. Vaccine 2006;24(Suppl 3):S42–S51.

174. Schiffman MH, Bauer HM, Hoover RN, et al. Epidemiologic evidence showing that human papillomavirus infection causes most cervical intraepithelial neoplasia. J Natl Cancer Inst 1993;85:958–964.

175. Demers GW, Espling E, Harry JB, et al. Abrogation of growth arrest signals by human papillomavirus type 16 E7 is mediated by sequences required for transformation. J Virol 1996;70:6862–6869.

176. Gage JR, Meyers C, Wettstein FO. The E7 proteins of the non-oncogenic human papillomavirus type 6b (HPV-6b) and of the oncogenic HPV-16 differ in retinoblastoma protein binding and other properties. J Virol 1990;64:723–730.

177. Munger K, Werness BA, Dyson N, et al. Complex formation of human papillomavirus E7 proteins with the retinoblastoma tumor suppressor gene product. EMBO J 1989;8: 4099–4105.

178. Demers GW, Foster SA, Halbert CL, et al. Growth arrest by induction of p53 in DNA damaged keratinocytes is bypassed by human papillomavirus 16 E7. Proc Natl Acad Sci U S A 1994;91:4382–4386.

179. Halbert CL, Demers GW, Galloway DA. The E6 and E7 genes of human papillomavirus type 6 have weak immortalizing activity in human epithelial cells. J Virol 1992;66:2125–2134.

180. Collins AS, Nakahara T, Do A, et al. Interactions with pocket proteins contribute to the role of human papillomavirus type 16 E7 in the papillomavirus life cycle. J Virol 2005;79: 14769–14780.

181. Banerjee NS, Genovese NJ, Noya F, et al. Conditionally activated E7 proteins of high-risk and low-risk human papillomaviruses induce S phase in postmitotic, differentiated human keratinocytes. J Virol 2006;80:6517–6524.

182. Zhang B, Chen W, Roman A. The E7 proteins of low- and high-risk human papillomaviruses share the ability to target the pRB family member p130 for degradation. Proc Natl Acad Sci U S A 2006;103:437–442.

CHAPTER 3

Human Papillomavirus Vaccine

Stanley A. Gall

KEY POINTS

- Current human papillomavirus (HPV) vaccines are prophylactic virus-like particle (VLP) vaccines that consist of recombinant L1 HPV capsid proteins reassembled into "viruslike" particles that are noninfectious and nononcogenic. They produce high levels of neutralizing antibodies.
- The vaccines have no effect on women who have already been infected by the particular HPV type. They will not make established lesions regress.
- The vaccine that is currently approved by the U.S. Food and Drug Administration (FDA) is the quadrivalent HPV vaccine against HPV types 6/11/16/18. The other vaccine that has been developed and is not yet FDA approved is a bivalent vaccine against HPV types 16/18.
- The quadrivalent HPV vaccine is made in yeast; the bivalent vaccine is made in Baculovirus. The vaccines also differ with respect to their adjuvant.
- Both vaccines show excellent efficacy in preventing HPV-related precancer of the cervix, vagina, and vulva. The quadrivalent vaccine also shows excellent efficacy in preventing genital warts.
- A comparative analysis of the efficiencies of each of the proprietary serologic tests is not available.
- The dosing schedule for the quadrivalent vaccine is 0, 2, and 6 months. The dosing schedule for the bivalent vaccine is 0, 1, and 6 months.
- The per-protocol efficacy of the quadrivalent HPV vaccine with regard to CIN 2,3 is 98%; with regard to external genital and vaginal lesions, 100%; and with regard to VIN 2,3 and ValN 2,3, 100%.
- The Advisory Committee on Immunization Practices (ACIP) recommends routine vaccination of females 11 to 12 years of age with three doses of quadrivalent HPV vaccine. The vaccine series can be started as young as 9 years of age at the discretion of the provider. The ACIP recommends vaccination of females 13 to 26 years of age who have not previously been vaccinated.
- Ideally the vaccine should be administered before onset of sexual activity, but females who are sexually active should still be vaccinated.
- Vaccination with quadrivalent HPV vaccine is recommended without knowing what HPV type caused the abnormal Pap test.
- Vaccination does not substitute for routine cervical cancer screening. Women should continue to undergo cervical cancer screening per standard of care.

Human papillomavirus (HPV) is a member of the Papovavirus class of viruses. More than 100 different genotypes are defined by differences in their L1 nucleotide sequence of the L1 protein. The genotypes have a predilection to cause disease in a defined anatomic location, but different genotypes can affect the same anatomic area, and the physical appearance of the lesion does not define the genotype. In the 1960s, it was assumed there was only one type of HPV and that variations were due to the anatomic site.[1] Soon, molecular biology techniques became available that demonstrated several types of HPV.[2,3] In the 1970s, zur Hausen and colleagues showed that cancer of the cervix was likely attributable to infection with a subset of HPV.[4] Subsequent development of technologies for cloning and sequencing genes showed that genetically distinct HPV could be found in many cancers and precancerous lesions.[5] Epidemiologic and molecular evidence has led to the conclusion that virtually all cases of cervical cancer as well as precursor lesions are attributable to infection with certain oncogenic HPV types.[6-8]

New information indicates oropharyngeal cancer is significantly associated with oral HPV 16 infection. HPV 16 deoxyribonucleic acid (DNA) was detected in 72% of 100 paraffin-embedded tumor specimens, and 64% of patients with cancer were seropositive for HPV 16 and proteins E6/E7.[9] HPV 6 and 11 can infect laryngeal epithelium and cause benign papillomas, and malignant degeneration does occur as a rare complication. Infection of the vulva with low-risk HPVs is known to occur and may cause benign genital condylomata. One subset of vulvar cancers occur in young women and have a basaloid histopathology, adjacent VIN, and risk factors related to sexual practices and are HPV associated.[10] High-risk HPV types 16, 31, and 33 are most often isolated from these vulvar carcinomas and their precursor lesions,[11] and these women have antibodies to E6 and E7 proteins.[12]

Although there is no convincing molecular evidence yet to explain why some genotypes are more or less oncogenic, it is agreed that *persistent infection with an oncogenic type is the hallmark of risk for cancer development.* The reason why certain HPV types are allowed to persist by the host may be due to host factors such as human leukocyte antigen

(HLA) and natural killer (NK) cell immunoglobulin receptor (KIR) polymorphisms[13] or viral gene products that block interferon host resistance mechanisms.[14] *Although all high-risk HPV types have some propensity for persistence, HPV 16 is the most important as it is present in 50% of cervical cancer cases worldwide. HPV 16 has the propensity for integration of viral genome into the host DNA, and persistent HPV 16 infection conveys a fivefold greater risk for development of malignancy than other HPV types.*[15]

EPIDEMIOLOGY AND TRANSMISSION

The average of sexual debut in the United States is 16.4 years, but at age 21, 74% of women will not have acquired HPV. It is also important to know that *60% of sexually active young women will acquire infection with one or more HPV within 5 years of sexual debut.* The risk of infection increases with the number of new sexual partners as well as with the total number of sexual partners and with the number of sexual partners of the current partner. The majority of infections in males and females are asymptomatic, but asymptomatic individuals seem to transmit infection as effectively as those with visible lesions.

It is common for HPV infections to last for weeks to months and then spontaneously resolve. This ability to clear HPV infections is probably the result of activation of cell-mediated immunity.[16] Cutaneous warts frequently undergo spontaneous regression, but patients with defects in cell-mediated immunity (CMI) have a high incidence of warts. There is a higher incidence of HPV-associated cancers in renal transplant patients.[17] These data suggest that the process of resolving HPV infection is due to immune-mediated responses including antibody recognizing confrontational determinants on the viral capsid[18] and T cell–mediated responses to viral nonstructural proteins.[19] Antibody to the viral capsid is of low level and appears late, if at all. Antibody to capsid protein is found in only 50% of persistently infected patients, thereby making serologic diagnosis of little value in making a diagnosis.

HUMAN PAPILLOMAVIRUS VACCINE DEVELOPMENT

The quest for a HPV cancer vaccine has progressed since the 1960s, when it was believed that there was only one HPV type, to the present day when approximately 40 oncogenic HPV types are known and HPV 16 and 18 are recognized as represented in 72% of the cervical cancers in the United States. *An ideal prophylactic vaccine should possess the following attributes:*

1. The vaccine should be safe because it will be given to many young individuals who would not be expected to develop cancer.
2. The vaccine should be effective in reducing HPV-induced clinical disease such as condyloma acuminata, cervical intraepithelial lesions, and cervical cancer.

3. The vaccine should not be difficult to administer and should not require a cold chain.
4. Protection should last many years because it is neither practical nor desirable to vaccinate frequently.

The goal of prophylactic vaccination is to generate the production of neutralizing antibodies to viral capsid proteins that will block the virus before it can enter the cell. Because HPV does not enter the systemic circulation but instead remains in the epidermis, antibodies that are capable of reaching the skin must be generated. Antibody induction has been demonstrated in the epithelium of the vagina following systemic immunization, indicating that antibodies cross the basement membrane.[20]

For a prophylactic vaccine to succeed, the obvious target antigens would need to be the capsid proteins because they are the only antigens accessible for a classical neutralizing antibody response that prevents infection. These antigens induce a strong, long-lasting, virus-neutralizing response. The work of Zhou et al. demonstrated that the HPV 16 L1 capsid proteins, when expressed in a recombinant system, form viruslike particles (VLPs) resembling native visions.[21] In cutaneous and oral mucosal animal Papillomavirus models, systemic vaccination with L1 VLPs can induce high titers of neutralizing antibodies that confer protection against experimental challenge of wild-type virus. This suggests that the effectiveness of L1 VLPs derives mainly from their capacity to induce high levels of neutralizing antibodies. Early phase clinical trials in humans with L1 VLPs indicated that the L1 VLPs are highly immunogenic, and antibody titers at least 40 times higher than those seen in natural infection were recorded.[22,23] Koutsky et al.[24] studied 2392 women 16 to 23 years of age in a double-blind, placebo-controlled trial. Subjects received three doses of placebo or HPV 16 VLP vaccine at 40 µgm per dose, at day 0, month 2, and month 6. Genital samples that were tested for HPV 16 DNA by polymerase chain reaction (PCR) were obtained at enrollment, 1 month after the third dose of vaccine, and every 6 months thereafter. Patients with abnormal cytology underwent colposcopy, biopsy, and HPV DNA sampling at the biopsy site. Serum was obtained for antibody measurement every 6 months. The primary endpoint was persistent HPV 16 infection obtained at two or more visits. The primary analysis was limited to women who were negative for HPV 16 DNA at 1 month after the third dose. Serum antibodies were measured by a competitive radioimmunoassay developed by Merck research laboratories and by the use of an HPV 16 enzyme-linked immunosorbent assay.[25]

The women were followed for median of 17.4 months after completing the three-dose vaccination regimen. The vaccine was 100% effective (95% confidence interval [CI] 0–100; P < 0.001) with the incidence of persistent HPV 16 infection being 3.8 per 100 woman-years at risk in the placebo group and 0 per 100 woman-years at risk in the vaccine group. All nine cases of HPV 16–related cervical intraepithelial neoplasia (CIN) occurred among placebo recipients. This study is considered pivotal in the clinical trial program, indicating that HPV VLPs can induce specific type-neutralizing antibodies and prevent not only CIN but also persistent HPV infection.

This study indicated that HPV 16 VLPs were able to induce neutralizing antibodies that would function as a conformational neutralizing epitope to provide protection against HPV infection. However, the amount of HPVs produced *in vitro* was limited and the quantity of HPV VLPs needed for vaccine production was large. With the successful synthesis and enhanced immunogenicity of recombinant hepatitis B virus surface antigen, the use of recombinant technology was suggested for the production of large quantities of HPV VLPs.[26,27] The use of prokaryotic techniques for producing large amino acids and proteins in native conformation needed to induce neutralizing antibodies against conformational viral capsid epitopes did not produce the desired product. The use of eukaryotic expression systems and a superior ability to clone genes using PCR techniques allowed expression of whole-length L1 capsid protein of HPV 16.[28] It was subsequently found that authentic-sequence L1 protein could fold naturally *in vitro*, which is necessary to induce neutralizing antibodies against conformational viral capsid epitopes.[29] Additional research extended the expression of HPV L1 capsid proteins to baculovirus and yeast.[30,31] This allowed large-scale expression and assembly of HPV L1 proteins into VLPs comprising 360 copies of the L1 protein. These VLPs are recognized by neutralizing antibody, and this has become the basis of the vaccines designated to prevent cervical cancer.[28]

The antibody response to HPV L1 capsid protein is type specific. Serology is important for determining the ability of HPV vaccines to induce protective antibodies and the longevity of these antibodies in the circulation. HPV antibody serology is performed in a limited number of expert laboratories, using different techniques. These include the enzyme-linked immunosorbent assays,[32] *in vivo* neutralization assays,[33] *in vitro* pseudo-neutralization assays, and multiplexed luminex assays.[34-36] Determination of antibodies against multiple HPV types simultaneously is preferred to running multiple separate tests. The multiple luminex assay is a competitive immunoassay measuring type-specific antibodies to neutralizing epitopes on HPV 6, 11, 16, and 18 simultaneously. A comparative analysis of the efficiencies of each of the proprietary serologic tests is not available. It is not known whether each technique measures the same conformational neutralizing antibody.

Clinical trials with two HPV vaccines are listed in Table 3-1. A quadrivalent HPV VLP vaccine (Gardasil, Merck, West Point, PA) with HPV 6, 11, 16, and 18 was licensed by the Food and Drug Administration (FDA) on June 8, 2006 and recommended by the Advisory Committee on Immunization Practices (ACIP) at the Centers for Disease Control (CDC) on June 29, 2006. *The quadrivalent HPV vaccine contains the following concentrations of VLPs from HPV 6, 11, 16, and 18: HPV 6, 20 μg; HPV 11, 40 μg; HPV 16, 40 μg; and HPV 18, 20 μg.*

The L1 protein for each HPV VLP type is expressed via a recombinant *Saccharomyce pombe* vector, and the product consists of purified L1 VLPs of HPV types 6, 11, 16, and 18.

The vaccine is reconstituted in an adjuvant of 225 μg of aluminum hydroxyphosphate sulfate (alum).

A candidate bivalent vaccine (Cervarix, GSK, Rixensart, Belgium) and supporting scientific data were submitted to the FDA for proposed licensure on March 29, 2007. *This bivalent candidate against HPV 16 and 18 contains the following concentrations of VLPs from HPV 16 and 18: HPV 16, 20 μg; and HPV 18, 20 μg.* Each type of VLP was produced on *Spodoptera trugiperda* and trichoplausia ni Hi-5 cell substitute with ASO4 adjuvant containing 500-μg aluminum hydroxide and 50-μg 3-deacylated monophosphoryl lipid A.

The criteria for accession to the clinical trials are different for the two vaccines. Each trial that has been published contained an intent-to-treat (ITT) group and a per-protocol efficacy (PPE) group with comparison to a matched placebo group. *The per-protocol analysis has the primary objective of evaluating vaccine efficacy in the prevention of infection with vaccine types or the development of CIN (low-grade squamous intraepithelial lesion [LSIL], high-grade squamous intraepithelial lesions [HSIL], or adenocarcinoma in situ [AIS]) associated with HPV 16 or 18. In the trials with the quadrivalent HPV vaccine, the prevention of genital warts was an added objective.* Case counting in the per-protocol analysis was started 1 month after administration of the third HPV dose. The quadrivalent vaccine was administered at 0, 2, and 6 months, and the bivalent vaccine was administered at 0, 1, and 6 months.

The publications of Harper[37,38] and Gall et al.[39] reported studies of bivalent (HPV 16 and HPV 18) L1 LVP vaccine administered in a randomized, double-blinded, placebo-controlled manner to girls and women aged 15 to 25 years. The three studies report on the same research population evaluated at 21 months,[37] 54 months,[38] and 67 months.[39] The objectives of the study were to assess vaccine efficacy against cytologic abnormalities and CIN as well as vaccine immunogenicity, safety, and tolerability. Eligibility for the study were girls and women aged 15 to 25 years who had no more than six lifetime sexual partners, no history of an abnormal Pap smear or ablative or excisional treatment of the cervix, and no ongoing treatment for condylomata acuminata. Additionally, the subjects had to be seronegative for HPV 16 and HPV 18 antibodies by ELISA and HPV DNA negative by PCR for 14 high-risk HPV types no more than 90 days before the study entry. The vaccine was administered on a 0-, 1-, and 6-month schedule, and assessment of immunogenicity was done at 0, 1, 6, 7, and 12 months and every 6 months thereafter. At study initiation, 1113 women were randomized, with 560 subjects receiving vaccine and 553 receiving placebo. The vaccine efficacy after 21 months of observation in the per-protocol analysis was 91.6% (95% CI, 64.5–98.0) against incident infection and 100% against persistent infection (47.0–100) with HPV 16/18. There was 100% efficacy against HPV 16/18 CIN 1+ lesions. Immunogenicity studies indicated that geometric mean titers for vaccine-induced antibodies were between 80 and 100 times greater than those seen in natural infections with HPV 16 or 18. Vaccine-induced

Table 3-1 Human Papillomavirus Clinical Trials

Author	Vaccine Q or B	Dosing Schedule; Subject Age Range	Follow-Up	Number of Subjects		Positive Endpoints		Vaccine Efficacy (%)	Confidence Interval	p Value
				V	PL	V	PL			
Koutsky[24]	HPV 16	0, 2, 6 months; 16–23 years	17.4	768	765	0	50	100	90–100	<0.001
Harper[37]	B	0, 1, 6 months; 15–25 years	21	560	553	HPV 16 = 220	HPV 18 = 111	95.2 91.2	64.0–99.4 51.7–98	<0.0001 <0.003
Villa[44]	Q	0, 2, 6 months; 16–23 years	30	HPV 6, 11: 214 HPV 16	HPV 18	0 16 3 21	1 9	100 86 89	68–100 54–97 21–100	
Mao[40]	HPV 16	0, 2, 6 months; 16–23 years	48	HPV 16 755	750	CIN 2,3 0 12	Infection 7 111	100 94	65–100 88–98	
Harper[38]	B	0, 1, 6 months; 15–25 years	54	HPV 16,18 393	383	1	28	96.9	81.3–99.9	<0.001
Future II[41]	Q	0, 2, 6 months; 15–25 years	36	5305	5260	1	42	98	86–100	
Garland[42]	Q	0, 2, 6 months; 16–24 years	36	2261	2279	0	60	100	94–100	
Joura[43]	Q	0, 2, 6 months; 16–26 years	48	7811	7785	0	15	100	72–100	
Gall[39]	B	0, 1, 6 months; 15–25 years	67	349	343	0	18	100	62–100	

Q, quadrivalent HPV vaccine; B, bivalent HPV vaccine; V, vaccine group; PL, placebo group; HPV, human papillomavirus.

titers remained elevated at 18 months and were still 10 to 16 times higher than those seen with natural HPV 16 or HPV 18 infections.

Harper et al.[38] reevaluated the data for the endpoints mentioned in the initial study after 4.5 years of follow-up. The vaccine group had 393 subjects with 383 in the placebo group. The vaccine efficacy against HPV 16 and HPV 18 endpoints included: incident infection 96.9% (95% CI, 81.3–99.9), persistent infection (12-month definition) 100% (33.6–100); and against CIN lesions associated with HPV 16/18, the vaccine was 100% effective (42.4–100). The immunogenicity of the vaccine remained impressive with a decline in the peak of the geometric mean titers (GMTs) at 1 month after the third vaccine dose to a stable plateau beginning at 18 months. GMTs were maintained at 17 times and 14 times at 51 to 53 months for HPV 16 and HPV 18, respectively. The safety profile remained excellent.

The subjects in this study were again evaluated at 5.5 years.[39] The per-protocol analysis included 349 women in the vaccine group and 343 women in the placebo group. High and sustained vaccine efficacy was demonstrated against HPV 16/18–related incident infection (98% CI, 89–100); persistent infection at 12 months (100% CI, 54–100). The combined analysis through the entire 5.5 years of follow-up showed 100% (62–100) vaccine efficacy against HPV 16/18–associated CIN 1+ and 100% (33–100) against CIN 2+ lesions (68% CI, 7–91) and cross protection against incident infection with HPV 45 (88%) and HPV 31 (52%).

The publication by Koutsky et al.[24] and the follow-up analysis by Mao[40] were the proof of concept study involving HPV 16 vaccine. The study populations were women age 16 to 23 years without prior abnormal Pap smears and no more than five lifetime male sex partners. HPV 16 L1 VLP was used as a monovalent vaccine and administered at a 0-, 2-, and 6-month interval. Subjects had thin-layer cytology and serologic samples at 0, 2, 6, and 7 months and every 6 months thereafter for 48 months. Case counting began 1 month after the third vaccine dose. The primary endpoint was persistent infection of HPV 16 in which HPV DNA was detected on two or more consecutive visits 4 or more months apart and a cervical biopsy showing CIN or cervical cancer with HPV 16 DNA in the biopsy sample and HPV 16 DNA in a swab or lavage sample.

The primary per-protocol efficacy analysis in 768 women who received HPV 16 L1 VLP vaccine compared with 765 women in the placebo group was 100% (90–100) (R < 0.001). There were 0/768 persistent HPV 16 infections in the vaccine group and 41/765 in the placebo group. The immunogenicity by GMT at month 7 showed HPV 16 antibodies 58.7 times as high as the GMT among women who demonstrated natural HPV 16 infections. A follow-up evaluation of the pattern with the Koutsky study[24] was published by Mao.[40] This study evaluated patients who received HPV 16 L1 VLP and were followed for 48 months. The end points for this study were taken from the per-protocol

efficacy group of 755 women compared with the placebo group of 750 women. Persistent HPV 16 infection was 7/755 in the vaccine group and 111/750 in the placebo group with a vaccine efficacy (VE) of 94% (88–98). CIN 1+ and CIN 2,3 lesions were 0/755 in the vaccine group and 27/755 in the placebo VE (100% CI, 84–100). High anti–HPV 16 GMT was observed after completion of the three-dose vaccination regimen. GMT stabilized at 18 months and exceeded GMT in placebo recipients.

Reports of three large studies using quadrivalent HPV vaccine in long-term efficacy studies regarding prevention of CIN, anogenital lesions, and vaginal and vulvar disease have been published.[41–43]

The Future II study[41] is a randomized, double-blind trial of 12167 women aged 15 to 26 years who received three doses of either quadrivalent HPV 6, 11, 16, 18 vaccine or placebo administered at 0, 2, and 6 months. The per-protocol analysis included 5305 women in the vaccine group and 5260 women in the placebo group. Women were eligible to participate if they were not pregnant, did not report abnormal results on a Pap smear, and had no more than four lifetime sex partners. First-day visit included a gynecologic exam and collection of cervical sample for Pap testing (liquid-based) and anogenital swabs of the labia, vulva, perineum, perianal, endocervical, and ectocervical areas for HPV DNA testing. Follow-up visits were done 1 and 6 months after the third vaccine injection and at months 24, 36, and 48. The primary endpoints were to analyze differences in HGSIL (CIN 2,3) in the vaccine and placebo group. The per-protocol analysis was conducted among subjects who had negative results on DNA and serology testing for HPV 16 or 18 at enrollment and remained DNA negative through 1 month after receiving the third vaccine dose. Case ascertainment started 1 month after the third dose. The per-protocol population included 4559 women in the vaccine group and 4408 women in the placebo group. *The results of the per-protocol analysis with regard to CIN 2,3 efficacy was 1/5305 in the vaccine group, and 42/5260 in the placebo group developed CIN 2,3, for a total per-protocol efficacy of 98% (86–100).* Among 1512 vaccinated women in the immunogenicity substudy, more than 99% had seroconversion to the relevant HPV types. At month 4, 96% of 986 subjects were seropositive to HPV 6; 97% of 953 were seropositive to HPV 11; 99% of 953 were seropositive to HPV 11; 99% of 953 were seropositive to HPV 16; and 68% of 1059 were seropositive to HPV 18. Despite a lower seropositivity rate for HPV 18, efficacy was maintained at 100%.

Pregnancy occurred in 1053 subjects in the vaccine group and 1106 in the placebo group in the Future II study.[41] When all phase III trials of quadrivalent vaccine were combined, 1396 subjects in the vaccine group (13%) and 1436 in the placebo group (16%) became pregnant, and outcomes were available for 82%. *The proportions of women with live births, difficulties with delivery, and spontaneous abortions were similar in the two groups.* Congenital anomalies were reported in 25/1396 (1.8%) women in the vaccine group and 22/1436 (1.5%) women in the placebo group.

These numbers are approximately 50% of the quoted anomaly rate of 3.5%.

A parallel study using the quadrivalent HPV vaccine or placebo was done to assess the efficacy of the quadrivalent HPV vaccine in preventing anogenital disease associated with HPV types 6, 11, 16, and 18.[42] The accession criteria were the same as in the previous study.[41] The endpoints for this study were comparison of vaccine and placebo patients regarding the incidence of genital warts, vulvar, or vaginal intraepithelial neoplasia or cancer and the incidence of CIN, AIS, or cancer associated with HPV 6, 11, 16, or 18. The per-protocol efficacy for external genital and vaginal lesions was evaluated in 2261 subjects in the vaccine group and 2279 subjects in the placebo group. *Evaluation showed that 0/2261 in the vaccine group and 60/2279 in the placebo group developed external genital and vaginal lesions, for a total per-protocol efficacy of 100% (94–100). CIN 1+ efficacy was 2/2667 in the vaccine group and 68/2684 in the placebo group (VE = 98% [92–100]).*

The third published report in this series described efficacy of the quadrivalent HPV L1 VLP vaccine against high-grade vulva and vaginal lesions.[43] A total of 18,174 women were enrolled in one of three double-blind, placebo-controlled, randomized trials[41,42,44] from 157 sites in 24 countries. Accession criteria was listed previously.[41] Per protocol susceptible population included 9087 women in the vaccine group and 9087 women in the placebo group. Evaluation showed 0/7811 in the vaccine group and 15/7285 in the placebo group were positive for HPV 16–related or HPV 18–related VIN 2/3 or VaIN 2/3 for a total per-protocol efficacy of 100% (72–100). *This study shows that quadrivalent HPV vaccine is 100% effective in preventing VIN 2/3 and VaIN 2/3 associated with HPV 16 and 18 according to the per-protocol analysis.*

In each of the clinical trials listed in Table 3-1, the subjects were young women aged 16 to 25 years who had fewer than six lifetime sex partners. Those women accessed were HPV DNA negative to the viral HPV types in the vaccine and were also HPV serologically negative. In addition, they needed to receive their vaccinations at the designated time. The patients adhering to the listed criteria were eligible to be included in the "per-protocol analysis."

HUMAN PAPILLOMAVIRUS VACCINE APPROVAL BY THE FOOD AND DRUG ADMINISTRATION

On June 8, 2006, the FDA licensed Gardasil (quadrivalent HPV 6/11/16/18) VLP L1 vaccine for prevention of diseases caused by HPV types 6, 11, 16, and 18, such as:

- Cervical cancer
- Genital warts (Condyloma acuminata) and the following precancerous or dysplastic lesions:
  - Cervical intraepithelial neoplasia (CIN) grade 1
  - Cervical intraepithelial neoplasia (CIN) grades 2 and 3

  - Cervical adenocarcinoma *in situ* (AIS)
  - Vulvar intraepithelial neoplasia (VIN) grades 2 and 3
  - Vaginal intraepithelial neoplasia (VaIN) grades 2 and 3

Furthermore, the FDA license was for girls and women aged 9 to 26 years, even though clinical trials with quadrivalent HPV vaccine were carried out primarily in women aged 16 to 26 years. Additional efficacy and immunologic studies are being performed in women older than age 26. Immunologic studies have been performed in girls and boys aged 11 to 15 years.[45] In 11- to 15-year-old girls, the antibody titers to vaccine HPV VLPs were higher than in the 15- to 26-year-old females, and because efficacy has been proven in 15- to 26-year-old females, the FDA determined, using immunologic bridging, that the 11- to 15-year-old female would be protected from infection with vaccine HPVs. Despite the antibody studies in males aged 11 to 15 years, which showed titers higher than girls at the same age, the FDA did not license the quadrivalent vaccine for males. Since the FDA action, other countries licensing Gardasil have had a gender-neutral recommendation (e.g., Canada, Mexico, Australia, New Zealand).

Additionally, both vaccine manufactures are currently conducting trials with HPV vaccines in women older than age 26. Preliminary data indicate the antibody response is robust in women aged 26 to 35, 35 to 45, and 45 to 55 years, but as would be expected with aging, with each 10-year increment, the peak titers are lower. As these trials mature and efficacy data are obtained, it is very likely the recommended age range will be expanded.[46]

HUMAN PAPILLOMAVIRUS VACCINE RECOMMENDATIONS BY THE ADVISORY COMMITTEE ON IMMUNIZATION PRACTICES

At the regular meeting of the ACIP on June 29, 2006, the committee voted on a number of recommendations regarding Gardasil (quadrivalent HPV 6/11/16/18 vaccine), which were published in *Morbidity and Mortality Weekly Report* (MMWR).[47]

The ACIP recommended routine vaccination of females 11 to 12 years of age with three doses of quadrivalent HPV vaccine. The vaccine series can be started as young as 9 years of age at the discretion of the provider. The age of 11 to 12 years chosen because the vaccine will be included in the group of vaccines administered to girls upon entry into junior high school, which is an opportune time as a physician's visit is already scheduled. Additional reasoning included (1) prevalent infection targeting high-risk groups was not possible, (2) modeling studies showed a greater impact with this age group, (3) vaccination should be done prior to sexual debut (age of onset of sexual intercourse in the United States is 16.4 years), (4) high antibody titers are achieved at this age, and (5) data through 5 years show no evidence of waning immunity, with ongoing studies monitoring duration of protection.

The ACIP recommended vaccination for females 13 to 26 years of age who have not previously been vaccinated.

The committee expressed the view that ideally the vaccine should be administered before onset of sexual activity, but females who are sexually active should still be vaccinated. Some sexually active females may not have full benefits of the vaccine because they may have been infected with vaccine HPV type (Table 3-2). It is well to remember that *only a small percentage are likely to have been infected with all four vaccine HPV types* (0.1% in Merck trials).[42] For those already infected with any vaccine type, the vaccine would provide protection against disease caused by other vaccine HPV types. It must be remembered that serologic studies underestimate cumulative incidence of HPV infection, as not all persons develop antibody after natural infection (as low as 60%). Additionally, detection of HPV DNA underestimates cumulative incidence and provides point prevalence estimates only, as most infections clear within 1 year.

Data from the quadrivalent HPV clinical trials indicate that 24.4% of 16- to 26-year-old females were positive for one vaccine type (Table 3-3) and that even at age 23, 76% of females entering the clinical trial were naïve to HPV 16 and 18 by PCR or serology.[42] This is strong evidence that vaccination of these women would be largely protective.

The ACIP also recommended no change in cervical cancer screening protocols. Vaccinated females could subsequently be infected with non-vaccine HPV types, and sexually active females could have been infected prior to vaccination. Furthermore, the ACIP stressed that *the decision to vaccinate should not be based on a HPV serologic test.*

The ACIP further recommended that *simultaneous administration of quadrivalent HPV vaccine can be given with other vaccines such as TdaP, MVC4, TIV, or HBV.* Clinical trials

Table 3-2 Percentage of North American Females 16–26 Years Naïve to Human Papillomavirus (HPV) 16 and 18 by Polymerase Chain Reaction or Serology, Quadrivalent HPV Trials

Age at Enrollment	Number (n)	Naïve to HPV 16 and 18 (%)
16	122	86
17	189	82
18	1022	86
19	1315	84
20	1119	81
21	890	76
22	693	77
≥23	581	76

From Garland, S, Avila MH, Wheeler CM, et al. Quadrivalent vaccine against human papillomavirus to prevent anogenital diseases. N Engl J Med 2007;356:1928–1943; and Joura EA, Leodolter S, Avila MH, et al. Efficacy of a quadrivalent prophylactic human papillomavirus (types 6, 11, 16, 18) L1 virus-like particle vaccine against high-grade vulva and vaginal lesions: a combined analysis of three randomized clinical trials. Lancet 2007;369:1693–1702.

Table 3-3 Positivity for Human Papillomavirus (HPV) 6, 11, 16, or 18 by Polymerase Chain Reaction on Serology, Females Aged 16–26 Years, North American Quadrivalent HPV Vaccine Trials

Positive to HPV 6, 11, 16, or 18	Number (n)	% Positive
PCR	5927	14.7
Serology	5966	15.6
PCR or serology	5933	24.4

From Garland, S, Avila MH, Wheeler CM, et al. Quadrivalent vaccine against human papillomavirus to prevent anogenital diseases. N Engl J Med 2007;356:1928–1943.
PCR, Polymerase chain reaction.
Note: 76% of women were naïve to all vaccine types. Less than 1% had evidence of infection to all four types. Among seropositive participants, 80% were positive for one type only.

indicate that immune responses when administering both HBV vaccine and quadrivalent HPV vaccine are noninferior when administering the vaccine at the same or different visits.

The following special situations arise in clinical practice and may add confusion:

1. History of abnormal Pap test. Vaccination with quadrivalent HPV vaccine is recommended without knowing what HPV type caused the abnormal Pap test. Data do not indicate the vaccine will have a therapeutic effect on active existing cervical lesions or HPV infection. It is also clear that infection with any of the 40 high- or low-risk genital HPV types is possible. The likelihood of infections with HPV 16/18 increases with severity of Pap results. Also, infections with all four HPV vaccine types is unlikely and the patient may not be infected with any vaccine type.

2. History of HPV DNA positive using high-risk Hybrid Capture II (HC 2) assay. In the patient with a positive HC 2 result, vaccination with quadrivalent HPV vaccine is recommended with the knowledge that infection with a HPV vaccine type could have occurred. However, a positive test indicates infection with any of the 13 high-risk types tested for the HC 2 assay, and specific types are not identified. Vaccination will provide protection against infection with HPV vaccine types not already acquired.

3. History of genital warts. Vaccination is recommended for the patient who has the presence or history of genital warts. The vaccine will have no therapeutic effect on existing warts or HPV infection. Individuals may not have had infection with both HPV 6 and 11 or with HPV-16,18. Vaccination would provide protection against infection with vaccine HPV types not already acquired.

4. Immunosuppressed persons. Vaccination of immunosuppressed persons is recommended. The vaccine is not a live-virus vaccine, but consists of VLPs without viral DNA. However, immune responses and vaccine efficacy might be less than in immunocompetent persons.

5. Lactating women. Lactating women may receive vaccine either as a primary series or a series that was initiated early in pregnancy and should be completed as soon as possible after delivery.

6. Pregnancy. Quadrivalent HPV vaccine was given a pregnancy category B rating by FDA. This is the only vaccine approved by the FDA to receive a pregnancy B categorization. At this time, the ACIP recommends that initiation of the quadrivalent HPV vaccine series be deferred until the completion of the pregnancy. If a woman is found to be pregnant after initiating the vaccine series, completion should be delayed until after the pregnancy. If the vaccine dose has been administered during pregnancy, there is no need for intervention. Quadrivalent HPV vaccine has not been casually associated with adverse outcomes of pregnancy or adverse events to the developing fetus.

A summary of known pregnancy outcomes in the phase III program for Gardasil is seen in Table 3-4.[41] It is of interest that despite the provision of contraceptives for women in this study, 10.7% of the vaccine group and 12.6% of the placebo group became pregnant during the trial. The outcomes and behavior among women in the two groups is similar, and the vaccine shows no adverse effect on pregnancy. Table 3-5 shows details of known pregnancy outcomes when women received quadrivalent vaccine or placebo within 30 days of pregnancy confirmation or receipt of the vaccine after 30 days of pregnancy (dated from the last menstrual period). Again, there is no difference between outcomes in the vaccine and placebo groups. Pregnancy outcomes relating to congenital anomalies are presented in Table 3-6. The 25 congenital anomalies occurring in the vaccine group are similar to 22 anomalies in the placebo group. If the vaccine was administered within 30 days of onset of pregnancy, 5 anomalies were reported in the vaccine group and 0 were reported in the placebo group. In reviewing the 5 anomalies, it is noted that there were no repeated anomalies in the entire report.[42]

HUMAN PAPILLOMAVIRUS VACCINES IN CLINICAL PRACTICE

The FDA has licensed quadrivalent HPV vaccine as safe and efficacious, and the ACIP has recommended the widespread use of this vaccine.[48] It is critically important that a program of education of the medical profession and the general public be accomplished. The general public is woefully ignorant of HPV disease, and many in the medical profession are not fully informed about the association between HPV and the disease it causes, particularly cervical cancer.[49]

A challenge is to instigate appropriate educational programs that would allow communities and political leaders to make intelligent decisions about vaccination against HPV infections. For developed countries, widespread use of HPV vaccines would most benefit lower socioeconomic groups who are least likely to take part in the current

Table 3-4 Summary of Pregnancies in the Phase II Program for Gardasil

	Gardasil (n = 10,419)	Placebo (n = 9120)
Subjects with pregnancies	1115	1151
Number of pregnancies	1244	1272
Pregnancies with either ongoing or unknown outcomes	258	263
Pregnancies with known outcomes	996	1018
Live births (% of pregnancies with known outcome)	621 (62)	611 (60)
Fetal loss (% of pregnancies with known outcomes)	375 (38)	407 (40)

From Garland, S, Avila MH, Wheeler CM, et al. Quadrivalent vaccine against human papillomavirus to prevent anogenital diseases. N Engl J Med 2007;356:1928–1943; and Future II Study Group. Quadrivalent vaccine against human papillomavirus to prevent high-grade cervical lesions. N Engl J Med 2007;356:1517–1527.

Table 3-5 Summary of Known Pregnancy Outcomes in the Phase III Program for Gardasil

	Gardasil	Placebo
Pregnancies with onset of pregnancy within 30 days of vaccination	112	115
Spontaneous loss	21 (18.8%)	26 (22.6%)
Elective termination	21 (18.8%)	23 (20.4%)
Live birth	70 (62.5%)	66 (57.4%)
Pregnancies with onset of pregnancy beyond 30 days of vaccination	879	898
Spontaneous loss	236 (26.9%)	237 (26.4%)
Elective termination	93 (10.6%)	117 (13.0%)
Live birth	549 (62.5%)	544 (60.6%)

From Garland, S, Avila MH, Wheeler CM, et al. Quadrivalent vaccine against human papillomavirus to prevent anogenital diseases. N Engl J Med 2007;356:1928–1943.

Table 3-6 Pregnancy Outcomes: Congenital Anomalies

	Gardasil Cases	Placebo Cases
Congenital anomalies	25	21
EGA ≤ 30 days	5*	0
EGA ≥ 30 days following vaccination	10	16

From Future II Study Group. Quadrivalent vaccine against human papillomavirus to prevent high-grade cervical lesions. N Engl J Med 2007;356:1517–1527
EGA, Estimated gestational age.
*Each of the 5 anomalies was different, with no repeats.

cervical cancer prevention programs. State Medicaid and private insurance companies should vigorously embrace this vaccine. The vaccine prevention results will be cost saving, not only in a monetary sense, but also in the reduction in stress involved with the treatment of HPV-caused disease.

REFERENCES

1. Rowson KE, Maky BW. Human Papova (wart) virus. Bacteriol Rev 1967;31:110–131.
2. Orth G, Favre M, Croissant O. Characterization of a new type of human papillomavirus that causes skin warts. J Virol 1977;24:108–120.
3. Gissman L, Pfister H, Zur Haussen H. Human papillomaviruses: characterization of four different isolates. J Virol 1982;44:393–400.
4. Zur Hausen H, deVilliers EM, Gissman L. Papillomavirus infections and human genital Cancer. Gynecol Oncol 1981;2(2pt2):S124–S128.
5. Durst M, Gissman L, Skenberg H, et al. A papillomavirus DNA from a cervical carcinoma and it's prevalence in cancer biopsy samples from different geographic regions. Proc Natl Acad Sci U S A 1988;80:3812–3815.
6. Bosch FX, Lorincz A, Munoz N, et al. The casual relation between human papillomaviruses and cervical cancer. J Clin Path 2002;55:244–265.
7. Walboomers JMN, Jacobs MV, Manos MN, et al. Human papillomavirus is a necessary cause of invasive cervical cancer worldwide. J Pathol 1999;189:12–19.
8. Munoz N, Bosch FX, de Sanjose S, et al. Epidemiological classification of human Papillomavirus types associated with cervical cancer. N Engl J Med 2003;348:518–527.
9. D'Souza G, Kreimer AR, Viscidi R, et al. Case-central study of human papillomavirus and orophryngeal cancer. N Engl J Med 2007;356:1944–1956.
10. Trimble C, Hildesherm A, Brinton L, et al. Heterogeneous etiology of squamous carcinoma of the vulva. Obstet Gynecol 1996;87:59–64.
11. Hillemans P, Wang X. Integration of HPV-16 and HPV-18 DNA in vulvar intraepithelial neoplasia. Gynecol Oncol 2006;100:276–282.
12. Sun Y, Hildesheim A, Brinton L, et al. Human papillomavirus-specific serologic response in vulvar neoplasia. Gynecol Oncol 1996;63:200–203.
13. Carrington M, Wang S, Martin MP, et al. Hiercerchy of resistance to cervical neoplasia mediated by combinations of immunoglobulins like receptor and human leukocyte antigen loci. J Exp Med 2005;201:1069–1075.
14. Tindle RW. Immune evasion in human papillomavirus-associated cervical cancer. Nature Rev Cancer 2002;2:59–65.
15. Schiffman M, Herrero R, De Salle R, et al. The carcinogenicity of human papillomavirus types reflects viral evolution. Virology 2005;337:76–84.
16. Doeberitz MK. Papillomaviruses in human disease. Part II: molecular biology and immunology of papillomavirus infection and carcinogenesis. Eur J Med 1992;1:485–492.
17. Penn I. Cancer of the anogenital region in renal transplant recipients. Cancer 1986;58:611–616.
18. Carter JJ, Koutsky LA, Hughes JP, et al. Comparison of human papillomavirus types 16, 18, and 6 capsid antibody responses following incident infection. J Infect Dis 2000;181:1911–1919.
19. Van Poelgeesst MI, Nijhuis ER, Kwappenberg KM, et al. Distinct regulation and impact of type 1 T-cell immunity against HPV 16 L1, E2 and E6 antigens during HPV-induced cervical infection and neoplasia. Int J Cancer 2006;118(3):675–683.
20. Bouvet JP, Belec L, Pives R, et al. Immunoglobulin G antibodies in human vaginal secretions after parenteral vaccinations. Infect Immunol 1994;62:3957–3961.
21. Zhou J, Sun XY, Stenzol DJ, et al. Expression of vaccine recombinant HPV 16: L1 and L2 ORF proteins in epithelial cells is sufficient for assembly of HPV virion-like particles. Virology 1991;185:251–257.
22. Zhand LF, Zhou J, Chen S, et al. HPV 66 virus-like particles are potent immunogens without adjuvant in man. Vaccine 2000;18:1051–1058.
23. Harro CP, Pany Y, Roden YS, et al. Safety and immunogenicity trial in adult volunteers of a human papillomavirus type 16, L1 virus-like particle. Natl Cancer Inst 2001;93:284–292.
24. Koutsky LA, Ault K, Wheeler CM, et al. A controlled trial of human papillomavirus type 16 vaccine. New Engl J Med 2002;347: 1645–1651.
25. Lowe RS, Brown DR, Bryant JT, et al. Human papillomavirus type 11 (HPV-11) neutralizing antibodies in the serum and genital mucosa secretions of African green monkeys immunized with HPV-11 virus-like particles expressed in yeast. J Infect Dis 1997;176:1144–1145.
26. McAleen WJ, Buynak EB, Maigettes RZ, et al. Human hepatitis B vaccine from recombinant yeast. Nature 1984;307:178–180.
27. Jilg W, Lorbeer B, Schmidt M, et al. Clinical evaluation of a recombinant hepatitis B vaccine. Lancet 1984;2:1174–1175.
28. Zhou J, Crawford L, McLean L, et al. Increased antibody response to human papillomavirus type 16 L1 protein expressed by recombinant vaccine virus lacking serine protease inhibitor genes. J Gen Virol 1990;71:2185–2190.
29. Zhou J, Sun XY, Stenzel DJ, et al. Expression of vaccinia recombinant HPV 16 L1 and L2 ORF proteins in epithelial cells is sufficient for assembly of HPV virion-like particles. Virology 1991;185:251–252.
30. Rose RC, Bonnez W, Reichman RC, et al. Expression of human papillomavirus type II L1 protein in insect cells in vivo and in-vitro assembly of virus-like particles. J Virol 1993;67:1936–1944.
31. Chen XS, Garcea RI, Goldberg L, et al. Structure of small virus-like particles assembled from the L1 protein of human papillomavirus 16. Mol Cell 2000;5:557–567.

32. Brown DR, Bryan JT, Schroeder JM, et al. Neutralization of human papillomavirus type II (HPV-II) by serum from women vaccinated with yeast-derived HPV-11 L1 virus-like particles correlation with competitive radioimmuno assay titer. J Infect Dis 2001;184:1183–1186.

33. Christensen ND, Dillner C, Eklund C, et al. Surface conformational and linear epitopes on HPV 16 and HPV 18 L1 virus-like particles as defined by monoclonal antibodies. Virology 1996;223:174–184.

34. Yeager MD, Aste-Amezaga M, Brown DR, et al. Neutralization of human papillomavirus (HPV) pseudovirions: a novel and efficient approach to detect and characterize HPV neutralizing antibodies. Virology 2000;278:570–577.

35. Opalka O, Lachman CE, MacMullen SA, et al. Simultaneous quantitation of antibodies to neutralizing antitropes on virus-like particles for human papillomavirus types 6, 11, 16, and 18 by a multiplexed huminex assay. Clin Diag Lab Immunol 2003;10:108–115.

36. Dias D, Van Doren J, Schlottman S, et al. Optimization and validation of a multiplexed luminex assay to quantify antibodies to neutralizing epitopes on human papillomaviruses 6, 11, 16, 18. Clin Diag Lab Immunol 2005;12:959–969.

37. Harper DM, Franco EL, Wheeler C, et al. Efficacy of a bivalent L1 virus-like particle vaccine in prevention of infection with human papillomavirus 16 and 18 in young women: a randomized controlled trial. Lancet 2004;364:1757–1765.

38. Harper TM, Franco EL, Wheeler C, et al. Sustained efficacy up to 4.5 years of a bivalent L1 virus-like particle vaccine against human papillomavirus types 16 and 18: follow up from a randomized control trial. Lancet 2006;367:1247–1255.

39. Gall SA, Teixeira J, Wheeler CN, et al. Extended follow-up through 5.5 years in women vaccinated with a prophylactic bivalent HPV 16 and HPV 18 L1 virus-like particle vaccine adjuvanted with ASO4. American Association for Cancer Research Annual Meeting. April 17, 2007. Los Angeles, CA.

40. Mao C, Koutsky LA, Ault K, et al. Efficacy of human papillomavirus 16 vaccine to present cervical intraepithelial neoplasia. Obstet Gynecol 2006;107:18–27.

41. Future II Study Group. Quadrivalent vaccine against human papillomavirus to prevent high-grade cervical lesions. N Engl J Med 2007;356:1517–1527.

42. Garland S, Avila MH, Wheeler CM, et al. Quadrivalent vaccine against human papillomavirus to prevent anogenital diseases. N Engl J Med 2007;356:1928–1943.

43. Joura EA, Leodolter S, Avila MH, et al. Efficacy of a quadrivalent prophylactic human papillomavirus (types 6, 11, 16, 18) L1 virus-like particle vaccine against high-grade vulva and vaginal lesions: a combined analysis of three randomized clinical trials. Lancet 2007;369:1693–1702.

44. Villa LL, Costa RLR, Petta CA, et al. A randomized, double-blind, placebo controlled efficacy trial of prophylactic quadrivalent human papillomavirus (types 6//11/16/18) L1 virus-like particle in young women. Lancet Oncol 2005;364:1752–1765.

45. Pedersen C, Petaja T, Strauss G, et al. Immunization of early adolescent females with human papillomavirus type 16 and 18 L1 virus-like particle vaccine containing ASO4-adjuvant. J Adolescent Health 2007;40:564–571.

46. Schwarz TF. Human papillomavirus (HPV) 16/18 L1 ASO4 virus-like particle (VLP) cervical cancer vaccine is immunogenic and well-tolerated 18 months after vaccination in women up to age 55 years. Annual Meeting of the American Society of Clinical Oncology. June 1-5, 2007. Chicago, IL.

47. Centers for Disease Control. Quadrivalent human papillomavirus vaccine. Recommendations of the Advisory Committee on Immunization Practices. MMWR 2007;56:RR2, 1–24.

48. Franco EL, Harper DM. Vaccination against human papillomavirus infection: a new paradigm in cervical cancer control. Vaccine. 2005;23:2388–2394.

49. Tjalma WA, Van Damne P. Is the public aware to accept a vaccination program against human papillomavirus? Vaccine 2005;23:3231.

CHAPTER 4

Cytology

4.1: Terminology in Cervical Cytology: The Bethesda System

Diane Davis Davey

KEY POINTS

▪ The Papanicolaou class system, first developed by Papanicolaou and Traut, had many variations and did not correspond to scientific advances in the knowledge of cervical carcinogenesis.

▪ The Bethesda System (TBS) was developed to provide a uniform terminology system that would lead to a clear set of management guidelines for patient care. TBS held workshops in 1988, 1991, and 2001.

▪ A satisfactory cervical cytology specimen should be properly labeled, accompanied by pertinent clinical information, and have adequate numbers of well-visualized and well-preserved squamous cells.

▪ Unsatisfactory specimens include those that are rejected by the laboratory for processing and those that are completely processed and evaluated by the laboratory but have either inadequate squamous cellularity or are largely obscured by blood, inflammation, or other factors. Women with unsatisfactory specimens should be scheduled for repeat cytology in 2 to 4 months unless there are clinical indications for other types of evaluation.

▪ TBS 2001 combined the *within-normal-limits* category and the *benign-cellular-changes* category into *negative-for-intraepithelial-lesion-or-malignancy (NILM)*. NILM is also used as a specific interpretation and more clearly denotes specimens as negative.

▪ Endometrial cells are reported in the *other* category in women age 40 and older; they may indicate increased risk for endometrial abnormalities in postmenopausal women but are generally associated with benign endometrial processes.

▪ Because the identification of organisms on a smear may reflect colonization rather than clinically significant infections, Bethesda 2001 changed the category of *infections* to *organisms*.

▪ Reactive and reparative changes refer to benign changes associated with inflammation, tissue injury, tissue repair, and other nonspecific causes. These changes are included under the overall heading of NILM, and descriptors are added after the NILM result.

▪ The two subcategories of ASC are *ASC-US* and *ASC-H*.

▪ *Atypical glandular cells of undetermined significance* was changed to *atypical glandular cells*, and the subcategory *atypical glandular cells, favor reactive* was eliminated. A separate category of *adenocarcinoma in situ* was introduced for those cases showing classic criteria.

Cervical cytology screening represents one of the major successes in cancer control and prevention. Dr. George Papanicolaou, a reproductive endocrinologist working with Dr. Herbert Traut, a gynecologist, is generally credited with developing the technique of evaluating cellular material from vaginal pool samples.[1] Dr. J. Ernest Ayre, a Canadian gynecologist, introduced direct sampling of the cervix by use of the wooden spatula.[2] Papanicolaou worked jointly with Dr. Charles Cameron, the first Medical and Scientific Director of the American Cancer Society, to promote cervical cancer screening in the United States 5 decades ago.[3]

A variety of reporting terminologies were used for the first 40 years.[4] Papanicolaou developed a reporting system composed of five classes; each specific class provided a level of concern about the presence of cancer cells. For example, class 1 smears were considered negative for cancer, and class 5 slides were considered positive. While simple in concept, the Papanicolaou class system had many variations and did not correspond to scientific advances in the knowledge of cervical carcinogenesis. Reagan encouraged use of the term *dysplasia* to designate pre-cancerous changes; dysplastic processes were further divided according to degree of abnormality and cell type.[5] Richart introduced cervical intra-epithelial neoplasia (CIN) terminology in the 1960s to promote the concept of a continuum of pre-cancerous lesions.[6] Both the dysplasia and CIN terminologies were primarily applied to histopathologic processes in the cervix but were also used to describe cytologic processes.

The Bethesda System (TBS) for reporting results of cervical cytology is now recognized as the most common reporting system for cervical cytology in the United States and many other countries.[7] *TBS was developed to provide a uniform terminology system that would lead to a clear set of management guidelines for patient care.* The first Bethesda conference consisted of an expert panel convened by the National Cancer Institute in 1988.[4] Two more workshops were held in 1991 and 2001 to address controversial topics, the role of new technologies, and scientific advances as related to terminology.[8,9] *One of the main innovations of TBS was the replacement of previous pre-cancerous terms with two levels of squamous intraepithelial lesion (SIL): low grade and high grade.*[4] The term *intraepithelial lesion* was used because many of these lesions regress, progression to invasive carcinoma cannot be predicted, and SIL can be used for squamous lesions anywhere in the lower genital tract. *Another innovation of TBS was the development of designations and criteria for specimen adequacy in cervical cytology.*[4,9]

According to the Clinical Laboratory Improvement Amendments of 1988, cytology laboratories must use descriptive terminology instead of a numerical class system in reporting cervical cytology results.[10] TBS is not mandated by federal regulations, but questionnaire surveys have documented widespread adoption of this reporting system. By 1998, more than 90% of laboratories in the United States were using the 1991 Bethesda System in its entirety or with slight modifications.[7]

TBS 2001 was finalized after several months of preparation. Nine forum groups, including clinicians, pathologists, cytotechnologists, and international members, developed draft recommendations that were posted on a dedicated Internet electronic board.[9] Any professional could provide input, and more than 1000 individual comments were posted on the board. Forty-four professional societies were cosponsors, and more than 400 participants attended the formal workshop meeting. TBS 2001 resulted in a published consensus terminology manuscript, a larger revised atlas, and an Internet educational site. The latter two were developed by a task force convened under the auspices of both the National Cancer Institute and the American Society of Cytopathology.[9,11,12]

GENERAL REPORTING CHANGES

Bethesda 2001 recommended that the heading of the cytology report be labeled either "interpretation" or "result" instead of "diagnosis" (Table 4.1-1). Workshop participants agreed that cervical cytology should be viewed as a "screening test, which in some instances may serve as a medical consultation by providing an interpretation that contributes to a diagnosis."[9] Another recommendation of Bethesda 2001 was that the type of cytology specimen, either smear or liquid-based preparation (LBP), be specified. Some management and screening guidelines differentiate the conventional smear from an LBP. The inclusion of recommendations in the cytology report was viewed by some clinicians as inappropriate in early versions of Bethesda, and Bethesda 2001 changed this section to *educational notes and suggestions*, which are optional.[9] These notes are to be directed to the provider and should be consistent with published clinical guidelines. Finally, any automated screening systems used by the laboratory should be specified in the report.[9] Ancillary test results including human papillomavirus (HPV) testing are ideally included in the cytology report, but if this is impossible in some laboratories, then they are included in a separate report.

SPECIMEN ADEQUACY

Routine evaluation of cervical cytology specimen adequacy is considered one of the most important quality assurance tools in cervical cancer screening.[9] Prior to TBS, most laboratories reported very few, if any, specimens as unsatisfactory for evaluation because there were no uniform criteria. Hence, many women with poor-quality specimens did not have repeat sampling performed. Routine reporting of a transformation zone component and other quality indicators was sporadic and variable in most locales.

The 1988 Bethesda System designated three adequacy categories: *satisfactory, less than optimal,* and *unsatisfactory.*[4] Unsatisfactory specimens included those with insufficient squamous cells and slides with extensive (>75%) obscuring inflammation, blood, or other factors. The *less-than-optimal* category included specimens lacking an endocervical/transformation zone (EC/TZ) component, as well as specimens

Table 4.1-1 Bethesda System for Reporting Cervical Cytology: 1991 versus 2001 Terminology

1991	2001
Specimen Type	
Not mentioned	Indicate conventional versus liquid-based preparation
Specimen Adequacy	**Specimen Adequacy**
Satisfactory for evaluation	Satisfactory for evaluation (describe presence or absence of endocervical T-zone component and any other quality indicators)
Satisfactory for evaluation but limited by (specify reason)	(Category eliminated*)
Unsatisfactory for evaluation (specify reason)	Unsatisfactory for evaluation (specify reason) Specimen may be processed and unsatisfactory or unprocessed
General Categorization (Optional)	
Within normal limits	NILM
Benign cellular changes; see descriptive diagnosis	(category eliminated†)

Epithelial cell abnormality; see descriptive diagnoses	Epithelial cell abnormality; see interpretation/result (specify squamous or glandular)
	Other (see interpretation/result)

Descriptive Diagnoses	**Interpretation/Result**
Within normal limits	*Negative for intraepithelial lesion or malignancy*
Benign cellular changes	*Negative for intraepithelial lesion or malignancy*

Infection
  Trichomonas vaginalis
  Fungal organisms morphologically consistent with *Candida* species
  Predominance of coccobacilli consistent with shift in vaginal flora
  Bacteria morphologically consistent with *Actinomyces* species
  Cellular changes associated with herpes simplex virus
  Other
Reactive changes
  Reactive cellular changes associated with inflammation (includes typical repair), atrophy with inflammation (atrophic vaginitis), radiation, intrauterine contraceptive device, or other
	Organisms
	  Trichomonas vaginalis
	  Fungal organisms morphologically consistent with *Candida* species
	  Shift in vaginal flora suggestive of bacterial vaginosis
	  Bacteria morphologically consistent with *Actinomyces* species
	  Cellular changes consistent with Herpes simplex virus
	  Other non-eoplastic findings (optional to report; list not inclusive)
	  Reactive cellular changes associated with inflammation (includes typical repair), radiation, intrauterine contraceptive device
	  Glandular cells status post hysterectomy
	  Atrophy

	Other Endometrial cells (in a woman $\geq$40 years of age)
Epithelial Cell Abnormalities	*Epithelial Cell Abnormalities*

Squamous cell
Atypical squamous cells of undetermined significance (qualify)
	Squamous cell
	Atypical squamous cells
	  Of undetermined significance
	  Cannot exclude high-grade squamous intraepithelial lesion

Low-grade squamous intraepithelial lesion encompassing human papillomavirus/mild dysplasia/CIN 1	Low-grade squamous intraepithelial lesion encompassing human papillomavirus/mild dysplasia/CIN 1
High-grade squamous intraepithelial lesion encompassing moderate and severe dysplasia, CIN 2, and CIN 3/CIS	encompassing moderate and severe dysplasia, CIN 2, and CIN 3/CIS With features suspicious for invasion (if invasion is suspected)
Squamous cell carcinoma	Squamous cell carcinoma
Glandular cell	Glandular cell
Endometrial cells, cytologically benign in postmenopausal woman	Category reported as other (above); specify if negative for SIL
Atypical glandular cells of undetermined significance, qualify	Atypical endocervical cells, endometrial cells, glandular cells
	Atypical glandular/endocervical cells, favor neoplastic
	Endocervical adenocarcinoma *in situ*

Endocervical adenocarcinoma
  Endometrial adenocarcinoma
  Extrauterine adenocarcinoma
  Adenocarcinoma not otherwise specified
	Adenocarcinoma
	  Endocervical
	  Endometrial
	  Extrauterine
	  Not otherwise specified

Other malignant neoplasms	*Other malignant neoplasms (specify)*

Homonal evaluation (applies to vaginal smears only)
  Hormonal pattern compatible with age and history
  Hormonal pattern incompatible with age and history
  Hormonal evaluation not possible because of (specify)
	(Category eliminated)

*These smears are categorized as satisfactory and quality indicators are described.
†These smears are categorized as either NILM if they are clearly negative or as ASC-US if an epithelial abnormality is suspected.
NILM, Negative for intraepithelial lesion or malignancy; *CIN,* cervical intraepithelial neoplasia; *CIS,* carcinoma *in situ.*

with partially obscuring inflammation, blood, or air-drying artifact. The *less-than-optimal* category was criticized as providing a negative connotation, and TBS 1991 renamed this intermediate category *satisfactory but limited by*.[8]

TBS 2001 made extensive revisions to specimen adequacy reporting.[9] The intermediate *satisfactory-but-limited-by* category was viewed as confusing and an oxymoron—was the specimen satisfactory or not? This led to widespread variation in patient follow-up, with some clinicians performing early repeat sampling and others ignoring the designation. Research papers on the importance of the EC/TZ component showed conflicting results, and there was no compelling data to show that all such patients should undergo early repeat.[13–15] Most SILs and carcinomas develop near the transformation zone, and cross-sectional studies generally showed that the subset of women with an EC/TZ component had a higher proportion of abnormal cytology results.[16] Yet, longitudinal studies failed to show that women lacking an EC/TZ component were at an increased risk for high-grade SIL (HSIL) and squamous carcinoma.[14,15] Thus TBS 2001 designates specimens with adequate squamous cells but lacking EC/TZ as satisfactory. Another problem with the earlier Bethesda criterion requiring more than 10% of the slide surface to have adequate squamous cells was that it was nearly impossible to apply on both conventional smears and new LBPs.[17]

TBS 2001 collapsed the three earlier categories of evaluation into two: *satisfactory* and *unsatisfactory*.[9] Other information, such as EC/TZ sampling, was to be provided through the use of quality indicators. Such quality indicators lead to increased awareness of adequacy by healthcare providers and promoted improved sampling devices, specimen collection, and laboratory processing. With the increasing incidence of adenocarcinoma and adenocarcinoma *in situ*, the implications of EC/TZ sampling may change in the future; the use of quality indicators provides flexibility in responding to new research studies.

Satisfactory Specimens

A satisfactory cervical cytology specimen should be properly labeled, accompanied by pertinent clinical information, and should have adequate numbers of well-visualized and preserved squamous cells (Figure 4.1-1). TBS 2001 provides differing cellularity for conventional smears and LBPs, recognizing that a smaller number of cells is required for a diagnostic specimen in LBPs because they have more random sampling of cellular constituents.[11] A satisfactory LBP should have a minimum of 5000 squamous cells, and the number can be reproducibly evaluated by estimates of representative fields.[18] A satisfactory conventional smear should have a minimum of 8000 to 12,000 squamous cells. Reference images are provided in the Bethesda atlas and web site for estimation of smear cellularity, and laboratories are instructed not to count individual cells.[11,12] Conventional smears may still be difficult to evaluate for cellularity given the lack of random distribution, but early studies suggest that the reference images promote greater reproducibility than the previous

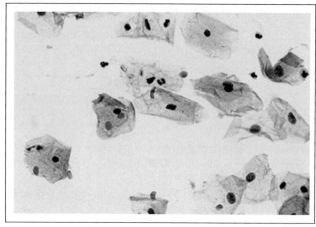

Figure 4.1-1 Superficial and intermediate squamous cells in satisfactory cervical smear. Note that the superficial cells have pink cytoplasm and a small nucleus about the size of a red cell. Intermediate squamous cells have a slightly larger nucleus and, in this stain, a slightly blue cytoplasm.

10% criterion.[19] The suggested minimum squamous cellularity criteria were based on preliminary data and could change if future studies suggest that different numbers are more appropriate.[11,20] Any specimen with abnormal cells is by definition "satisfactory for evaluation."

A statement about the presence or absence of an EC/TZ component is provided as a quality indicator immediately following the satisfactory designation. An adequate EC/TZ component is defined as a minimum of 10 well-preserved endocervical or squamous metaplastic cells, individual or in clusters.[11] Inclusion of a statement is unnecessary if the specimen shows HSIL or cancer. In situations that lead to atrophy, differentiating metaplastic specimens from parabasal cells can be impossible, and laboratories may comment that the present of an EC/TZ component cannot be reliably determined. Other quality indicator statements, such as partially obscuring inflammation, may also be added. Specimens with 50% to 75% of cells obscured are considered partially obscured but still qualify as satisfactory specimens because data have not shown that these factors are associated with false-negative reports.[21,22] Cervical LBPs are less likely to have obscuring or air-drying quality indicators. Some laboratories may designate an LBP with estimated 5000 to 20,000 as borderline cellularity.[11]

Criteria for specimen adequacy were developed for cervical cytology screening specimens and generally do not apply in other situations. Vaginal specimens and those performed in women following radiation and chemotherapy for gynecologic malignancies may have lower cellularity and still be considered satisfactory. The laboratory is instructed to consider patient history and risk factors in evaluation of such specimens.

Unsatisfactory Specimens

Laboratories should provide the reason for designating a cervical cytology specimen as unsatisfactory. Unsatisfactory specimens include those that are rejected by the laboratory for processing because they are received unlabeled, broken beyond repair, or contain an LBP that has leaked from the container. The majority of unsatisfactory specimens are completely processed and evaluated by the laboratory but have either inadequate squamous cellularity (as defined previously) or are largely (>75%) obscured by blood, inflammation, or other factors. The average unsatisfactory reporting rate is 0.5% to 1.5%.[23] Ransdell et al. reported a two-institution retrospective study prior to TBS 2001 and found that 0.3% of specimens were unsatisfactory.[24] Unsatisfactory specimens were more likely to be from high-risk or symptomatic patients, and significantly more had SIL or cancer on follow-up than those with satisfactory specimens. Many of these smears associated with abnormal outcome were obscured. Since TBS 2001, the most common reason for unsatisfactory specimens is insufficient squamous cellularity, especially when LBPs are used (Figure 4.1-2). The implications of scant cellularity for patient follow-up are not as well understood and may change with future research.[25]

Management According to Specimen Adequacy

The American Society for Colposcopy and Cervical Pathology (ASCCP) convened a task force that issued follow-up guidelines according to specimen adequacy designation (Figure 4.1-3).[26] *Generally, most women with specimens lacking an EC/TZ component and those with partially obscuring factors should be scheduled for an annual repeat cytology screen. Certain women with an abnormal cytology history, an abnormal examination, or inadequate previous screening may be considered for an early 6-month repeat. Pregnant women can be scheduled for a postpartum repeat specimen. Women with unsatisfactory specimens should be scheduled for repeat cytology in 2 to 4 months unless there are clinical indications for other types of evaluation or it is determined that the cytology can be repeated in 1 year.*

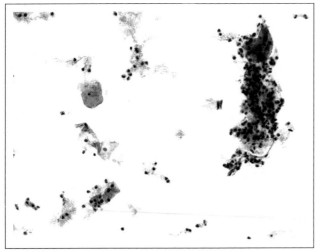

Figure 4.1-2 Unsatisfactory liquid-based preparation. A few squamous cells are present, but there are fewer than the 5000 recommended minimum. The abundant blood and inflammation shown may dilute liquid-based preparations and obscure squamous cells.

Women exhibiting repeatedly unsatisfactory obscured specimens and those with unexplained bleeding or cervical lesions should be considered for colposcopy.[26]

SPECIMEN CATEGORIZATION

General categorization of cervical cytology reports is an optional component that allows clinics to triage reports. In the earlier versions of TBS, there were three general categories: *within normal limits, benign cellular changes,* and *epithelial abnormalities.*[4,8] *Benign cellular changes* included microbial infections, reactive and reparative changes, and other benign processes. The *benign-cellular-changes* category was criticized because it was confusing: was the specimen negative or not? Furthermore, laboratory criteria for reporting this category varied tremendously, and patient follow-up strategies were not well defined.[27]

TBS 2001 combined the *within-normal-limits* and the *benign-cellular-changes* categories into the *negative-for-intraepithelial-lesion-or-malignancy (NILM)* category.[9] NILM is also used as a specific interpretation and more clearly denotes specimens as negative. Additional descriptive entries that were previously included in the *benign cellular changes* category are provided below the NILM interpretation.[11] These entries include organisms, atrophic changes, reactive cellular changes, changes associated with radiotherapy, and lymphocytic cervicitis, and they are discussed later.

Other Categories and Reporting of Endometrial Cells

TBS 2001 added a third category for processes that do not fit the NILM or the epithelial abnormality category. The most common use of this category is to report cytologically benign–appearing endometrial cells in a woman 40 years of age or older.[11] Laboratories are also advised to add a statement that the specimen is negative for SIL. In prior versions of TBS, endometrial cells were reported in postmenopausal women as a type of epithelial abnormality. However, laboratories were often not aware of a woman's menopausal status and other risk factors. Endometrial cells in women aged 40 and older may indicate increased risk for endometrial abnormalities, especially if the women are postmenopausal, but the cells are generally associated with benign endometrial processes, including irregular cycling and polyps.[28–30] Postmenopausal women with endometrial cells generally should be evaluated, and the use of hormonal therapy generally does not affect management. Women older than age 40 who are still having regular menstrual cycles are unlikely to have endometrial pathology, even if cells are present in the second half of the cycle and clinical correlation is suggested.[29] Endometrial cell reporting is not a sensitive indicator of endometrial pathology.[11]

Exfoliated endometrial cell clusters include both glandular and stromal cells, and they generally are three-dimensional with small nuclei.[11] Double contoured clusters of cells are common during the menstrual cycle. Endometrial cells

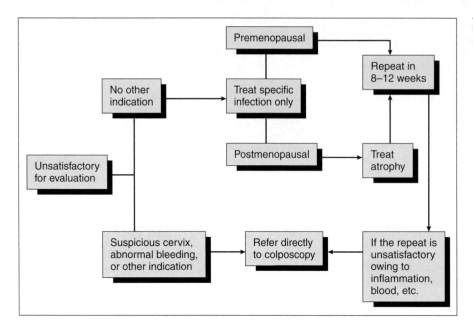

sampled directly from the lower uterine segment, isolated histiocytes, and stromal cells do not have the same significance as exfoliated endometrial cells and should not be reported.[29]

Organisms

Bethesda 2001 changed the category of *infections* to *organisms*, recognizing that some organisms reflect colonization instead of clinically significant infections. The presence of organisms is reported as a descriptor along either the NILM result or a specific epithelial abnormality. Reporting organisms is not the main focus of cytology screening, and cervical cytology is often less sensitive than cultures or other testing modalities.[31–33] Molecular probes have been developed for trichomonas, candida, and *Gardnerella vaginalis* but are not widely used because of cost. However, organism reporting by cytology may provide clinically relevant information for many women. Clinicians are encouraged to contact laboratories about their expectations for reporting organisms. The specific organisms included in the Bethesda 2001 menu and their main features are shown in the following figures:

Trichomonas vaginalis (Figure 4.1-4): Pear- or oval-shaped cyanophilic organism, 15 to 30 microns, vesicular pale nucleus, eosinophilic cytoplasmic granules often seen, may see flagella in LBP, may have associated Leptothrix bacteria. They may be confused with cytoplasmic fragments or macrophages if strict criteria are not used. Can confirm with wet mount, culture, or molecular probe.[34]

Fungal organisms morphologically consistent with *Candida* spp. (Figure 4.1-5): 3- to 7-micron budding years, pseudohyphae with variable staining, may see epithelial cells speared by pseudohyphae. Cytology is less sensitive than culture or molecular probe.[35]

Shift in flora suggestive of bacterial vaginosis (Figure 4.1-6): Bethesda 2001 changed the terminology from the

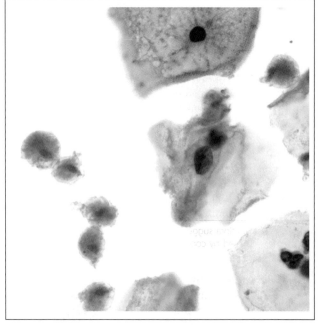

Figure 4.1-4 Trichomonas vaginalis organisms with pale nuclei adjacent to squamous cells.

previous descriptor *predominance of coccobacilli consistent with shift in vaginal flora* so that the current term is more reflective of the clinical diagnosis of bacterial vaginosis. Shows filmy background of small coccobacilli with individual squamous cells covered by a layer of bacteria, obscuring the cell membrane (clue cell).[11] Lactobacilli, the normal flora, are lacking. Cytology sensitivity is variable; the combination of vaginal pH, characteristic discharge, amine-odor whiff test, and wet-mount specimen analyzed for clue cells is often done in clinic settings.[31,33] The presence of 20% or more clue cells on cervical cytology correlates well with clinic testing.[36]

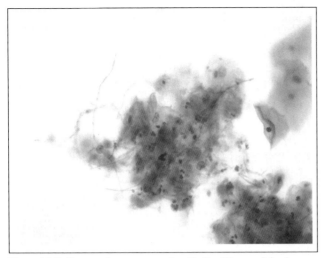

Figure 4.1-5 Clusters of squamous cells with *Candida* pseudohyphae spearing squamous cells.

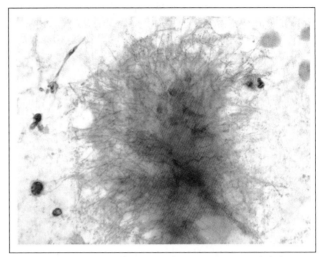

Figure 4.1-7 Actinomyces filamentous bacteria seen as tangled clumps in 37-year-old woman with an intrauterine device.

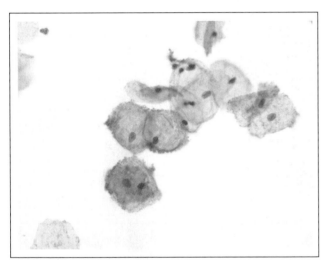

Figure 4.1-6 Shift in flora suggestive of bacterial vaginosis showing squamous cells covered by coccobacilli that obscure the cell borders.

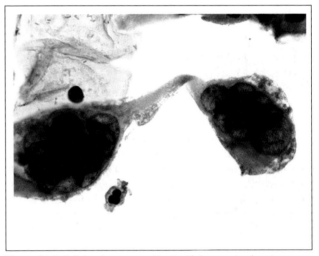

Figure 4.1-8 Cellular changes consistent with herpes simplex virus: multinucleated squamous cells with molded nuclei and ground glass appearance.

Bacteria morphologically consistent with *Actinomyces* spp. (Figure 4.1-7): Filamentous bacteria in tangled clumps seen as cotton ball clusters. Filaments have a radial pattern, an irregular woolly appearance, and are often swollen at the periphery.[11] Actinomyces is strongly associated with the presence of an intrauterine contraceptive device (IUD) or other foreign object and can lead to pelvic abscess formation.

Cellular changes consistent with herpes simplex virus (Figure 4.1-8): Intranuclear viral particles lead to a ground-glass appearance and enhanced nuclear envelope with margination of chromatin, dense eosinophilic intranuclear inclusions surrounded by halo are variably present, multinucleated epithelial cells with molded nuclei are frequent but not always present.[11] Viral changes need to be distinguished from reactive and neoplastic nuclear changes. Cytology is less sensitive than culture, and molecular probes (polymerase chain reaction [PCR]) may offer the highest sensitivity.[32,37]

REACTIVE CELLULAR CHANGES

Reactive and reparative changes refer to benign changes associated with inflammation, tissue injury, tissue repair, IUDs, radiation, and other nonspecific causes.[38] These descriptors are added after the NILM result, and reporting rates and policies may vary among laboratories.[27]

Reactive changes include nuclear enlargement, generally 1.5 to 2 times the normal size, and binucleation or multinucleation[11] (Figure 4.1-9). Chromatin is variable but usually pale with only minimal, if any, hyperchromasia. Nucleoli may be prominent. Cytoplasm may show vacuoles, perinuclear halos, and polychromasia. Repair shows similar features, but cells are present in orderly monolayer sheets with streaming polarity. Radiation causes exaggerated reparative changes with more bizarre cell shapes, more nuclear size variability, more frequent cytoplasmic vacuoles, and polychromasia.

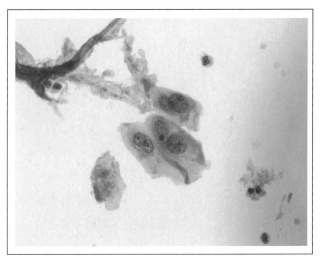

Figure 4.1-9 Reactive squamous cells have enlarged nuclei with visible chromocenters or nucleoli and may be binucleated or multinucleated.

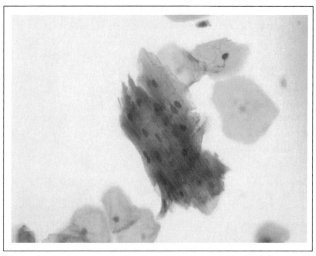

Figure 4.1-11 Parakeratosis showing clusters or individual miniature keratinized cells with small nuclei.

Atrophy with or without inflammation (atrophic vaginitis) has parabasal cells that may show nuclear enlargement but generally show a bland chromatin pattern (Figure 4.1-10). Degenerative changes may mimic parakeratosis.[11] The background is often granular with inflammation and blue blobs representing either mucin or degenerated cells. If an epithelial abnormality cannot be excluded, these changes are reported as atypical, and the patient can be managed by HPV triage testing or by repeat cytology.

Parakeratosis and hyperkeratosis represent miniature and anucleate squamous cells, respectively (Figure 4.1-11). *Such changes usually represent a benign or reactive finding but may be present on the surface of an epithelial abnormality.*[11] If the parakeratosis is described as atypical or pleomorphic, but no diagnostic epithelial changes are seen, the patient should be managed as if she had atypical squamous cells. Vulvar contamination of the specimen may introduce anucleate squamous cells, but such contaminating cells generally do

not produce thick plaques of squamous cells. Clinical correlation with exam findings and history is suggested.

Tubal metaplasia is a common normal finding and is usually identified by the presence of terminal bars and cilia (Figure 4.1-12). If the latter are not seen, such groups may be designated as atypical glandular cells because of cell crowding, pseudostratification, and nuclear changes. With IUDs, glandular cells with enlarged nuclei and prominent cytoplasmic vacuoles that compress the nucleus may be observed.[11] Nucleoli, degenerative changes, and calcific debris may be present, and these cellular changes may be difficult to

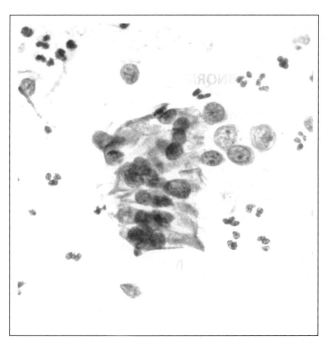

Figure 4.1-12 An example of tubal metaplasia showing organized clusters of glandular cells with terminal bars and cilia *(seen on right side of group)*. The groups may appear crowded or atypical because of pseudostratification of cells and slight nuclear hyperchromasia.

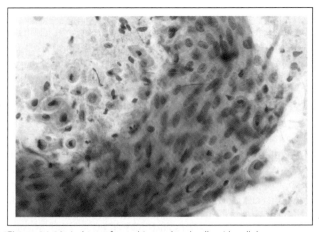

Figure 4.1-10 A sheet of atrophic parabasal cells with cellular degeneration and orange pyknotic cells. In atrophic vaginitis, the background usually contains granular debris.

distinguish from atypical glandular cells or HSIL. Removal of the IUD may be necessary if there is any question as to the nature of the changes.

A report of glandular cells following a hysterectomy consists of endocervical type cells or other types of benign-appearing glandular cells. These may be the result of glandular adenosis, prolapsed fallopian tube tissue, remaining cervical tissue, metaplasia, colonic fistula, or other etiologies.[11] Clinical correlation is suggested, especially if the patient has a history of adenocarcinoma. In previous versions of Bethesda, sometimes such cells were included in the atypical glandular cells category.

Reactive and reparative changes are among the least reproducible in Bethesda 2001,[39,40] and, according to federal regulations, any report with the terms *reactive* or *reparative* must be confirmed by a pathologist.[27] *Some cases with reactive changes may be overcalled as an epithelial abnormality by some observers (false-positive result), and, of more significance, some epithelial abnormalities may be misinterpreted as reactive (false-negative result).*[39] Laboratories also vary considerably in use of terms such as *inflammation* and *inflammatory changes*, and the presence of inflammation alone probably has little significance in terms of cancer risk. High-risk women with marked inflammation are more likely to have a specific infection, and the presence of sexually transmitted infections could indicate increased risk status for SIL.[41,42] One study showed that women with reactive cellular changes may be at slightly increased risk for an epithelial abnormality,[43] and another on benign cellular changes found little risk, especially in women with negative history.[38] There are no existing evidence-based consensus guidelines for evaluation of reactive/reparative results. *Clinical correlation is suggested, and colposcopy may be useful if there are repeated reactive/reparative results, marked obscuring inflammation, or unexplained symptoms.*[42]

EPITHELIAL ABNORMALITIES

Atypical Squamous Cells

The *atypical squamous cells (ASC)* category has been controversial since its inception because it represents the largest number of epithelial abnormalities in most laboratories.[23] Interpretation of atypical cellular changes is also rather subjective, with considerable interobserver variability.[44,45] The large expense involved in clinical management led to a large National Cancer Institute randomized multicenter trial, the results of which have shaped current ASC management guidelines.[46,47] Some participants at Bethesda 2001 favored elimination of the ASC category, but it was recognized that cervical cytology would have lower sensitivity if many ASC cases were reclassified as negative, and this would not be acceptable to the public.[9,48] *While the relative risk for a single ASC case is low (5-20% will have a high-grade lesion, and 0.1% will have cancer), the high number of ASC cases means that a considerable number of high-grade lesions will originate from an ASC cytology report.*[9,47,49]

Earlier versions of the Bethesda System defined ASC as an equivocal category for cellular changes "that are more marked than those attributable to reactive changes but that quantitatively or qualitatively fall short of a definitive diagnosis of SIL."[9] Laboratories also qualified many such cases to indicate whether a reactive or premalignant process was favored. Bethesda 2001 attempted to narrow the definitions and criteria for ASC and eliminated the *ASC, favor reactive,* subcategory.[9,11] Only cases in which SIL is suspected should be classified as ASC, while other likely reactive cases should be downgraded to negative as appropriate. *The two subcategories of ASC are of undetermined significance (ASC-US) and cannot exclude HSIL (ASC-H). The median reporting rates for ASC-US and ASC-H are 3.9% and 0.2%, respectively.*[23] However, these reporting rates will vary considerably according to patient population and risk factors. The ASC: SIL ratio is less variable, and the median ratio is 1.4, with 90% of laboratories reporting ratios of 2.9 or less.[23]

ASC-US accounts for >90% of ASC cases, and the cytologic features are suggestive of low-grade SIL (LSIL) but are either qualitatively or quantitatively insufficient. Cellular changes include nuclear enlargement 2.5 to 3 times normal, slightly increased nuclear to cytoplasmic ratio, and only mild nuclear hyperchromasia and other nuclear abnormalities[11] (Figure 4.1-13). Benign nuclear enlargement may occur in the menopausal and perimenopausal age group and may be difficult to distinguish from ASC-US.[50] Appropriate management strategies for ASC-US include HPV DNA triage (preferred for liquid cytology specimens), two repeat cytology examinations, or colposcopic examination[47] (see Chapter 11).

ASC-H specimens account for around 5% of ASC cases, and they have cytologic features suggestive of HSIL but are not definitive. Cells are generally the size of metaplastic cells and may occur singly or in small groups (Figure 4.1-14). There is

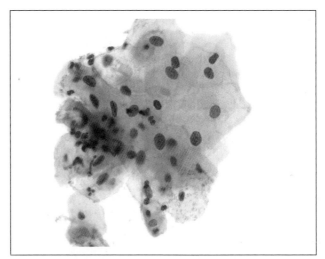

Figure 4.1-13 Atypical squamous cells of undetermined significance with enlarged, slightly hyperchromatic nuclei in a liquid-based preparation from a 47-year-old woman. Initial colposcopy revealed cervical intraepithelial neoplasia (CIN) 1, but later biopsies showed CIN 2.

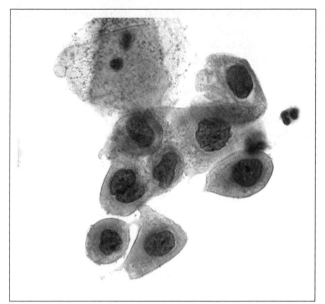

Figure 4.1-14 Liquid-based preparation showing atypical squamous cells; cannot exclude high-grade squamous intraepithelial lesion. The metaplastic squamous cells have enlarged irregular nuclei with increased nuclear:cytoplasmic ratio. These changes were insufficient both quantitatively and qualitatively to report as high-grade squamous intraepithelial lesion (HSIL), but follow-up biopsies showed a high-grade cervical intraepithelial neoplasia (CIN).

nuclear enlargement 1.5 to 2.5 times normal and mild nuclear changes. Some ASC-H cases were described as atypical metaplasia in the past. *The recommended management is colposcopy (see Chapter 11), as at least 35% of these women will have high-grade lesions on follow-up in most studies.*[47,51–54] A much higher percentage will have positive HPV test results (67–86%) than in the ASC-US subcategory, making HPV DNA triage unhelpful in these women.[53,54]

Squamous Intraepithelial Lesions and Carcinoma

Bethesda 2001 discussed various options for the SIL category, from merging all levels of SIL to subdividing into three categories.[9] The two-tiered separation of SILs into low- and high-grade categories has been controversial since its inception in 1988. Studies have shown that CIN 2 has a more benign natural history than CIN 3, and CIN 2 management may have greater similarity to CIN 1 than to CIN 3 management in some countries. The two-tiered structure therefore provides less information to clinicians. However, HSIL lesions cannot be reproducibly divided into CIN 2 and CIN 3 by different pathologists and laboratories. Consequently no significant change was made in SIL terminology. Nevertheless, some laboratories may choose to qualify some HSIL cases as either CIN 2 or CIN 3.[55] This may facilitate cytologic–histologic correlation exercises for individual patients. One example where this may be helpful is in a teenage girl who might be followed conservatively with HSIL/CIN 2 on cytology and CIN 1 on biopsy. Some cases of HSIL may be qualified *with features suspicious for invasion* when there are

incomplete cytologic criteria for invasive squamous carcinoma.[11] There was no consensus on histopathology terminology as this was felt to be outside the purview of the Bethesda 2001 cytology workshop.

LSIL is characterized by nuclear enlargement more than 3 times normal, variable hyperchromasia and other nuclear changes, and koilocytotic change consisting of perinuclear cavitation and peripheral dense rim of cytoplasm (Figure 4.1-15). Not all LSIL cells will show all features, but cells with koilocytosis must show at least some nuclear abnormalities to qualify as LSIL.[11] Cell size is usually large with abundant cytoplasm so that nuclear: cytoplasmic ratio is only slightly increased. The median laboratory reporting rate for LSIL was 2.1% in 2003.[23]

HSIL cells are generally smaller and less mature, and cells may occur singly or in aggregates. Nuclear:cytoplasmic ratio is higher than in LSIL, and nuclear hyperchromasia and irregular nuclear membranes are observed (Figure 4.1-16). Cytoplasm is often scant but may vary from lacy to dense or keratinized. Squamous carcinoma may be difficult to separate from HSIL on cytology specimens, but it shows in addition one or more of the following characteristics: tumor diathesis in background, pleomorphic cells, irregular chromatin pattern with clearing, and prominent nucleoli. The median HSIL and cancer reporting rate is about 0.5%.[23]

A minority of cases will be difficult to subclassify as either LSIL or HSIL, and some may be reported as SIL of indeterminate grade.[11] Such cases often have few cells with indeterminate features, poorly preserved cells, or predominantly LSIL with a few cases worrisome for HSIL.[11,56] Many of these cases may be CIN 2 or difficult to classify on biopsy.[56] LSIL is certainly more reproducible than ASC, with 68% of LSIL cases confirmed by the ALTS pathology quality control group, as compared with 43% of ASC-US cases.[45] However, *even when SIL slides are referenced by expert pathologists and have correlating biopsies, there is still considerable interobserver variation. About 10% to 15% of individual*

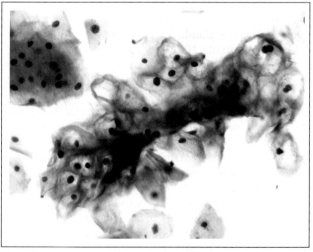

Figure 4.1-15 Liquid-based preparation showing low-grade squamous intraepithelial lesion. Several koilocytes with slightly enlarged hyperchromatic nuclei are observed with distinct perinuclear haloes. A few binucleate cells are present in upper right.

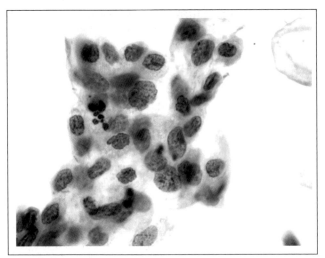

Figure 4.1-16 Liquid-based preparation showing high-grade squamous intraepithelial lesion consistent with cervical intraepithelial neoplasia (CIN) 3. The dysplastic cell cluster shows overlapping cells with high nuclear: cytoplasmic ratio and irregular nuclei with coarse chromatin.

responses were discrepant between LSIL and HSIL in the College of American Pathologists Interlaboratory Comparison program,[57] and about 20% of all SIL slides never achieve field validation required for proficiency testing.[58,59]

Glandular Abnormalities

Cervical cytology is mainly a screening test for squamous lesions and should not be considered reliable for detection of adenocarcinomas, especially those of endometrial origin. Adenocarcinoma *in situ* of the cervix is increasing in incidence, and cytology screening appears to be less effective in decreasing cervical adenocarcinoma mortality than for squamous carcinoma and its precursors.[60] This is probably related to both sampling issues and cytologic presentation. Many adenocarcinomas are diagnosed only after the patient is evaluated for a coexistent squamous lesion.

Terminology for glandular abnormalities was extensively modified by Bethesda 2001. The category *atypical glandular cells of undetermined significance* was changed to *atypical glandular cells (AGC)* to avoid confusion with ASC-US.[9] The subcategory *atypical glandular cells, favor reactive* was eliminated as it provided mixed messages, and many patients received insufficient follow-up. *The AGC category represents a high-risk group, as about 10% to 40% of women will have significant lesions or carcinoma on follow-up studies.*[47,61,62] Many of these lesions turn out to be HSIL or squamous carcinoma and reflect the difficulty in classifying crowded cell clusters. Fortunately, the median reporting rate of AGC is much lower than for ASC-US, about 0.2 %.[23] Because AGC represents a high-risk category, histologic follow-up is recommended for all women, and specific management depends on the age of the woman and the glandular cell type.[47]

Laboratories are encouraged to specify AGC cell type as to endometrial versus endocervical origin, but it is recognized that this may not always be possible.[63] Interobserver reproducibility for the general AGC category is poor.[64] A separate category of *adenocarcinoma in situ (AIS)* was introduced for those cases showing classic criteria. Such cases have a much higher positive-predictive value for AIS than other AGC cases,[65] but it is recognized that many histologically proven AIS cases will not be classified reproducibly as such on cervical cytology.[66] Participants at Bethesda 2001 debated whether earlier preneoplastic processes could be recognized and classified on cytology, but there was no convincing evidence for endocervical dysplasia on histology. Atypical glandular/endocervical cells may be reported when there is a higher level of concern but not all AIS criteria are met. There is no additional subcategorization for atypical endometrial cells.

Atypical endocervical cells are characterized by crowded strips and sheets of cells with enlarged hyperchromatic nuclei as well as an increased nuclear:cytoplasmic ratio. (Figure 4.1-17) Some cells may have small nucleoli. AIS shows more well-developed glandular architecture and abnormal cellular features, including crowded hyperchromatic columnar cells, rosettes, and feathering; mitoses and apoptotic bodies are commonly observed.[11] Atypical glandular cells, favor neoplastic, show intermediate atypia with incomplete features of AIS. Atypical endometrial cells occur in small clusters and show enlarged nuclei compared with benign endometrial cells; small nucleoli may be observed.

Invasive adenocarcinomas show considerable overlap with atypical glandular cells but tend to show features of invasion, including tumor diathesis, macronucleoli, and irregular chromatin clearing (Figure 4.1-18). Well-differentiated adenocarcinomas of both the endometrium and endocervix may be classified as AGC and even as *other, endometrial cells.*

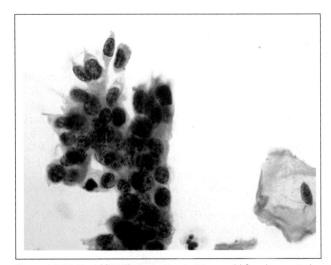

Figure 4.1-17 Liquid-based preparation in 18-year-old female reported as atypical endocervical cells. Note crowded glandular cluster with hyperchromatic nuclei and feathering appearance at edge *(upper left)*. Follow-up biopsies revealed adenocarcinoma *in situ* (AIS) and cervical intraepithelial neoplasia (CIN) 2.

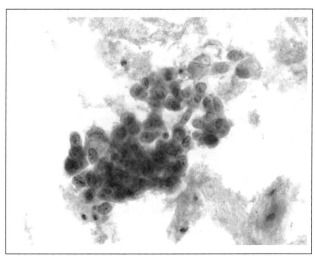

Figure 4.1-18 Recurrent invasive endometrial adenocarcinoma in liquid vaginal cytology of 76-year-old woman. Note necrotic diathesis in background.

ACKNOWLEDGMENTS

Certain sections of the chapter, including figures from the first edition, were reused with permission. A special thank you to Joseph Novak, M.D., Pathologist, Columbia–St. Mary's Hospital, Milwaukee, WI for his help in obtaining some of the images used in this chapter.

REFERENCES

1. Papanicolaou GN, Traut HF. The diagnostic value of vaginal smears in carcinoma of the uterus. Am J Obstet Gynecol 1941; 42:193–205.
2. Ayre JE. Selective cytology smear for diagnosis of cancer. Am J Obstet Gynecol 1947;53:609–617.
3. Koss LG. Cervical (Pap) smear: New directions. Cancer 1993; 71:1406–1412.
4. National Cancer Institute Workshop. The 1988 Bethesda System for reporting cervical/vaginal cytologic diagnoses. JAMA 1989;262:931–934.
5. Reagan JW, Seidemann IL, Saracusa Y. The cellular morphology of carcinoma in situ and dysplasia or atypical hyperplasia of the uterine cervix. Cancer 1953;6:224–234.
6. Richart RM. Natural history of cervical intraepithelial neoplasia. Clin Obstet Gynecol 1967;10:748–784.
7. Davey DD, Woodhouse S, Styer P, et al. Atypical epithelial cells and specimen adequacy: Current laboratory practices of participants in the College of American Pathologists Interlaboratory Comparison Program in Cervicovaginal Cytology. Arch Pathol Lab Med 2000;124:203–211.
8. The Bethesda System for reporting cervical/vaginal cytologic diagnoses. Report of the 1991 Bethesda Workshop. JAMA 1992;267:1892.
9. Solomon D, Davey DD, Kurman R, et al. The 2001 Bethesda System: Terminology for reporting results of cervical cytology. JAMA 2002;287:2114–9.
10. Davey DD. Cervical cytology classification and the Bethesda System (review). Cancer J 2003;9:327–334.
11. Solomon D, Nayar R (eds). The Bethesda System for Reporting Cervical Cytology, ed 2. New York: Springer Verlag, 2004. p 1–156.
12. www.cytopathology.org/NIH/ (accessed May 12, 2006).
13. Baer A, Kiviat NB, Kulasingam S, et al. Liquid-based Papanicolaou smears without a transformation zone component: Should clinicians worry? Obstet Gynecol 2002;99:1053–1059.
14. Bos AB, van Ballegooijen M, van den Akker-van Marle ME, et al. Endocervical status is not predictive of the incidence of cervical cancer in the years after negative smears. Am J Clin Pathol 2001;115:851–855.
15. Mitchell HS. Longitudinal analysis of histologic high-grade disease after negative cervical cytology according to endocervical status. Cancer (Cancer Cytopathol) 2001;93:237–240.
16. Martin-Hirsch P, Lilford R, Jarvis G, Kitchener HC. Efficacy of cervical smear collection devices: A systematic review and meta-analysis. Lancet 1999;354:1763–1770.
17. Renshaw AA, Friedman MM, Rahemtulla A, et al. Accuracy and reproducibility of estimating the adequacy of the squamous component of cervicovaginal smears. Am J Clin Pathol 1999;111:38–42.
18. Haroon S, Samayoa L, Witzke D, Davey DD. Reproducibility of cervicovaginal ThinPrep cellularity assessment. Diagn Cytopathol 2002;26:19–21.
19. Sheffield MF, Simsir A, Talley L, et al. Interobserver variability in assessing adequacy of the squamous component in conventional cervicovaginal smears. Am J Clin Pathol 2003;119:367–373.
20. Studeman KD, Ioffe OB, Puszkiewicz J, et al. Effect of cellularity on the sensitivity of detecting squamous lesions in liquid-based cervical cytology. Acta Cytol 2003;47:605–610.
21. Mitchell H, Medley G. Differences between Papanicolaou smears with correct and incorrect diagnoses. Cytopathology 1995;6:368–375.
22. O'Sullivan JP, A'Hern RP, Chapman PA, et al. A case-control study of true-positive versus false-negative cervical smears in women with cervical intraepithelial neoplasia (CIN) III. Cytopathology 1998;9:155–161.
23. Davey DD, Neal MH, Wilbur DC, et al. Bethesda 2001 implementation and reporting rates: 2003 practices of participants in the College of American Pathologists Interlaboratory Comparison Program in Cervicovaginal Cytology. Arch Pathol Lab Med 2004;128;1224–9.
24. Ransdell JS, Davey DD, Zaleski S. Clinicopathologic correlation of the unsatisfactory Papanicolaou smear. Cancer (Cancer Cytopathol) 1997;81:139–143.
25. Adams AL, Gidley J, Roberson J, et al. Clinical significance of unsatisfactory conventional Pap smears owing to inadequate squamous cellularity defined by the Bethesda 2001 criterion. Am J Clin Pathol 2005;123:738–43.
26. Davey DD, Austin RM, Birdsong G, et al. ASCCP patient management guidelines: Pap test specimen adequacy and quality indicators. J Low Genit Tract Dis 2002;6:195–199.
27. Moriarty AT, Young NA. The four R's: Reactive/repair, reporting, and regulations. Diagn Cytopathol 2003;29:1–3.
28. Browne TJ, Genest DR, Cibas ES. The clinical significance of benign-appearing endometrial cells on a Papanicolaou test in women 40 years or older. Am J Clin Pathol 2005;124:834–7.
29. Greenspan DL, Cardillo M, Davey DD, et al. Endometrial cells and cervical cytology: Review of cytological features and clinical assessment. J Low Genit Tract Dis 2006;10:111–122.
30. Simsir A, Carter W, Elgert P, Cangiarella J. Reporting endometrial cells in women 40 years and older: Assessing the clinical usefulness of Bethesda 2001. Am J Clin Pathol 2005;123:571–5.

31. Owen MK, Clenney TL. Management of vaginitis. Am Fam Physician 2004;70:2125–32.

32. Sulak PJ. Sexually transmitted diseases. Sem Rep Med 2003;21:399–413.

33. Tokyol C, Aktepe OC, Cevrioğlu AS, Altindiş M, Dilek FH. Bacterial vaginosis: Comparison of Pap smear and microbiological test results. Mod Pathol 2004;17:857–60.

34. Caliendo AM, Jordan JA, Green AM, et al. Real-time PCR improves detection of Trichomonas vaginalis infection compared with culture using self-collected vaginal swabs. Infect Dis Obstet Gynecol 2005;13:145–150.

35. Trama JP, Mordechai E, Adelson ME. Detection and identification of Candida species associated with Candida vaginitis by real-time PCR and pyrosequencing. Mol Cell Probes 2005;19:145–152.

36. Discacciati MG, Simoes JA, Amaral RG, et al. Presence of 20% of more clue cells: An accurate criterion for the diagnosis of bacterial vaginosis in Papanicolaou cervical smears. Diagn Cytopathol 2006;34:272–276.

37. Strick LB, Wald A. Diagnostics for herpes simplex virus: Is PCR the new gold standard? Mol Diagn Ther 2006;10:17–28.

38. Malik SN, Wilkinson EJ, Drew PA, Hardt NS. Benign cellular changes in Pap smears: Causes and significance. Acta Cytol 2001;45:5–8.

39. Colgan TJ, Woodhouse SL, Styer PE, et al. Reparative changes and the false positive/false negative Pap smear: A study from the College of American Pathologists Interlaboratory Comparison in Cervicovaginal Cytology. Arch Path Lab Med 2001;125:134–140.

40. Renshaw AA, Davey DD, Birdsong GG, et al. Precision in gynecologic cytologic interpretation: A study from the College of American Pathologists Interlaboratory Comparison Program in Cervicovaginal Cytology. Arch Pathol Lab Med 2003;127:1413–20.

41. Eckert LO, Koutsky LA, Kiviat NB, et al. The inflammatory Papanicolaou smear: What does it mean? Obstet Gynecol 1995;86:360–6.

42. Seçkin NC, Turhan NÖ, Özmen S, et al. Routine colposcopic evaluation of patients with persistent inflammatory cellular changes on Pap smear. Int J Gynecol Obstet 1997;59:25–9.

43. Barr Soofer S, Sidawy MK. Reactive cellular changes: Is there an increased risk for squamous intraepithelial lesions. Cancer (Cancer Cytopathol) 1997;81:144–7.

44. Davey DD. Cytopathology update on atypical squamous cells. J Low Genit Tract Dis 2005;9:124–9.

45. Stoler MH, Schiffman M, for the Atypical Squamous Cells of Undetermined Significance-Low-Grade Squamous Intraepithelial Lesion Triage Study (ALTS) group. Interobserver reproducibility of cervical cytologic and histologic interpretations: Realistic estimates from the ASCUS-LSIL triage study. JAMA 2001;285:1500–5.

46. Solomon D, Schiffman M, Tarone R, for the ALTS Group. Comparison of three management strategies for patients with atypical squamous cells of undetermined significance: Baseline results from a randomized trial. J Natl Cancer Inst 2001; 93:293–9.

47. Wright TC, Cox JT, Massad LS, et al. 2001 Consensus guidelines for the management of women with cervical cytological abnormalities. JAMA 2002;287:2120–9.

48. Pitman MB, Cibas ES, Powers CN, et al. Reducing or eliminating use of the category of atypical squamous cells of undetermined significance decreases the diagnostic accuracy of the Papanicoloau smear. Cancer (Cancer Cytopathol) 2002; 96:128–34.

49. Kinney WK, Manos MM, Hurley LB, Ransley JE. Where's the high-grade cervical neoplasia? The importance of minimally abnormal Papanicolaou diagnoses. Obstet Gynecol 1998; 91:973–6.

50. Cibas ES, Browne TJ, Bassichis MH, Lee KR. Enlarged squamous cell nuclei in cervical cytologic specimens from perimenopausal women ("PM cells"): A cause of ASC overdiagnosis. Am J Clin Pathol 2005;124:58–61.

51. Alli PM, Ali SZ. Atypical squamous cells of undetermined significance—rule out high-grade squamous intraepithelial lesion: Cytopathology characteristics and clinical correlates. Diagn Cytopathol 2003;28:308–12.

52. Louro AP, Roberson J, Eltoum I, Chhieng DC. Atypical squamous cells, cannot exclude high-grade squamous intraepithelial lesion: A follow-up study of conventional and liquid-based preparations in a high-risk population. Am J Clin Pathol 2003;120:392–7.

53. Sherman ME, Solomon D, Schiffman M, for the ALTS group. A comparison of equivocal LSIL and equivocal HSIL cervical cytology in the ASCUS LSIL Triage Study. Am J Clin Pathol 2001;116:386–94.

54. Srodon M, Parry Dilworth H, Ronnett BM. Atypical squamous cells, cannot exclude high-grade squamous intraepithelial lesion: Diagnostic performance, human papillomavirus testing, and follow-up results. Cancer (Cancer Cytopathol) 2006;108:32–8.

55. Howell LP, Zhou H, Wu W, Davis R. Significance of subclassifying high-grade squamous intraepithelial lesions into moderate dysplasia/CIN II versus severe dysplasia/CIN III/CIS in the Bethesda System terminology. Diagn Cytopathol 2004;30:362–6.

56. Adams KC, Absher KJ, Brill YM, et al. Reproducibility of subclassification of squamous intraepithelial lesions: Conventional versus ThinPrep Paps. J Low Genit Tract Dis 2003;7:203–8.

57. Woodhouse SL, Stastny JF, Styer PE, et al. Interobserver variability in subclassification of squamous intraepithelial lesions: Results of the College of American Pathologists Interlaboratory Comparison Program in Cervicovaginal Cytology. Arch Pathol Lab Med 1999;123:1079–84.

58. Renshaw AA, Wang E, Mody DR, et al. Measuring the significance of field validation in the College of American Pathologists Interlaboratory Comparison Program in Cervicovaginal Cytology: How good are the experts? Arch Pathol Lab Med 2005;129:609–13.

59. Renshaw AA, Mody DR, Styer P, et al. Papanicolaou tests with mixed high-grade and low-grade squamous intraepithelial lesion features: Distinct performance in the College of American Pathologists Interlaboratory Comparison Program in Cervicovaginal Cytopathology. Arch Pathol Lab Med 2006; 130:456–9.

60. Sherman ME, Wang SS, Cerreon J, Devesa SS. Mortality trends for cervical squamous and adenocarcinoma in the United States: Relation to incidence and survival. Cancer 2005;103:1258–64.

61. Chhieng DC, Gallaspy S, Yang H, et al. Women with atypical glandular cells: A long-term follow-up study in a high-risk population. Am J Clin Pathol 2004;122:575–9.

62. Ronnett BM, Manos MM, Ransley JE, et al. Atypical glandular cells of undetermined significance (AGUS): Cytopathologic features, histopathologic results, and human papillomavirus DNA detection. Hum Pathol 1999;30:816–25.

63. Krane JF, Lee KR, Sun D, et al. Atypical glandular cells of undetermined significance: Outcome predictions based on human papillomavirus testing. Am J Clin Pathol 2004;121:87–92.

64. Lee KR, Darragh TM, Joste NE, et al. Atypical glandular cells of undetermined significance (AGUS): Interobserver reproducibility in cervical smears and corresponding thin-layer preparations. Am J Clin Pathol 2002;117:96–102.

65. Roberts JM, Thurloe JK, Biro C, et al. Follow-up of cytologic predictions of endocervical glandular abnormalities: Histologic outcomes in 123 cases. J Low Genit Tract Dis 2005;9:71–7.

66. Renshaw AA, Mody DR, Lozano RL, et al. Detection of adenocarcinoma in situ of the cervix in Papanicolaou tests: Comparison of diagnostic accuracy with other high-grade lesions. Arch Pathol Lab Med 2004;128:153–7.

4.2: Conventional Cytology

Peter A. Drew • Edward J. Wilkinson

KEY POINTS

▪ The dramatic reduction of the incidence and mortality rates of cervical cancer occurred during the era of conventional Pap test screening.

▪ The conventional Pap test has excellent specificity and adequate but less-than-optimal sensitivity.

▪ In less than 10 years since its introduction to clinical use in 1996, liquid-based cervical cytology has captured over 85% of the U.S. cervical cancer screening market.

▪ Use of the conventional Pap test does not necessarily preclude reflex human papillomavirus (HPV) testing. An additional cervical sample can be obtained for reflex testing concurrent with the Pap test collection.

▪ Food and Drug Administration (FDA)–approved automated screening of conventional Pap tests is available.

▪ Effort should be made to schedule women for Pap tests between menstrual periods. Women should avoid use of intravaginal medications, tampons, and douches for 48 hours prior to obtaining the Pap test. Women should also abstain from sexual intercourse for 48 hours prior to cervical sampling.

▪ For conventional cytology, the combined use of the Ayre spatula with the endocervical brush, the cervical broom, or other sampling methods that sample the transformation zone (the immediately adjacent epithelium and endocervix), are likely to be satisfactory for interpretation.

▪ Inadequate sampling and sample transfer are the major causes of conventional Pap test false-negative results, accounting for up to two thirds of false-negative cases. The remaining one third of cases is due to screening and/or interpretive errors.

THE HISTORY OF THE PAP TEST

The Conventional Pap Test

In 1928 Dr. George N. Papanicolaou, a PhD biologist and anatomist working in Cornell Medical College in the laboratory of Dr. Charles Stockard, reported the observation of dysplastic/malignant cells in women with cervical carcinoma by sampling vaginal smears. This observation evolved from his study of endocrine function by evaluation of the cytologic changes in vaginal smears. The detection of neoplastic cells in women with cervical carcinoma was presented at the Third Race Betterment Conference in Battle Creek, Michigan in January 1928.[1] His work was historically concurrent with the work of Aurel Babes, a physician and gynecologist working in the Romanian Cancer Institute. Dr. Babes published his pioneering work, *Identifying Cancer in the Cervix Through Scrapings*, in the Presse Medicale, a French medical journal, in April, 1928.[2] He had presented this work in early 1927 to the Romanian Society of Gynecology.[3] Although Babes's publication preceded Papanicolaou's, it is not often cited, perhaps because of his lack of subsequent publications in this area.

Subsequently, Papanicolaou, working with Dr. Herbert Traut, a gynecologist, identified cells of both invasive cervical cancer and preinvasive cervical neoplastic lesions. This finding led to the concept that cervical cancer may be preceded by a latent, preinvasive lesion. Furthermore, the preinvasive lesion could be detected by cervical cytology and treated at a curable stage. Thus the groundwork was laid for the application of cervical cytology as a possible screening test for cervical cancer.[4]

This test, developed by Drs. Papanicolaou and Traut, is now known as the conventional Pap smear or Pap test. Only a few refinements to the conventional Pap test have occurred over the years. In 1947 Dr. J. Ernest Ayre introduced a contoured cervical spatula to improve cellular collection from the cervical transformation zone.[5] Later, the endocervical brush was added to improve detection of endocervical lesions.

Cervical cancer screening using the conventional Pap test began in the 1940s.[6] Although it was never evaluated in a controlled, prospective study, today few people question its efficacy as a screening test for cervical cancer. *Since the initiation of mass screening programs in the United States in the 1970s, there has been a 50% decrease in the incidence of cervical cancer and a 70% decrease in deaths due to cervical cancer.* Before the introduction of screening, cervical cancer was a leading cause of cancer-related death in women. Today, in the United States, cervical cancer does not even rank in the top 10 by site.[7] *In all populations where Pap test screening was established, the mortality rate for cervical cancer dropped precipitously.* Relative high- and low-risk areas developed based on access to Pap test screening programs.[8] For the individual woman, not having Pap test screening became a highly significant independent risk factor for developing cervical cancer.[9] In short, the Pap test has been the most cost-effective cancer reduction program ever devised.

The era between the 1970s and the mid-1990s might be considered the "golden age" of conventional cytology. During this period the conventional Pap test was the preeminent and uncontested method of choice for cervical cancer screening. It was during this era, however, that some very real problems with the Pap test were recognized. Some high-volume, low-cost laboratories were poorly regulated and encouraged excessive productivity at the expense of accuracy. As a result, these laboratories had unacceptably high false-negative rates, leading to cervical cancer screening failures.[10] Government intervention followed and culminated in an amendment to the Clinical Laboratories Improvement Act (CLIA) in 1988. *CLIA 1988 established cytotechnologist workload screening limits and instituted performance standards for laboratories and laboratory professionals. CLIA 1988 also mandated a 10% rescreening of Pap tests initially screened as normal, and cytotechnologists were required to undergo remediation training if they were found to have clinically significant underdiagnoses.*[11]

Liquid-Based Cervical Cytology

Recognition of the problems associated with the Pap test led to attempts to develop new technology, including automated screeners, in order to reduce the need for labor-intensive manual screening. Liquid-based cervical cytology preparations were developed to provide a better platform for automated screeners. As an added benefit, studies showed that some liquid-based cytology systems had superior sensitivity for the detection of squamous intraepithelial lesions (SIL) compared with the conventional Pap test.[12–14]

Liquid-based cervical cytology was first introduced in 1996 as an FDA-approved alternative to conventional Pap tests (ThinPrep). SurePath and MonoPrep liquid-based cervical cytology systems subsequently obtained FDA approval in 1999 and 2006, respectively. Claimed advantages of liquid-based cervical cytology systems varied by manufacturer. All liquid-based systems claim to have more superior specimen quality than conventional cytology, and some liquid-based systems claim to have improved test sensitivity.[12–14] Better suitability for automated screening and the ability to do ancillary molecular human papillomavirus (HPV) testing made liquid-based cervical cytology testing attractive to both laboratories and clinicians. Despite added cost, liquid-based cervical cytology was quickly embraced by the U.S. medical community. *In less than 10 years since its introduction, liquid-based cytology has captured over 85% of the U.S. market.* The United Kingdom has recently mandated that liquid-based testing be used for cervical cancer screening. The switch to liquid-based testing will be phased in over a 5-year period.[15] For a more detailed discussion of liquid-based cytology, see Chapter 4.3.

Human Papillomavirus Testing

Another notable development in cervical cancer screening was the introduction of high-risk HPV deoxyribonucleic acid (DNA) molecular testing in the management of patients with cervical epithelial abnormalities. Principally used as reflex testing for the management of women with a cytology interpretation of atypical squamous cells of undetermined significance (ASC-US), high-risk HPV DNA testing can also replace or supplement cytology for follow-up testing in certain circumstances. *The major advantage of high-risk HPV DNA testing is its high sensitivity for detecting squamous cervical carcinomas and its precursors.*[16] Its use in conjunction with cervical cytology is outlined in the 2001 and 2006 Consensus Guidelines for the Management of Women with Cervical Cytological Abnormalities.[17] The ThinPrep liquid-based cervical cytology system has FDA approval for adjunctive HPV testing. In the case of an ASC-US interpretation, the remaining sample can be used for high-risk HPV testing. It is important to note, however, that the use of the conventional Pap test does not preclude reflex HPV testing. The clinician may simply elect to concurrently collect an additional cervical sample for reflex HPV testing (see Digene.com [*www.digene.com/healthcare healthcare_hpvtest_01.html*]). For a more detailed discussion of HPV DNA testing, see Chapter 5.1.

Automated Screening

As previously noted, liquid-based cytology was originally developed as a platform to facilitate automated screening. Currently, there are two FDA-approved automated cervical cytology screening systems in use in the United States: Cytyc Corporation's ThinPrep Imaging System (see Chapter 4.3 for discussion of Cytyc's imaging system) and TriPath Imaging's FocalPoint Primary Screening System. The latter system can be used in the initial screening of conventional Pap tests as well as TriPath Imaging's liquid-based SurePath slides. The device can detect cellular abnormalities and, through the use of algorithms, assigns each slide a score. The score ranks slides according to the probability of an abnormality. FocalPoint can identify up to 25% of slides that do not need further review. The remaining 75% of slides are screened manually. FocalPoint also identifies 15% of the manually screened slides to undergo a second manual review based on a score indicating that they have the highest probability of being abnormal. This 15% can be substituted for the federally mandated requirement of a 10% rescreening of negative slides.[18]

FocalPoint is not approved for the screening of slides from "high-risk" women. In addition, performance standards have not been established for endometrial cells in postmenopausal women, reactive changes associated with radiation and atrophy, and some rare malignant tumors.[18] Studies regarding the accuracy of FocalPoint vary. The studies show that FocalPoint is equivalent or superior in accuracy to standard manual cervical cytology screening practice.[19,20]

Despite the success of the Pap test and the subsequent advances in cervical cancer screening, cervical cancer has not been eliminated in the United States. In 2005 an estimated 10,370 women were diagnosed with cervical cancer, and approximately 3710 women died of cervical cancer.[21] Approximately 60% of women diagnosed with cervical cancer in the United States either never had a Pap test or did not have a Pap test in the past 5 years.[22] Worldwide, cervical cancer is the second most common cancer in women. Cervical cancer is the most common cancer in women in many developing countries that lack screening programs.[23] Countries with health systems that cannot absorb the added cost of liquid-based testing will probably rely on the conventional Pap test for cervical cancer screening.

PERFORMING THE CONVENTIONAL PAP TEST

Patient Preparation Before Cervical Cytologic Sampling

Prior to having the patient come to the office for a Pap test, the American Society of Cytopathology and the American Cancer Society advise that the patient should take several actions to optimize cervical cytologic sampling (see American Society of Cytopathology 2001 Guidelines [*www.cytolpathology.org/guidelines/cervical-cytologyiii.php*]). These steps are as follows: *Efforts should be made not to schedule the clinic visit during the onset of the menstrual period and preferably not during the menstrual period. Women should refrain from intercourse for approximately 48 hours prior to cytologic examination. Women should avoid the use of tampons, vaginal creams, contraceptive foams or jellies, or other vaginal medications for 48 hours prior to the test.*

It is recognized that some patients, in spite of their best scheduling efforts, may arrive in the office during a menstrual period. It is possible to perform a cervical cytologic sampling in a patient during her menses; however, the sample may be somewhat limited by the presence of blood or relative hypocellularity. For some patients it is not practical or reasonable to simply reschedule the examination. In that case every effort should be made to obtain the best cytologic sample possible and to avoid as much blood as possible when collecting and preparing the smear.

Sampling/Collection

Although the initial Pap test as described by Drs. Papanicolaou and Traut employed sampling of the vaginal pool, the introduction of the Ayre spatula for scraping the cervical transformation zone substantially contributed to the value of cervical cytology. *Cervical cytologic sampling requires circumferential sampling of the cervical transformation zone, including the ectocervical squamous mucosa immediately adjacent to the transformation zone and the endocervical mucosa immediately superior to the transformation zone.* It is important to recognize that vaginal cytologic sampling is not of value in screening for cervical neoplasia and should not be included in the cervical cytologic sample. The vaginal sample often has a substantial inflammatory cell component and many benign superficial squamous cells that often obscure the cervical cytologic sample. If there is concern about vaginal neoplasia, as in women with prior in utero diethylstilbestrol (DES) exposure, separate four-quadrant sampling of the vaginal mucosa should be performed. The four vaginal cytologic samples also should be submitted separately from the cervical cytologic sample.[24–26] For a more detailed discussion of DES exposure, see Chapter 20.

Thorough sampling of the cervical transformation zone can be accomplished through the use of proper cervical cytologic sampling devices, such as an extended-tip spatula to sample the transformation zone and adjacent squamous mucosa and an endocervical brush device to sample the endocervix (Figure 4.2-1). This combined sampling technique has demonstrated the lowest false-negative rate of available conventional sampling methods.[27–30] *Both wood and plastic spatulas are available, and both are acceptable for cytologic sampling.* The plastic spatula may have some advantages in liquid-based systems because cells detach more easily from plastic than they do from wood.

The use of the endocervical brush requires that the brush be inserted into the endocervix but not into the endometrial cavity.

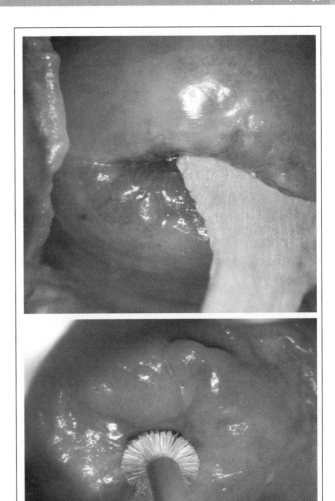

Figure 4.2-1 Cervical sampling with spatula and brush.

This usually requires that the brush be inserted into the endocervix until the junction of the bristles of the brush with the end of the handle is approximately even with the external os. Once inserted, *the brush should be rotated 180 degrees (one-half turn) in the endocervical canal.* Additional rotations are usually not necessary to adequately sample the endocervix near the squamo–columnar junction, and *excessive rotations may produce undesirable bleeding that can obscure the cytologic sample.*

The manufacturer does not recommended the endocervical brush for use in pregnant women because the brush has a stiff center support, usually made of thin wire, and the device could theoretically perforate the amniotic sac. However, *a published study on the use of the endocervical brushes in pregnant women has reported no complications* in one series.[31] An alternative for pregnant women is to use a saline-moistened swab rather than brush to sample the endocervical canal. Moistening the swab with sterile saline is necessary before use because a dry swab will desiccate the cells if the material is not adequately moist.

Pregnant women, especially after the second trimester, will usually have a visible transformation zone, and careful sampling with a spatula alone will usually sample the transformation zone adequately. The swab device does not collect the same number of cells as one would expect with a brush. *For routine sampling in the nonpregnant patient, the swab is not the preferred endocervical sampling device.*[32]

There are a number of devices that have been developed for cervical cellular sampling, and these can be reviewed in other texts. Cervical broom devices are attractive because they are a single instrument and, when used properly, simultaneously sample the endocervix, the transformation zone, and the ectocervix. A separate endocervical cytologic sample is not needed. *The broom is also approved for use in pregnant women.* The broom is used by inserting the longer central portion of the broom into the endocervical os and applying gentle pressure to cervix so the bristles bend. *The broom is then rotated in a single direction (clockwise or counterclockwise) for five complete rotations.* Rotating the broom into two different directions usually collects fewer cells. When the device is used for conventional cytology, the sample is applied to the properly labeled glass slide by simply swabbing the broom device onto the glass slide, followed by prompt fixation of the slide. The broom device is also applicable to liquid-based cytology and can either be rinsed in the preservative solution (ThinPrep), or the broom can be removed from the handle and placed into the fixative solution (SurePath).

Application of the Cellular Material to the Slide

Unlike liquid-based cytology, conventional cytology requires the clinician to manually prepare the sample. Although there are many methods used for this procedure, the following procedure has been demonstrated to have excellent results. A slide is properly labeled on its frosted section with the patient's name and any other identifier using a number-two pencil. The specimen is then obtained using an Ayre spatula and an endocervical cytobrush. *The endocervical brush sample is rolled at right angles to the long axis of the slide near the frosted end, covering less than one third of the slide with several rolls of the brush* (Figure 4.2-2). *The spatula sample is then quickly applied to the remaining portion of the slide, usually at least the remaining two thirds, through a rotating motion of the cervical sampling face of the spatula across the glass slide* (see Figure 4.2-2). Immediately after preparing the smear with the spatula, the slide should be rapidly fixed with a spray fixative or placed into 95% ethanol. *It is important that the applied cellular material does not air dry.* The endocervical brush component will dry more slowly than the spatula component, and that is why it is applied first.[33]

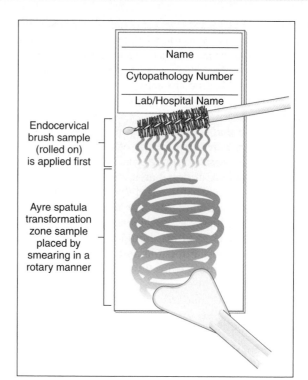

Figure 4.2-2 Recommended technique for the manual application of cellular material to the glass slide.

EVALUATION OF THE CONVENTIONAL PAP TEST AS A SCREENING TECHNIQUE

The Ideal Screening Test

Cervical cancer is a disease that is especially well suited for a preventive screening test. Prevalence rates for potentially developing cervical cancer are high.

Progression to invasive cervical cancer is associated with high morbidity and mortality rates. Cervical cancer typically is preceded by a relatively long latent, preinvasive phase that can be detected by cervical cytology, treated, and cured. The Pap test is the nearly ideal screening test because it is inexpensive, easy to administer, well tolerated, and poses no significant risk to the patient.

Pap Test Quality

Despite the acknowledged limitations of conventional cytology, *only 0.3% to 0.5% of specimens are considered unsatisfactory for interpretation.*[34] Over 15% of Pap tests, however, are limited in quality because of obscuring blood, inflammation, or thick cellular areas.[19,35]

Test Sensitivity and Specificity

For the detection of cervical cancer and its precursors, conventional cytology has a high test specificity (range, 79–100%, mean, 95%) and an acceptable test sensitivity (range, 30–80%, mean, 47%).[36]

Although the test sensitivity is acceptable, it is not optimal. *The false-negative rate associated with the conventional Pap test has been recognized as one of its major weaknesses as a screening test parameter.*

A false-negative cervical cytologic report is a negative report when a patient has a cervical carcinoma or high-grade cervical intraepithelial neoplasia. The false-negative rates are primarily due to sampling issues where the abnormal cells are not placed on the slide or are otherwise not submitted for microscopic examination. *Sampling issues are estimated to account for approximately two thirds of false-negative cervical cytologic reports. Sampling issues are most commonly related to inadequate scraping of the cervical transformation zone of the cervix, where the vast majority of cervical neoplastic lesions occur.* Sometimes inflammatory exudate, blood, lubricants, and thick cellular areas can obscure potentially diagnostic cells on the slide. Some neoplastic cells may be too cohesive and are resistant to sampling by scraping. It is also recognized that collected cells might be retained on the sampling device or devices and not placed onto the slide or into the sampling solution submitted for cytologic evaluation. It is also possible that cells might be lost from the slide once applied because of suboptimum fixation or lack of cohesiveness of the neoplastic cells to the glass slide.[37]

False-negative errors related to a failure to identify diagnostic cells on cervical cytology slides have to do with two key issues: screening or interpretation. Screening errors occur when the cytotechnologist evaluating the slide fails to identify abnormal cells that are present. *Screening errors account for slightly less than one third of false-negative cases.* Interpretative errors occur when the abnormal cells identified are not recognized as dysplastic/malignant cells. Interpretative errors may result from either the cytotechnologist or the cytopathologist not recognizing the cells in question. *Interpretative errors account for the smallest percentage of false-negative results associated with the Pap test.*[38]

Patient compliance issues can significantly affect the accuracy of the Pap test. *Sensitivity can be greatly improved by repeat testing at recommended regular intervals.* In addition, the negative-predictive value of the test improves with each sequential negative result. *A woman's risk of developing cervical cancer is significantly decreased in proportion to the number of negative tests she has had. In one study, one negative Pap test decreased the risk by 48%. A woman with five or more negative tests had virtually eliminated the risk of not identifying cervical cancer (a negative predictive value approaching 100%).*[39]

Cost

One of the criteria for an ideal screening test is that it must be inexpensive. Certainly the conventional Pap test is inexpensive. Liquid-based cervical cytology, HPV reflex testing, and automated screening add value but also add significant cost to cervical screening. To some extent, improved test sensitivity has the potential to partially offset added costs by safely allowing an increase in the testing interval. Improved test accuracy could reduce unnecessary referrals for colposcopy.

The cost of automated screening could also be partially offset by increases in productivity.

CYTOLOGIC NUANCES ASSOCIATED WITH THE PAP TEST

The Pap test can detect all types of epithelial abnormalities, including atypical squamous cells, low-grade squamous intraepithelial cells, high-grade squamous intraepithelial cells, squamous cell carcinoma, atypical glandular cells, and cervical adenocarcinoma (Figure 4.2-3). Both conventional Pap tests and liquid-based cytology can detect specific cervical infections, such as candida, actinomyces, trichomonas vaginalis, and herpes simplex virus.

When liquid-based cervical cytology was first introduced in 1996, it was recognized that certain nuances existed in the interpretation of these preparations that differed from conventional tests. In order to adapt to these nuances in interpretation, *cytotechnologists and pathologists needed additional training before liquid-based tests could be used in their clinical laboratories.*

Now that over 85% of the U.S. cervical screening market is using liquid-based preparations, cytotechnologists- and pathologists-in-training may need added training in interpreting conventional cytology. Novices to the conventional Pap test will have to adjust to test artifacts, such as thick cellular areas, obscuring blood, inflammation, and air drying artifact. In addition, *dysplastic cells on conventional tests tend to have darker "smudged" nuclei compared with the dysplastic cells of liquid-based slides* (Figure 4.2-4). *Diagnostic cells may be concentrated in certain areas of the slide and unevenly distributed, in contrast to the more random distribution of abnormal cells seen on liquid-based slides.* This concentration of diagnostic cells can actually be a helpful artifact, readily identified by the experienced cytotechnologist (Figure 4.2-5).

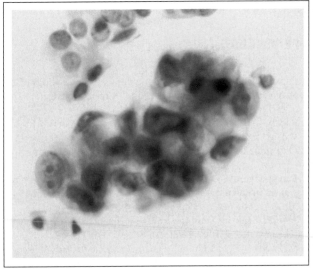

Figure 4.2-3 Conventional Pap test showing abnormal glandular cells consistent with adenocarcinoma.

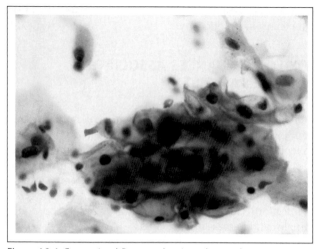

Figure 4.2-4 Conventional Pap test showing a low-grade squamous intraepithelial lesion. Note that the nuclei have a "dark smudgy" appearance, a characteristic degenerative change.

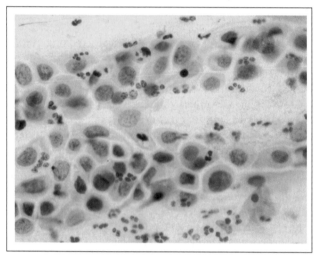

Figure 4.2-5 Conventional Pap test showing a high-grade squamous intraepithelial lesion. Note the linear array of diagnostic cells, a helpful artifact of manual test preparation.

REFERENCES

1. Papanicolaou GN. New Cancer Diagnosis in Proceedings of 3rd Race Betterment Conference. Battle Creek, Michigan 1928: 528–534.
2. Babes A. Diagnostic du cancer du col uterin par les frottes. Presse Med 1928;29:451–454.
3. O'Connor DM. A brief history of lower genital tract screening. J Lower Gen Tract Dis 2007;11(3):182–188.
4. Papanicolaou GN, Traut HF. The diagnostic value of vaginal smears in carcinoma of the uterus. Am J Obstet Gynecol 1941; 42:193–206.
5. Ayre JE. Selective cytology smear for diagnosis of cancer. Am J Obstet Gynecol 1947;53:609–617.
6. McSweeney DJ, McKay DG. Uterine cancer: Its early detection by simple screening methods. N Engl J Med 1948;238:867–870.
7. Greenlee RT, Murray T, Bolden S, et al. Cancer statistics, 2000. CA Cancer J Clin 2000;50:7–33.
8. Cramer DW. The role of cervical cytology in the declining morbidity and mortality of cervical cancer. Cancer 1974;34: 2018–2027.
9. Clarke EA, Anderson TW. Does screening by Pap smears help prevent cervical cancer? A case control study. Lancet 1979;2:1–4.
10. Bogdanich W. Lax laboratories. The Pap test misses much cervical cancer through labs' errors. The Wall Street Journal, November 2, 1987:section 1A.
11. Clinical Laboratory Improvement Amendments of 1988 (CLIA 88) (Public Law 100–578). Fed Register 1990;55:9538.
12. Bernstein SJ, Sanchez-Ramos L, Ndubisi B. Liquid-based cervical cytologic smear study and conventional Papanicolaou smears: A metaanalysis of prospective studies comparing cytologic diagnosis and sample adequacy. Am J Obstet Gynecol 2001:185:308–317.
13. Abulafia O, Pezzullo JC, Sherer DM. Performance of ThinPrep liquid-based cervical cytology in comparison with conventionally prepared Papanicolaou smears: A quantitative survey. Gynecol Oncol 2003;90:137–144.
14. Limaye A, Conner AJ, Huang X, et al. Comparative analysis of conventional Papanicolaou tests and a fluid-based thin-layer method. Arch Pathol Lab Med 2003;127:200–204.
15. NHS. NHS cervical screening programme. Available at *cancerscreening.nhs.uk/cervical/*
16. Solomon D, Schiffman M, Tarone R, ALTS Study Group. Comparison of three management strategies for patients with atypical squamous cells of undetermined significance baseline results from a randomized trial. JNCI 2001;93:293–299.
17. Wright TC Jr, Massad LS, Dunton CJ, Spitzer M, Wilkinson EJ, Solomon D; for the 2006 ASCCP-Sponsored Consensus Conference. 2006 consensus guidelines for the management of women with abnormal cervical screening tests. J Low Genit Tract Dis. 2007 Oct;11(4):201–22.
18. Wojcik EM, Booth CN. Automation in cervical cytology. Pathol Case Reviews 2005;10(3):138–143.
19. Bishop JW, Bigner SH, Cologen TJ, et al. Multicenter masked evaluation of AutoCyte PREP thinlayers with matched conventional smears including initial biopsy results. Acta Cytol 1998;42(1):189–197.
20. Australian Health Technology Advisory Council. Review of Automated and Semi-Automated Cervical Screening Devices. Canberra, Australia: Commonwealth Department of Health and Family Services, 1998.
21. American Cancer Society (ACS). Cancer Prevention and Early Detection. Facts and Figures, 2005.
22. McCrory DC, Matcher DB, Bastian L, et al. Evaluation of cervical cytology. AHCPR Publication No. 99-E010. Rockville, Maryland: Agency for Health Care Policy and Research, February 1999.
23. Parkin DM, Pisani P, Ferlay J. Global Cancer Statistics, CA Cancer J Clin 1999;49:33–64.
24. Anderson B, Watring WG, Edinger DD, et al. Development of DES-associated clear-cell carcinoma: The importance of regular screening. Obstet Gynecol 1979;53:293–299.
25. Tedeschi CA, Rubin M, Krumholz BA. Six cases of women with diethylstilbestrol in utero demonstrating long-term manifestations and current evaluation guidelines. J Lower Gen Tract Dis 2005;9:11–18.
26. Kaufman RH, Adam E. Findings in female offspring of women exposed in utero to diethylstilbestrol. Obstet Gynecol 2002; 99:197–200.
27. Saslow D, Runowicz CD, Solomon D, et al. American Cancer Society guidelines for the early detection of cervical neoplasia and cancer. CA: A Cancer Journal for Clinicians 2002;52:342–362.

28. Alons-van Kordelaar JJ, Boon ME. Diagnostic accuracy of squamous cervical lesions studied in spatula-cytobrush smears. Acta Cytol 1988;32:801–804.

29. Chakrabarti S, Guijon JC, Paraskevas M. Brush vs. spatula for cervical smears: Histologic correlation with concurrent biopsies. Acta Cytol 1994;38:315–318.

30. Boon ME, de Graaff Guilloud JC, Rietveld WJ. Analysis of five sampling methods for the preparation of cervical smears. Acta Cytol 1989;33:843–848.

31. Orr JW, Barrett JM, Orr PF, et al. The efficacy and safety of the cytobrush during pregnancy. Gynecol Oncol 1992;44:260–262.

32. Martin-Hirsch P, Lilford R, Jarvis G, et al. Efficacy of cervical-smear collection devices: A systematic review and meta-analysis. Lancet 1999;354:1763–1770.

33. Rubio CA. The false negative smear. II. The trapping effect of collecting instruments. Obstet Gynecol 1977;49:576–580.

34. Ransdell JS, Davey DD, Zaleski S. Clinicopathologic correlation of the unsatisfactory Papanicolaou smear. Cancer 1997;81:139–143.

35. Bolick DR, Hellman DJ. Laboratory implementation and efficacy assessment of the ThinPrep cervical cancer screening system. Acta Cytol 1998;42:209–213.

36. Nanda K, McCrory DC, Myers ER, et al. Accuracy of the Papanicolaou test in screening for and follow-up of cervical cytologic abnormalities: A systemic review. Ann Intern Med 2000;132:810–819.

37. McGoogan E, Colgan TJ, Ramzy I, et al. Cell preparation methods and criteria for sample adequacy. IAC Task Force summary. Acta Cytologica 1998;42:25–32.

38. DeMay RM. Cytopathology of false negatives preceding cervical carcinoma. Am J Obstet Gynecol 1996;175:1110–1113.

39. Lynge E, Poll P. Incidence of cervical cancer following negative smear: A cohort study of Maribo County, Denmark. Am J Epidemiol 1986;124:345–352.

4.3: Thin-Layer, Liquid-Based Cytology

Juan Felix

Liquid-based cytology allows Pap specimens to be collected into a liquid solution, machine processed into monolayer preparations on a glass slide, and prescreened by a computerized image analysis system. The residual, unused sample is available to perform ancillary molecular testing, including a variety of preordered or reflex examinations. The bulk of ancillary testing has been reflex testing for human papillomavirus (HPV) of cytology interpreted as atypical squamous cells of undetermined significance (ASC-US); however, other ancillary testing from a liquid-based medium is rapidly gaining acceptance. Examples include sexually transmitted infections, such as chlamydia and gonorrhea, as well as testing for genetic conditions, such as cystic fibrosis mutations.

The changes brought about by liquid-based cytology have increased diagnostic sensitivity and specificity over the conventional Pap test while maintaining cost neutrality to the health system. In addition, the increment in productivity achieved by computer-based imaging has temporarily eliminated the imminent workforce gap caused by the reduction in the number of cytotechnologists in the United States.

BACKGROUND

Dr. George Papanicolaou introduced cervical cytology into clinical practice circa 1940.[1] In 1945 the Pap smear received the endorsement of the American Cancer Society (ACS) as an effective method for the prevention of cervical cancer. The significant reduction in the incidence and mortality of cervical cancer in the United States, Canada, and Western Europe in the last 50 years has been largely credited to the widespread implementation of cervical cytology screening programs.[2–5] The ingenious technique of collecting exfoliated cells from the cervix, placing them on a glass slide, and examining them under the microscope has remained largely unchanged for over 50 years. It was only in the 1980s when a combination of events spurred a reevaluation of the efficacy of the conventional Pap smear method. An explosion of technology in the field culminated in the introduction of liquid-based, thin-layer cytology.

The U.S. Air Force reported the first documented incident of deficiencies in gynecologic cytology laboratories. Allegations claiming inaccuracies in Pap smear diagnoses performed by a contract laboratory between 1972 and 1977 resulted in an investigation by government agencies. These investigations led to the discovery of large numbers of under-diagnoses on Air Force personnel and their dependents, which were largely attributed to poor regulation of laboratory personnel and their large workloads.[6] In 1987 a highly publicized investigative report published in the *Wall*

Street Journal denounced the egregious practices of a few cytology laboratories in the Eastern United States.[7] The report *exposed the policies of several high-volume, low-cost laboratories that encouraged excessive productivity from their screening cytotechnologists at the cost of accuracy.* Similar problems had been documented in other laboratories but had not received such widespread attention.[8] Spurred on by public outcry, further government investigations into these and other allegations led to the recommended guidelines for the practice of cytology that culminated in an amendment to the Clinical Laboratory Improvement Act (CLIA) in 1988.[9] CLIA 1988 established workload limits on cytotechnologists, which included limits on the number of slides that can be screened daily, and it instituted performance standards for both laboratories and laboratory professionals. *CLIA regulations limit the number of cytology slides that a cytotechnologist may screen in a 24-hour period to 100. They mandate screening of no less than 10% of slides that were initially interpreted as normal by a cytotechnologist. They also mandate remediation of cytotechnologists when they make clinically significant under-diagnoses.*

In subsequent years, numerous studies evaluated the sensitivity of conventional cervical cytology. The sensitivity of the conventional Pap smear ranged from 31% to 89%, depending on the design, population, and endpoint of the study.[10–19] Of note, in the three series in which the cause of a false-negative result was investigated, careful rescreening of the slides showed that screening errors were less common than errors of sampling.[11,12,19] These data suggested that the limitations of conventional cytology were related to more than just poor laboratory practice or the human error of cytotechnologists. Systematic evaluation of conventional cytology culminated with the publication of two meta-analyses of the world's literature.[20,21] *Both these studies demonstrated that the sensitivity of conventional cytology was less than 50% for the detection of cervical cancer precursors.*

The regulations imposed by CLIA presented laboratory directors with an unending list of challenges. Workload limitations increased demands for cytotechnologists. As costs and the number of Pap smears increased, reimbursements and the number of cytotechnologists decreased. This put tremendous strain on the system. Temporary relief resulted from decreasing the number of slides per patient by combining the cervical, endocervical, and vaginal samples onto a single slide. This was done despite a paucity of data proving equal efficacy of this approach, compared with the submission of multiple slides.[22] Despite these measures, the prospect of being unable to cope with the demands for screening cervical cytology in the future was alarming. Advances in image analysis and increased speed of computer processors allowed for the development of computerized instruments that could assist or even replace cytotechnologists in the tedious task of screening Pap smears. Although several efforts were undertaken to design equipment that would evaluate conventional cytology, there were still limitations (sampling and preparation) inherent in a conventionally prepared slide that posed insurmountable impediments to computer analysis.

LIMITATIONS OF CONVENTIONAL CYTOLOGY

The efficacy of cervical cytology is based on the presumption that if an abnormality exists on the cervix, it will be collected by the Pap smear device and transferred onto the glass slide. This presupposes that an adequate number of the abnormal cells are transferred. Hutchinson et al. examined the first of these premises and showed that commonly used collection devices for cervical cytology collected between 600,000 and 1.2 million cervical epithelial cells but that less than 20% of the collected cells were transferred onto the glass slide (Figure 4.3–1).[23] The failure to transfer most of the epithelial-cell sample to the slide provided a viable explanation for the high false-negative rates reported in the previously mentioned studies. *Particularly disturbing was the realization that the transfer of cells to the glass slide is a random event and is therefore statistically subject to error if the population of abnormal cells is not homogeneously distributed throughout the specimen.*

Preparation of conventional cytology by the clinician is a highly variable and poorly controlled technique. Optimal application of cells onto a glass slide should be done in a systematic fashion in order to evenly spread the epithelial cells across the entire surface of the slide and maximize the transfer of cells while minimizing clumping. Furthermore, the transfer of cells onto the slide must be done rapidly in order to promptly fix the specimen and avoid air-drying or degeneration of the cells. In addition to these technical challenges,

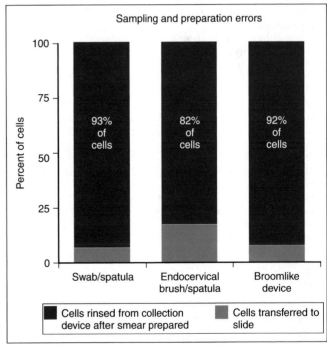

Figure 4.3-1 Each bar in this graph shows the total number of cells collected by the three most common cervical sampling devices: the Ayres spatula and cotton swab, the Ayres spatula and endocervical brush, and the broom device. The portion of the sample that adheres to the glass slide is represented in green, whereas the portion in blue remains on the device and is destined to be discarded.

uncontrollable variables exist that affect the optimization of conventional cytology. Inflammatory cells and blood compete for available space on the glass slide. In extreme cases, the inflammatory cells or blood could replace or obscure the epithelial cells, creating an impediment to visual analysis (Figure 4.3-2). Finally, inflamed epithelial cells and normal epithelial cells in the late luteal phase may form thick three-dimensional aggregates that obscure visualization of the diagnostic cells (Figure 4.3-3). Studies evaluating the adequacy of conventional cytology report that more than 15% of all Pap smears are limited because of the presence of obscuring blood, inflammation, or thick areas of overlapping epithelial cells.[23,24]

The stated limitations of conventional cytology were believed to pose obstacles to the successful development of a computer-assisted screening device. Inherent limitations needed to be overcome in order to create computer-assisted technology that was superior to the method of conventional cytology.

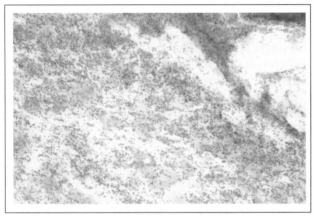

Figure 4.3-2 Photomicrograph of a conventional Pap smear showing numerous red blood cells and inflammatory cells that overlie the cervical epithelial cells, obstructing a clear vision of cellular detail (×100).

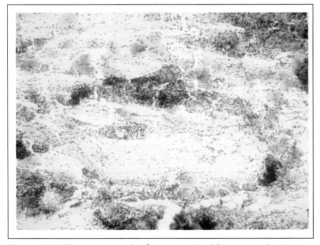

Figure 4.3-3 Photomicrograph of a conventional Pap smear showing aggregation of epithelial cells. Some aggregates are associated with inflammatory cells, whereas other areas are composed of only aggregates of epithelial cells (×100).

PRINCIPLES OF EFFICACY OF LIQUID-BASED CYTOLOGY

The liquid-based technology was developed to address the following five major limitations of conventional cytology: failure to capture the entire specimen obtained from the patient, inadequate specimen fixation, non-random distribution of abnormal cells in the sample, obscuring elements, and technical variability in the quality of the smear. The collection of cells directly into a liquid fixative addresses the first two limitations. If proper technique is observed, the vast majority of the cells retrieved by the sampling devices are rinsed into the liquid media, capturing virtually the entire sample obtained from the patient into the vial. In addition, by immersing the cervical collection device into the liquid fixative, the cells are fixed instantly, avoiding the damaging contact with the dry slide and minimizing postcollection degeneration and air-drying.

Mechanical mixing of the cells follows placement of cells into liquid fixative. Although the different products that utilize the liquid-based technology have different methods of mixing, the principle is the same. Mixing of the cells creates a homogenous sample in which abnormal cells, if present, are evenly distributed throughout the liquid. Specimen homogeneity minimizes false-negative results, seen in conventional cytology as a result of non-randomly distributed abnormal cells. Sample homogeneity is critical because conventional cytology does not capture the entire cell sample collected from the patient, but rather will contain only a relatively small aliquot of the cells. Hutchinson et al. demonstrated the efficacy of this process by producing multiple slides from abnormal samples and identifying abnormal cells in virtually all the slides.[25] The effect of liquid collection and sample mixing appears to afford a consistent identification of abnormal cells regardless of the liquid-based method used. Khalbuss et al. used a modified electric toothbrush to mix liquid-fixed residual cells obtained from conventional cytology collection. Slides were produced by simple cytocentrifugation onto glass slides. Despite the simplicity of the procedure, diagnostic equivalency to the conventionally prepared Pap smear was demonstrated.[26]

The other limitations of conventional cytology, obscuring elements and thick sample, are handled differently by the liquid-based products currently available. ThinPrep (Cytyc, a subsidiary of Hologic, Bedford MA) utilizes a polycarbonate cylinder that holds a membrane with an 8-micron pore size to mix and subsequently suction the liquid media. As the collection fluid of the sample passes through this semipermeable barrier, the membrane traps epithelial cells and infectious organisms but allows much of the debris and some inflammatory cells to pass. When the pressure sensor determines that sufficient epithelial cells are accumulated on the membrane, the suction is discontinued, and the membrane is placed against the glass slide to allow for the transfer of cells. The residual, unused sample is available to perform ancillary molecular testing.

The AutoCyte Prep (TriPath, a subsidiary of Becton Dickinson Company, Franklin Lakes NJ) utilizes a liquid gradient onto which the sample is layered following vigorous vortexing. The sample and gradient are then centrifuged. The gradient preferentially concentrates epithelial cells, partially depleting the extraneous material, blood, and inflammatory cells. An aliquot of this filtrate is then robotically pipetted onto a chamber, and the sample is allowed to settle by gravity onto the slide. Both ThinPrep and AutoCyte techniques result in consistent, thin-layer preparations of epithelial cells that are depleted of extraneous elements. Both products produce circular areas containing 50,000 to 75,000 cells per slide.

EFFICACY OF LIQUID-BASED, THIN-LAYER TECHNOLOGY

The efficacy of liquid-based, thin-layer cytology has been assessed through numerous clinical trials. Two types of study designs are used in most of the published studies: the split-sample design and the intended use, direct-to-vial design. The studies of split-samples utilize a single sample collection design. A sample is prepared by conventional cytology method. The residual material remaining on the collection device is then rinsed in collection media and sent for thin-layer preparation. This study design suffers from a bias in favor of conventional cytology, which is prepared first and may deplete the remaining sample of cells for thin-layer preparation. In the intended use, direct-to-vial design, the cervical sample is directly deposited into the liquid collection media. Conventional cytology controls are obtained from matched populations of historical control subjects. There are numerous inherent biases in the direct-to-vial method. These include differences in the studied populations, election bias on the basis of ability to afford a more expensive technology, and selection of high-risk women to a test perceived to have superior sensitivity. To date, no prospective randomized trials comparing these technologies with conventional cytology have been conducted. Despite these limitations, the studies include an excess of 500,000 women with the preponderance of data, indicating a significant benefit of liquid-based, thin-layer cytology over conventional cytology in the detection of cervical cancer precursors and in the improvement of specimen adequacy.

Early clinical studies comparing ThinPrep and AutoCyte Prep (formerly known as Cyto-Rich) were performed on initial versions of the devices that subsequently underwent significant modifications. These studies will not be reviewed in detail, as the tested devices were replaced with newer versions, and those newer versions are the only ones that are clinically available. The importance of these early trials was in the demonstration of diagnostic equivalence to conventional cytology despite the adverse bias introduced by the split sample study design.[19,22,27-36]

Most of the more recent studies use versions of the automated devices approved by the Food and Drug Administration (FDA) and are reviewed and summarized in Tables 4.3-1 through 4.3-4. The studies are divided into split-sample and intended-use direct-to-vial design. Examination of the data revealed that liquid-based cytology outperformed conventional cytology in the detection of cervical cancer precursors. In fact, only one study failed to find more squamous intraepithelial lesions (SILs) on the liquid-based slides than on the conventional smears, demonstrating a nonsignificant 3% decrease in the detection of SIL.[35] The equivalent or superior performance of the liquid-based, thin-layer method is particularly impressive in the split-sample studies when the conventional smear failed to show SIL that was subsequently identified on the residual cells. The range of improvement afforded by liquid-based cytology in the split-sample study was between 6% and 110% with ThinPrep technology and 3% to 137% with AutoCyte Prep technology (Tables 4.3-1 and 4.3-3). In summary, the improvement shown in these studies was 15% with ThinPrep[23,37-41] and 18% with AutoCyte Prep.[27,35,43-45]

Because the direct-to-vial studies using ThinPrep revealed such marked improvements in the detection of SIL, it was suspected that the increase in diagnoses of SIL might have resulted from "overcalls" by overzealous cytopathologists rather that true detection of abnormalities. A summary of the direct-to-vial studies for ThinPrep showed a 140%

Table 4.3-1 Performance of ThinPrep in Split-sample studies

Reference	No. of Cases	Conv. SIL	TP SIL	% Increase	ASC-US TP	ASC-US Conv.	Unsatisfactory TP	Unsatisfactory Conv.	SBLB TP	SBLB Conv.
Lee, 1996	6,747	8.0%	9.4%	18.4%	7.7%	7.4%	1.6%	1.9%	27.8%	19.8%
Roberts, 1997	35,560	2.0%	2.3%	11.7%	N/A	N/A	3.5%	0.7%	8.3%	20.0%
Corkill, 1998	1,583	2.7%	5.6%	109.5%	3.7%	5.1%	N/A	N/A	2.2%	0.3%
Shield, 1999	300	7.0%	8.3%	19.1%	N/A	N/A	17.3%	6.3%	N/A	15.3%
Wang, 1999	972	4.4%	6.0%	34.9%	N/A	N/A	N/A	N/A	N/A	N/A
Hutchinson, 1999	8,636	4.9%	5.2%	6.0%	1.8%	7.5%	N/A	N/A	N/A	N/A

Conv=conventional
TP=ThinPrep
SBLB=satisfactory but limited by

Table 4.3-2 Performance of ThinPrep in Direct-to-vial Studies

Reference	No. of Cases Conv./TP	Conv. SIL	TP SIL	Increase	ASC-US Conv.	TP	Unsatisfactory Conv.	TP	SBLB Conv.	TP
Weintraub, 1997	13,067/18,247	1.0%	2.9%	190%	1.6%	2.7%	0.7%	0.3%	30.9%	10.9%
Papillo, 1998	18,569/8,541	1.6%	2.5%	56%	9.0%	6.6%	0.2%	0.4%	4.8%	4.4%
Bolick, 1998	39,408/10,694	1.1%	2.9%	164%	2.3%	2.9%	1.0%	0.3%	17.8%	11.6%
Dupree, 1998	22,323/19,351	1.2%	1.7%	40%	4.9%	4.6%	2.0%	3.8%	N/A	N/A
Guidos, 1999	5,423/9,583	1.3%	4.7%	262%	2.0%	3.4%	1.2%	0.5%	21.4%	0.7%
Carpenter, 1999	5,000/2,727	7.7%	10.5%	36%	12.5%	6.9%	0.6%	0.3%	19.4%	10.5%
Diaz-Rosario, 2000	74,756/56,339	1.8%	3.2%	79%	4.8%	4.5%	0.2%	0.7%	22.0%	18.7%
Weintraub, 2000	129,619/39,455	0.6%	2.3%	141%	1.5%	2.4%	0.3%	0.2%	27.8%	8.1%

Table 4.3-3 Performance of Auto-Cyte Prep in Split-sample Studies

Reference	No. of Cases	Conv. SIL	Prep SIL	Increase	ASC-US Conv.	Prep	Unsatisfactory Conv.	Prep	SBLB Conv.	Prep
Vassilakos, 1996	560	3.8%	4.6%	24%	12.9%	7.7%	5.4%	3.8%	28.3%	8.4%
Takahashi, 1997	2,000	3.5%	3.4%	-3%	1.1%	4.6%	N/A	N/A	N/A	N/A
Wilbur, 1997	286	4.2%	9.1%	117%	13.6%	13.3%	3.5%	1.1%	30%	16%
Bishop, 1998	8,983	5.2%	5.9%	13%	6.2%	6.0%	1.0%	0.6%	28.1%	15.8%
Kunz, 1998	554	1.4%	3.4%	137%	9.6%	3.3%	19%	12%	N/A	N/A
Minge, 2000	14,539	4.4%	5.8%	32%	6.9%	5.9%	0.9%	0.6%	N/A	N/A

Table 4.3-4 Performance of the Auto-Cyte Prep in Direct-to-vial Studies

Reference	No. of Cases Conv. / Prep	Conv. SIL	Prep SIL	Increase	ASC-US Conv.	Prep	Unsatisfactory Conv.	Prep	SBLB Conv.	Prep
Vassilakos, 1998	15,402/32,655	1.1%	3.6%	224%	3.7%	1.6%	1.9%	0.4%	13.4%	2.7%
Vassilakos, 1999	88,569/111,358	2.0%	3.2%	63%	3.0%	1.2%	1.5%	0.2%	4.6%	1.2%
Vassilakos, 2000	19,923/81,120	1.2%	3.4%	283%	3.5%	1.9%	N/A	N/A	N/A	N/A
Tench, 2000	10,367/2,231	1.0%	1.7%	67%	3.8%	5.5%	2.9%	0.4%	31%	16%

improvement in the detection of SIL over the historical conventional cytology controls[24,46–52] (Table 4.3-2).

A summary of the direct-to-vial studies for AutoCyte Prep is similar with a more than 200% increase in the detection of SIL over historic conventional controls[53–56] (Table 4.3-4). Of note, three of the four direct-to-vial AutoCyte Prep studies used manual pipetting to produce the slides rather than the FDA-approved instrument.[54,55] However, the one direct-to-vial study of AutoCyte Prep that utilized the FDA-approved instrument and procedure showed a 67% increase in the detection of SIL.[53]

Confirmation that this increase in SIL is true detection rather than "overcall" by cytopathologists can be found in several studies in which subsets of women with histology follow-up is available. Papillo et al. found a statistically significant increase in the specificity of a diagnosis of SIL on ThinPrep (81%) over conventional cytology (72%).[50] Diaz-Rosario et al. found equivalent specificity between ThinPrep (74%) and conventional cytology (79%), as determined by biopsy-proven cervical intraepithelial neoplasia (CIN).[47] Finally, Hutchinson et al. presented histology correlation data from a population-based study in Costa Rica.[23] Biopsy correlation results in this study showed that the specificity of the ThinPrep diagnosis was 85.4% compared with 88.8% for conventional cytology. In all three studies, the higher sensitivity combined with the specificity demonstrated a significant increase in the detection of biopsy-proven CIN. These data strongly support the FDA labeling that ThinPrep is superior to conventional cytology for the detection of true cervical cancer precursor lesions.

Although less data exist for AutoCyte Prep, two reports comment on biopsy correlation. Vassilakos et al. reported a statistically significant improvement in the correlation between the AutoCyte Prep diagnosis and biopsy result when compared with conventional cytology.[56] The improvement in correlation was particularly notable among cases diagnosed as high-grade squamous intraepithelial lesion (HSIL) by the AutoCyte Prep method, with 90% of biopsies confirming the diagnosis. Finally, Tench et al. reported a preliminary biopsy correlation of 30 cases using AutoCyte Prep. The biopsy-confirmed CIN diagnoses in 26 of the 30 cases suggested adequate specificity.

Another concern regarding liquid-based thin-layer technology was the increase in the diagnosis of ASC-US in several studies. Although many series reported an absolute decrease in the frequency of ASC-US, all the series reported a decrease in the ASC-US:SIL ratio. This parameter is considered more representative of performance because the detection of more disease will be accompanied by the detection of all cytological abnormalities, including ASC-US. There was also increased detection of atypical glandular cells of undetermined significance (AGC-US). Ashfaq et al. reported a significant improvement in the detection of adenocarcinoma of the cervix using ThinPrep, with a 65% decrease in the false-negative rate of the same diagnosis over conventional cytology as well as a 64% increase in the specificity of a diagnosis of AGC-US or adenocarcinoma.[57]

THIN-LAYER–BASED COMPUTER-ASSISTED SCREENING

Computer-assisted screening devices have been shown to reduce the incidence of false-negative cytology when used in a quality control mode to rescreen cases with a diagnosis of *negative for intraepithelial lesion and malignancy*.[58,59] Currently there are two FDA-approved systems that utilize computer-assisted screening of cervical cytology: the AutoPap 300 and the ThinPrep Imaging System. These two systems take dramatically different approaches to the automated processing of cervical cytology.

The AutoPap 300 uses a "black box" model, by which all slides eligible for screening are processed through the instrument. During processing, the instrument identifies a subset of slides at lowest risk for containing an abnormality. This subset includes 20% to 25% of the slides processed, and they are designated as normal and not requiring further interpretation by cytotechnologists. The remaining slides are scored based on the likelihood of containing an abnormality, and they are distributed to cytotechnologists for screening and interpretation.

The ThinPrep Imaging System identifies all slides acceptable for screening and records the coordinates of the 22 areas on the slide most likely to contain an abnormality.

All the slides are then placed on a computer-controlled microscope and are screened by a cytotechnologist who is directed to these 22 most likely areas. The cytotechnologist assesses whether the slide is normal or abnormal and if a pathologist should review the slide. The cytotechnologist saves time by focusing only on the 22 fields rather than the usual average of 120 fields per slide. This reduction in effort and the inherent sensitivity of the instrument is thought to be responsible for the reported increase in sensitivity of the system. A secondary benefit is that cytotechnologists can screen more slides with less fatigue than they could under the previously mandated CLIA limits. This increase in efficiency has made it possible for laboratories to meet workload requirements without increasing the number of cytotechnologists.[60]

There are few clinical trials evaluating the expanded use of the AutoPap 300 system. and these are in the early phases of study. In a series of 583 patients, Takahashi et al. found that an interactive computer analysis system, the AutoCyte Screen, yielded a false-negative rate of only 1.8% (detecting 55 of 56 diagnoses of SIL) while triaging only 21% of cases to pathologist review.[61] In a series of 1676 thin-layer preparations, Bishop et al. reported that the AutoCyte Screen showed improved sensitivity in the detection of SIL, with the computer-assisted screening yielding 98% sensitivity, compared with 89% sensitivity for manual screening alone.[62] Although larger clinical trials are needed, these early results offer promise for an improvement in screening sensitivity while reducing human effort and time utilization. To this date the AutoPap 300 remains largely underutilized by laboratories. Unresolved issues regarding the definition of the *high-risk patient*, the unacceptability of many slides read by the device, and the increase in cost and lower reimbursement by insurance carriers have delayed the widespread acceptance of this technology.

The ThinPrep Imaging System (TIS) was approved by the FDA in June 2003. Data presented to the FDA showed that by using TIS, the cytotechnologist achieved equivalence in the diagnosis of HSIL and low-grade SIL (LSIL) while screening 200 slides per day, when compared with manually screening 80 slides per day. Based on this data, the FDA allowed cytotechnologists to screen up to 200 slides a day using the TIS. Subsequent to FDA approval, several studies have reported increased detection rates using the TIS, compared with manual screening of ThinPrep slides.[63–66] The TIS increased the sensitivity of the detection of HSIL while maintaining the rate of biopsy-confirmed abnormalities.[60] In this study cytotechnologists also increased their average daily throughput of slides from 75 to 115 using TIS.

MOLECULAR TESTING OUT OF RESIDUAL MATERIAL LEFT IN THE VIAL

An unexpected benefit of liquid-based, thin-layer technology was that abundant cellular material remained in the vial following the production of the slide. It is estimated that on the average, 10% or less of the cellular material is used to make the diagnostic slide. With the advancement of molecular testing, biologists began using the residual material to test for the presence of infectious organisms. To date successful out-of-vial testing has been demonstrated for HPV, chlamydia, and herpes simplex virus (HSV). *The ability to detect infections in the residual volume of the collection fluid offers numerous opportunities, including the simplification of collection and minimization of routing errors from multiple samples.* Another benefit of this adjunct technology is the ability to perform HPV deoxyribonucleic acid (DNA) testing in women with a cytological diagnosis of ASC-US. Results of two large clinical trials have shown that detection of high-risk HPV DNA using the Hybrid Capture (HC) 2 assay effectively separates women with ASC-US into two groups: those with an increased risk of having high-grade CIN (CIN 2,3) and those at a decreased risk of harboring high-grade CIN.[44,67] The HPV test using the HC 2 test can be performed by separately collecting a sample of cells into a transport media or by using the residual cell sample from the liquid-based cytology sample. The latter choice offers the option of reflex testing (automatically testing the samples of women with ASC-US without the necessity of additional clinic visits). If the testing shows the presence of high-risk HPV DNA, colposcopy is recommended. Women who test negative for high-risk HPV DNA can return to annual screening. More details about the management of women with ASC-US smears can be found in Chapter 11.

CYTOLOGICAL CRITERIA

Microscopic evaluation of liquid-based, thin-layer slides differs from the examination of conventionally prepared Pap smears. The appearance of the material on the slide differs from conventionally prepared cytology because of a reduction in obscuring inflammation and blood, and because the slides are produced by a touch prep, they lack a smearing pattern (Figure 4.3-4). The obliteration of this pattern initially worried cytotechnologists who relied on these features to assist in the identification of abnormalities. Similarly the excellent fixation of the cells produced clear, crisp-appearing nuclei that lacked degenerative changes. Cytotechnologists relied on these degenerative changes to highlight extremely dark nuclei that help to identify abnormalities. However, most agreed that the benefits of a better-fixed sample without obstructing debris greatly outweigh any detriments. The large body of clinical data shows that with minimal retraining, cytotechnologists increased their detection of abnormalities using liquid-based technology.

Optimal fixation minimizes degenerative nuclear changes, so abnormal cells will often lack degenerative hyperchromasia (Figure 4.3-5). Instead the nuclei will appear euchromatic but will still demonstrate the marked nuclear irregularities that characterize dysplasia (Figure 4.3-6). Although the machine-made touch prep eradicates the smear pattern, the evenly dispersed epithelial cell layers allow the abnormal cells to be seen against a clear background. The abnormal

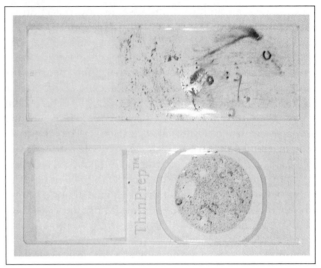

Figure 4.3-4 Comparison of the appearance of conventional Pap smear versus a machine-made thin-layer preparation. Note the uniformity in the distribution of cells throughout the machine-made slide *(bottom)* compared with the streaking and aggregating of cellular material seen in the conventional Pap smear *(top)*.

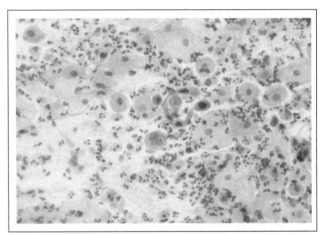

Figure 4.3-5 Conventional Pap smear revealing abnormal squamous cells. The nuclei show dark chromatin, revealing little internal detail. This "smudged" appearance of the chromatin is characteristic of degenerative change (×200).

cells are not obscured by inflammation or hidden by sheets of normal epithelial cells (Figure 4.3-7).

Low-Grade Squamous Intraepithelial Lesions

LSIL is most prevalent in women in their early-reproductive age (ages 16–26) or at the onset of sexual activity.[9,68–70] The cytologic diagnosis of LSIL is made upon the identification of abnormal squamous cells whose cell size is equivalent to a normal superficial or intermediate cell (Figure 4.3-8). Diagnostic abnormalities include enlargement of the nucleus, irregularity of the nuclear membrane, and irregular chromatin distribution. Additional features that aid in the diagnosis include hyperchromasia as well as cavitation of the cytoplasm immediately surrounding the nucleus to

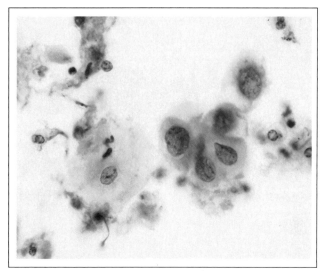

Figure 4.3-6 A ThinPrep Pap test showing a high-grade squamous intraepithelial lesion (HSIL). Note that although hyperchromasia is slight to absent, the chromatin is irregularly distributed, and the nuclear outlines are markedly irregular, ensuring the abnormal diagnosis (×600).

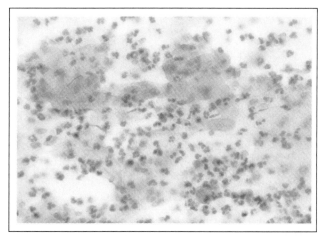

Figure 4.3-7 A conventional Pap smear showing several abnormal squamous cells among normal epithelial cells, inflammatory cells, and blood. Scrutiny of the abnormal cells, once identified, reveals a diagnosis of a high-grade squamous intraepithelial lesion (HSIL) (×400).

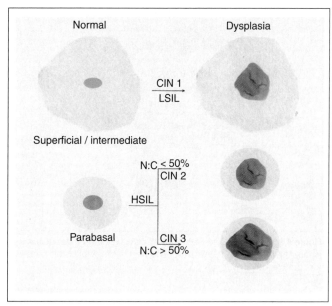

Figure 4.3-8 The cytologic diagnosis of a low-grade squamous intraepithelial lesion *(LSIL)* is made upon the identification of abnormal squamous cells whose cell size is equivalent to a normal superficial or intermediate cell. *CIN,* cervical intraepithelial neoplasia; *N:C,* nuclear:cytoplasmic ratio; *HSIL,* high-grade squamous intraepithelial lesion.

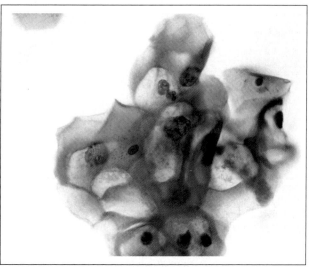

Figure 4.3-9 A ThinPrep Pap test showing a low-grade squamous intraepithelial lesion (LSIL). Note the clarity of both cytoplasmic and nuclear detail afforded by the liquid fixation as well as the absence of extraneous material (×600).

form a well-demarcated internal cytoplasmic border. The latter cytoplasmic changes, commonly referred to as koilocytosis, should not be equated to LSIL in the absence of the diagnostic nuclear features. *Liquid-based cytology enhances both the nuclear irregularities and chromatin pattern seen in LSIL, and more importantly, it highlights the cytoplasmic cavity, enhancing the true internal border of the koilocytic clearing* (Figures 4.3-9, 4.3-10). When findings are inconclusive, the diagnosis of ASC-US should be considered (see following).

High-Grade Squamous Intraepithelial Lesions

HSIL is most prevalent in women in their mid-to-late reproductive years (ages 26–48), although it can be seen at any age following the onset of sexual activity.[3,69,71] The cytological diagnosis of HSIL relies on the presence of abnormal

squamous cells that are smaller than those seen in low-grade lesions. The average size of a high-grade squamous cell is equivalent to that of a normal parabasal cell. Diagnostic abnormalities include nuclear enlargement, a marked increase in nuclear:cytoplasmic ratio, irregularity of the nuclear membrane, and irregular chromatin distribution (see Figure 4.3-8). Marked hyperchromasia and abnormal nuclear shapes are also commonly encountered. *Although liquid-based cytology reduces degenerative hyperchromasia, it does not affect hyperchromasia caused by aneuploidy* (Figures 4.3-11, 4.3-12, 4.3-13, and 4.3-14). *The enhancement brought*

73

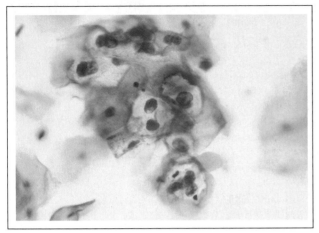

Figure 4.3-10 An AutoCyte Prep Pap test showing a low-grade squamous intraepithelial lesion (LSIL). Note the sharpness of the cytoplasmic borders forming the koilocytic cavity and the excellent nuclear detail (×600).

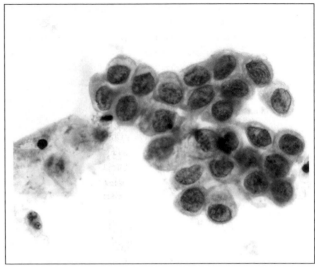

Figure 4.3-12 A ThinPrep Pap test showing a high-grade squamous intraepithelial lesion (HSIL). This cluster of HSIL represents a true syncytium of abnormal cells. The individual nuclei are easily distinguishable, as are the nuclear irregularities and irregular chromatin distribution (×600).

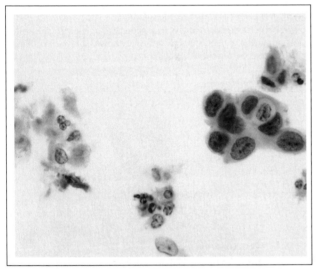

Figure 4.3-11 A ThinPrep Prep Pap test showing a high-grade squamous intraepithelial lesion (HSIL). Note that although marked hyperchromasia is present, nuclear detail is preserved, indicating the true rather than degenerative nature of the increase in chromatin (×600).

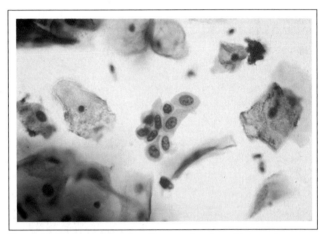

Figure 4.3-13 An AutoCyte Prep Pap test showing a high-grade squamous intraepithelial lesion (HSIL). The abnormal cells are easily identified among normal epithelial cells. The absence of debris, inflammatory cells, and blood greatly facilitate their identification (×200).

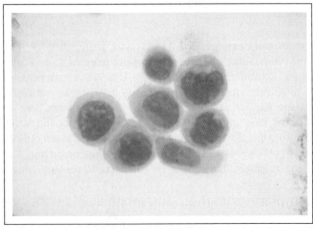

Figure 4.3-14 An AutoCyte Prep Pap test showing a high-grade squamous intraepithelial lesion (HSIL). Note the readily identifiable nuclear convolutions seen in these abnormal nuclei. Nuclear convolutions and irregularities are expected with liquid-based fixation (×600).

about by the optimal fixation of liquid-based slides increases the likelihood that abnormal high-grade cells will exhibit identifiable nuclear irregularities not seen in benign mimics.

Atypical Squamous Cells of Undetermined Significance

The diagnosis of ASC-US is an undesirable but inevitable diagnosis that results from the morphological variability of squamous cells in different physiological and pathological states. While inevitable, the frequency of the ASC-US diagnosis should be minimized.[1] The percentage of women with a cytologic diagnosis of ASC-US who harbor biopsy-proven CIN 2,3 is generally accepted to be around 20%.[3,45] Importantly, some series show that the absolute number of high-grade (HG)–CIN lesions identified in women with ASC-US is greater than the number identified in women with HSIL.[2,28] While criteria exist to separate most cervical cancer precursor lesions from lesions that are reactive in nature, no single criterion or combination of criteria will effectively do so in all cases. The category of ASC-US is therefore reserved for lesions in which a clear distinction between reactive and neoplastic cells cannot be made. *Some studies have shown that liquid-based cytology reduces the proportion of ASC-US diagnoses based on improvements in both the fixation and slide quality. Improved slide quality allows for more cases to be correctly classified as either normal or SIL* (Figures 4.3-15, 4.3-16).

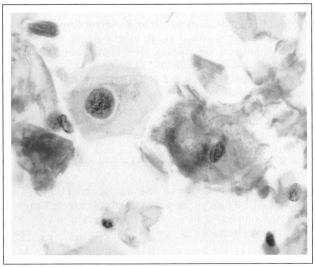

Figure 4.3-15 An AutoCyte Prep Pap test showing atypical squamous cells of undetermined significance (ASC-US). The nuclear enlargement and increase in chromatin content mark this cell as abnormal. The absence of nuclear convolutions or irregularities and the presence of a small nucleolus puts into question the diagnosis of squamous intraepithelial lesion (SIL) (×600).

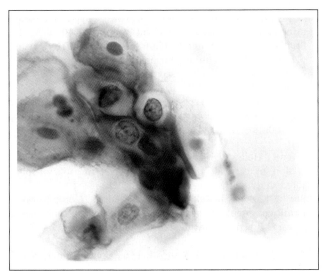

Figure 4.3-16 A ThinPrep Prep Pap test showing atypical squamous cells of undetermined significance (ASC-US). Again, the nuclear enlargement and cytoplasmic cavitation suggests squamous intraepithelial lesion (SIL); however, the finely distributed, delicate chromatin and absence of nuclear irregularities place it in the ASC-US category (×600).

CYTOLOGY OF CERVICAL ADENOCARCINOMA

Glandular lesions of the cervix are not as easily detected as squamous lesions on cytologic examination.[72] Reasons cited for the decreased sensitivity of the cytology for glandular lesions are the subtle nature of the cytologic features of early cervical adenocarcinoma.[73] *Liquid-based thin-layer technology has proven superior to conventional cytology for the diagnosis of adenocarcinoma. The even dispersal of normal cells and excellent preservation of glandular clusters contrast sharply with the appearance of cervical adenocarcinoma. The cytologic characteristics of cervical adenocarcinoma include abundant glandular cellular material, marked crowding of endocervical glandular cells within clusters, architectural aberrations of glandular groups, and cytologic atypia*[73] (Figures 4.3-17, 4.3-18, and 4.3-19). In a retrospective study of cervical

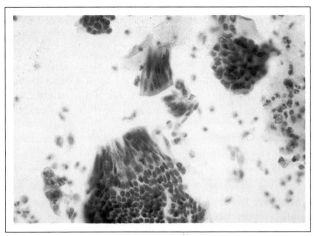

Figure 4.3-17 An AutoCyte Prep Pap test showing abnormal endocervical glandular aggregates. The cells show marked crowding, stratification, and nuclear enlargement. Findings are indicative of cervical adenocarcinoma *in situ* (AIS) (×200).

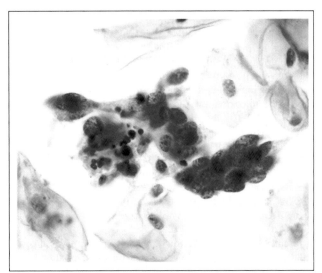

Figure 4.3-18 A ThinPrep Pap test showing abnormal endocervical glandular cells showing marked nuclear enlargement, hyperchromasia, and nuclear crowding. The cells have lost their orderly relationship to each other, a characteristic of adenocarcinoma *in situ* (AIS) (×600).

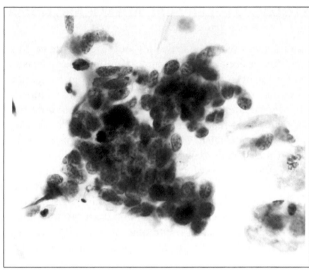

Figure 4.3-19 A ThinPrep Pap test showing abnormal endocervical glandular cells. The aggregate shows crowding and peripheral loss of polarity of the nuclei (feathering), characteristic of adenocarcinoma *in situ* (AIS) (×600).

adenocarcinoma, Ashfaq et al. showed both a higher sensitivity and higher specificity in the diagnosis of adenocarcinoma using ThinPrep compared with conventional cytology.[58]

REFERENCES

1. Widra EA, Dookhan D, Jordan A, et al. Evaluation of the atypical cytologic smear. Validity of the 1991 Bethesda System. J Reprod Med 1994;39:682–684.
2. Benedet JL, Anderson GH. Cervical intraepithelial neoplasia in British Columbia: A comprehensive program for detection, diagnosis, and treatment. Gynecol Oncol 1981;12;280–291.
3. Cramer DW. The role of cervical cytology in the declining morbidity and mortality of cervical cancer. Cancer 1974;34:2018–2027.
4. Laara E, Day NE, Hakama M. Trends in mortality from cervical cancer in the Nordic countries: Association with organised screening programmes. Lancet 1987;1:1247–1249.
5. Macgregor JE, Moss S, Parkin DM, Day NE. Cervical cancer screening in north-east Scotland. IARC Sci Publ 1986;76:25–36.
6. New Papanicolaou test suggested for Air Force dependents. US Med 1978:1.
7. Bogdanich W. The Pap test misses much cervical cancer through labs' errors. Wall Street Journal 1987:1.
8. Chapman B. Crisis in Newport. CAP Today 1994;8:26–33.
9. Meisels A. Cytologic diagnosis of human papillomavirus. Influence of age and pregnancy stage. Acta Cytol 1992;36:80–82.
10. Giles JA, Hudson E, Crow J, et al. Colposcopic assessment of the accuracy of cervical cytology screening. Br Med J (Clin Res Ed) 1988;296:1099–1102.
11. Joseph MG, Cragg F, Wright VC, et al. Cyto-histological correlates in a colposcopic clinic: A 1-year prospective study. Diagn Cytopathol 1991;7:477–481.
12. Kristensen GB, Skyggebjerg KD, Hølund B, et al. Analysis of cervical smears obtained within three years of the diagnosis of invasive cervical cancer. Acta Cytol 1991;35:47–50.
13. MacCormac L, Lew W, King G, Allen PW. Gynaecological cytology screening in South Australia: A 23-year experience. Med J Aust 1988;149:530–536.
14. Mitchell H, Medley G, Giles G. Cervical cancers diagnosed after negative results on cervical cytology: Perspective in the 1980s. BMI 1990;300:1622–1626.
15. Plott AE, Martin FJ, Cheek SW, et al. Measuring screening skills in gynecologic cytology. Results of voluntary self-assessment. Acta Cytol 1987;31:911–923.
16. Soost HJ, Lange HJ, Lehmacher W. Ruffing-Kullmann B. The validation of cervical cytology. Sensitivity, specificity and predictive values. Acta Cytol 1991;35:8–14.
17. van der Graaf Y, Vooijs GP, Gaillard HL, Go DM. Screening errors in cervical cytologic screening. Acta Cytol 1987;31:434–438.
18. Yobs AR, Plott AE, Hicklin MD, et al. Retrospective evaluation of gynecologic cytodiagnosis. II. Interlaboratory reproducibility as shown in rescreening large consecutive samples of reported cases. Acta Cytol 1987;31:900–910.
19. Hutchinson ML, Cassin CM, Ball HG. The efficacy of an automated preparation device for cervical cytology. Am J Clin Pathol 1991;96:300–305.
20. Fahey MT, Irwig L, Macaskill P. Meta-analysis of Pap test accuracy. Am J Epidemiol 1995;141:680–689.
22. Hutchinson ML, Agarwal P, Denault T, et al. A new look at cervical cytology. ThinPrep multicenter trial results. Acta Cytol 1992;36:499–504.
23. Hutchinson ML, Zahniser DJ, Sherman ME, et al. Utility of liquid-based cytology for cervical carcinoma screening: Results of a population-based study conducted in a region of Costa Rica with a high incidence of cervical carcinoma. Cancer 1999;87:48–55.
24. Bishop JW, Bigner SH, Colgan TJ, et al. Multicenter masked evaluation of AutoCyte PREP thin layers with matched conventional smears. Including initial biopsy results. Acta Cytol 1998;42:189–197.
25. Bolick DR, Hellman DJ. Laboratory implementation and efficacy assessment of ThinPrep cervical cancer screening system. Acta Cytol 1998;42:209–213.
26. Hutchinson ML, Isenstein LM, Goodman A, et al. Homogeneous sampling accounts for the increased diagnostic accuracy using ThinPrep Processor. Am J Clin Pathol 1994;101:215–219.
27. Khalbuss WE, Rudomina D, Kauff ND, et al. SpinThin, a simple, inexpensive technique for preparation of thin-layer cervical cytology from liquid-based specimens: Data on 791 cases. Cancer 2000;90:135–142.
28. Aponte-Cipriani SL, Teplitz C, Rorat E, et al. Cervical smears prepared by an automated device versus the conventional method. A comparative analysis. Acta Cytol 1995;39:623–630.
29. Awen C, Hathway S, Eddy W, et al. Efficacy of ThinPrep preparation of cervical smears: A 1,000-case, investigator-sponsored study. Diagn Cytopathol 1994;11:33–37.
30. Bur M, Knowles K, Pekow P, Corral O, et al., Comparison of ThinPrep preparations with conventional cervicovaginal smears. Practical considerations. Acta Cytol 1995;39:631–642.
31. Ferenczy A, Robitaille J, Franco E, et al. Conventional cervical cytologic smears vs. ThinPrep smears. A paired comparison study on cervical cytology. Acta Cytol 1996;40:1136–1142.
32. Geyer JW, Hancock F, Carrico C, Kirkpatrick M. Preliminary evaluation of Cyto-Rich: An improved automated cytology preparation. Diagn Cytopathol 1993;9:417–422.

33. Laverty CR, Thurloe JK, Redman NL, Farnsworth A. An Australian trial of ThinPrep: A new cytopreparatory technique. Cytopathol 1995;6:140–148.

34. McGoogan E, Reith A. Would monolayers provide more representative samples and improved preparations for cervical screening? Overview and evaluation of systems available. Acta Cytol 1996;40:107–119.

35. Sprenger E, Schwarzmann P, Kirkpatrick M, et al. The false-negative rate in cervical cytology. Comparison of monolayers to conventional smears. Acta Cytol 1996;40:81–89.

36. Takahashi M, Naito M. Application of the CytoRich monolayer preparation system for cervical cytology. A prelude to automated primary screening. Acta Cytol 1997;41:1785–1789.

37. Wilbur DC, Cibas ES, Merritt S, et al. ThinPrep Processor. Clinical trials demonstrate an increased detection rate of abnormal cervical cytologic specimens. Am J Clin Pathol 1994;101:209–214.

38. Corkill, M., Knapp, D, and Hutchinson, ML. Improved accuracy for cervical cytology with the ThinPrep method and the endocervical brush-spatula collection procedure. J Lower Gen Tract 1988;167:466–469.

39. Lee KR, Ashfaq R, Birdsong GG, et al. Comparison of conventional Papanicolaou smears and a fluid-based, thin-layer system for cervical cancer screening. Obstet Gynecol 1997;90:278–284.

40. Roberts JM, Gurley AM, Thurloe JK, et al. Evaluation of ThinPrep Pap test as an adjunct to conventional cytology. Med J Aust 1997;167:466–469.

41. Shield PW, Nolan GR, Phillips GE, Cummings MC. Improving cervical cytology screening in a remote, high risk population. Med J Aust 1999;170:255–258.

42. Wang TY, Chen HS, Yang YC, Tsou MC. Comparison of fluid-based, thin-layer processing and conventional Papanicolaou methods for uterine cervical cytology. J Formos Med Assoc 1999;98:500–505.

43. Kunz J, Rondez R, Yoshizaki C, et al. Comparison of conventional PAP smears with thin layer specimen (liquid-based PAP test) and correlation with cytopathological findings with HPV status using the hybrid capture system. Schweiz Rundsch Med Prax 1998;87:1434–1440.

44. Minge L, Fleming M, VanGeem T, Bishop JW. AutoCyte Prep system vs. conventional cervical cytology. Comparison based on 2,156 cases. J Reprod Med 2000;45:179–184.

45. Vassilakos P, Cossali D, Albe X, et al. Efficacy of monolayer preparations for cervical cytology: Emphasis on suboptimal specimens. Acta Cytol 1996;40:496–500.

46. Wilbur DC, Facik MS, Rutkowski MA, et al., Clinical trials of the CytoRich specimen-preparation device for cervical cytology. Preliminary results. Acta Cytol 1997;41:24–29.

47. Carpenter AB, Davey DD. ThinPrep Pap Test: Performance and biopsy follow-up in a university hospital. Cancer 1999;87:105–112.

48. Diaz-Rosario LA, Kabawat SE. Performance of a fluid-based, thin-layer Papanicolaou smear method in the clinical setting of an independent laboratory and an outpatient screening population in New England. Arch Pathol Lab Med 1999;123:817–821.

49. Dupree WB, Suprun HZ, Beckwith DG, et al. The promise and risk of a new technology: The Lehigh Valley Hospital's experience with liquid-based cervical cytology. Cancer 1998;84:202–207.

50. Guidos BJ, Selvaggi SM. Use of the Thin Prep Pap Test in clinical practice. Diagn Cytopathol 1999;20:70–73.

51. Papillo JL, Zarka MA, St. John TL. Evaluation of ThinPrep Pap test in clinical practice. A seven-month, 16,314-case experience in northern Vermont. Acta Cytol 1998;42:203–208.

52. Weintraub J. The coming revolution in cervical cytology: A pathologist's guide for the clinician. Gynecol Obstet 1997;5:2–6.

53. Weintraub J, Morabia A. Efficacy of a liquid-based thin layer method for cervical cancer screening in a population with a low incidence of cervical cancer. Diagn Cytopathol 2000;22:52–59.

54. Tench W. Preliminary assessment of the AutoCyte PREP. Direct-to-vial performance. J Reprod Med 2000;45:912–916.

55. Vassilakos P, Griffin S, Megevand E, Campana A. CytoRich liquid-based cervical cytologic test. Screening results in a routine cytopathology service. Acta Cytol 1998;42:198–202.

56. Vassilakos P, Saurel J, Rondez R. Direct-to-vial use of the AutoCyte PREP liquid-based preparation for cervical-vaginal specimens in three European laboratories. Acta Cytol 1999;43:65–68.

57. Vassilakos P, Schwartz D, de Marval F, et al. Biopsy-based comparison of liquid-based, thin-layer preparations to conventional cytology. J Reprod Med 2000;45:11–16.

58. Ashfaq R, Gibbons D, Vela C, et al. ThinPrep Pap Test. Accuracy for glandular disease. Acta Cytol 1999;43:81–85.

59. Duggan MA. Papnet-assisted, primary screening of cervico-vaginal smears. Eur J Gynaecol Oncol 2000;21:35–42.

60. Wilbur DC, Prey MU, Miller WM, et al. Detection of high grade squamous intraepithelial lesions and tumors using the AutoPap System: Results of a primary screening clinical trial. Cancer 1999;87:354–358.

61. Felix J, Li A, Wang G, Gunn SW, et al. The performance of an image directed cytology system for detecting cervical cancer precursors in a screening population in California. Int J Gynecol Cancer 2006;16:757.

62. Takahashi M, Kimura M, Akagi A, Naitoh M. AutoCyte SCREEN interactive automated primary cytology screening system. A preliminary evaluation. Acta Cytol 1998;42:185–188.

63. Bishop JW, Kaufman RH, Taylor DA. Multicenter comparison of manual and automated screening of AutoCyte gynecologic preparations. Acta Cytol 1999; 43:34–38.

64. Chivukula M, Saad R, Elishaev E, et al. Introduction of the Thin Prep Imaging Systemtrade mark (TIS): Experience in a high volume academic practice. Cytojournal 2007;4:6.

65. Dziura B, Quinn S, Richard K. Performance of an imaging system vs. manual screening in the detection of squamous intraepithelial lesions of the uterine cervix. Acta Cytol 2006;50:309–311.

66. Lozano R. Comparison of computer-assisted and manual screening of cervical cytology. Gynecol Oncol 2007;104:134–138.

67. Miller FS, Nagel LE, Kenny-Moynihan MB. Implementation of the ThinPrep(R) imaging system in a high-volume metropolitan laboratory. Diagn Cytopathol 2007;35:213–217.

68. Solomon D, Schiffman M, Tarone R. Comparison of three management strategies for patients with atypical squamous cells of undetermined significance: Baseline results from a randomized trial. J Natl Cancer Inst 2001;93:293–299.

69. Burghardt E. Early histological diagnosis of cervical cancer. Maj Problems Obstet Gynecol 1973;6:1–401.

70. Carson HJ, DeMay RM. The mode ages of women with cervical dysplasia. Obstet Gynecol 1993;82:430–434.
71. Luthra UK, Prabhakar AK, Seth P, et al. Natural history of pre-cancerous and early cancerous lesions of the uterine cervix. Acta Cytol 1987;31:226–234.
72. Fabiani G, Pittino M, D'Aietti V, et al. Cervical dysplasias. Comparative study of the cytological picture, anatomo-pathologic and age stage. Minerva Gynecol 1987;39:629–632.
73. Raab SS. Can glandular lesions be diagnosed in Pap smear cytology? Diagn Cytopathol 2000;23:127–133.
74. Biscotti CV, Gero MA, Toddy SM, et al. Endocervical adenocarcinoma in situ: An analysis of cellular features. Diagn Cytopathol 1997;17:326–332.

CHAPTER 5

Adjunctive Testing

5.1: Human Papillomavirus Testing

Attila T. Lorincz

KEY POINTS

- HPV testing can detect 30% to 100% more cervical precancers than conventional cytology and 20% to 50% more precancers than liquid-based cytology.
- Women with a persistently positive HPV test should be evaluated carefully for the possibility of occult high-grade cervical intraepithelial neoplasia (CIN) or cancer despite a colposcopic impression of benign epithelium or minimal abnormality.
- In general, an adequate sample for cytology is also an adequate sample for HPV testing.
- Hybrid Capture 2 (HC 2) is an *in vitro*, solution hybridization, signal amplification–based test for detecting DNA and ribonucleic acid (RNA) targets. HC 2 can detect 13 different oncogenic HPV types that represent virtually all important cervical cancer–causing HPV types known worldwide. The test has demonstrated highly reproducible results among study sites.
- In polymerase chain reaction (PCR), the target DNA is selectively amplified by enzymatic means through repeated cycles of denaturation, primer hybridization, and primer extension. The numbers of amplicons rise almost exponentially. After 30 to 40 cycles, more than 1 billion amplicon copies of the original target DNA may be produced.
- *In situ* hybridization (ISH) is less sensitive than PCR or HC 2. The test shows its highest sensitivity and best clinical benefit as a confirmatory test on equivocal biopsies of low-grade squamous intraepithelial lesion (LSIL).
- Typically, 10% to 30% of CIN 2 and CIN 3 and cancer are negative by ISH but positive by PCR and HC 2.
- One reason for poor agreement among accurate HPV DNA tests may be the subjectivity of histopathology that can result in underdiagnosis or overdiagnosis of the biopsy.
- HPV triage of atypical squamous cells of undetermined significance (ASC-US) is clinically useful at all ages, but HPV screening in normal populations should be reserved for women older than 30 years.
- Reflex HPV-based triage of ASC-US detects 90% to 96% of high-grade CIN (HG-CIN), compared with 75% to 85% for a repeat liquid-based cytology.
- In normal screening settings, cytology is slightly more specific than HPV DNA testing for the presence of high-grade cervical disease.

The human papillomavirus (HPV) genome is a small, double-stranded, circular deoxyribonucleic acid (DNA) that consists of three important functional regions[1]: (1) a noncoding upstream regulatory region (URR); (2) an early (E) region that codes for oncoproteins and regulatory proteins (the E6 and E7 oncoproteins are of most interest because, in the carcinogenic HPV types, these proteins antagonize the functions of cellular tumor suppressor proteins, including p53 and RB, respectively); and (3) a late (L) region that codes for two capsid proteins.[1] L1 being the key protein of interest in the new HPV virus-like particle (VLP) prophylactic vaccines.[2] *HPV types are classified by DNA sequence comparison of the L1 region.* A novel HPV type is defined as any complete genomic clone that shares less than 90% nucleotide sequence identity with any other known type. The list of characterized HPV types continues to grow and could eventually number in the several hundreds.[3] Mucosatropic HPV are most often sexually transmitted, and the main sites of infection are genital, anal, oral, and nasopharyngeal skin; these types (Table 5.1-1) cause the majority of clinically important HPV disease, including warts, papules, diverse flat lesions, and cervical, anal, vulvar, vaginal, penile, oral, tonsillar, and other assorted carcinomas. Nearly 100% of cervical cancers and precancers have detectable HPV DNA, almost all of which are high risk (HR) or intermediate risk (IR) HPV types.[4]

Exposure to HPV typically produces a sexually transmitted infection (STI) and may progress to a clinically apparent sexually transmitted disease (STD) such as genital warts and various flat lesions. A large majority (>90%) of these HPV STI and STD spontaneously resolve within 2 years. The STD and carcinogenic effects of HR- and IR-HPV (collectively called *carcinogenic HPV*) are temporally quite distinct and may be confounded by co-infection of low-risk (LR) types such as HPV 6 and 11 that predominantly cause genital warts. A minority of HR-IR–HPV infections persists over a span of 5 to 20 years, and these are the true cancer precursors. *Persistent infection with HR-IR–HPV is a necessary step in the development of certain cancers.*[4] Thus *the clinical*

Table 5.1-1 Human Papillomavirus Screening Tests Should Detect All High Risk and Most Intermediate Risk Types

HR- and IR-HPV*
16, 18, *26*, 31, 33, 35, 39, 45, 51, 52, *53*, 56, 58, 59, *66*, 68, *73, 82*

LR-HPV*
6, 11, *40*, 42, 43, 44, *54, 61, 70, 72, 81*

HPV, Human papillomavirus; *HR*, high risk; *IR*, intermediate risk; *LR*, low risk.
*For routine clinical use HPV infections should be identified only at relevant viral load levels. HPV types that are set in italics are not part of the probe sets in the HC 2 test but some infections are detected as a result of cross-reactivity. Many of the italicized HR-IR HPVs should be considered for addition to next generation HPV tests. HPV types 16, 18, and 45 are considered HR while the remaining HPVs are the IR types. The LR HPV indicated are a partial listing.

negative predictive value (NPV) of a highly accurate and well-validated HPV DNA test can reach 99.95%.[4-6]

CERVICAL CANCER SCREENING

In 2002 there were an estimated 493,000 worldwide cases of cervical cancer and 273,000 deaths.[7] Widespread implementation of cervical cytology screening has produced a dramatic reduction in cervical cancer incidence and deaths in many developed countries. Unfortunately *cervical cancer remains the second leading cause of cancer-related female deaths in resource-poor regions of the world.*[8]

Because HPV infection precedes the appearance of neoplastic disease by many years,[9,10] HPV DNA testing offers the possibility of further large reductions in cancer incidence if implemented wisely and widely. Some of the recognized uses of HPV DNA testing include the management of women with Papanicolaou (Pap) cytology showing atypical squamous cells of undetermined significance (ASC-US), follow-up after treatment as a test of cure, and the routine population-based screening of at-risk women.[11-16]

A strong impetus driving the clinical adoption of HPV testing is recognition that Pap cytology is prone to irreducible errors.[17-19] *HPV testing can detect 30% to 100% more cervical precancers compared with conventional cytology and 20% to 50% more precancers than liquid-based Pap cytology.* HPV testing has an equivalent or superior specificity to cytology for ASC-US triage but is 5% to 10% less specific than cytology in general population screening applications.[11,13,14,20] An important confounder of clinical performance assessment is the inadequacy of the gold standard. Even in experienced hands, colposcopy may not find the most significant disease in as many as 30% of cases.[21-24] Thus HPV testing can help colposcopists more accurately define a cervix lacking neoplastic changes: a colposcopically normal–appearing cervix that is negative by a highly sensitive HPV DNA test such as Hybrid Capture II (HC 2, Digene, a Qiagen Company Gaithersburg, Md.) or by a clinically validated HPV polymerase chain reaction (PCR) test is very unlikely to harbor occult disease. Conversely, *if the HPV test is persistently positive for carcinogenic HPV types, the colposcopist should be careful to rule out occult high-grade cervical intraepithelial neoplasia*

(HG-CIN) or cancer, even if the colposcopic impression is of benign epithelium or minimal abnormality.

There is growing interest in the potential clinical applications of HPV genotyping related to the recognition that some oncogenic HPV types may be more carcinogenic that others. For example, the HR-HPV types 16, 18, and 45 (in combination associated with 70% to 80% of invasive cervical cancer) have been reported to have elevated odds ratios for cancer as compared with the IR-HPV types. HR-HPVs appear to cause infections with an apparently elevated predisposition to HG-CIN, especially CIN 3 (predominantly HPV 16), cervical squamous carcinomas (mostly HPV 16), and adenocarcinomas (equally HPV 16 and HPV 18 with some HPV 45).[25-31]

One of the evolving clinical roles for HPV genotyping is to test cytologically normal women initially positive by an HPV carcinogenic screening test to determine whether there is infection by HPV 16, 18, or 45. These women may need more vigilant follow-up, including the possibility of prompt referral to colposcopy, whereas women infected by only IR-HPVs may be deferred to a repeat HPV and cytology test in 1 year.[26,27,32]

TYPES OF PROBE TESTS

Probe tests can be *in vitro* or *in situ* hybridization (ISH) tests. The tests can be subdivided into three broad groups: (1) nonamplified tests, (2) target amplification–based tests, and (3) signal amplification–based tests.

An important consideration for every type of test is the collection of a good clinical specimen. Although it is quite easy to collect exfoliated cells for use in HC 2 or PCR, there is nevertheless a need for some training and care. *The general rule is that a good sample for cytology is also a good sample for HPV DNA testing.* Specimens for HPV DNA testing may be collected into special media, such as Specimen Transport Medium (STM, Digene), PreservCyt (PC, Cytyc, a subsidiary of Hologic, Bedford, MA), or CytoRich (Tripath, a subsidiary of Becton Dickinson Company, Franklin Lakes, NJ). In the case of exfoliated cervical cells collected into PC medium for a ThinPrep cytology test (Figure 5.1-1), a 2-mL aliquot can be processed for HC 2 HPV DNA testing by a simple procedure that involves centrifugation of the cells into a pellet or by using a newer filtration procedure that reduces the labor requirements.[33] When a clinician desires an HPV test to accompany conventional cytology, it is necessary to collect a separate specimen into a vial of STM with a specially designed cone-shaped brush (Figure 5.1-2).

When HC 2 HPV testing is done on the residual specimen from a liquid-based cytology test, it is expected that 2% to 5% of residual specimens will be reported as "quantity not sufficient" (QNS) for HPV DNA testing. QNS is indicated if the PC vial has less than 4 mL of liquid after processing for cytology. However, even in these cases an HC 2 test can be performed if at least 1 mL is available. Under such circumstances, positive results are valid, but negative results may not be valid and collection of an

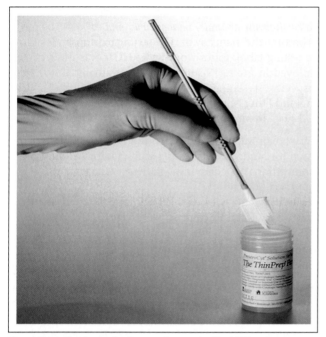

Figure 5.1-1 Specimens for Pap cytology and reflex HPV testing may be collected into a liquid cytology medium such as PreservCyt by employing a broom *(shown)* or a spatula and brush combination.

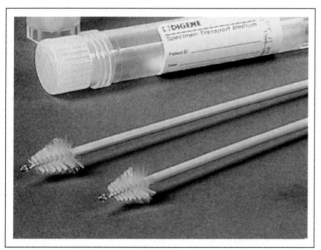

Figure 5.1-2 Hybrid Capture HPV test cervical sampler, a cone-shaped brush for collecting a specimen of exfoliated cells from the uterine cervix. After clearing the cervical transformation zone of mucus, the brush is inserted into the os until the large outer bristles are barely visible. The brush is turned slowly counterclockwise for three full turns and slowly removed. It is placed into the liquid in the accompanying transport tube. The shaft is broken at the marked score line, and the tube is capped for shipping to the HPV testing laboratory.

additional specimen is advisable. This creates a dilemma because it may require the affected women to return in order to obtain additional specimens for testing.

The cause of QNS specimens is usually related to: (1) adequacy of sampling of the cervix, (2) adequacy of transfer of cells from the sampling instruments to the PC vials, or (3) other laboratory technical issues. The reason behind this inadequate

sampling can be explained through an understanding of the mechanism by which the liquid-based cytology specimen is produced. After collecting a clinical specimen into liquid medium, the cells are separated from the preservative and collected onto a micropore filter. The process of filtration is terminated when a sufficient number of cells have been collected on the filter, leaving the remaining preservative solution for ancillary testing. If an inadequate number of cells are present in the preservative solution due to poor collection or specimen transfer, the process of filtration is not terminated in time, leaving very little preservative solution for use in ancillary testing. One way of avoiding these QNS issues is to remove a 2 mL "PreQuot" for HPV testing before the specimen is submitted for cytology. Another is to collect a separate specimen into a vial of STM with a specially designed, cone-shaped brush. This is especially recommended when the specimen is to be used for primary screening. A related issue is the possibility that the liquid volume in the collection vial may be adequate (usually the case with STM specimens) to conduct an HPV test but the specimen may nevertheless be inadequate for HPV testing because of the presence of assay inhibitors. HC 2 does not suffer from inhibition, but this issue is of concern for PCR, necessitating the performance of an inhibition assessment, which usually involves the amplification of a cellular gene such as β-globin or the use of a special added internal control nucleic acid target. A flow cell analysis for cell subsets has been proposed as a way to reduce the risk of Pap or HPV test failures due to inadequate cellularity.[34]

Hybrid Capture II

The most common commercially available HPV test used for clinical purposes is HC 2, an *in vitro,* solution hybridization, signal amplification–based test for detecting DNA or RNA targets (Figure 5.1-3). *HC 2 can detect at least 13 different carcinogenic HPV types that represent virtually all important cancer-causing HPV types known worldwide.* The test is formatted as a solution hybridization of RNA probes with HPV DNA genomic targets coupled to an immunologically based back end, similar to an enzyme-linked immunosorbent assay (ELISA).[35] Table 5.1-2 shows the temporal sequence of steps in the HC 2 test. Long, unlabeled, single-stranded RNA probe manufactured by *in vitro* transcription is used in the test to hybridize the HPV DNA genome that may be present in the clinical specimen; the entire genome of the virus is the target. Then antibody conjugate reactive to RNA-DNA hybrid is supplied and recognizes multiple short stretches of RNA-DNA hybrid in a specific but non–sequence-dependent manner, such that hundreds of antibodies can coat a single genomic hybrid of HPV DNA. Each immobilized alkaline phosphatase enzyme catalyzes the dephosphorylation of numerous molecules of a chemiluminescent dioxetane substrate, producing a steady stream of photons that are counted by the photomultiplier tube of a luminometer (Figure 5.1-4).

HC 2 has the capability for quantitation of DNA targets over a four log range; however, the test is usually regarded

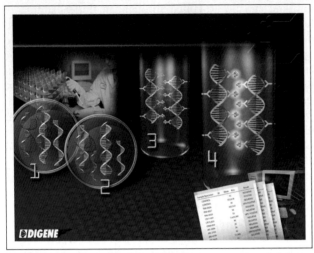

Figure 5.1-3 The key steps of the Hybrid Capture procedure. *1*, Release and denature nucleic acids. *2*, Hybridize single-stranded RNA probe with target nucleic acid. *3*, Capture RNA:DNA hybrids onto a solid phase. *4*, Allow reaction of captured hybrids with multiple antibody conjugates and detect the enhanced chemiluminescent signal.

Table 5.1-2 Hybrid Capture 2 Procedure

Assay Step	Time	Temperature
Sample denaturation	45 min	65°C
Hybridization with full genomic RNA probes	1 hr	65°C
Capture on the surface of plate coated with RNA:DNA antibody	1 hr	Ambient
Detection react with reagent 1 alkaline phosphatase RNA:DNA antibody conjugate	30 min	Ambient
Wash (six times)	3–5 min	Ambient
Detection react with reagent 2 chemiluminescent substrate	15 min	Ambient
Read in plate luminometer	3 min	Ambient
Total time	~4.5 hr	

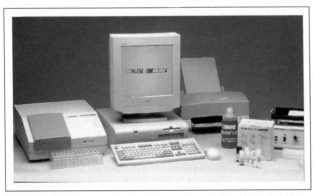

Figure 5.1-4 Equipment for detecting reaction results of the HC 2 test. The luminometer is the low instrument on the left.

as semi-quantitative.[11,35,36] *Numerous studies have shown HC 2 to be clinically accurate, reproducible, and robust,*[37] hence, it has become the mainstay of HPV testing in thousands of routine testing laboratories worldwide. HC 2 was the HPV test employed in the ALTS study and in essentially all the large prospective screening studies worldwide to date.[20] The U.S. Food and Drug Administration (FDA) indications for use of HC 2 may be summarized as follows:

- In women 30 years and older, the HC 2 test can be used for adjunctive screening with cytology (liquid or conventional) to determine patient management (primary screening)
- To test patients with ASC-US cytology to determine the need for referral to colposcopy (triage)

Polymerase Chain Reaction

Target-amplified tests create extra copies of the desired target sequence (Figure 5.1-5) by an enzymatic polymerization process that copies the original DNA or RNA. *In PCR,*[38] *the target DNA is selectively amplified through repeated cycles of temperature changes that facilitate denaturation, primer hybridization, and primer extension by DNA polymerase (e.g., Taq polymerase) to produce amplicons, the numbers of which rise almost exponentially.* After 30 to 40 PCR cycles, as few as 10 initial HPV DNA molecules within a few thousand cells in a portion of a biopsy, a cell smear, or a liquid cytology aliquot can be turned into billions of identical amplicon copies. PCR is a remarkably flexible procedure and has been used to detect HPV DNA in a diversity of specimen types

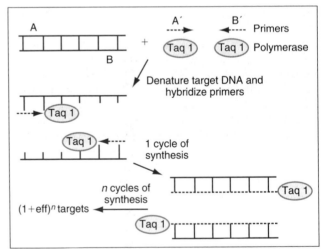

Figure 5.1-5 Performance of one cycle of PCR synthesis. Double-stranded target DNA is denatured by heating to approximately 100°C and then cooled to 50° to 70°C, to allow the two primers (A' and B') to hybridize specifically to their complementary DNA target sequences (A and B), usually a few hundred nucleotides apart. The primers direct synthesis of new DNA toward each other by means of a polymerase enzyme such as Taq 1, converting the initial two DNA target strands into four target strands, upon which another full PCR cycle can be performed. After *n* cycles, one double-stranded target will become $(1 + \text{eff})^n$ double-stranded amplicons (or targets), where *n* is the number of PCR cycles and eff is the efficiency of the amplification, a number between 0 and 1. In an ideal PCR with 100% efficiency, eff = 1. Usually, the value of *eff* is 0.7 to 0.8.

including fresh or fixed exfoliated cell preparations and biopsies, such as cytology and sections of paraffin-embedded tissue biopsies from CIN and cervical cancer. Diverse ways are available to detect the PCR amplicons. For example, amplicons may be spotted and immobilized on membranes, or they may be electrophoresed in gels to resolve molecules of various sizes. In gel-based procedures, detection may be accomplished by fluorescent dye (e.g., ethidium bromide, cyber green) staining followed by photography or direct digitization of the gels or photographs. For added sensitivity and specificity, the amplicons may be treated like targets and hybridized with probes in dot blot, Southern blot, ELISA or microarray formats.[38]

Two currently popular HPV genotyping PCR formats are line blots and microchips in which type-specific capture probes are arrayed onto a solid surface such as a membrane or silica-based support and the amplicons are captured. Immobilization of amplicons allows the other reactants to be eliminated by washing, after which the purified amplicons can be detected by direct fluorescence or by a multitude of enzymatically generated signals.[38] This general approach allows for rapid and flexible genotyping for single or multiple infections, because each HPV type or combination of types present in a specimen can be visually or digitally read from the solid support based on the pattern of colored bands.

A newer method that shows much promise is to attach discrete oligonucleotide capture probes to differentially dyed 5.5-μm polystyrene beads in a set called a liquid bead array system. For example, there may be a special bead with a capture oligonucleotide for HPV 16 and another one for HPV 18.[39] The Luminex x-MAP system (Luminex Corporation, Austin, Tex.) is a liquid bead array analysis procedure capable of up to 100-multiplex discrimination in a homogeneous format. In one variation of this procedure, the PCR reactions from clinical specimens of interest are performed with at least one primer that is labeled with biotin. Amplicons from discrete PCR reactions are then hybridized, each in a separate tube, with a mixture of beads. Thus certain amplicons if present (e.g., an HPV 16 amplicon) hybridize to their specifically designed bead (HPV 16 capture bead) but not to other bead types. Hybridized amplicons are then reacted with a phycoerythrin-streptavidin conjugate that localizes the phycoerythrin dye to the beads with the attached biotinylated hybrids. The mixture of beads is then passed linearly through a flow cell and interrogated by a red and a green laser. The red laser determines the identity of each bead as it passes by the detector, and the green laser excites any phycoerythrin that may be attached to the bead to allow simultaneous detection of a positive signal (Figure 5.1-6).

Many real-time detection versions of PCR (Figure 5.1-7) have become very popular in recent years. One common method is the TaqMan test.[38,40] In this method, signal is generated during the PCR reaction by degradation of a TaqMan signal oligonucleotide probe. The probe in its dark state contains a fluorescent molecule usually attached to one of the nucleotide bases that is juxtaposed with a similarly attached quenching molecule. As a PCR reaction proceeds, the initially dark signal oligonucleotide hybridized to the target in a region between

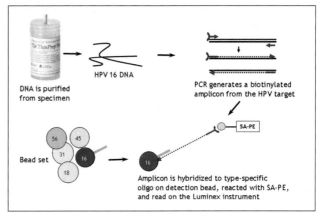

Figure 5.1-6 Detection of HPV by a PCR liquid bead array. In one version of this procedure, HPV DNA is purified from clinical specimens by a standard silica microsphere protocol. PCR is conducted employing GP+ primers (indicated by the blue arrows) where one member of the primer pair is biotinylated (indicated by the arc). After PCR amplification, the biotinylated amplicon strands are hybridized to partner-capture oligonucleotides on members of the bead array (HPV 16 capture oligo shown as a green line). Signal generation is accomplished by specific reaction and attachment of streptavidin-phycoerythrin (SA-PE) to biotin moieties on the amplicon-oligo-beads. Completed bead arrays are then passed through a Luminex instrument, where each bead type in the set is identified and signals are enumerated.

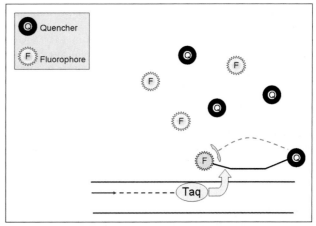

Figure 5.1-7 TaqMan PCR, a real-time detection test with quantitative capability. Target is revealed when quenched fluorophores (quenching is indicated by the arc and the dotted grey line attached to the quencher moiety) are released by the Taq exonuclease activity from the proximity of the quencher during the PCR process. Increasing amounts of fluorophores build up during each cycle and, when irradiated by light of a specific wavelength, they emit light of a longer wavelength that can be quantitated.

the two primers is digested by the Taq polymerase exonuclease activity, in which process the quencher is separated from close proximity to the fluorophore. These released fluorophores are then excited by an appropriate wavelength of incident light, and the longer wavelengths emitted are read by a modified fluorescent reader.

The most commonly employed PCR primers are directed to the conserved HPV L region. Four such sets of primers are the consensus primer pair MY09/MY11 (the MY set)[41]; the general primers GP5/GP6[42]; the PGMY primers, which are a family of related primers[43]; and the SPF primers.[44] Other sets of primers have been reported in the literature, such as consensus E1 primers[45] and type-specific E6 primers.[46] The MY primers produce a PCR amplicon of approximately 450 nucleotides in length, whereas the GP primer pair produces an amplicon of approximately 140 nucleotides from an area of L1 that overlaps with the MY region. Debate continues as to which HPV PCR method is better. Primer sets that produce smaller amplicon sizes (GP, PGMY, and SPF) are better for amplification of targets from paraffin-embedded sections, because the longer MY amplicons are not synthesized as efficiently owing to formalin cross-linking in the tissue. The SPF primers seem to have a very high analytic sensitivity, perhaps greater than that of the other primer systems, but important questions remain about their relatively diminished specificity and clinical utility.

Theoretically it is possible to make PCR ever more sensitive by combining optimized target amplification with newer highly sensitive signal amplification. In a research setting, this may be desirable. *Generally, ultra-high sensitivity is not needed in the clinical context for HPV detection, as excessive sensitivity can quickly become a liability that markedly reduces the utility of the results owing to concerns over contamination (analytic false positives)[47,48] or detection of true but inconsequential amounts of HPV DNA (clinical false positives).[49,50]*

In Situ Hybridization (ISH)

ISH is usually applied to histology sections or cell smears and can provide excellent morphologic detail of tissue or cellular contents[51] (Figure 5.1-8a to 5.1-8c). Thin tissue sections or cells are permeabilized by a gentle process involving enzymes, detergents, or both so that small pores permit access of probes to the nucleus.[51] Hybridization of probe to target occurs within the permeabilized nuclei or other organelles. Morphology is often very good, but there may be some loss of detail depending on the harshness of the procedure (especially the permeabilization steps), the type of tissue, and the method of tissue fixation. Neutral-buffered 10% formalin is a particularly good tissue fixative that is compatible with ISH.

Because ISH is so different from *in vitro* tests, it is difficult to make direct comparisons. A disadvantage of ISH is that it is relatively labor intensive and does not lend itself readily to high throughput manual testing or automation. As performed in most laboratories, *ISH is less sensitive than PCR or HC 2. The test shows its highest clinical sensitivity and best utility as a confirmatory test on equivocal biopsies of suspected LSIL or other warty conditions.* The presence of a nuclear HPV signal assists in confirmation of the nature of the lesion (Figure 5.1-9ab). HG-CIN and cancer may have low levels of HPV per cell and biopsies are often negative by ISH, which usually requires 5 or 10 genomes or more per cell to show a positive result. *Typically, 10% to 30% of cancers and HG-CIN positive by HC 2 or PCR are negative by ISH.*[52–54] ISH can be enhanced by sophisticated fluorescence-based confocal microscopy with digitized image detection and computer enhancement.

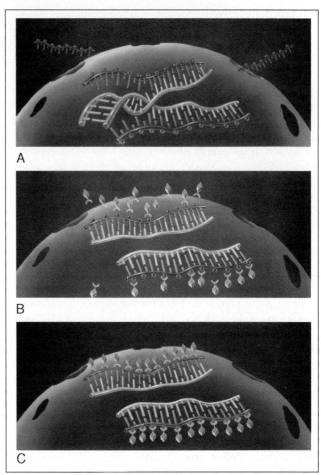

Figure 5.1-8 Key steps in the *in situ* hybridization procedure. **A**, Probes are drifting into the cell nucleus through pores created by detergent and/or protease treatment. The probe molecules are starting to hybridize with a partially unraveled HPV DNA target in the cell nucleus. **B**, Two probe molecules have fully formed hybrids with each strand of an original target duplex. Enzyme molecules *(diamonds with curved attachments)* are starting to attach to the hybrids via the label on the probes (one example might be biotins on the probes binding streptavidin-conjugated alkaline phosphatase). **C**, Fully decorated hybrids containing numerous enzymes per hybrid. These enzymes will then catalyze deposition of colored precipitates that will stain the nuclei of HPV-infected cells, as shown in Figure 5.1-9.

A signal-amplified version of ISH that employs tyramide deposition to enhance the signal is sometimes called the *CARD-ISH test.*[55] CARD-ISH can achieve a sensitivity of one copy of HPV per cell, and the method is excellent for research purposes. Despite the obvious attraction of high sensitivity, CARD-ISH is a finicky and difficult procedure for routine use and requires special expertise and care to avoid nonspecific staining.

Another limitation of ISH is that it may show cross-reactivity among HPV types. In particular, some versions that employ biotin-labeled DNA probes can be misleading for type determination, especially in the hands of inexperienced users. Careful attention to reagent preparation, hybridization and washing conditions, and slide interpretation can overcome most problems and provide accurate typing.

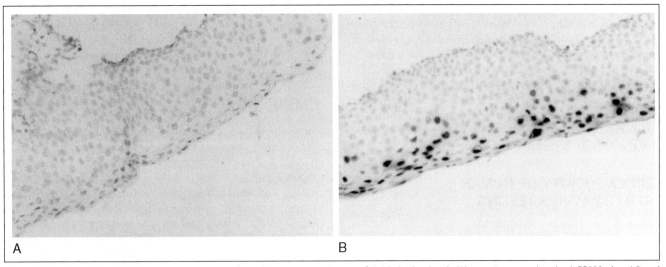

Figure 5.1-9 An *in situ* hybridization showing sections from the same tissue biopsy of CIN hybridized with **(A)** negative control probe (pBR322 plasmid) and **(B)** HPV probe. The positive reaction can be seen by the darkly stained nuclei of the superficial epithelial cells.

TEST VALIDATION

Many papers on HPV testing are limited by insufficient details on clinical validation. Of particular importance is the difference between clinical and analytic performance. Analytic sensitivity often refers to a lower limit of detection, usually reported as a genome or copy number per milliliter or per aliquot. Some authors define analytic sensitivity as the proportion of test-positive specimens among all specimens that contain the target of interest. Clinical sensitivity typically refers to the detection of a specific disease endpoint such as HG-CIN; this parameter is reported as a proportion or a percentage. As may be obvious from the preceding statement, there is a substantial danger of confusion if the various measurement terms are not specified adequately. As there is an HPV viral load of approximately 50,000 or more HPV genomes per mL of clinical specimen in the vast majority of high-grade CIN, the analytically more sensitive tests that can detect well below this level may not confer any clinical advantage over tests that are designed to detect HPV viral load at more relevant levels.[50] Furthermore, some analytically ultrasensitive tests appear to be less sensitive than generally presumed due to issues such as inhibition effects, genome deletions, and others. On the other hand, a test that has too much analytic sensitivity may produce poor clinical specificity if it detects low levels of viral DNA not related to clinical disease or risk of cancer. Diagnostic test performance predicted from theoretic considerations is an inadequate indicator of actual real-world performance. The complexity of carcinogenesis and HPV natural history make it imperative that tests for HPV intended for routine clinical use undergo extensive clinical validation studies in realistic-use settings.

The literature reveals a substantial variation in the reported performance of HPV probe tests relative to each other and to histology. In many studies, the HC 2 and PCR tests show excellent sensitivity and specificity for detecting disease.[11,56–59] In other studies, the correlations are not as good.[59,60] There are many possible reasons for these variations; for example, HC 2 is prone to cross-reactivity,[61,62] whereas PCR is prone to inhibitory substances. These inhibitors can totally or partially interfere with the amplification step and thus produce lower clinical sensitivity than anticipated. With HC 2, inhibition is not of concern; this fact may be responsible in part for the observations from many screening studies that HC 2 identifies a greater percentage of HPV-positive HG-CIN and cervical cancer than PCR.[59] Although HC 2 appears to have better performance than (non-commercial) "home brew" PCR tests, initial data from some commercially available PCR kits appear promising. In the past, many versions of HPV PCR tests were associated with an elevation in the proportion of false-positive specimens. This problem has lessened somewhat in recent years through the implementation of stringent contamination control procedures and better understanding of test cutoff determination; however, in some instances a lower clinical sensitivity has been the trade-off.

Specimen adequacy is critical to avoid false-negative results in both HC 2 and PCR. During the clinical examination, some essential elements to consider are proper access to potential HG-CIN lesions that may be buried deep inside the endocervical canal, especially in older women. Brush devices are better at cutting through mucus or other material to access HPV-infected cells. Carefully standardized sampling should be learned by every clinician attempting to use HPV tests in screening and patient management. Dacron swabs are not optimal but may be acceptable for self-sampling or for use in pregnant women.

Another reason for poor agreement between accurate HPV DNA tests and histology may be related to subjectivity of the histopathology.[17] CIN 2 is often categorized with CIN 3 into the single category of HG-CIN. Occasional errors of reading on histology may inadvertently elevate CIN 1 into CIN 2, allowing CIN 1 to be falsely incorporated into the HG-CIN diagnosis. Although most CIN 1 lesions are infected by carcinogenic HPVs, some are caused by LR-HPV types; if such a CIN 1 is accidentally assigned to the HG-CIN group, the result will be an apparent false-negative for a probe test that detects only carcinogenic HPV types. In some instances, variants of immature squamous metaplasia (usually HPV negative) or other artifacts may be misread as CIN 2 or CIN 3.

CLINICAL UTILITY OF HUMAN PAPILLOMAVIRUS TESTING

Carcinogenic HPV types are strong determinants of cervical cancer. *The relative risk for cervical cancer in infected women is almost a hundredfold higher that in uninfected women.*[4,25] HPV is highly prevalent in young, sexually active populations, with an incidence of up to 20%.[63,64] Infection is mostly transient with a mean duration of about 8 months for LR-HPV types and 13 months for carcinogenic HPV types. In a minority of infected individuals, carcinogenic HPV types become persistent and predispose the women to cancer 10 to 40 years later.

In light of these facts and, in particular, of the frequent occurrence of HPV infection in young women who are at lowest risk for neoplastic disease, it is apparent that HPV testing should be applied differentially at different ages. *With respect to the triage of women with ASC-US Pap smears, HPV testing has a good positive predictive value at all ages, and the very high (>99%) negative predictive value of the HPV test can reassure clinicians and women who test HPV negative that there is a very low probability of missed disease.*[13–15,68] *Most HPV screening strategies call for HPV DNA testing in women older than 30 years, although some authors have recently suggested that the test may have clinical utility in screening women starting at age 25.*[66,67]

As a triage tool for women with ASC-US Pap tests, the HC 2 test was employed in the ALTS study and other important ASC-US cytology triage studies involving cumulatively more than 5000 women, with final disease diagnoses totaling more than 500 cases of HG-CIN.[20] *The results showed that reflex or immediate HPV-based triage had a significantly improved clinical sensitivity of 90% to 96%, compared with 75% to 85% for the repeat cytology. The specificity of the HC 2 HPV test was equivalent to or better than cytology.*

HPV testing can be used in a number of situations to provide clinicians with information on potential alternative management strategies for patients with previous abnormal diagnoses. These other uses include: (1) follow-up after treatment as a "test of cure"[16,69–71]; (2) resolution of discordant cytology, colposcopy, and histology findings[72]; and (3) as a reassurance tool in combination with colposcopy to more effectively rule out the possibility of missed disease.[21–24]

HPV testing has been employed in more than 15 large population screening trials in various countries, with a combined total of more than 200,000 women. Most investigations enrolled between 5000 and 15,000 women; these included studies in the United Kingdom,[73] Germany,[6] France,[5] The Netherlands,[74] Switzerland,[75] Finland,[76] Canada[77], Costa Rica,[11] Mexico,[78] South Africa,[79] China,[22] and Italy.[80] The studies all concluded that HPV DNA testing was much more sensitive in detecting HG-CIN and cancer than cervical cytology, although the latter was almost always the more specific test. *The median screening sensitivity of HPV testing combined with cytology for detecting women with HG-CIN and invasive cancer was 100% (range 76% to 100%), compared with 68% (range 38% to 94%) for the conventional cytology.* The Italian study by Ronco et al.[80] is of particular interest because it was the first randomized control trial (RCT) of HPV testing and included 16,706 women in the HPV arm and 16,658 in the cytology control arm. Ronco et al. demonstrated that when screening women over the age of 30 years, HPV testing detected 97% of HG-CIN versus only 74% for the liquid-based cytology. The specificity for HPV testing was similar to that of cytology: 93% and 95% respectively.

HUMAN PAPILLOMAVIRUS DNA POSITIVITY AND RISK OF FUTURE CERVICAL INTRAEPITHELIAL NEOPLASIA 2,3 AND CANCER

HPV testing can also identify women at risk for prevalent and future high-grade CIN. At the Kaiser Permanente clinics in Portland, Oregon, a cohort study followed about 23,000 women over a period of 10 years. Tests for oncogenic HPV DNA were conducted on cervicovaginal lavage specimens collected at baseline in 1989, and then the women were followed by routine annually scheduled cervical cytology. After 10 years of follow-up, all accumulated data were examined.[9] Among the group of women with normal or minimally abnormal cytologies, 171 cases of CIN 3 were detected over the 10-year period. Of these cases, only 33% had an abnormal cytology (>ASC-US) at or close to the baseline. The rest of the HG-CIN was subsequently discovered or developed over the ensuing 10 years and was detected by repeat Pap testing and colposcopy. In contrast, just one baseline positive HR-HPV test identified a population of at-risk women in whom two-thirds of the CIN 3 cases developed.

Studies by various authors demonstrated that women persistently infected by HR-HPV were at high risk for the development of CIN 2,3.[9,10,81–83] A recent cohort study conducted in Copenhagen, Denmark[10] extended these observations and arrived at conclusions similar to those of the Portland study. The Copenhagen study also provides data on women positive for HR-HPV on two separate occasions. Specifically, a cohort of younger women (8656 subjects; age range 22–33 years) and a smaller cohort of older women (1578 subjects; age range 40–50 years) were enrolled in the study and asked to provide a specimen for HPV DNA testing. The

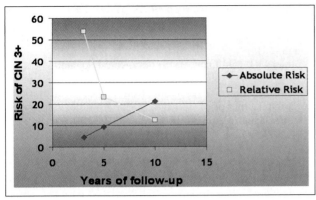

Figure 5.1-10 Absolute and relative risk of CIN 3 or more severe disease (CIN 3+) during 10-year follow-up of cytologically negative older women as a function of carcinogenic HPV positivity. (From Kjaer S, Hogdall E, Frederiksen K, et al. The absolute risk of cervical abnormalities in high-risk human papillomavirus-positive, cytologically normal women over a 10-year period. Cancer Res 2006;66:10630–10636.)

women were followed through the Danish Pathology Data Bank, and the development of HG-CIN was compared among subsets with different test results. The absolute risk of CIN 3 or cancer (CIN 3+) within 10 years among the cytologically normal younger women with a positive HPV test was 13.6% (10.9–16.2), whereas the absolute risk was 21.2% (2.7–36.1) among older women (Figure 5.1-10). Among younger women who were also positive for carcinogenic HPV at 2 years before baseline, the 10-year risk of CIN 3+ was 18% (14.6–21.5). The authors suggested that even a single positive HPV test in cytologically negative women is substantially predictive of HG-CIN and suggest that HC 2 testing may help stratify women into different risk categories.

Cost-modeling studies have indicated that HPV testing by means of a cocktail of 13 or 14 (HC 2 probe B set plus HPV 66) carcinogenic types is a more effective means of managing women with ASC-US Pap smears[84] and is also cost effective for general population screening.[85] The drop in specificity of HPV testing combined with cytology can be accommodated quite well in current screening programs by extending the screening intervals.[86,87]

FUTURE DIRECTIONS

Approximately ten million HPV DNA tests are conducted in the United States annually as of this writing, and it appears that incorporation of HPV testing into routine clinical practice continues to increase. Although HPV testing is also conducted in Europe and other countries, it is used less commonly. Fully automated instruments are in development that should make routine HPV testing for triage and screening more accurate, less expensive, and more broadly available. HPV testing may be conducted in conjunction with the cervical cytology. In other situations HPV testing may be a superior alternative to cervical cytology, especially

in countries that lack sufficient numbers of qualified cyto-technicians or the resources to install automated image screeners. Self-sampling for HPV shows potential value as a new avenue in difficult screening situations.[65,78] Among populations where cytology screening programs do not exist due to patient resistance or poor access to care, there might be better coverage and compliance if specimens could be self-collected and submitted to HPV testing laboratories from the privacy of a patient's home. The cytology interval might also be extended to 3 years or more if supplemented by a home HPV test in the intervening years.

There has been reluctance in some medical quarters to employ HPV testing for routine screening because most infections do not progress to cancer. Thus there is concern that this may lead to excessive and costly interventions and lead to negative psychologic consequences for patients; these concerns are especially acute in Europe. The best age cutoff for HPV mass screening by HPV testing also continues to be debated. Most clinicians believe the ideal age is between 25 and 35 years. However, even with this age stratification there is a clear need for additional improvement in the specificity of HPV tests.

One way to achieve this specificity is through the use of reflex tests. Many novel reflex tests are under investigation to follow an initial HPV DNA positive result. These include: (1) HPV genotyping, (2) HPV viral load, (3) HPV RNA expression, and (4) p16 and other marker panels. HPV genotyping is a front-runner among these potential triage tests, as discussed previously. Women infected with HPV 16 and 18 in particular appear to warrant careful clinical attention and follow-up regardless of concurrent cytology results. It may be possible to further stratify women according to risk for cancer on the basis of the levels E6 and/or E7 expression, although adequate clinical data in support of this strategy are still lacking. Some investigators have suggested that testing for protein markers such as p16, MCM family members, EGFR, cyclins, and others may complement or even replace the need for HPV testing.[88] However, none of these markers has been validated, and we must await appropriate clinical data before reliance on such markers can be recommended. Preliminary data reveal that none of the markers are as sensitive for detection of high-grade squamous intraepithelial lesions (HSIL) as HPV DNA testing[89] and in some cases may also be less specific.[90] It is possible that protein markers may need to be used in larger panels to reach adequate sensitivity if the specificity of such tests is not too low.

HPV viral load may be a useful triage test, but the data so far are inconsistent and no definitive understanding has emerged. It is clear that HPV viral load is higher in women with prevalent CIN than in HPV-positive women who do not have detectable prevalent CIN; however, it does not appear to be possible to clearly distinguish women with HG-CIN versus LG-CIN on the basis of viral load because there is a great overlap between these categories. It may be possible to distinguish a subset of HPV-positive women at lower risk for prevalent HG-CIN,[91] but more data are needed to substantiate this approach. It is also unclear whether cytologically normal women with higher viral loads have a greater long-term risk for incident HG-CIN than women who have lower viral loads and whether HPV genotype modulates the relationship.[92]

REFERENCES

1. Lorincz A. Human papillomaviruses. In: Lennette EH, Lennette DA, Lennette ET (eds). Diagnostic Procedures for Viral, Rickettsial, and Chlamydial Infections. Washington, DC: American Public Health Association, 1995, pp 465–480.

2. Franco EL, Harper DM. Vaccination against human papillomavirus infection: A new paradigm in cervical cancer control. Vaccine 2005;23:2388–2394.

3. de Villiers E-M, Fauquet C, Broker TR, et al. Classification of papillomaviruses. Virology 2004;324:17–27.

4. Bosch FX, Lorincz A, Munoz N, et al. The causal relation between human papillomavirus and cervical cancer. J Clin Pathol 2002;55:244–265.

5. Clavel C, Masure M, Bory J-P, et al. Human papillomavirus testing in primary screening for the detection of high-grade cervical lesions: A study of 7932 women. Br J Cancer 2001;84: 1616–1623.

6. Petry K-U, Menton S, Menton M, van Loenen-Frosch F, et al. Inclusion of HPV testing in routine cervical cancer screening for women above 29 years in Germany: Results for 8468 patients. Br J Cancer 2003;88:1570–1577.

7. Sankaranarayanan R, Ferlay J. Worldwide burden of gynaecological cancer: The size of the problem. Best Pract Res Clin Obstet Gynaecol 2006;20:207–225.

8. Monsonego J. HPV infections and cervical cancer prevention. Priorities and new directions. Highlights of EUROGIN 2004 International Expert Meeting, Nice, France, October 21–23, 2004. Gynecol Oncol 2005;96:830–839.

9. Sherman ME, Lorincz AT, Scott DR, et al. Baseline cytology, human papillomavirus testing, and risk for cervical neoplasia: A 10-year cohort analysis. J Natl Cancer Inst 2003;95:46–52.

10. Kjaer S, Hogdall E, Frederiksen K, et al. The absolute risk of cervical abnormalities in high-risk human papillomavirus-positive, cytologically normal women over a 10-year period. Cancer Res 2006;66:10630–10636.

11. Schiffman M, Herrero R, Hildesheim A, et al. HPV DNA testing in cervical cancer screening: Results from women in a high-risk province of Costa Rica. J Am Med Assoc 2000;283:87–93.

12. Lorincz AT, Schiffman MH, Jaffurs WJ, et al. Temporal associations of human papillomavirus infection with cervical cytologic abnormalities. Am J Obstet Gynecol 1990;162:645–651.

13. Cox JT, Lorincz AT, Schiffman MH, et al. Human papillomavirus testing by hybrid capture appears to be useful in triaging women with a cytologic diagnosis of atypical squamous cells of undetermined significance. Am J Obstet Gynecol 1995; 172:946–954.

14. Manos MM, Kinney WK, Hurley LB, et al. Identifying women with cervical neoplasia: using human papillomavirus DNA testing for equivocal Papanicolaou results. J Am Med Assoc 1999;281:1605–1610.

15. Solomon D, Schiffman M, Tarone R, for the ALTS Group. Comparison of three management strategies for patients with Atypical Squamous Cells of Undetermined Significance (ASCUS): baseline results from a randomized trial. J Natl Cancer Inst 2001;93:293–299.

16. Zielinski GD, Bais AG, Helmerhorst THJ, et al. HPV testing and monitoring of women after treatment of CIN 3: Review of the literature and meta-analysis. Obstet Gynecol Surv 2004;59: 543–553.

17. Stoler MH, Schiffman M, for the Atypical Squamous Cells of Undetermined Significance—Low-grade Squamous Intraepithelial Lesion Triage Study (ALTS) Group. Interobserver reproducibility of cervical cytologic and histologic interpretations: Realistic estimates from the ASCUS-LSIL Triage Study. J Am Med Assoc 2001;285:1500–1505.

18. Sherman ME, Schiffman MH, Lorincz AT, et al. Toward objective quality assurance in cervical cytopathology: Correlation of cytopathologic diagnoses with detection of high-risk human papillomavirus types. Am J Clin Pathol 1994;102:182–187.

19. Fahey MT, Irwig L, Macaskill P. Meta-analysis of Pap test accuracy. Am J Epidemiol 1995;141:680–689.

20. Lorincz AT, Richart RM. Human papillomavirus DNA testing as an adjunct to cytology in cervical screening programs. Arch Pathol Lab Med 2003;127:959–968.

21. Guido R, Schiffman M, Solomon D, et al, for the ASCUS LSIL Triage Study (ALTS) Group. Postcolposcopy management strategies for women referred with low-grade squamous intraepithelial lesions or human papillomavirus DNA-positive atypical squamous cells of undetermined significance: A two-year prospective study. Am J Obstet Gynecol 2003;188:1401–1405.

22. Belinson J, Qiao YL, Pretorius R, et al. Shanxi Province cervical cancer screening study: A cross-sectional comparative trial of multiple techniques to detect cervical neoplasia. Gynecol Oncol 2001;83:439–444.

23. Gage JC, Hanson VW, Abbey K, et al. Number of cervical biopsies and sensitivity of colposcopy. Obstet Gynecol 2006;108: 264–272.

24. Pretorius RG, Zhang W-H, Belinson JL, et al. Colposcopically directed biopsy, random cervical biopsy, and endocervical curettage in the diagnosis of cervical intraepithelial neoplasia II or worse. Am J Obstet Gynecol 2004;191:430–434.

25. Lorincz AT, Reid R, Jenson AB, et al. Human papillomavirus infection of the cervix: Relative risk associations of 15 common anogenital types. Obstet Gynecol 1992;79:328–337.

26. Khan MJ, Castle PE, Lorincz AT, et al. The elevated 10-year risk of cervical precancer and cancer in women with human papillomavirus (HPV) type 16 or 18 and the possible utility of type-specific HPV testing in clinical practice. J Natl Cancer Inst 2005;97:1072–1079.

27. Castle PE, Solomon D, Schiffman M, et al, for the ALTS Group. Human papillomavirus type 16 infections and 2-year absolute risk of cervical precancer in women with equivocal or mild cytologic abnormalities. J Natl Cancer Inst 2005;97:1066– 1071.

28. Clifford GM, Rana RK, Franceschi S, et al. Human papillomavirus genotype distribution in low-grade cervical lesions: Comparison by geographic region and with cervical cancer. Cancer Epidemiol Biomarkers Prev 2005;14:1157–1164.

29. Ferguson AW, Svoboda-Newman SM, Frank TS. Analysis of human papillomavirus infection and molecular alterations in adenocarcinoma of the cervix. Mod Pathol 1998;11:11–18.

30. Castellsague X, Diaz M, de Sanjose S, et al. Worldwide human papillomavirus etiology of cervical adenocarcinoma and its cofactors: Implications for screening and prevention. J Natl Cancer Inst 2006;98:303–315.

31. Pirog EC, Kleter B, Olgac S, et al. Prevalence of human papillomavirus DNA in different histological subtypes of cervical adenocarcinoma. Am J Pathol 2000;157:1055–1062.

32. Khan MJ, Partridge EE, Wang SS, et al, for the Atypical Squamous Cells of Undetermined Significance—Low-Grade Squamous Intraepithelial Lesion Triage Study (ALTS) Group. Socioeconomic status and the risk of cervical intraepithelial neoplasia grade 3 among oncogenic human papillomavirus DNA-positive women with equivocal or mildly abnormal cytology. Cancer 2005;104:61–70.

33. Castle PE, Garcia-Meijide M, Holladay EB, et al. A novel filtration-based processing method of liquid cytology specimens for human papillomavirus DNA testing by Hybrid Capture II. Am J Clin Pathol 2005;123:250–255.

34. Grundhoefer D, Patterson BK. Determination of liquid-based cervical cytology specimen adequacy using cellular light scatter and flow cytometry. Cytometry (Communications in Clinical Cytometry) 2001;46:340–344.

35. Lorincz AT. Hybrid Capture method for detection of human papillomavirus DNA in clinical specimens: A tool for clinical management of equivocal Pap smears and for population screening. J Obstet Gynaecol Res 1996;22:629–636.

36. Nindl I, Lorincz A, Mielzynska I, et al. Human papillomavirus detection in cervical intraepithelial neoplasia by the second-generation hybrid capture microplate test, comparing two different cervical specimen collection methods. Clin Diagn Virol 1998;10:49–56.

37. Carozzi FM, Del Mistro A, Confortini M, et al. Reproducibility of HPV DNA testing by Hybrid Capture 2 in a screening setting: Intralaboratory and interlaboratory quality control in seven laboratories participating in the same clinical trial. Am J Clin Pathol 2005;124:1–6.

38. Brink AATP, Snijders PJF, Meijer CJLM. Target amplification-based techniques. In: Lorincz A (ed). Nucleic Acid Testing for Human Disease. Boca Raton, FL: CRC Press, 2006, pp 3–18.

39. Schmitt M, Bravo IG, Snijders PJF, et al. Bead-based multiplex genotyping of human papillomaviruses. J Clin Microbiol 2006;44:504–512.

40. Josefsson A, Livak K, Gyllensten U. Detection and quantitation of human papillomavirus by using the fluorescent 5′ exonuclease assay. J Clin Microbiol 1999;37:490–496.

41. Ting Y, Manos MM. Detection and typing of genital human papillomaviruses. In: Innis MA, Gelfand DH, Sninsky JJ, et al (eds). PCR Protocols: A Guide to Methods and Applications. San Diego: Academic Press, 1990, pp 356–367.

42. van den Brule AJC, Meijer CJLM, Bakels V, et al. Rapid detection of human papillomavirus in cervical scrapes by combined general primer-mediated and type-specific polymerase chain reaction. J Clin Microbiol 1990;28:2739–2743.

43. Gravitt PE, Peyton CL, Alessi TQ, et al. Improved amplification of genital human papillomaviruses. J Clin Microbiol 2000;38:357–361.

44. Quint WGV, Scholte G, van Doorn LJ, et al. Comparative analysis of human papillomavirus infections in cervical scrapes and biopsy specimens by general SPF10 PCR and HPV genotyping. J Pathol 2001;194:51–58.

45. Gregoire L, Arella M, Campione-Piccardo J, et al. Amplification of human papillomavirus DNA sequences by using conserved primers. J Clin Microbiol 1989;27:2660–2665.

46. Shibata DK, Arnheim N, Martin WJ. Detection of human papilloma virus in paraffin-embedded tissue using the polymerase chain reaction. J Exp Med 1988;167:225–230.

47. Kwok S, Higuchi R. Avoiding false positives with PCR. Nature 1989;339:237–238.

48. Tidy J, Farrell PJ. Retraction: Human papillomavirus subtype 16b. Lancet 1989;2:1535.

49. Hinchliffe SA, van Velzen D, Korporaal H, et al. Transience of cervical HPV infection in sexually active, young women with normal cervicovaginal cytology. Br J Cancer 1995;72:943–945.

50. Snijders PJF, van den Brule AJC, Meijer CJLM. The clinical relevance of human papillomavirus testing: Relationship between analytical and clinical sensitivity. J Pathol 2003;201:1–6.

51. Qian X, Lloyd RV. In situ hybridization. In: Lorincz A (ed). Nucleic Acid Testing for Human Disease. Boca Raton, FL: CRC Press, 2006, pp 113–138.

52. Hesselink AT, van den Brule AJC, Brink AATP, et al. Comparison of Hybrid Capture 2 with in situ hybridization for the detection of high-risk human papillomavirus in liquid-based cervical samples. Cancer Cytopathol 2004;102:11–18.

53. Bewtra C, Xie Q, Soundararajan S, et al. Genital human papillomavirus testing by in situ hybridization in liquid atypical cytologic materials and follow-up biopsies. Acta Cytol 2005;49:127–131.

54. Davis-Devine S, Day SJ, Freund GG. Test performance comparison of Inform HPV and Hybrid Capture 2 high-risk HPV DNA tests using the SurePath liquid-based Pap test as the collection method. Am J Clin Pathol 2005;124:24–30.

55. Poddighe PJ, Bulten J, Kerstens HMJ, et al. Human papilloma virus detection by in situ hybridisation signal amplification based on biotinylated tyramine deposition. J Clin Pathol Mol Pathol 1996;49:M340–M344.

56. Bosch FX, Manos MM, Munoz N, et al. Prevalence of human papillomavirus in cervical cancer: A worldwide perspective. J Natl Cancer Inst 1995;87:796–802.

57. Hesselink AT, Bulkmans NWJ, Berkhof J, et al. Cross-sectional comparison of an automated Hybrid Capture 2 assay and the consensus GP5+/6+ PCR method in a population-based cervical screening program. J Clin Microbiol 2006;44:3680–3685.

58. Kulasingam SL, Hughes JP, Kiviat NB, et al. Evaluation of human papillomavirus testing in primary screening for cervical abnormalities: Comparison of sensitivity, specificity, and frequency of referral. J Am Med Assoc 2002;288:1749–1757.

59. Lorincz AT, Smith JS. Sexually transmissible viral pathogens: Human papillomaviruses and herpes simplex viruses. In: Lorincz A (ed). Nucleic Acid Testing for Human Disease. Boca Raton, FL: CRC Press, 2006, pp 243–299.

60. Cuzick J, Beverley E, Ho L, et al. HPV testing in primary screening of older women. Br J Cancer 1999;81:554–558.

61. Terry G, Ho L, Londesborough P, et al. Detection of high-risk HPV types by the Hybrid Capture 2 test. J Med Virol 2001;65:155–162.

62. Castle PE, Schiffman M, Burk RD, et al. Restricted cross-reactivity of Hybrid Capture 2 with non-oncogenic human papillomavirus types. Cancer Epidemiol Biomarkers Prev 2002;11:1394–1399.

63. Ho GYF, Bierman R, Beardsley L, et al. Natural history of cervicovaginal papillomavirus infection in young women. N Engl J Med 1998;338:423–428.

64. Franco EL, Villa LL, Sobrinho JP, et al. Epidemiology of acquisition and clearance of cervical human papillomavirus infection in women from a high-risk area for cervical cancer. J Infect Dis 1999;180:1415–1423.

65. Belinson JL, Qiao YL, Pretorius RG, et al. Shanxi Province cervical cancer screening study II: Self-sampling for high-risk human papillomavirus compared to direct sampling for human papillomavirus and liquid-based cervical cytology. Int J Gynecol Cancer 2003;13:819–826.

66. Ronco G, Giorgi-Rossi P, Carozzi F, et al. Human papillomavirus testing and liquid-based cytology in primary

screening of women younger than 35 years: Results at recruitment for a randomised controlled trial. Lancet Oncol 2006;7: 547–555.

67. Kitchener HC, Almonte M, Wheeler P, et al. HPV testing in routine cervical screening: Cross sectional data from the ARTISTIC trial. Br J Cancer 2006;95:56–61.

68. Arbyn M, Buntinix F, Van Ranst M, et al. Virological versus cytologic triage of women with equivocal Pap smears: A meta-analysis of the accuracy to detect high grade intraepithelial neoplasia. J Natl Cancer Inst 2004;96:280–293.

69. Bollen LJM, Tjong-A-Hung SP, van der Velden J, et al. Clearance of cervical human papillomavirus infection by treatment for cervical dysplasia. Sex Transm Dis 1997;24:456–460.

70. Elfgren K, Bistoletti P, Dillner L, et al. Conization for cervical intraepithelial neoplasia is followed by disappearance of human papillomavirus deoxyribonucleic acid and a decline in serum and cervical mucus antibodies against human papillomavirus antigens. Am J Obstet Gynecol 1996;174: 937–942.

71. Alonso I, Torne A, Puig-Tintore LM, et al. Pre- and post-conization high-risk HPV testing predicts residual/recurrent disease in patients treated for CIN 2-3. Gynecol Oncol 2006; 103:631–636.

72. Fait G, Daniel Y, Kupferminc MJ, et al. Does typing of human papillomavirus assist in the triage of women with repeated low-grade, cervical cytologic abnormalities? Gynecol Oncol 1998;70:319–322.

73. Cuzick J, Szarewski A, Cubie H, et al. Management of women who test positive for high-risk types of human papillomavirus: The HART study. Lancet 2003;362:1871–1876.

74. Bulkmans NWJ, Rozendaal L, Voorhorst FJ, et al. Long-term protective effect of high-risk human papillomavirus testing in population-based cervical screening. Br J Cancer 2005;92: 1800–1802.

75. Bigras G, de Marval F. The probability for a Pap test to be abnormal is directly proportional to HPV viral load: Results from a Swiss study comparing HPV testing and liquid-based cytology to detect cervical cancer precursors in 12 842 women. Br J Cancer 2005;93:575–581.

76. Nieminen P, Vuorma S, Viikki M, et al. Comparison of HPV test *versus* conventional and automation-assisted Pap screening as potential screening tools for preventing cervical cancer. Br J Obstet Gynecol 2004;111:842–848.

77. Ratnam S, Franco EL, Ferenczy A. Human papillomavirus testing for primary screening of cervical cancer precursors. Cancer Epidemiol Biomarkers Prev 2000;9:945–951.

78. Salmeron J, Lazcano-Ponce E, Lorincz A, et al. Comparison of HPV-based assays with Papanicolaou smears for cervical cancer screening in Morelos State, Mexico. Cancer Causes Control 2003;14:505–512.

79. Kuhn L, Denny L, Pollack A, et al. Human papillomavirus DNA testing for cervical cancer screening in low-resource settings. J Natl Cancer Inst 2000;92:818–825.

80. Ronco G, Segnan N, Giorgi-Rossi P, et al. Human papillomavirus testing and liquid-based cytology: Results at recruitment from the new technologies for cervical cancer randomized controlled trial. J Natl Cancer Inst 2006;98:765–774.

81. Bory J-P, Cucherousset J, Lorenzato M, et al. Recurrent human papillomavirus infection detected with the hybrid capture II assay selects women with normal cervical smears at risk for developing high grade cervical lesions: A longitudinal study of 3091 women. Int J Cancer 2002;102:519–525.

82. Rozendaal L, Westerga J, van der Linden JC, et al. PCR based high risk HPV testing is superior to neural network based screening for predicting incident CIN III in women with normal cytology and borderline changes. J Clin Pathol 2000;53:606–611.

83. Dalstein V, Riethmuller D, Pretet J-L, et al. Persistence and load of high-risk HPV are predictors for development of high-grade cervical lesions: A longitudinal French cohort study. Int J Cancer 2003;106:396–403.

84. Kulasingam SL, Kim JJ, Lawrence WF, et al. Cost-effectiveness analysis based on the Atypical Squamous Cells of Undetermined Significance/Low-Grade Squamous Intraepithelial Lesion Triage Study (ALTS). J Natl Cancer Inst 2006;98:92–100.

85. Goldie SJ, Gaffikin L, Goldhaber-Fiebert JD, et al. Cost-effectiveness of cervical-cancer screening in five developing countries. N Engl J Med 2005;353:2158–2168.

86. Mandelblatt J, Lawrence W, Yi B, et al. The balance of harms, benefits, and costs of screening for cervical cancer in older women: The case for continued screening. Arch Intern Med 2004;164:245–247.

87. Mandelblatt JS, Lawrence WF, Womack SM, et al. Benefits and costs of using HPV testing to screen for cervical cancer. J Am Med Assoc 2002;287:2372–2381.

88. von Knebel Doeberitz M. New markers for cervical dysplasia to visualise the genomic chaos created by aberrant oncogenic papillomavirus infections. Eur J Cancer 2002;38:2229–2242.

89. Holladay EB, Logan S, Arnold J, et al. A comparison of the clinical utility of p16(INK4a) immunolocalization with the presence of human papillomavirus by hybrid capture 2 for the detection of cervical dysplasia/neoplasia. Cancer Cytopathol 2006;108:451–461.

90. Ekalaksananan T, Pientong C, Sriamporn S, et al. Usefulness of combining testing for p16 protein and human papillomavirus (HPV) in cervical carcinoma screening. Gynecol Oncol 2006; 103:62–66.

91. Snijders PJF, Hogewoning CJA, Hesselink AT, et al. Determination of viral load thresholds in cervical scrapings to rule out CIN 3 in HPV 16, 18, 31 and 33-positive women with normal cytology. Int J Cancer 2006;119:1102–1107.

92. Lorincz AT, Castle PE, Sherman ME, et al. Viral load of human papillomavirus and risk of CIN3 or cervical cancer. Lancet 2002;360:228–229.

5.2: Cervical Screening with In Vivo and *In Vitro* Modalities: Speculoscopy Combined with Cytology

Neal M. Lonky

KEY POINTS

- Adding an adjunctive visualization technique to routine Papanicolaou (Pap) smear screening identifies more patients with dysplastic cervical lesions (that cytology had missed), but with an increase in the number of patients referred for colposcopy who are subsequently found to have a normal colposcopy or biopsy. However, it is not possible to tell whether the false-positive rate is truly due to false-negative colposcopy.
- False-negative Pap smears may be due to failure of the neoplastic lesions to exfoliate, examiner error, or laboratory error.
- Speculoscopy visualizes the cervix with blue-white chemiluminescent illumination and low-power, portable magnification following the application of dilute acetic acid.
- The sensitivity and specificity of screening with chemiluminescence were superior when compared with those of projected incandescent or halogen illumination, with a lower false-positive rate.
- Colposcopy is a more sensitive test than speculoscopy for very small lesions.
- When examiners are trained to distinguish sharp acetowhite lesions from look-alike faint lesions with indistinct borders, they are less apt to identify benign lesions as suspicious under chemiluminescent illumination.
- A positive speculoscopy result is defined as the presence of at least one acetowhite lesion that appears bright and distinct with at least one sharply marginated border on the cervix or vagina.
- A negative speculoscopy is one in which the cervix or lower genital tract is devoid of any sharply marginated acetowhite lesion and the cervix coloration is uniformly pink with a bluish hue. Faint lesions with indistinct borders should be considered negative and often represent benign areas of squamous metaplasia or inflammation.
- A combined visual-cytologic test (PapSure) is positive when either the speculoscopy result or the cytology result is abnormal, and it is negative when both are normal.
- The physical properties of chemiluminescent light that are thought to be responsible for disclosing lesions under the epithelial surface are low energy, diffuse light emission, intravaginal placement of the light, proximity to the cervical mucosa, and ideal color spectrum that contrasts tissues with differing reflective indices.
- When one discovers ulcerations, erosions, or vascularized areas that are suspicious for cancer, the presence or absence of acetowhite change is of secondary importance. The examiner should be sure to biopsy the lesion to establish the diagnosis as soon as possible.
- Speculoscopy aids in identifying women with neoplastic lesions, because it does not rely on exfoliation or *in vitro* laboratory analysis.
- It may be possible to widen screening intervals for women who are screen negative for the PapSure procedure.

EVOLUTION OF VISUALIZATION OF THE CERVIX AND LOWER GENITAL TRACT FROM A DIAGNOSTIC TO A SCREENING ROLE

Performing colposcopy involves a significant investment of clinician time and financial expenditures. Colposcopy requires special training, is expensive, and is not available in many clinical settings. Therefore it has not been used during routine screening. If colposcopy was widely available and cost-effective, it might have an added benefit when used in tandem with the Papanicolaou (Pap) smear as a part of routine screening. However, *all visual inspection techniques, including colposcopy, are limited to examination of the areas that are overtly visible, making adequate evaluation of the endocervical canal problematic.* Cervical cytology remains useful in the discovery of endocervical and small lesions not visible to the unaided eye of the examiner.

As it is currently used, colposcopy is a diagnostic tool to direct biopsies for women whose screening test was abnormal. However, visual tests may have a role in *screening*. When visual tests are used in screening they are simplified, eliminating consideration of vascular patterns and tissue characteristics and leading to a dichotomous "positive" or "negative" result.

To appreciate the value of tissue visualization in the screening process, one must understand that screening tests are not fully diagnostic of the underlying histologic grade. They identify women at risk for having cervical dysplasia or cancer but require a further test to make the final diagnosis. Furthermore, to properly evaluate the value of a screening test, the disease it is trying to identify (all women with precursor lesions or just those with high-grade disease or early invasive carcinoma) must be clearly defined.

ENHANCED SCREENING WITH CERVICAL VISUALIZATION: EVIDENCE-BASED ANALYSIS

Acetic acid denatures nuclear proteins and dehydrates cellular cytoplasm, causing tissues with increased nuclear:cytoplasmic ratios to reflect projected white light and appear white. This effect can also be appreciated during magnified or unaided (naked eye) examinations following the application of 4% to 6% acetic acid. This has been the basis for screening women for cervical disease (predominantly in underdeveloped countries where Pap smear programs are not feasible) using a procedure that has been called "downstaging" by some.[1-3] The appearance of well-demarcated acetowhite cervical lesions in women undergoing screening for cervical cancer correlates with underlying cervical neoplasia, but this correlation is not perfect. In the study by Van Le et al.,[1] nurse practitioners, physicians, and physician assistants screened women with downstaging and Pap smears. Eighty-five additional patients (with negative Pap smears) were referred for colposcopy based on the presence of acetowhite cervical lesions seen during screening. Thirty-five of 85 (41%) patients had dysplasia on directed biopsies. The number of women screened, which included those 85 additional referrals, was not reported; therefore the number of women referred for colposcopy who were subsequently found to have normal findings could not be calculated.

A study from the University of Zimbabwe/JHPIEGO Cervical Cancer Project[4] studied 2203 screening patients referred for colposcopy with either abnormal cytology or visual inspection and downstaging. Downstaging (called "visual inspection following acetic acid" [VIA] in this study) detected 76.7% (95% confidence interval [CI], 70.3–82.3%) of the cervical cancer precursor lesions. *Adding visualization identified more patients with dysplastic cervical lesions that cytology had missed, but with an increase in the number of patients referred for colposcopy who were subsequently found to have a normal colposcopy or biopsy.* Because "screen-negative" women were not evaluated with colposcopy and biopsy, true sensitivity and specificity were not determined.

Slawson et al.[3] evaluated 2872 women without a previous history of cervical disease who were eligible for screening. Each patient was evaluated by conventional cytology and downstaging as previously defined. Of the 140 cases of biopsy-proven cervical intraepithelial neoplasia (CIN) discovered (prevalence 4.9%), 33 (24%) were discovered solely because of abnormal downstaging (Pap smear was negative). A recent multicenter study from India and Africa demonstrated that the sensitivity, specificity, and predictive values of visual inspection following acetic acid or following the application of Lugol's iodine (VILI) are comparable to what is reported regarding conventional cervical cytologic screening in industrialized countries.[5]

False-positive visual screening cases may occur for two major reasons. Benign conditions such as inflammatory atypia or immature metaplasia may turn white after the application of dilute acetic acid, or the biopsy may be misdirected. In both instances, the clinician may conclude that the visual screen was false positive, but in the second scenario this false-positive result is due to examiner error. This conclusion is supported by three studies[6-8] in which patients had directed biopsies for presumed high-grade visually suspicious lesions, followed immediately by electrosurgical loop excision of the entire transformation zone. In at least a third of the cases, the loop excision specimen documented a more severe change than did the directed

biopsy. *The false-positive rate of any screening tool is dependent on the ability of the "gold standard" diagnostic test (colposcopically directed biopsy) to detect all the disease. The failure of colposcopy to detect all the disease may increase the false-positive rate of the screening test.* Recent evidence suggests that colposcopic biopsy is not as sensitive as previously thought.[9,10] The practice of obtaining additional biopsies may aid in the correct identification of all the disease present and limit the false-positive rate. This supports the suggestion that the false-positive rate of visual screening may be lower than reported. Finally, *any screening test studied in populations where the results are truly subjective (visual screening and interpretation by the bedside clinician) and the prevalence of disease is low will be prone to findings of low specificity and positive predictive values.*

OVERCOMING THE LIMITATIONS OF THE CONVENTIONAL PAP SMEAR

Although the performance of exfoliative cytology has improved our ability to indirectly identify cervical neoplasia, it has limitations. One study documents a high false-negative rate (50%) of a single conventional Pap smear examination.[11] Enhancements to the conventional Pap smear, such as thin-layer preparations and computerized Pap smear reading, resulted in improved collection, fixation, and inspection steps of this *in vitro* process. However, there is evidence that some cervical lesions are not represented in the cellular specimen submitted to the laboratory. This may be due to failure of these neoplastic lesions to exfoliate,[12] examiner error, or laboratory error. Some lesions that cannot be detected with cytology-based screening (both cytopathologic analysis and human papillomavirus [HPV] testing) may be visualized.[13,14] However, some lesions in the endocervical canal cannot be visualized and can only be accessed for sampling through cytologic brushing. The most sensitive screening procedure to detect both types of lesions (those detectable only through visualization and those detectable only through exfoliative cytology) would seem to be one that combines visual (in vivo) and laboratory cytology–based (in vivo) methodologies. *The objective is to increase the sensitivity of a single examination without reducing test accuracy through loss of specificity or referring an excessive number of patients for colposcopy, which might make the test too impractical or too expensive.*

MAGNIFIED VISUALIZATION WITH CHEMILUMINESCENCE: SPECULOSCOPY AND THE EVIDENCE-BASED LITERATURE

Speculoscopy visualizes the cervix with blue-white chemiluminescent illumination and low-power, portable magnification (4–6× magnification loupe or monocular) following the application of dilute (4–6%) acetic acid. Speculoscopy differs from colposcopy in that it uses the unique spectral frequency, placement, and energy emitted from the chemiluminescent light source. In two studies where the chemiluminescent light source was compared with magnified inspection using projected white- and blue-filtered, incandescent illumination of the cervix (PIL), speculoscopy disclosed more biopsy-proven dysplastic lesions of the cervix than did PIL.[15,16] In more than 10,000 published cases from a wide array of clinical settings and examiners (colposcopists, non-colposcopists, physicians, and nurse clinicians), the addition of speculoscopy to conventional cytology resulted in a greater than twofold increase in sensitivity (from 40.7% for the Pap smear alone to 92.2% using the combined approach). This involved the detection of all grades of cervical dysplasia or malignancy.[17]

Screening with the combination of speculoscopy and conventional cytology has been studied prospectively. The first multicenter study was specifically designed to include colposcopy for all study participants. Mann et al. reported on 243 screening patients (no history of cervical or vaginal pathology or treatment) from 12 clinical sites.[18] All patients had both a screening Pap smear and speculoscopy. The Pap smear detected 9 of 29 (31%) women with cervical dysplasia or condyloma, whereas the combination of the Pap smear and speculoscopy (called "magnified chemiluminescent illumination" in that study) detected 24 of 29 cases (83%) (p < 0.001). The negative predictive value of the combined visual-cytologic test was 99%. Polatti et al. replicated this study design in Italy, where 600 patients were screened.[19] Colposcopy was performed in all participants, and colposcopically directed biopsy was used to establish the tissue diagnosis. The Pap smear alone detected 23.7% of cervical dysplasia or carcinoma, whereas the combination of Pap smear and speculoscopy increased the detection rate to 78.8%. Cytology failed to detect about one third of biopsy-proven, high-grade CIN that was discovered by speculoscopy alone (10 of 33 cases). Although the majority of the false-negative Pap smears represented low-grade disease, one third of the cases were high grade.

In a larger study by Wertlake et al., the question of examiner expertise was addressed.[20] More than 180 practitioners, including physicians and non-physicians (most were not colposcopy trained), evaluated 5692 screening patients (as previously defined). Only women with a positive screening test were referred for colposcopic evaluation; therefore the true sensitivity and specificity could not be determined. Of the women screened who completed the protocol, speculoscopy alone (patients with negative Pap smear results) detected 11 of 32 cases of high-grade dysplasia and 154 of 191 low-grade dysplasias. Once again, one third of the high-grade dysplasias would have been missed if speculoscopy were omitted during screening. *The authors concluded that combined visual-cytologic screening is appropriate for all clinicians currently performing the conventional Pap smear procedure, not just colposcopists.*

When evaluating visual screening adjuncts, the increase in sensitivity must be balanced against the propensity for referring healthy women for colposcopy (false positive) because of an abnormal screening test. According to

published data, *screening with chemiluminescence (as opposed to other light sources) imparts the lowest false-positive rate. False-positive rates ranged from 6% to 8% in most series, as compared with studies using projected non-chemiluminescent light sources with false-positive rates of 10% to 20%.*[18–20] Photographic documentation and inspection of the cervix (cervicography), which employs magnification and projected illumination, exhibited lower sensitivity and a higher false-positive rate.[21] When speculoscopy is added to conventional cytology, one can expect the specificity of screening to decrease from 95% to the range of 80% to 85%. If speculoscopy was removed from the screening setting and compared directly with colposcopy for higher-risk women already referred for colposcopy, examiners were twice as likely to false-positive suspicious lesions with colposcopy as compared with speculoscopy.[22]

Colposcopy is a more sensitive test than speculoscopy for very small lesions. When examiners are trained to distinguish sharp acetowhite lesions from "look-alike" faint lesions with indistinct borders, they are less apt to identify benign lesions as suspicious under chemiluminescent illumination, making speculoscopy more suitable for screening than colposcopy. Finally, in populations with a low prevalence of CIN, the screening test may exhibit a low positive predictive value and high false-positive rate. Two such studies by Yu and Boonklit, in which the prevalence of CIN in the population was very low, documented impressive increases in sensitivity in detecting CIN when speculscopy was added to cytology, with a concomitant decrease in the positive predictive value.[23,24]

SPECULOSCOPY AS PART OF THE PAPSURE PROCEDURE: INDICATIONS FOR USE AND METHOD OF PROCEDURE

Speculoscopy may be added as a screening adjunct whenever a patient is having a Pap smear for cervical cancer screening. The chemiluminescent Speculite light source and other tools needed to perform speculoscopy are shown in Figure 5.2-1. The examiner may choose a monocular or binocular, low-power magnification loupe to visualize the cervix and vagina during the inspection phase of the procedure. *The Speculite device (capsule of chemiluminescent chemicals) is activated by bending the outer capsule, which fractures a more brittle inner capsule, allowing chemicals to intermix* (Figure 5.2-2). The Speculite capsule should be shaken vigorously for 10 to 15 seconds, allowing the chemicals to mix and activating the blue-white chemiluminescent illumination (Figure 5.2-3). *The Speculite is then attached to the inner, middle aspect of the upper blade of the vaginal speculum using double-sided tape* (Figure 5.2-4). Following insertion of the vaginal speculum and gross inspection, an endocervical and exocervical Pap smear specimen is collected, and the tissues are then *rinsed with a dilute (4–6%) acetic acid solution. The ambient room light is dimmed or extinguished.* To avoid a completely dark room environment, the examiner may leave a light source

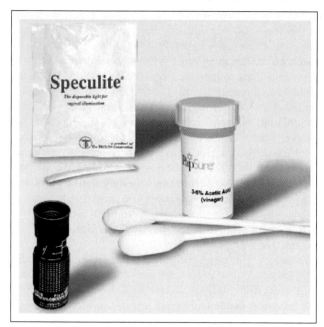

Figure 5.2-1 Speculoscopy requires the foil packet containing the Speculite, dilute acetic acid solution, and 4–6× magnification.

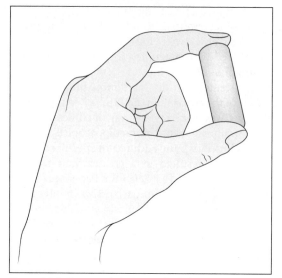

Figure 5.2-3 The capsule is vigorously shaken to intermix the chemicals to accelerate the chemical reaction and create bright light.

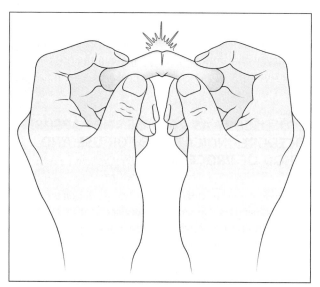

Figure 5.2-2 To activate the chemiluminescent light, the outer flexible capsule is bent to fracture the brittle inner capsule, thereby mixing the chemicals and creating blue-white light.

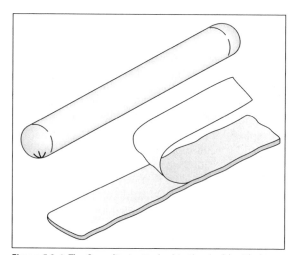

Figure 5.2-4 The Speculite is attached to the double-sided tape. The other side is attached to the inner aspect of the upper speculum blade.

illuminated in the corner of the room or a window shade drawn to allow only a small amount of ambient room light. The unique blue-white illumination can be noted in Figure 5.2-5.

The appearance of intravaginal structures is improved using chemiluminescent light energy, compared with using projected conventional light. *The tissues appear brighter, and visualization of the landmarks needed to evaluate the cervix and vagina is facilitated when the room light is dimmed or extinguished.* The cervix and vagina are inspected for the presence of exophytic or endophytic lesions, acetowhite epithelium, ulcers, or masses and changes associated with cervical cancer or its precursors. Vascular abnormalities may be distinguished, but owing to the low-power magnification and low-energy light source, *they are not specifically used to grade lesions already seen under Speculite illumination.*

The results are interpreted as either positive or negative. *A positive speculoscopy result is defined as the presence of at least one acetowhite lesion that appears bright and distinct with at least one sharply marginated border on the cervix or vagina. The lesions may stand out from the surrounding dark-red or blue-tinged normal epithelium that does not reflect the chemiluminescent light. A negative speculoscopy result is one in which the cervix or lower genital tract is devoid of any sharply*

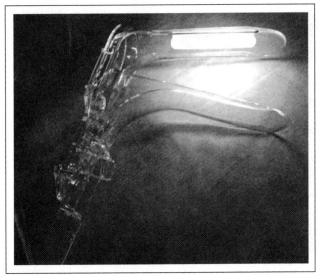

Figure 5.2-5 Speculoscopy is ideally performed in a setting with low ambient room light. This permits the lesions to become faintly luminescent and be more easily visualized.

marginated acetowhite lesion and the cervix coloration is uniformly pink with a bluish hue. Faint lesions with indistinct borders should be considered negative and often represent benign areas of squamous metaplasia or inflammation.

Figure 5.2-6A demonstrates a negative speculoscopy result in which the cervix shows a normal transformation zone devoid of lesions. Light reflection can be easily distinguished from true lesions because they appear glossy and change shape when depressed with a cotton-tipped applicator. Figure 5.2-6B shows a negative result as well. Figure 5.2-7A also shows a negative speculoscopy result, but there is an indistinct lesion with an indistict border at 3 o'clock. Metaplastic or inflammatory lesions appear as indistinct, faint, acetowhite changes and differ from dysplasia that appears sharp and well demarcated. Figure 5.2-7B shows the corresponding colpophotograph. Figures 5.2-8 and 5.2-9A

demonstrate positive speculoscopy results with at least one sharply marginated lesion. Figure 5.2-9A can be compared with the corresponding colpophotograph in Figure 5.2-9B showing a mosaic pattern. Positive speculoscopy and colposcopy results are compared in Figure 5.2-10. The lesions are larger and more numerous under speculoscopy. This may be due to the lower energy of the speculoscopy light source permitting a lower reflectivity and a higher tissue penetration. The biopsies from the anterior and posterior cervix showed CIN 2 and CIN 3 in this case. A combined visual-cytologic test (PapSure) is positive when either the speculoscopy result or the cytology result is abnormal, and it is negative when both results are normal.

CHEMILUMINESCENCE: PROPERTIES THAT ENHANCE THE DETECTION OF TRUE CERVICAL NEOPLASIA

Two studies have shown that simply filtering projected incandescent illumination (with a blue or green filter) toward the cervical portio will not duplicate the ability of chemiluminescence to disclose CIN lesions.[15,16] In these studies, the sensitivity and specificity of screening with chemiluminescence were superior when compared with those of projected incandescent or halogen illumination, with a lower false-positive rate.

The physical properties of chemiluminescent light that are thought to be responsible for disclosing lesions under the epithelial surface are *low energy, diffuse light emission, intravaginal placement of the light, proximity to the cervical mucosa, and ideal color spectrum that contrasts tissues with differing reflective indices.* When using the intravaginal chemiluminescent light capsule, the following pitfalls and remedies exist:

1. Instead of projecting light toward the cervical portio, the light capsule should be attached to the inner upper speculum blade. *This is akin to "lighting the room" from the ceiling as opposed to projecting light from the "doorway" to*

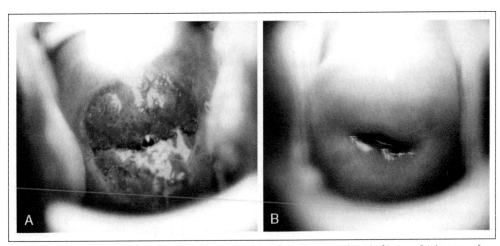

Figure 5.2-6 **A,** Cervix under speculoscopy with a normal transformation zone devoid of lesions. Bright areas of reflection appear glossy and deform or disappear when depressed with a cotton-tipped applicator. **B,** Normal cervix without lesions appears uniform and is pink-blue in color under speculoscopy. No well-demarcated lesions are seen.

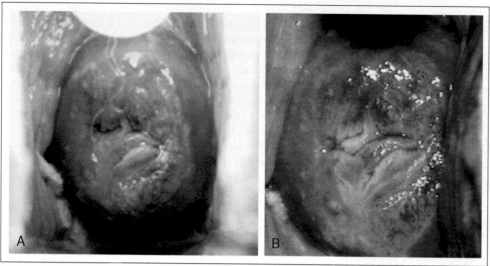

Figure 5.2-7 A, This cervix represents a variant of normal. A small area of metaplasia at 3 o'clock is faintly acetowhite, but the margins are poorly defined or have fuzzy borders. This would be a look-alike, potentially false-positive examination to the untrained examiner. **B,** The same cervix during colposcopy appears normal. No suspicious lesions are seen.

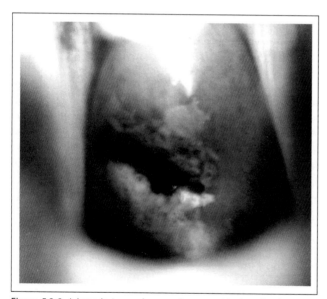

Figure 5.2-8 A large lesion under speculoscopy with sharp borders defines a positive screening examination.

view the object at the distal end. The bar of light may reflect off the moist mucosal surface. The reflection takes on a glossy appearance and may be distinguished from a true cervical lesion if the clinician gently rotates the speculum or depresses the area with a moist cotton-tipped applicator. True lesions should remain white and uniform, whereas light reflection will change in shape and appearance or may entirely disappear when the speculum and light are moved or the tissue is depressed.

2. Women with *a large cervix or acentric portio may obstruct the light and may require manipulation of the speculum or the cervix to achieve adequate visualization.* Replacement of the light onto the lower speculum blade may be necessary if the cervix is displaced anteriorly.

3. *Neoplastic lesions appear to have an opaque or matte surface texture,* whereas light reflection appears quite shiny or glossy in appearance.

4. *The borders of neoplastic lesions are sharp, whereas lesions with indistinct borders more likely represent metaplastic or inflammatory changes.* Nabothian cysts are more rounded and also exhibit indistinct borders.

5. When one discovers ulcerations, erosions, or vascularized areas that are suspicious for cancer, the presence or absence of acetowhite change is of secondary importance. The examiner should biopsy the lesion to establish the diagnosis.

INTERPRETATION AND TRIAGE OF PAPSURE SCREENING RESULTS

The PapSure examination uses two modalities to evaluate a woman's risk for cervical or lower genital tract neoplasia: the results of *in vitro* cytologic data and the result of in vivo visual inspection. Table 5.2-1 shows the potential findings based on the data obtained with two tests. *A positive Pap smear is defined as evidence of a low-grade squamous intraepithelial lesion (LSIL) or a higher-grade abnormality.* The presence of atypical glandular cells of undetermined significance (AGC-US) should also be defined as abnormal in this management algorithm.

In Table 5.2-1, *women in group A should be referred for colposcopy* by virtue of the Pap smear abnormality alone, and speculoscopy does not add new information regarding their risk status. *Women in group B also require colposcopy,* but experience shows that they comprise the smallest referral group. If dysplasia is found, these patients usually have

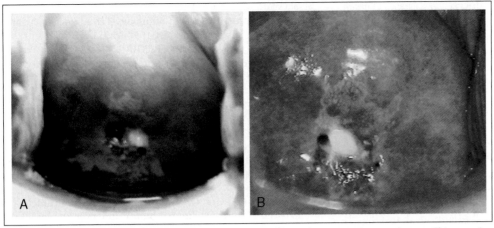

Figure 5.2-9 A, A bright, well-demarcated lesion on the anterior lip can be seen under speculoscopy. This screening test is positive. **B,** The same cervix under colposcopy is also positive with a suspicious lesion near 12 o'clock. Owing to the high-power illumination and magnification, mosaic can be appreciated and serves as the landmark for a directed biopsy. The biopsy showed high-grade dysplasia.

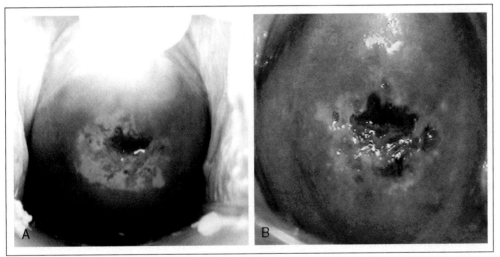

Figure 5.2-10 Photograph of a neoplastic lesion seen under speculoscopy **(A)** and colposcopy **(B)**. The lesions are larger and more numerous under speculoscopy owing to the lower-energy light source and deeper tissue penetration. These were low-grade lesions on biopsy.

Table 5.2-1 Combined Visual/Cytologic Examination Using Speculoscopy and Cytology (PapSure)*

Group	Pap Smear Result	Speculoscopy Result	PapSure Result
A	+	+	+
B	−	−	+
C	−	+	+
D	−	−	−
E	ASC-US	+	Consider high risk
F	ASC-US	−	Consider low risk

Pap, Papanicolaou; *ASC-US*, atypical squamous cells of undetermined significance; +, positive; −, negative.
*It may be possible to widen screening intervals for women who are "screen negative" for the PapSure procedure. Colposcopy may be advised for patients with positive or high-risk PapSure results.

small lesions on the portio or endocervical disease. *Women in group C are newly discovered to be at risk because they have positive speculoscopy despite negative Pap smear results.* If colposcopy is performed within a few weeks, biopsies show CIN 1 or worse in over 60% of cases. Research has shown that colposcopy may be safely deferred for 6 months in women deemed reliable for follow-up who are otherwise low risk. In women with persistent speculoscopic lesions 6 months later, the yield of colposcopic biopsy increased to more than 90%.[25] All the cases of high-grade dysplasia missed by the Pap smear should be discovered in group C, except for the remote case of isolated endocervical disease. *Women in group D receive negative evaluations on both cytology and speculoscopy.* This provides reassurance to patients because the negative predictive value is more than 99%. It may be possible to widen screening intervals for women who are screen negative for the PapSure procedure. Groups E and F demonstrate the value of speculoscopy in the triage of patients with atypical squamous cells of undetermined significance (ASC-US) Pap smears.

In a study in which all women received speculoscopy, conventional cytology, and colposcopy, Massad et al. found that in those with ASC-US results, 53% had lesions seen under speculoscopy, and 96% of women with positive speculoscopy had positive colposcopy. In addition, 97% of all patients with biopsy-proven intraepithelial neoplasia were correctly identified.[26] The remaining 3% of cases with ASC-US results, negative speculoscopy, and positive colposcopy showed biopsies no worse than CIN 1. This study suggests that performing primary PapSure examinations could assist in effective triage when ASC-US Pap smear results are encountered (without requiring an additional clinic visit or laboratory HPV test).

IMPACT ON COST-EFFECTIVENESS OF SCREENING

Speculoscopy can be effectively performed by all clinicians currently performing Pap smears with an improvement in screening sensitivity of 200% to 300%.[20, 27] The added cost of the equipment and added service (approximately $20–25 per examination) is offset by the improvement in sensitivity (cost per case of CIN or cancer detected). Speculoscopy may be used as a triage tool in women with ASC-US cytology to reduce unnecessary colposcopic referral.[26] *A study comparing conventional cytology performed annually with PapSure performed biannually showed PapSure to be cost-effective while reducing the cervical cancer prevalence and death rate using a Markov prediction model.*[28]

REFERENCES

1. Van Le L, Broekhuizen F, Janzer-Steele R, et al. Acetic acid visualization of the cervix to detect cervical dysplasia. Obstet Gynecol 1993;81:293–295.
2. Nene B, Deshpande S, Jayant K, et al. Early detection of cervical cancer by visual inspection: A population-based study in rural India. Int J Cancer 1996;68:770–773.
3. Slawson D, Bennett J, Herman J. Are Papanicolaou smears enough? Acetic acid washes of the cervix as adjunctive therapy: A HARNET study. J Fam Pract 1992;35:271–277.
4. University of Zimbabwe/JHPIEGO Cervical Cancer Project. Visual inspection with acetic acid for cervical-cancer screening: Test qualities in a primary-care setting. Lancet 1999;353: 869–873.
5. Sankaranarayanan R, Basu P, Wesley RS, et al. Accuracy of visual screening for cervical neoplasia: Results from an IARC multicenter study in India and Africa. Int J Cancer 2004; 110:907–914.
6. Buxton E, Luesley D, Shafi M, et al. Colposcopically directed punch biopsy: A potentially misleading investigation. Br J Obstet Gynecol 1991;98:1273–1276.
7. Chappatte O, Byrne D, Raju K, et al. Histological differences between colposcopic-directed biopsy and loop excision of the transformation zone (LETZ): A cause for concern. Gynecol Oncol 1991;43:46–50.
8. Massad L, Halperin C, Bitterman P. Correlation between colposcopically directed biopsy and cervical loop excision. Gynecol Oncol 1996;60:400–403.
9. Pretorius RG, Kim RJ, Belinson JL, et al. Inflation of sensitivity of cervical cancer screening tests secondary to correlated error in colposcopy. J Low Genit Tract Dis 2006;10:5–9.
10. Gage JC, Hanson VW, Abbey K, et al, and the ASCUS LSIL Triage Study (ALTS) Group. Number of cervical biopsies and sensitivity of colposcopy. Obstet Gynecol 2006;108: 264–272.
11. Agency for Health Care Policy and Research. Evidence Report/Technology Assessment No. 5, Evaluation of Cervical Cytology, AHCPR Publication No. 99-E010, Rockville, MD, January 1999.
12. Felix JC, Lonky NM, Tamura K, et al. Aberrant expression of E-cadherin in cervical intraepithelial neoplasia correlates with a false-negative Papnicolaou smear. Am J Obstet Gynecol 2002;186:1308–1314.
13. Lonky NM, Felix JC, Naidu YM, et al. Triage of atypical squamous cells of undetermined significance with Hybrid Capture II: colposcopy and histologic human papillomaviurs correlation. Obstet Gynecol 2003;101:481–489.
14. Lonky NM, Felix J, Tsadik GW, et al. False-negative hybrid capture II results related to altered adhesion molecule distribution in women with atypical squamous cells pap smear results and tissue-based human papilloma-virus positive high-grade cervical intraepithelial neoplasia. J Low Genit Tract Dis 2004;8: 285–291.
15. Lonky N, Edwards G. Comparison of chemiluminescent light versus incandescent light in the visualization of acetowhite epithelium. Am J Gynecol Health 1992;6:11–15.
16. Suneja A, Mahishee, Agarwal N, et al. Comparison of magnified chemiluminescent examination with incandescent light examination and colposcopy for detection of cervical neoplasia. Indian J Cancer 1998;35:81–87.
17. U.S. Food and Drug Administration: Monograph: Papanicolaou Smear Plus Speculoscopy, Rockville, MD, 1997.
18. Mann W, Lonky N, Massad S, et al. Papanicolaou smear screening augmented by a magnified chemiluminescent exam. Int J Gynecol Obstet 1993;43:289–296.
19. Polatti F, Giunta P, Migliora P, et al. Speculoscopy combined with Pap smear in the cervical-vaginal screening. Current Obstet Gynecol 1994;3:178–180.
20. Wertlake P, Francus K, Newkirk G, et al. Effectiveness of the Papanicolaou smear and speculoscopy as compared with the Papanicolaou smear alone: A community-based clinical trial. Obstet Gynecol 1997;90:421–427.

21. Baldauf JJ, Dreyfus M, Ritter J, et al. Cervicography. Does it improve cervical cancer screening? Acta Cytol 1997;41: 295–301.

22. Lonky N, Mann W, Massad L, et al. Ability of visual tests to predict underlying cervical neoplasia. J Reprod Med 1995;40: 530–536.

23. Yu BK, Kuo BI, Yen MS, et al. Eur J Gynaecol Oncol 2003;24: 495–499.

24. Boonlikit S, Supakarapongkul W, Preuksaritanond N, et al. Screening of cervical neoplasia by using Pap smear with speculoscopy compared with Pap smear alone. J Med Assoc Thai 2005;88:138–144.

25. Parham GP, Andrews NR, Lee ML. Comparison of immediate and deferred colposcopy in a cervical screening program. Obstet Gynecol 2000;95:340–344.

26. Massad L, Lonky N, Mutch D, et al. Use of speculoscopy in the evaluation of women with atypical Papanicolaou smears. J Repro Med 1993;38:163–169.

27. Edwards G, Rutkowski C, Palmer C. Cervical cancer screening with Papanicolaou smear plus speculoscopy by nurse practitioners in a health maintenance organization. J Low Gen Tract Dis 1997;3:141–147.

28. Taylor L, Sorensen S, Ray N, et al. Cost-effectiveness of the conventional Pap smear test with a new adjunct to cytological screening for squamous cell carcinoma of the uterine cervix and its precursors. Arch Fam Med 2000;9:713–721.

CHAPTER 6

Principles and Technique of the Colposcopic Exam

Barbara S. Apgar • Gregory L. Brotzman • Mary M. Rubin

KEY POINTS

- The main role of colposcopy is to locate abnormal-appearing epithelium and to direct biopsies to areas in which cervical intraepithelial neoplasia (CIN) 2,3 or invasive cancer is suspected.
- Because the ability of histology to define the true level of disease is dependent on a properly prepared, colposcopically directed biopsy, the histologic interpretation is only as accurate as the skill of the colposcopist in interpreting the colposcopic findings and properly directing the biopsy.
- As many as 40% of patients are lost to follow-up. Transportation, childcare, work, fear, and preoccupation with busy life routines have been identified as barriers to recommended follow-up care.
- The green filter absorbs certain wavelengths of light, making the red color of the vessels appear blacker and sharpening the contrast with the surrounding epithelium.
- The colposcopic image on video colposcopes is two-dimensional rather than three-dimensional, making assessment of the contour and density of the lesion more difficult.
- In order to achieve an adequate acetowhite reaction in nonkeratinized epithelium, the dilute acetic acid or vinegar must be left in contact with the tissue until the reaction has maximally evolved.
- Dilute Lugol's solution stains normal squamous epithelium a dark, mahogany color, indicating that glycogen is present in the cells. The absence of staining denotes a nonglycogenated state that may represent benign or abnormal epithelium.
- Monsel's solution and silver nitrate will interfere with biopsy interpretation and should not be applied until after all the biopsies are performed.
- Taking more biopsies, rather than fewer, ensures that the most appropriate site is sampled and that histology reflects the most serious pathology.
- The value of a routine endocervical curettage (ECC) is controversial, and it may be reserved for selected patients such as those in whom the transformation zone is not fully visualized, those who were previously treated, those at high risk for recurrent disease, and before treatment with ablative therapy.
- ECC is contraindicated in the pregnant patient.
- Although a large biopsy cannot be taken with a small-jawed biopsy instrument, a large-jawed biopsy instrument need not take only large biopsies. A small biopsy can be taken using only the tip of the jaw.
- Demographic information, clinical findings, and recommendations for follow-up visits or referral should be included in the colposcopic record.

The colposcopic examination involves the systematic evaluation of the lower genital tract, with special emphasis on the superficial epithelium and blood vessels of the underlying stroma. Although the term *colposcopy* specifically refers to the cervix, it is broadly used to mean the magnified illumination of the entire lower female genital system, including the vulva, vagina, and cervix. Specific terms such as *vulvoscopy*, *vaginoscopy*, and even *high-resolution anoscopy* are also used. *The main role of colposcopy is to locate abnormal-appearing epithelium and to direct biopsies to areas in which cervical intraepithelial neoplasia (CIN) 2,3 or invasive cancer is suspected.*[1] Colposcopy allows the examiner to identify specific colposcopic features that distinguish normal from abnormal findings and to form an impression as to whether the features are benign or indicate the presence of preinvasive or invasive disease. It has been traditionally held that if the colposcopic examination is performed according to acceptable protocols and is guided by a colposcopic assessment method that grades colposcopic findings according to severity,[2] an accurate histologic diagnosis can be obtained. Recent data from the ALTS trial call this paradigm into question. Relying solely on a grading system for detection of the most serious abnormalities may unfortunately fail to sample the most serious disease. In order to detect the most abnormal lesions and secure the most accurate histology, a change in the traditional colposcopic method must occur.[3]

The traditional role of cervical cytologic screening has been to identify women with abnormalities and direct them to diagnostic testing including colposcopy and colposcopically directed biopsy. The conventional approach of screening cytology, triage colposcopy, and diagnostic histology has been successful in reducing the rate of cervical cancer.[4] Following the publication of the 2001 American Society of Colposcopy and Cervical Pathology (ASCCP) Consensus Guidelines for the management of cervical cytologic abnormalities, colposcopy remained the recommended triage for all cytologic abnormalities except for atypical squamous cells of undetermined significance (ASC-US). By being more efficient and cost-effective for identifying CN 2,3 than repeat cytology or immediate colposcopy, human papillomavirus (HPV) deoxyribonucleic acid (DNA) testing became the preferred method of triage for ASC-US.[5]

The sensitivity and specificity of colposcopy compares favorably with other diagnostic testing methods. For distinguishing normal cervix from all other diagnoses, the individual estimations of sensitivity of colposcopy (87–99%) were high, whereas specificity was lower (23–87%).[6] *High-grade lesions were better separated from low-grade lesions than low-grade lesions from the normal cervix.* The higher sensitivity and lower specificity may be explained by the overinterpretation of low-grade lesions. The likelihood ratios showed much higher shifts between low- and high-grade lesions than between normal cervix and low-grade lesions.[6] *Colposcopy appears to be more accurate for identifying high-grade than lower-grade disease.*[7] Another study agreed that it was more difficult to separate cervices with biopsy-proven metaplasia from those with CIN 1.[8] Eight percent of women with biopsy-proven CN 2,3 retain a colposcopic impression of metaplasia without characteristics of high-grade disease. Additionally, colposcopic assessment of the severity of cervical disease (colposcopic impression) is significantly associated with the subsequent histology. However, the strength of the correlation or agreement between colposcopic impression and histology remains poor (k = 0.20).[9] Although colposcopy was sensitive for identifying the presence of cervical disease, a colposcopic impression of a high-grade lesion identified only 56% of actual histologic high-grade disease. Exact correlation between colposcopic impression and biopsy results was relatively uncommon, existing in only 37% of women. Results agreed within one grade, however, in 75% of the women. Colposcopic impression more often overestimated (40%) than underestimated (23%) the severity of disease. The positive predictive value of agreement of high-grade colposocpic impression with high-grade histology was only 39%.[9] In the ALTS trial, only 54.8% of women who had a final diagnosis of CIN 3 had a colposcopically directed biopsy > CIN 2 at baseline or in the 2-year follow-up period.[10,11]

Colposcopy is subject to interobserver variability. The ability of a colposcopy quality control group (ALTS) to agree on the colposcopic impression of digitalized cervical images was fair, and the k values were poor.[12] The group showed fair rates of agreement (84–89.3%) on the modified Reid colposcopic index, and *k* values were poor.[0.23–0.28] The group also showed poor to fair *k* scores and fair agreement (71%) for estimation of lesion size and image quality. However, poor image quality may have contributed to the disappointing *k* scores.

Each time a colposcopic examination is performed, the principles of practice are the same: exclude the presence of invasive disease, and, if indicated, select the most appropriate sites for biopsy. The accurate interpretation of the colposcopic findings is basic to the decision of whether or not to perform a biopsy. The ability to accurately direct a biopsy to the areas of greatest abnormality is dependent on the expertise of the colposcopist.[7] *Because the ability of histology to define the true level of disease is dependent on a properly directed biopsy, the histologic interpretation is only as accurate as the skill of the colposcopist in interpreting the colposcopic findings correctly by accurately biopsying all abnormal-appearing lesions.*

The cornerstone of colposcopic practice is a systematic approach that includes correlation of cytology, histology, and the colposcopic impression.[13]

No technology is currently available that has replaced the need for rigorous colposcopic training to identify abnormal lower genital tract abnormalities. Computer imaging systems[14] need validation before they can be used as alternatives or substitutes for colposcopy. Preliminary data suggest these systems may detect more high-grade lesions than colposcopy alone, but this will have to be demonstrated in further studies.[15]

TRAINING IN COLPOSCOPY

The ASCCP (www.asccp.org/member/mentorship.shtml) recommends a three-tied approach for training in colposcopy that includes completion of a didactic program, a mentorship program, and an examination to document colposcopic proficiency. The first tier is the didactic program completed either during a U.S. accredited residency program or through an ACCME-accredited basic colposcopy course. The second tier consists of a mentorship where colposcopy skills are evaluated by a more experienced colposcopist who is an ASCCP-approved mentor. The mentee documents a minimum of 25 consecutive supervised colposcopic examinations on women with abnormal cervical cytology. Three of the colposcopies should be of high-grade findings. The third tier includes cognitive and pattern recognition skills testing through the Colposcopy Mentorship Program examination. The ASCCP also encourages utilization of self-learning modules for maintenance of colposcopic skills. There is no national certification for colposcopy. A national survey of obstetric and family medicine residency programs revealed that, as a group, 73% of programs surveyed report having a formal colposcopy curriculum in place.[16]

PREPARATION FOR INITIATION OF COLPOSCOPY SERVICES

The equipment and supplies needed to perform colposcopy are listed in Tables 6-1 to 6-3. Consideration should also be given to the physical space where the colposcopy will be performed. A cramped examination room similar to that used for routine examinations may not have sufficient space for all the additional equipment needed to perform colposcopy and may hinder the ability to comfortably and efficiently examine both routine patients and those undergoing colposcopic examination.

The choice of a cytology-pathology laboratory is also an important one. Ideally, the laboratory and the pathologist should be accessible to the colposcopist for discussion of cases and correlation of findings. *The colposcopist should speak with the pathologist and agree about the transmission of specimens, the interpretation of reports, and the consultation guidelines should questions arise. The pathologist and colposcopist should also come to a clear understanding about the classification systems that will be used for cytologic and histologic*

Table 6-1 General Equipment for Colposcopy

Examination room
Examination table, preferably with adjustable height and heel cushions
Stand or surgical table for supplies
Examination gloves of various sizes, including latex-free gloves
Various-sized specula (Graves', Pedersen's)—metal reusable or plastic disposable
Container for dirty surgical instruments (preferably rubber)
Autoclave for equipment and supplies
Disinfectant solution containing 2% glutaraldehyde

Table 6-2 Colposcopic Equipment

Colposcope with extra light bulbs
Optional attachments for colposcope (camera, video, teaching head, television monitor, videocassette recorder, digital archival system)
Punch biopsy forceps
Endocervical curette
Endocervical specula of various sizes
Cervical hook
Ring or sponge forceps
Needle holder (long handle)
Surgical scissors (long handle)
Anoscope, clear plastic

Table 6-3 Specific Supplies for the Colposcopic Examination

Monsel's solution (ferric subsulfate) dehydrated to thick paste
Diluted (quarter- or half-strength) Lugol's iodine solution
3–5% acetic acid (or vinegar) in small container
Small containers for individual patient use
Silver nitrate sticks
Large cotton swabs and small cotton-tipped applicators
Toothpicks
Gauze pads (4 × 4)
Disposable pads for placement under patient's buttocks
Lens paper for cleaning optical pieces
Glass slide equipment if using conventional cytology
Buffered formalin or other laboratory preservative
Liquid-based cytology supplies
Suture material, various sizes
Local anesthetic (1% lidocaine) with and without epinephrine
Dental syringe with spinal needle and anesthesia cartridges or regular needles and syringes and needle extender

interpretation, what the terminology means, and the clinical implication of a particular cytologic diagnosis. This will help avoid misguided therapeutic decisions related to misunderstandings between the pathologist and the colposcopist.

Competent nursing or medical assistant support is critical in making the colposcopic examination successful. Ideally the assistant and the colposcopist share a similar philosophy about colposcopic practice and general care of the patient. The medical assistant can check the equipment and supplies before each examination, ensuring that supplies are replenished and equipment is available and in good working order. The medical assistant is also a working bridge between the patient and the colposcopist.

The colposcopist should develop a new or adapt an existing colposcopic record that contains basic medicolegal documentation (see Appendices 6-1 to 6-4 for examples of forms). The demographic and colposcopic findings can be included on the same form or on separate ones. If informed consent is to be obtained, the legal office of the institution will generally approve the forms. In addition to record documentation, a procedure for patient notification should be

developed. *Patients who are lost to follow-up may not receive appropriate and recommended treatment and fail to benefit from the clinician's screening and diagnostic efforts.*

It has been shown that there are many barriers to the compliance of patients returning for requested follow-up visits. *Reports indicate that as many as 40% of patients are lost to follow-up.*[17] Among the barriers that have been identified are transportation, childcare, work, fear, and preoccupation with busy life routines. Patient lack of understanding about the seriousness of the problem has also been studied.[18] Other researchers have found that compliance with follow-up is more closely correlated with the severity of the disease at the time of colposcopy than with an understanding of the disease process.[19] The authors suggest that greater compliance after colposcopy may be gained by improving the identification of noncompliant patients when they schedule nongynecologic visits.

SPECIFIC EQUIPMENT FOR THE COLPOSCOPIC EXAMINATION

Colposcope

As a procedure, colposcopy has been available since the 1920s, when the colposcope was little more than an inexpensive, optically modified binocular with an illuminator on the upper surface.[20] By the 1930s, colposcopy was widely used in central Europe. After cervical cytologic screening was introduced, the colposcopic examination became a secondary verification technique, even in Europe where the method was first introduced. It was not until the 1970s that colposcopy became an accepted procedure for the verification of cytologic findings in the United States. Colposcopy is now accepted worldwide as the most studied method for detection of cervical neoplasia and intraepithelial precursors.

The modern optical colposcope is a binocular microscope with a built-in light source and a converging objective lens attached to a support appliance. *It provides magnification and illumination for colposcopic assessment of the target tissue* (Figure 6-1). Each optical colposcope is equipped with binocular lenses and optical tubes with individual diopter settings (Figure 6-2). If desired, the diopters can be set to individually correct the refractive error of each of the colposcopist's eyes so that eyeglasses are unnecessary during the procedure. If eyeglasses are not worn, the rubber appliances on the eyepieces can produce a seal between the eyes and the binocular tubes, thereby blocking out extraneous light. Other colposcopists prefer to wear their glasses during the procedure and peel back the rubber appliances on the

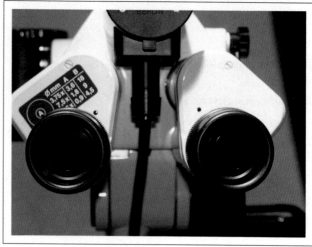

Figure 6-2 Close-up of binocular eyepieces. Each eyepiece can be turned to the right or left to allow for individual eye adjustments to provide a crisp focus.

eyepieces. The interpupillary distance can be individually adjusted so that a clear stereoscopic image is displayed (Figure 6-3A,B).

The colposcope has a fixed focal distance determined by the objective lens; that is, the working distance between the lens and the target tissue. *Most colposcopes have a focal length of around 300 mm. If the focal distance is too short, there will be limited room to maneuver instruments in front of the lens. If the focal length is too long, the colposcopist will be too far from the target tissue to comfortably perform the examination.*

Most colposcopes are equipped with the capability for fine and coarse focusing. As long as the colposcope is at its fixed focal length, the target tissue should be in relatively good focus. Coarse focus can always be achieved by simply moving the entire colposcope. Finer-focus capability can be achieved by turning the fine focus knob (Figures 6-4 and 6-5). Some colposcopes can achieve par-focal capability so that the focus remains throughout all magnification levels. To obtain par focus, the focus must first be achieved under high magnification.

Colposcopes typically provide the capability for variable magnification. Less expensive colposcopes may be equipped with a single, fixed magnification. Most colposcopists will find them unacceptable for precise examination of the target tissues. Some colposcopes have a mechanism to change magnifications through separate discrete steps (Figure 6-6), whereas others are able to zoom through low, medium, and high magnification levels without going through individual steps of magnification (see Figure 6-4). Low-power magnification (2–6×) is typically used for examination of the vulva and of male genitalia; medium power (8–15×) is generally used for examination of the vulva, vagina, and cervix; and high power (15–25×) is especially helpful for assessing the fine detail of vessel patterns, specifically atypical vessels. Changing the magnification will alter the diameter of the field of vision; *the higher the magnification, the smaller the field of vision and lesser the illumination of the target*

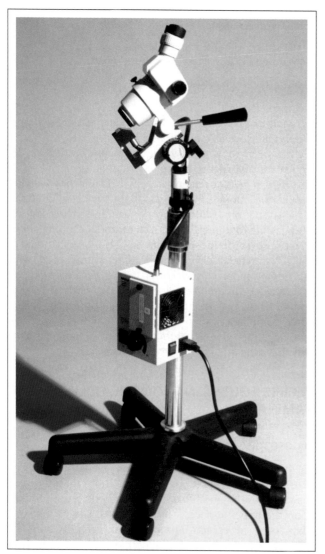

Figure 6-1 Colposcope on a rolling stand.

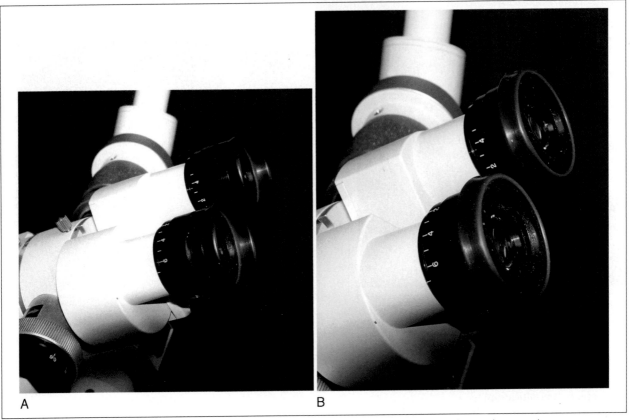

A   B

Figure 6-3 A, Eyeshields flipped up for those who do not wear eyeglasses. **B,** Eyeshields flipped down so that eyeglasses can be worn.

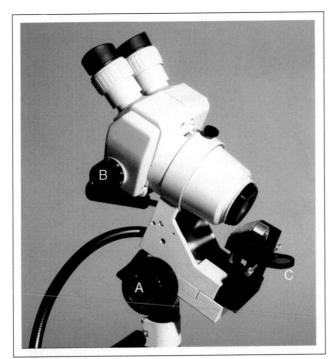

Figure 6-4 A, Close-up of the colposcope head with the fine-focus knob noted at the base of the head *(A)* and the zoom focus noted near the oculars *(B)*. The green filter *(C)* flips up to provide green-light examination of the target tissue.

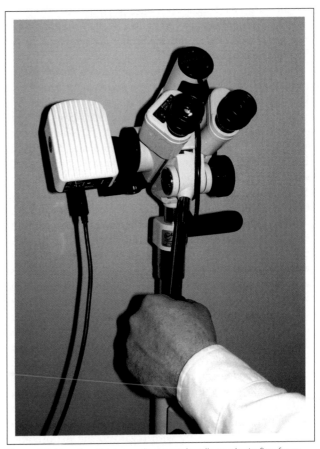

Figure 6-5 Use of a stick-type adjustment handle to obtain fine focus.

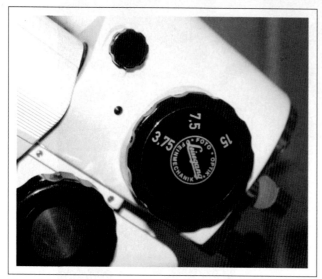

Figure 6-6 Close-up of the colposcope with preset, discrete, variable focus settings.

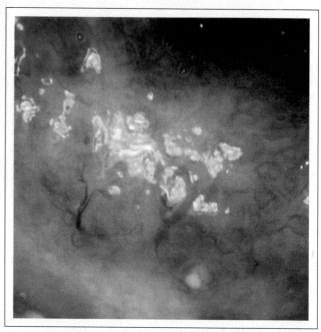

Figure 6-7 Use of a green filter to delineate blood vessel patterns.

tissue. Most modern colposcopes provide a totally illuminated field at low magnification.

Colposcopes are equipped with a green (red-free) filter that serves to enhance the fine detail of the vascular pattern of the target epithelium (see Figure 6-4). The light may need to be increased while the green filter is being used. *The green filter absorbs certain wavelengths of light, making the red color of the vessels appear blacker and sharpening the contrast with the surrounding epithelium* (Figure 6-7).

The light source on the colposcope may be incandescent, tungsten, xenon, or halogen. The halogen light provides a bright light that is excellent for photography.

The colposcope head and stand rest on a base. Various types of stands are available, including rolling, swivel (joystick-type), or swing arm (Figures 6-8 and 6-9). With some colposcopes, the swing arm is attached directly to the examination table or the wall. However, having this type of setup limits the use of the colposcope to just one room, which may not serve the needs of every practice.

Until the introduction of video colposcopy, the basic technique of optical colposcopy had not changed significantly. Video colposcopy is a new method of providing magnification and illumination without use of binocular eyepieces. The system includes a video colposcope and a high-resolution video monitor.[21] The colposcopic image is viewed on a video monitor in a manner similar to laparoscopy (Figures 6-10 and 6-11). *One major drawback to the video colposcope is that the colposcopic image on the video monitor is a two-dimensional rather than a three-dimensional image, making assessment of the contour and density of the lesion more difficult.*

It may take some time for a colposcopist to adjust from standard colposcopy to video colposcopy. The adjustment phase is required to allow for the development of new psychomotor skills, especially with regard to the performance

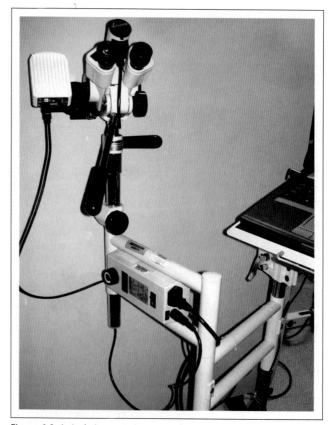

Figure 6-8 Articulating or swing-arm colposcope stand.

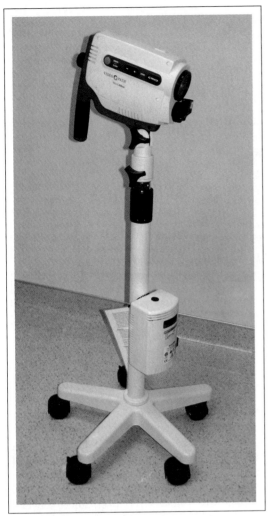

Figure 6-9 A rolling base with a videoscope head.

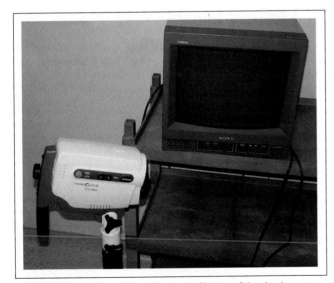

Figure 6-10 A videoscope and monitor. Unlike a traditional colposcope, the image is viewed via the monitor instead of through the binoculars.

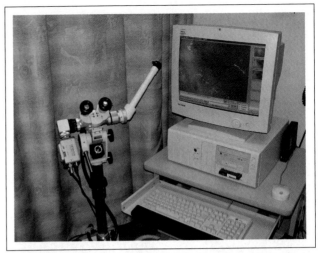

Figure 6-11 A traditional colposcope fitted with a video camera, allowing the examination to be viewed through the binoculars as well as on the monitor.

of the directed biopsy.[22] In one study, colposcopists were able to assess the grade of colposcopic change equally well with both the optical and video colposcopes. In this comparison, the nonstereoscopic video monitor did not appear to hinder contour assessment and depth perception. However, there were more unsatisfactory colposcopic examinations of the endocervical canal with the video colposcope. The rates of agreement of colposcopic impression were not significantly different between the two colposcopes. However, colposcopists using the two systems preferred visualization, assessment, and sampling through the optical colposcope and judged it to be *easier*.

Photographic, Video, and Image Management Systems

Many colposcopes will offer a camera option for taking photographs, most of which, until recently, have involved the use of 35-mm cameras and a special (and expensive) L-shaped adapter called a *C-mount* (Figure 6-12). The user will quickly discover that obtaining quality photographs using these cameras is more of an art than an exact science. Advanatages include high-quality slides that can be used for teaching. Disadvantages include the additional costs of film purchase and processing.

More recent developments include various video attachment add-ons or systems (Figure 6-13) or pure videoscopes (see Figure 6-10). Video viewing during colposcopy can be valuable for patient education and can also be used as an alternative to using a teaching tube attachment on colposcopes during training (Figure 6-14). There is ongoing debate on the advisability of recording photographic or video clip documentation during a colposcopy or treatment due to medicolegal concerns. If obtaining still or video images, written consent should be included in the basic colposcopy consent process or with a separate consent so that patients are aware in advance of the video recording.

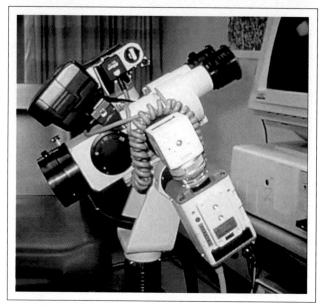

Figure 6-12 A colposcope with a 35-mm camera attached via a C-mount adapter that can be used for cervical photography.

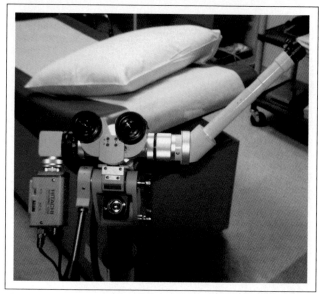

Figure 6-14 A colposcope with a teaching tube attachment. A beam splitter allows the viewer to see exactly what the colposcope operator is seeing.

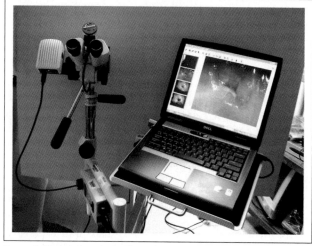

Figure 6-13 A colposcope with a video camera attached, allowing the examination to be viewed through the binoculars as well as on the monitor. This system also allows image capture for review at a later time.

As technology advances, computers play a more active role in the colposcopy clinic, not just in acquisition of digital images but also in data management. A few of the currently available management systems include the Cooper Surgical CerviPATH system (Trumbull, CT) and the Welch Allyn Colposcopy Image Management System (Skaneateles Falls, NY). All systems incorporate video input, digital still-screen shots, and the ability to input various types of demographic information allowing for image review, comparison with prior examination findings, and electronic transmission of images to offsite locations. Some systems have patient management capability including letter generation, scheduling, and actual topographic mapping of lesions for monitoring regression or progression. The costs of these systems vary but range from $15,000 to $30,000.

Cerviscope

Another means of obtaining cervical images independent of a standard or video colposcope is with the use of a cerviscope. The cerviscope was developed in 1980 by Dr. Adolf Stafl, a colposcopist and photographer at the Medical College of Wisconsin. The original function of the instrument was as an adjunct to the Pap smear to avoid missing cervical lesions. Although this function has been effectively supplanted by the use of HPV DNA testing for cytologic triage and primary screening, the cerviscope remains a useful tool for obtaining excellent-quality cervical photographs, also referred to as *cervigrams.** The cerviscope is a 35-mm camera with a fixed focal-distance telephoto macrolens, illumination source, and a strobe flash mounted on a hand-held platform* (Figure 6-15). Following placement of an intravaginal speculum, the cervix is visualized, cleaned with dry gauze, and moistened with dilute acetic acid. The cervicoscope achieves its focus on the cervix by moving the instrument back and forth. Once focus is obtained, a picture is taken. Optimal photographic results are achieved with the use of Ektachrome color slide film. All settings are preset so as to provide consistency in image quality.

Taking a Cervigram Picture

The cervigram is normally taken after the Pap smear has been obtained (Figure 6-16). It is important to ensure that there is a clear and unobstructed view of the entire cervix and that the cervix is centered in the image field. The cervix

---

*Editor's note: Many of the high-quality colposcopic images in this text are cervigrams.

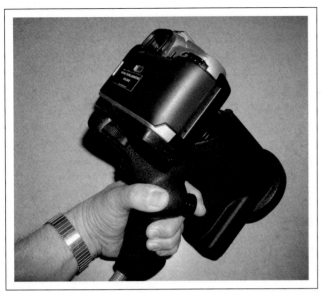

Figure 6-15 A cerviscope is held with the left hand. The shutter-release button is activated by the left index finger to take a picture.

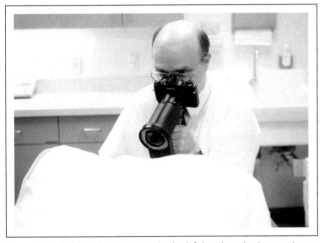

Figure 6-16 Holding the cerviscope in the left hand to obtain a cervigram. Focusing is accomplished by leaning slightly forward or backward.

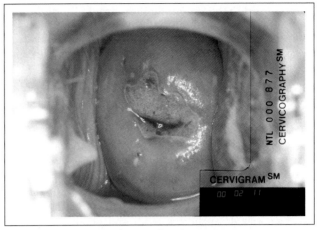

Figure 6-17 A cervigram of a normal cervix.

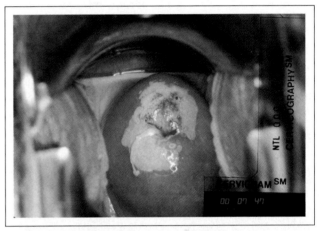

Figure 6-18 A cervigram of a large, low-grade lesion.

light is attached to the colposcope by a bracket (Figure 6-19). Using the camera flash and the macrolens function to obtain a magnified view of the cervix, digital images are obtained and can be downloaded to a computer for viewing. From this

is generously soaked with vinegar or dilute acetic acid for about 30 seconds, and two cervigrams are taken. The procedure normally adds less than 2 minutes to the examination time. The slides that are subsequently produced can be viewed with a slide projector or scanned into a digital format (Figure 6-17 and 6-18). *The cerviscope camera produces consistent, high-resolution, panoramic photographic images of the lower genital tract. These high-quality images can be used for lesion documentation, colposcopy training, and the testing and monitoring of colposcopic skills.*

A digital alternative to use of a tradional cerviscope is a digital cerviscope described by Dr. Adolf Stafl.[23] A digital cerviscope can be assembled using a 5-megapixel or higher digital camera, a CLA4 lens adapter tube, and a macroconverter lens with a high-intensity light for focusing. The focusing

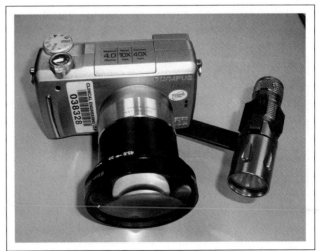

Figure 6-19 A digital cerviscope with a macrolens to allow for close-ups and a focusing light to allow the camera to focus properly.

author's (GB) perspective, the image quality is significantly more variable than with the traditional cerviscope, resulting in images that resemble those obtained with camera attachments of the past. Results will vary greatly depending upon the operator's technique and experience.

Instruments for Colposcopy

Punch Biopsy Forceps

Many punch biopsy forceps are available and, over time, each colposcopist will select a favorite one to use. *Most of the biopsy instruments are named after the designer or manufacturer (Tischler, Burke, Kevorkian, and Eppendorfer), and each obtains a slightly different-shaped specimen. The Tischler forceps has a single anchoring tooth and obtains a rounded* specimen (Figure 6-20). The Kevorkian forcep has alligator teeth on the anchoring edge and obtains a square specimen (Figure 6-21). A Baby Tischler forceps retrieves a smaller specimen with potentially less bleeding at the biopsy site (Figure 6-22). All the punch biopsy forceps are constructed with a handle shank and a biopsy tip or head. The jaws of the head consist of an anchoring device and a cutting edge. Some of the shanks can be rotated 360 degrees so that the entire instrument does not have to be rotated during the procedure.

Endocervical Curettes

Endocervical curettes are long, stainless steel rods consisting of a finger-grip handle and a head or tip with a slightly upturned cutting

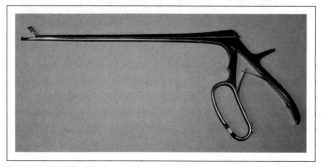

Figure 6-20 A Tischler biopsy forceps.

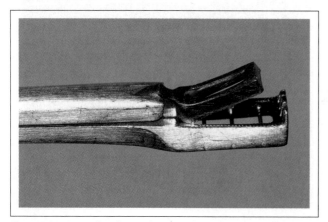

Figure 6-21 A Kevorkian biopsy forceps with a square jaw and a row of teeth on the lower jaw.

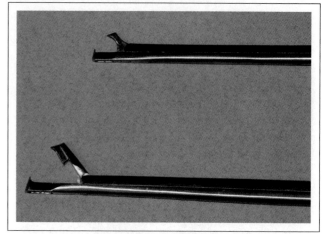

Figure 6-22 Comparison of the differences in biopsy tip size of a baby Tischler *(top)* and a regular Tischler *(bottom).*

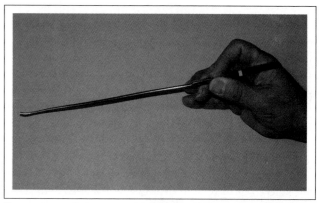

Figure 6-23 Endocervical curette without a basket.

edge (Figure 6-23). Only one edge of the tip is a sharp cutting edge. The other edge is dull and is not used as a cutting surface. The cutting edge of the tip is on the same plane as the finger hold on the handle. The head or tip is made with or without a basket. If a basket is present, the sample collected in the basket may prove difficult to remove.

Cervical Hooks

A long surgical hook can be used to "pucker" the tissue so a biopsy sample can be obtained (Figure 6-24). *A hook is especially helpful if the biopsy surface is flat and the punch biopsy forceps cannot be adequately anchored on the tissue.* A skin hook can prevent the tissue from slipping away from the biopsy forceps. The bend of the hook should not be too acute; otherwise it will be impossible to grasp the tissue. The tip of the hook should not be too sharp lest the tissue be torn during the sampling procedure. It is rare that a hook will be needed on the cervical epithelium. More often, the hook is used to visualize the rugae or lesions in the vagina.

Endocervical Speculum

It is occasionally necessary to visualize the endocervical canal, either because a lesion extends into the canal or because the transformation zone is not fully visualized.

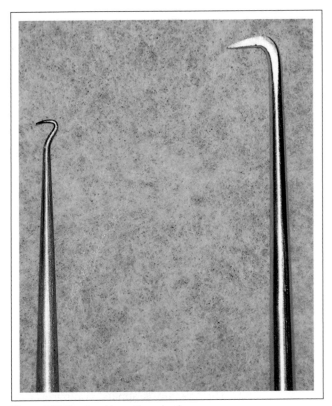

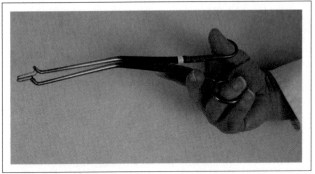

Figure 6-25 An endocervical speculum is held in a palm-up manner. If held palm down, the back of the hand can obstruct the colposcopic view.

Figure 6-24 Small and large tissue hooks.

In one report, unsatisfactory colposcopy was noted to occur in approximately 1% to 5% of colposcopic examinations.[24] Others have reported that 10% to 15% of premenopausal women younger than 45 years will have an unsatisfactory colposcopic examination.[25] Postmenopausal women may have even higher percentages of unsatisfactory colposcopy because the squamocolumnar junction is located deep in the endocervical canal. *Adequate visualization of the entire transformation zone may be facilitated by the use of an endocervical speculum* (Figure 6–25). Additionally, the instrument can be used to examine the endocervical canal for polyps or other lesions. The endocervical speculum is placed into the external os and then opened gently (Figure 6-26). The blades of the endocervical speculum are available in regular and narrow or thin sizes, with the thin blades designed specifically for nulliparous or stenotic cervices (Figure 6-27).

Vaginal Sidewall Retractors

The vaginal sidewalls may obscure visualization of the cervix during the colposcopic examination. *Vaginal sidewall retraction is usually unnecessary, but when the vaginal walls are lax and redundant, the ability to retract the sidewall may allow the colposcopist to complete an otherwise impossible examination.* Vaginal retractors are specially designed to fit inside the speculum and open with a ratchet mechanism (Figure 6-28). The hinges of the speculum, however, may prevent complete separation of the retractor paddles, such that the colposcopist may be unable to achieve the desired visualization of the cervix. Another option is to place a condom or the finger of an examination glove over the speculum blades so that when the speculum is opened, the vaginal walls will be retracted. After the tip is cut off, the condom or latex

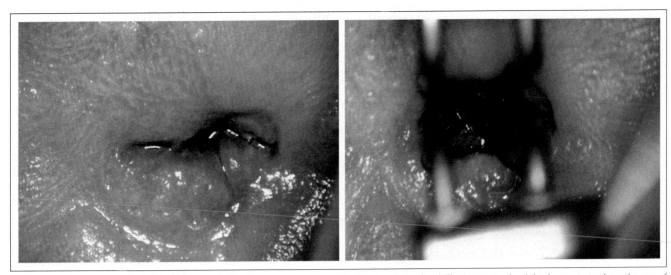

Figure 6-26 The image on the left is a post-cryotherapy treatment cervix, and the SCJ is not visualized. The image on the right demonstrates how the use of an endocervical speculum allows visualization of the SCJ.

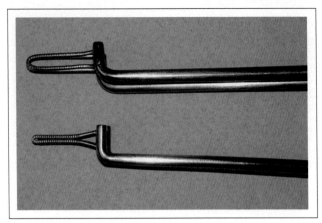

Figure 6-27 Close-up of tips of a Kogan endocervical speculum. A regular-blade endocervical speculum is on top, and the thin-line speculum used for a narrowed cervical os is on the bottom.

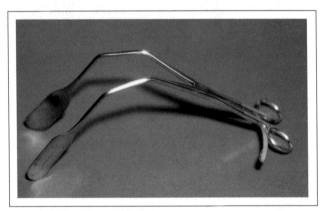

Figure 6-28 Lateral vaginal wall retractor.

finger is placed over the closed blades of the speculum (Figures 6-29 and 6-30). In some situations, especially if the patient is obese, it is difficult to open the speculum with the latex finger or condom in place, and extra hand strength is required.

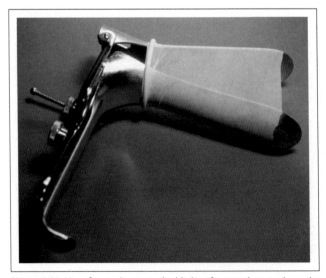

Figure 6-29 Use of a condom over the blades of a speculum can keep the vaginal walls from obscuring the cervix during colposcopy.

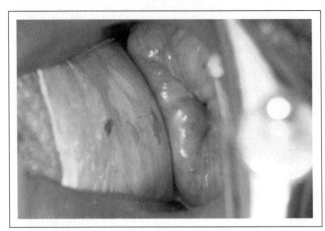

Figure 6-30 Example of the use of a condom over the blades of a speculum to improve visibility. Previously the view of the cervix was completely obscured by the collapsed vaginal side walls.

Supplies for Colposcopy

Dilute Acetic Acid or Vinegar

Colposcopy of the cervix is performed after the application of dilute (3–5%) acetic acid or vinegar. The resulting "acetowhiteness" of the epithelium may indicate a benign or neoplastic process. The solution is applied copiously with gauze sponges, large cotton-tipped swabs, or a spray bottle. *To achieve an acetowhite reaction in nonkeratinized epithelium, the 3% to 5% acetic acid must be left in contact with the tissue until the reaction is maximally expressed.* During the examination, reapplication of the dilute acetic acid may be necessary to maintain the acetowhite effect. The vessel patterns may be more prominent as the acetowhite reaction begins to fade. The solution may cause discomfort, especially if the patient has a vaginal infection. Allergic reactions are rare, but irritation may occur.

Aqueous Lugol's Solution

Iodine solution is diluted to quarter-strength or half-strength to obtain Lugol's solution. Lugol's solution is unstable on the shelf and should be replaced every 3 to 6 months. Although the dilute solution may produce less drying effect and irritation than full-strength iodine produces, some patients are particularly sensitive. Some will even have an intense allergic reaction. *Patients should always be queried about previous allergic reactions to iodine before Lugol's solution is applied. Lugol's solution stains normal mature nonkeratonized squamous epithelium a dark, mahogany color, indicating that glycogen is present in the cells. The absence of staining* denotes a nonglycogenated state or a keratinized surface (Figure 6-31). Squamous metaplasia may exhibit variegated staining, whereas columnar epithelium stains a mustard-yellow color (see Chapter 10).

Monsel's Solution

Monsel's (ferric subsulfate) solution (Figure 6-32) is used to achieve hemostasis after a cervical biopsy. In its original consistency the solution is too thin to be useful.

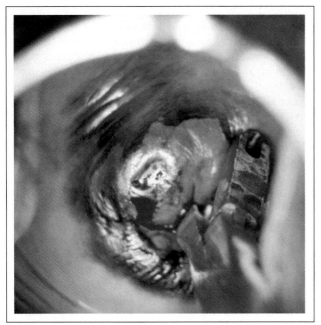

Figure 6-31 Area on the anterior lip of the cervix that rejects iodine. A biopsy forceps is about to sample this area of a low-grade lesion.

The solution becomes more effective when it is allowed to dehydrate in the open air until it becomes more thickened. This is achieved by pouring Monsel's solution into a clean urine container and setting it on a shelf with an open lid for approximately 1 week, stirring it every few days with a tongue blade. It will change from its initial dark-drown color to a mustard-yellow color due to oxidation. Once it is the consistency of syrup, the lid is placed on the container. If the consistency becomes too thick (to the consistency of a paste), it becomes less effective. If it dehydrates even more, it will solidfy and become unusable. Adding a few milliliters of the solution from the stock bottle to the cup and stirring it with a tongue blade should restore it to its proper consistency. Heating the solution by running the closed container under hot water may help to mix the old and new solutions. When Monsel's solution is needed, a small amount of the thickened solution is poured into a medication-dispensing cup, keeping the main container free of contamination. If thickened Monsel's solution is needed quickly, a small amount of Monsel's solution can be placed from the stock bottle into a glass beaker (one-third full), and the uncovered beaker is *cooked* in the microwave on high at 30-second intervals until the correct consistency is achieved after stirring with a wooden tongue blade. The thickened Monsel's solution is allowed to cool and subsequently poured into a clean urine container cup. The lid is applied, and Monsel's solution is ready to use on an urgent basis.

After the biopsy is completed, thickened Monsel's and/or pressure are applied directly to the biopsy site with a small cotton-tipped applicator (Figure 6-33). When hemostasis is difficult to achieve, the applicator should be held on the biopsy site for a few minutes. *Monsel's solution*

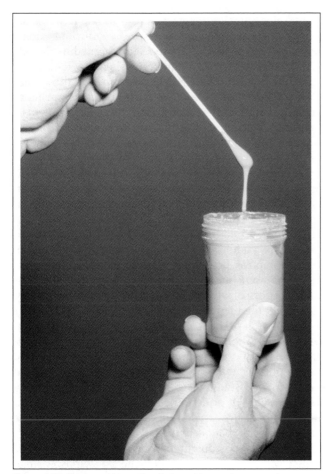

Figure 6-32 Thickened Monsel's solution with a molasses consistency.

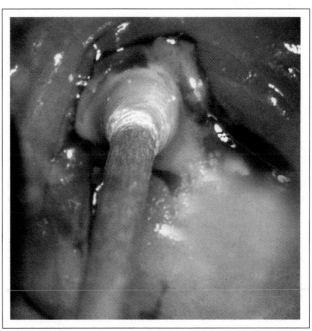

Figure 6-33 The application of Monsel's solution to a cervical biopsy site by a cotton-tipped applicator using gentle pressure to obtain hemostasis.

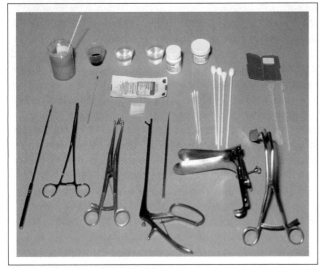

Figure 6-34 Supply and equipment setup for colposcopy. Starting at the left upper corner of the figure, the supplies shown are Monsel's solution, iodine, saline, 5% acetic acid, benzocaine gel, specimen container, silver nitrate sticks, hemostatic gauze, 1- × 1-inch paper towel squares, small and large cotton-tipped applicators, Pap smear supplies, lateral wall retractor, speculum, cervical hook, biopsy forceps, endocervical speculum, ring forceps, and endocervical curette.

will interfere with biopsy interpretation and should not be applied until after all the samples are taken.[26] Excessive Monsel's solution should be removed from the vagina before the speculum is removed. The patient should be warned that Monsel's solution may produce a charcoal-like vaginal discharge for several days.

Silver Nitrate

Silver nitrate sticks can be used for hemostasis. They are especially helpful if they are placed directly in the center of the biopsy site. The patient may experience more irritation or burning with silver nitrate than with Monsel's solution. As with Monsel's solution, the silver nitrate will interfere with biopsy interpretation and should be applied only after all biopsies are completed.

See Figure 6-34 for an example of colposcopy equipment and a supply tray.

COLPOSCOPICALLY DIRECTED BIOPSY

The colposcopist must consider many important aspects when performing colposcopically directed biopsies. The speculum should be opened as wide as the patient can tolerate, using both the bottom pin and the side pin on the speculum. Colposcopic assessment is aided by using a grading or assessment system to identify the most severe lesion or lesions requiring biopsy. Grading systems (see Chapter 10) promote the inspection of several colposcopic features including degree of acetowhiteness, lesion margin, blood vessels, and, with the Reid's scoring system, the addition of Lugol's iodine staining, The indices of margin, acetowhiteness, and blood vessels were prospectively evaluated in a

randomized study to determine their performance in clinical practice.[27] The degree of acetowhiteness was the only feature significantly associated with any CIN or CIN 2,3. For detection of CIN 2,3, a strong acetowhite change had a sensitivity and specificity of 28% and 98%, respectively, with a negative predictive value of 74%. Recent data suggest that not all lesions may be critically identified by a grading system that includes color, margin, and vessels.[28] The three colposcoopic signs of color, margin, and vessels were not individually sensitive for detecting CIN 3. It is noteworthy that a maximum score of 2 for color, margin, and vessels on the Reid's scale was insensitive in detecting ≥ CIN 3. Assessment of vessel findings was slightly more sensitive but less specific than color and margin status at predicting ≥ CIN 3 at a maximum score of 2.

It has been suggested that low- and high-grade lesions are found significantly more often in the anterior and posterior locations of the cervix, suggesting that CIN is not randomly distributed on the ectocervix.[29] The author concluded that these areas exhibited more serious colposcopic features and were not chosen simply because of ease of biopsy in these areas. Data from ALTS also demonstrated that acetowhite areas are more common on the anterior and posterior lips of the cervix than at the 3- and 9-o'clock positions. On further analysis, the excess of acetowhitening at the 12- and 6-o'clock positions was attributable entirely to an excess that could be seen if CIN or HPV infection were absent.[1] Because the same uneven distribution of acetowhiteness was present in women with normal histology, the evidence is weak that more CIN is located at the 12- and 6-o'clock positions. These regions tend to look more acetowhite even if CIN or HPV is absent. Given these data, it follows that the 12- and 6-o'clock quadrants are more frequently biopsied than the 3- and 9-o'clock quadrants.[1] From this observation, evidence was lacking that a biopsy taken from the more frequently biopsied sites was more or less likely to reveal high-grade histology.

Grading systems are not the only step in the process of ensuring that the most abnormal area is biopsied. The abnormal area(s) may be too small to be detected in complex lesions.[3] Detection of these subtle lesions requires taking more than one biopsy in the area of the most severe lesion. Taking additional biopsies in other abnormal areas may also improve detection.[3] Whether the person performing the biopsy is an inexperienced or advanced colposcopist, detection of abnormalities is best accomplished by more rather than fewer biopsies.

The question of the role of random biopsies has recently been raised. Although not endorsed by all expert colposcopists, the premise is intriguing and deserves further study to determine its ability to increase detection of high-grade lesions. In one study all colposcopically detected lesions were biopsied.[30] If no lesion was identified in a quadrant, a random biopsy was performed at the squamocolumnar junction (SCJ) in that quadrant and an ECC was performed. Although all colposcopies were satisfactory, only 57% of women with ≥ CIN 2 were detected by colposcopically directed biopsy. Adding a random biopsy in a quadrant where no lesion was identified increased the proportion of $\geq$ CIN 2 detected from 57.1% to 94.5%. Disease detected by random biopsy was smaller and of lower grade than that detected by colposcopically directed biopsy. The yield of $\geq$ CIN 2 per random biopsy for women with high-grade squamous intraepithelial lesion (HSIL) or cancer was 17.6% compared with 3.6% and 1.7% in women who had low-grade squamous intraepithelial lesion (LSIL) or were HPV positive/ASC-US, respectively.

When performing multiple biopsies, the clinician should order the biopsy sites from posterior to anterior to prevent blood from flowing onto other lesions and obscuring subsequent sample sites. Local anesthetic is not usually required for biopsy of the cervix or the upper to middle third of the vagina. It is usually necessary if the distal third of the vagina or the vulva is biopsied. Some clinicians have found it beneficial to use topical anesthetic, but at least one study offered some evidence that it is ineffective.[31]

The highest-grade lesions are likely to be found closest to the SCJ. When the lesion extends into the endocervical canal, an attempt should be made to manipulate the cervix to sample the proximal aspect of the lesion. The value of routine endocervical curettage (ECC) is controversial. *Those advocating ECC at the time of colposcopy see it as insurance that invasive cancer is not present, although adding ECC to the evaluation of women with satisfactory colposcopy did not improve diagnostic accuracy.* Some authors conclude that a positive ECC in women with satisfactory colposcopy is most likely due to contamination.[32] In one study, 5.5% of women with satisfactory coloposcopy had a positive ECC as their only biopsy showing $\geq$ CIN 2.[32] *Some colposcopists reserve an ECC for selected patients such as those in whom the transformation zone is not fully visualized, those who have been previously treated, those at high risk for recurrent disease, and those to be treated with ablative therapy. ECC is always contraindicated in the pregnant patient. Whether to perform ECC before or after the cervical biopsies is a matter of style rather than correct technique.* Performing the ECC first under colposcopic guidance allows the colposcopist to avoid inadvertently contaminating the ECC with tissue from an ectocervical lesion. This is important when the colposcopy is otherwise satisfactory and the presence of a positive ECC would indicate the need for a deeper excisional procedure rather than an ablative procedure or a shallower excision. However, once done, the ECC may cause bleeding that can obscure the remaining lesions and interfere with properly directing the biopsy. Ultimately, the colposcopic examination will determine order of biopsy and ECC.

When the desired biopsy site is found in the vagina, the difficulty of obtaining a biopsy is increased because the tubular configuration of the vagina does not allow a perpendicular approach to the lesion. The biopsy may be facilitated by slowly withdrawing the speculum and creating a ridge or fold, enabling the clinician to securely grasp the desired site for biopsy. A surgical hook may assist in grasping the tissue.

The choice of a punch biopsy instrument is usually one of personal preference. It is important to realize that the size of the jaws should not dictate the size of the biopsy. Although a large biopsy cannot be taken with a small-jawed biopsy instrument, a large-jawed biopsy instrument need not take only large biopsies. A small biopsy can be taken using only the tip of the jaw. In some cases, however, the specific punch biopsy forceps needed to perform colposcopic biopsy is dependent on the size and location of the lesion. If there is concern about microinvasion or frank invasion, a larger punch biopsy forceps with a wider-opening jaw, such as the Tischler forceps, may be necessary to obtain a sample of adequate depth. If the sample is too small and superficial, the pathologist may not be able to rule out invasion. A biopsy forceps with a small basket, such as the baby Tischler forceps, may enable adequate sampling of a lesion extending into the narrow endocervical canal. If the basket of the forceps is larger than the cervical os, it is impossible to enter the endocervical canal.

Small lesions can often be completely excised. In many cases, the exact area to be biopsied in a large, uniformly abnormal lesion may not be critical. However, when ulceration is present, the colposcopist should attempt to sample an edge of intact epithelium, as well as a portion of the ulcerative bed to more accurately establish the diagnosis.

At times, it is difficult to securely grasp the tissue with the punch biopsy forceps. Depending on the location of the lesion and the configuration of the biopsy forceps, the jaw of the instrument may slide off the tissue, or the cutting edge will not be able to touch the surface of the lesion. Occasionally, the angle required for the cutting edge of the forceps to contact the tissue cannot be achieved within the limited confines of the speculum. It may be easier to turn the biopsy forceps upside down, allowing the longer cutting edge to reach the tissue with less of an angle. Occasionally, a tenaculum or hook is needed to mobilize the cervix or tent the tissue to obtain the sample.[33]

A colposcopist who finds it necessary to locate the biopsy site with the colposcope and then push the colposcope aside and obtain the sample without the benefit of magnification and illumination has not sufficiently mastered the skills of colposcopy and may benefit from more direct supervision. This approach can lead to inadequate sampling, underdiagnosis, and inappropriate treatment. The difficulty may be related to the lack of binocular vision caused by the failure to correct for the refractive error of each of the colposcopist's eyes by setting the diopters of the colposcope individually or the adjusting the interpupillary distance of the colposcope so that a clear stereoscopic image is displayed. The biopsy sites should be visualized with the colposcope on completion of the procedure to ensure that the desired area was sampled.[34]

The biopsy forceps should be kept closed until withdrawn from the vagina to avoid dropping the small specimen before it is deposited in the specimen container. Occasionally, if a small basket forceps is used, a small specimen will pass right through the basket. It is important to verify that the specimen is present in the basket before applying pressure to the biopsy site to control the bleeding. The specimen will sometimes be found on the blade of the speculum and can be easily retrieved and deposited in the appropriate specimen container, rather than lost in the trash on a cotton swab. The basket may also be empty when a complete cut through the tissue has not been achieved. One small edge of the specimen may still be attached at the biopsy site. This usually occurs when the punch biopsy forceps is *dull*. In truth, as most biopsy forceps cut with a scissor cut (forcing the tissue between the upper and lower blades of the instrument) rather than with a knife cut (cutting with the sharpness of a single blade), the dullness of an instrument is usually due to a microscopically bent or misaligned blade rather than one that needs sharpening. In fact, sharpening the blade may damage it. Instruments that are not cutting properly are best returned to the manufacturer for repair rather than being sharpened by a local vendor.

The biopsy sample should be removed from the biopsy punch with a toothpick and placed in preservative. Care should be taken not to crush or overmanipulate the specimen, and it should be placed immediately in the preservative to avoid air-drying. Both situations can lead to difficulty in interpretation and diagnosis.[35]

The need to biopsy multiple sites warrants a word of caution about the application of hemostatic agents. All samples should be obtained before applying Monsel's solution or silver nitrate. The caustic nature of these chemicals can interfere with the histologic reading of the sample.[26] Immediate pressure after each biopsy with a large cotton swab will also decrease blood loss and may obviate the need for additional hemostatic agents.

Ideally, the colposcopist should place each biopsy in a separate, labeled container. This enables the colposcopist to correlate the colposcopic impression with the cytologic and histologic results. The grade and location of the lesion can affect the choice of treatment. However, the cost considerations of separate pathology charges for each specimen may obviate the use of this approach. Labeling the specimen containers is critical, and *it is the colposcopist's responsibility to ensure that all samples are correctly labeled before they are removed from the examination room for transport to the laboratory.*

TECHNIQUE OF COLPOSCOPIC EXAMINATION

1. The supplies and equipment are checked before the examination is begun.
2. The proper documentation forms are labled with the patient's identifying information and if applicable, informed consent is obtained.
3. The patient is placed in the dorsal lithotomy position and properly draped.
4. The colposcopist sits comfortably at the colposcope, the interpupillary distance of the binoculars and the diopters are set, and the colposcope is turned on.
5. Depending on the indications for the colposcopy, the vulva may be inspected with the colposcope. Three to five percent acetic acid or vinegar may be used to enhance the epithelial findings. If an abnormal area is

identified, vulvar biopsy may be performed at this time. Some colposcopists defer colposcopy and biopsy of the vulva until the end of the examination.

6. The largest size of intravaginal speculum that the patient can comfortably tolerate is placed in the vagina.
7. If necessary, vaginal sidewall retraction is achieved with a vaginal retractor placed inside the speculum or by a condom or latex-gloved finger applied over the speculum blades *(the tip of condom or glove must be cut off)*.
8. The cervix must be adequately visualized. Gentle wiping of mucus may be necessary. If the cervix is not in a satisfactory position and it is impossible to view the cervix, moistened, rolled-up gauze pads can be placed in the fornix with ring forceps.
9. If applicable, cytologic sampling is performed. If bleeding follows, applying gentle pressure to the bleeding site or in the endocervical canal with a cotton-tipped applicator will usually stop the bleeding. Monsel's solution should not be applied at this time.
10. The cervix is viewed with white light (and saline, if it is dry) under low power (4–8×) magnification. Gross findings and the presence of leukoplakia are noted.
11. The vessel pattern is evaluated with the green filter. The vessels are examined under low and high magnification. Three to five percent acetic acid should not be applied until after the vessel pattern is assessed.
12. A copious amount of 3% to 5% acetic acid (or vinegar) is applied to the cervix with saturated cotton swabs, gauze, cotton balls on a ring forceps, or a spray bottle. Excessive rubbing or patting of the cervix should be avoided. Gently placing the cotton balls, gauze, or swabs on the cervix and allowing the solution to thoroughly soak the tissue avoids unnecessary abrasions or bleeding. Another approach is to apply the vinegar with a spray-mist bottle. A second application of dilute acetic acid or vinegar should follow the first application to ensure an appropriate acetowhite reaction. Once the cervix is thoroughly soaked, excess mucus can be more easily removed.
13. The cervix is assessed for epithelial findings after the dilute acetic acid application (acetowhite reaction) with low, intermediate, and high magnification. The acetowhite reaction will begin to fade slowly or quickly depending on the severity of the epithelial abnormality. As the acetowhite reaction fades, the vessel patterns (mosaic and punctation) become more distinct because of the contrast with the surrounding tissue. If vessel patterns are present, they should be examined under high-power magnification. Use of the green filter again may confirm vessel patterns after the acetowhite reaction has faded.
14. The normal and abnormal epithelial and blood vessel patterns should be mentally mapped because it will be necessary to recall the findings when it is time to complete the documentation forms.
15. If the patient is not allergic to iodine, the cervix may be stained with dilute Lugol's solution. An assessment of

the epithelial patterns is dependent on the interaction between cellular glycogen and iodine. Lugol's solution can have a drying effect on the vagina, and it will stain the patient's underclothing. Not all colposcopists use Lugol's solution on with every colposcopic examination.

16. If applicable, endocervical sampling is accomplished with an endocervical curette or cytobrush. The curette is held like a pencil and inserted through the external os, and the entire endocervical canal is sampled with definitive strokes. Care should be taken not to contaminate the sample with ectocervical lesions. While it is in the endocervical canal, the sample is spun onto the tip of the curette, and the curette is removed straight from the canal. A cytobrush or ring forceps can be used to remove the remainder of the sample from the canal. The entire sample is placed in fixative, and the specimen bottle is labeled with patient identification.

17. If applicable, colposcopically directed biopsies are performed. The biopsy site(s) is/are selected, and the sample is obtained with the cervical biopsy punch. The anchoring edge of the biopsy punch firmly grasps the tissue so that the lesion will not slip away while the biopsy is performed. The posterior surface of the cervix is biopsied first to prevent blood obscuring the biopsy site. The sample should not be pulled from the biopsy site but should be cleanly cut. Additional samples are obtained from other identified sites. If the tooth of the biopsy punch cannot anchor the tissue, a skin hook is used to create a fold of tissue around which the jaws of the punch can close. The cervix is checked to make sure all biopsies have been successfully obtained. The biopsy specimens are removed from the biopsy punch and placed in fixative. The specimen bottles are labeled with the patient identification information.

18. Thickened Monsel's solution is applied to achieve hemostasis after all the biopsies are obtained. Occasionally, only pressure will be required. The Monsel's solution should contact the actual tissue rather than only the blood oozing from the biopsy site. Silver nitrate sticks can also be used. Excessive blood and Monsel's solution should be cleaned from the fornices with a cotton swab before the speculum is removed to avoid postcolposcopy discharge.

19. The vagina is inspected as the speculum is removed. Application of dilute Lugol's solution is helpful to delineate abnormal epithelium. If Lugol's solution is not used, the vagina should be grossly inspected as the speculum is removed. A skin hook can be used to visualize between and around the vaginal rugae.

20. If applicable, vulvar biopsy can be accomplished at this time.

21. The patient is informed about the preliminary colposcopic impression. She is also instructed about the mechanism and time frame for reporting her results. Educational material may be distributed before she leaves the office.

22. The specimens are checked to ensure that patient identification has been properly applied. Laboratory forms are completed, and the specimen is prepared for transportation to the laboratory.

23. The documentation forms are completed. The cervical diagram should indicate satisfactory or unsatisfactory colposcopy and the presence of normal and abnormal findings, and location of colposcopically directed biopsies.

24. The colposcope is cleaned and the supplies replenished. Surgical instruments are prepared for sterilization.

DOCUMENTATION OF COLPOSCOPIC FINDINGS

Documentation of clinical findings is an important part of the systematic colposcopic procedure. It is recommended that the colposcopic record be an independent part of the patient's chart and that it be readily retrievable. Consideration should be given to preprinting the colposcopic record forms so that all information is completed in a systematic manner at the time of each examination. Demographic information, clinical findings, and recommendations for follow-up visits or referrals should all be included in the colposcopic record (Tables 6-4 to 6-6). The demographic information should include name, address, and telephone number of the patient (or contact person); date of last menstrual period; pertinent sexual history; menstrual history; and current contraceptive methods, if applicable. The clinician should then obtain a history of the current complaint, including a history of previous abnormal Pap tests, a history of previous STDs, and a history of STDs in sexual partners (see Appendices 6-1 to 6-4 for examples of forms).

In recording the clinical findings, the location of the SCJ and the external os should be identified on the diagram of the cervix. The colposcopic impressions of both normal and abnormal findings on the cervix, vulva, vagina, and rectum should be displayed on the colposcopic record. These include acetowhite epithelium, leukoplakia, mosaic, punctation, and atypical vessels.

The clinician should record any cytologic specimens or cultures that were obtained or biopsies that were performed at the time of colposcopy. The record of colposcopic findings should include a statement about whether the transformation zone was fully visualized, whether invasive cancer was suspected, and whether all the abnormal lesions were visualized in their entirety. Finally, the recommendations for follow-up visits or referrals are recorded, including the return visit interval. If the patient fails to return for the appropriate follow-up visit(s), the method of notification should be recorded. If all attempts to reach the patient fail, a registered letter should be sent, with documentation of the mailing placed in the medical record.

Table 6-7 lists the steps and the expected findings for site-specific colposcopy of the cervix, vagina, and vulva.

Table 6-4 Site-Specific Colposcopy: Cervix

Steps in Colposcopic Assessment of the Cervix	Specific Observations at This Step of the Examination	
	Normal Findings	**Abnormal Findings**
1. Clean the cervix with normal saline.*	Mature squamous and columnar epithelia	Leukoplakia Polyps Nabothian cysts
2. Assess the cervix with a green filter before the application of 3–5% acetic acid.*		Abnormal vessel patterns. Atypical vessels
3. Assess the cervix after the application of 3–5% acetic acid.	Gland openings Squamous metaplasia Squamocolumnar junction Nonspecific acetowhite changes	Condyloma acuminatum Acetowhite changes specific for preinvasive disease Low and high grade disease Cervical carcinoma Abnormal vascular patterns Atypical vessels Ulcerations
4. Assess the cervix after the application of diluted Lugol's iodine solution.*	Dark, mahogany staining (glycogenated epithelium)	Nonstaining (nonglycogenated epithelium) Variegated (nonglycogenated epithelium)
5. Perform endocervical sampling* (ECC, cytobrush).		
6. Perform colposcopic-directed biopsy* (cervical biopsy punch).		
7. Achieve hemostasis (direct pressure, Monsel's solution, silver nitrate).*		

ECC, Endocervical curettage.
*Not required.

Table 6-5 Site-Specific Colposcopy: Vagina

Steps in Colposcopic Assessment of the Vagina	Specific Observations at This Step of the Examination	
	Normal Findings	**Abnormal Findings**
1. Clean the vagina with saline* and assess.	Squamous epithelium (no glands)	Adenosis and other DES morphology Vaginal polyps Vaginal cysts Vaginal ulcerations
2. Assess the vagina with a green filter before the application of 3–5% acetic acid.*		Abnormal vascular patterns (punctation) Atypical vessels Patches of superficial erosions ("strawberry spots" caused by trichomoniasis)
3. Assess the vagina after the application of 3–5% acetic acid.	Nonspecific acetowhite epithelium	Acetowhite epithelium specific for preinvasive or invasive disease VaIN (low and high grade) Vaginal carcinoma
4. Assess the vagina after the application of diluted Lugol's iodine solution.	Dark, mahogany staining (glycogenated epithelium)	Nonstaining (nonglycogenated epithelium) Variegated (nonglycogenated epithelium)
5. Perform colposcopic-directed biopsy* (vaginal biopsy punch, local anesthesia, excision).		
6. Achieve hemostasis* (pressure, Monsel's solution, silver nitrate).		

DES, Diethylstilbestrol; *VaIN,* vaginal intraepithelial neoplasia.
*Not required.

Table 6-6 Site-Specific Colposcopy: Vulva

Steps in Colposcopic Assessment of the Vulva	Specific Observations at This Step of the Examination	
	Normal Findings	**Abnormal Findings**
1. Assess before the application of 3%–5% acetic acid.	Hart's line Hair-bearing and non–hair-bearing squamous epithelium Sebaceous hyperplasia	Benign epithelial abnormalities (lichen sclerosus, lichen planus, psoriasis, dermatitis) Lentigo maligna Bartholin's cyst/abscess Epithelial cysts
2. Assess with 3% acetic acid.	Micropapillomatosis labialis Nonspecific acetowhite epithelium	Condyloma acuminatum Acetowhite epithelium specific for preinvasive disease or invasion VIN Vulvar carcinoma
3. Perform colposcopic-directed biopsy* (local anesthesia, punch, or excision).		
4. Achieve hemostasis (direct pressure, Monsel's solution [small amount, wipe away excess]).		
5. Apply protective dressing.*		

VIN, Vulvar intraepithelial neoplasia.
*Not required.

Table 6-7 Documentation, Laboratory Forms, and Patient Education

Colposcopic record

Demographic form if it is separate from the colposcopic record

Informed consent

Laboratory forms for cytopathology and surgical pathology

General laboratory forms (DNA or cultures, B-hCG, wet smear preparation)

Preoperative and postoperative patient information sheets

3 × 5 card for "tickler" file if there is no computer database

Patient reminder card, addressed at clinic visit

Educational brochures

B-hCG, Beta-human chorionic gonadotropin.

REFERENCES

1. Guido RS, Jeronimo J, Schiffman M, et al, for the ALTS Group. The distribution of neoplasia arising on the cervix: Results from the ALTS trial. Am J Obstet Gynecol 2005;193:1331–1337.
2. Reid R, Scalzi P. Genital warts and cervical cancer. VII. An improved colposcopic index for differentiating benign papilloma viral infections from high-grade cervical intraepithelial neoplasia. Am J Obstet Gynecol 1985;153:611–618.
3. Jeronimo J, Schiffman M. Colposcopy at a crossroads. Am J Obstet Gynecol 2006;195:349–353.
4. ACOG Practice Bulletin. Management of abnormal cervical cytology and histology. Obstet Gynecol 2005;106:645–664.
5. Wright TC, Cox JT, Massad LS, et al. 2001 Consensus Guidelines for the management of women with cervical cytological abnormalities. J Am Med Assoc 2002;287:2120–2129.
6. Folen Mitchel MF, Schottenfeld D, Tortolero-Lne G, et al. Colposcopy for the diagnosis of squamous intraepithelial lesions: a meta-analysis. Obstet Gynecol 1998;91:626–631.
7. Hopman EH, Kenemans P, Helmerhorst TJ. Positive predictive rate of colposcopic examination of the cervix uteri: an overview of the literature. Obstet Gynecol Surv 1998;53:97–106.
8. Sheshadri V, O'Connor D. The agreement of colposcopic grading as compared to directed biopsy results. J Lower Genital Tract Dis 1999;3:150–154.
9. Massad LS, Collins YC. Strength of correlations between colposcopic impression and biopsy histology. Gynecol Oncol 2003;89:424–428.
10. ASCUS-LSIL Triage Study (ALTS) Group. A randomized trial on the management of low-grade squamous intraepithelial lesion cytology interpretations. Am J Obstet Gynecol 2003;188:1393–1400.
11. ASCUS-LSIL Triage Study (ALTS) Group. Results of a randomized trial on the management of cytology interpretations of atypical squamous cells of undetermined significance. Am J Obstet Gynecol 2003;188:1383–1392.
12. Ferris DG, Litaker M, for the ALTS Group. Interobserver agreement for colposcopy quality control using digitalized colposcopic images during the ALTS Trial. J Lower Genital Tract Dis 2005;9:29–35.
13. Skehan M, Soutter WP, Lim K, et al. Reliability of colposcopy and directed punch biopsy. Br J Obstet Gynecol 1990;97:811–816.

14. Drezek RA, Richards-Kortum R, Brewer MA, et al. Optical imaging of the cervix. Cancer 2003;98(9 Suppl):2015–2127.

15. Huh WK, Cestero RM, Garcia FA, et al. Optical detection of high-grade cervical intraepithelial neoplasia in vivo: results of a 604-patient study. Am J Obstet Gynecol 2004;190:1249–1257.

16. Spitzer M, Apgar B, Brotzman GL, et al. Residency training in colposcopy: a survey of program directors in obstetrics and gynecology and family medicine. Am J Obstet Gynecol 2001;185:507–513.

17. Laedtke TW, Dignan M. Compliance with therapy for cervical dysplasia among women of low socioeconomic status. South Med J 1992;8:5–8.

18. Lerman C, Hanjani P, Caputo C, et al. Telephone counseling improves adherence to colposcopy among lower-income minority women. J Clin Oncol 1992;80:330–333.

19. Gold MA, Dunton CJ, Macones GA, et al. Knowledge base as a predictory of follow-up compliance after colposcopy. J Lower Genital Tract Dis 1997;1:132–135.

20. Ferenczy A, Hilgarth M, Jenny J, et al. The place of colposcopy and related systems in gynecologic practice and research. J Reprod Med 1988;33:737–738.

21. Ferris DG: Video colposcopy. J Lower Genital Tract Dis 1997;1:15–18.

22. Ferris DG, Ho TH, Guijon F, et al. A comparison of colposcopy using optical and video colposcopes. J Lower Genital Tract Dis 2000;4:65–71.

23. Stafl A. Presentation on digital cerviscope. 2006 ASCCP Biennial Meeting, Las Vegas, NV, March 2006.

24. Yandell RB, Hannigan EV, Dinh TV, et al. Avoiding conization for inadequate colposcopy: suggestions for conservative therapy. J Reprod Med 1996;4:135–139.

25. Rochelson B, Krumholtz B. The "unsatisfactory" colposcopy examination. J Reprod Med 1983;28:131–136.

26. Spitzer M, Chernys AE. Monsel's solution-induced artifact in the uterine cervix. Am J Obstet Gynecol 1996;175:1204–1207.

27. Shaw E, Sellors J, Kaczorowski J. Prospective evaluation of colposcopic features in predicing cervical intraepithelial neoplasia: degree of acetowhite change most important. J Lower Tract Dis 2003;7:6–10.

28. Ferris DG, Litaker MS, for the ALTS Group. Prediction of cervical histologic results using an abbreviated Reid Colposcopic Index during ALTS. Am J Obstet Gynecol 2006;194:704–710.

29. Allard JE, Rodriquez M, Rocca M, et al. Biopsy site selection during colposcopy and distribution of cervical intraepithelial neoplasia. J Lower Tract Dis 2005;9:36–39.

30. Pretorius RG, Zhang WH, Belinson JL, et al. Colposcopically directed biopsy, random cervical biopsy, and endocervical curettage in the diagnosis of cervical intraepithelial neoplasia II or worse. Am J Obstet Gynecol 2004;191:430–434.

31. Ferris D, Harper D, Callahan B, et al. The efficacy of topical benzocaine gel for providing anesthesia prior to cervical biopsy and endocervical curettage. J Lower Genital Tract Dis 1997;1:221–225.

32. Spirtos NM, Schaerth JB, d'Ablaing G, et al. A critical evaluation of the endocervical curettage. Obstet Gynecol 1987;70:729–733.

33. Burghardt E. The colposcopic examination. In: Burghardt E, Pickel H, Girardi F (eds). Colposcopy-Cervical Pathology Textbook and Atlas, ed 2. New York: Georg Thieme Verlag, 1991, p 125.

34. Burke L, Antonioli D, Ducatman B. Instrumentation and biopsy technique. In: Burke L, Antonioli D, Ducatman B (eds). Colposcopy Text and Atlas. Norwalk, CT: Appleton and Lange, 1991, p 7.

35. Kolstadt P, Stafl A. Diagnostic criteria. In: Kolstadt P, Stafl A (eds). Atlas of Colposcopy, ed 2. Baltimore: University Park Press, 1977, p 23.

Appendix 6-1

Colposcopy Form

Patient ID#:_____

Examiner Name(s):_____ Date:_____ Primary Care Physician:_____

Reason(s) for colposcopy:_____
_____

Colposcopic Findings: LK—leukoplakia, WE—white epithelium, PN—punctation, MO—mosaic, AV—atypical vessel, SCJ—squamocolumnar junction, X—biopsy sites

Pap smear done: _____ Yes _____ No

_____ ECC _____ Biopsy of _____ Cervix _____ Vagina _____ Vulva _____ HPV testing _____ Wet prep

Other_____

Colposcopy findings:

*Vulva, vagina, perineum, perianal area normal: _____ Yes _____ No

   If no, describe: _____

*Entire SCJ seen: _____ Yes _____ No

*Limits of lesion seen: _____ Yes _____ No _____ NA

*Invasive cancer seen: _____ Yes _____ No

Colposcopic Diagnosis: _____

Cytology Diagnosis: _____

Biopsy Diagnosis: _____

Final Impression:

_____ Low-grade CIN

_____ High-grade CIN

_____ Invasive carcinoma

_____ Condyloma acuminatum

_____ Ectropion

_____ Squamous metaplasia

_____ Endocervical polyp_____Endometrial polyp

_____ Other _____

_____ Remarks: _____

Results and plan discussed with patient: Yes   No

by_____ Phone_____Letter_____ other (   ) Date:_____

Treatment options discussed, including:

_____LEEP_____ LEEP cone _____ Laser _____Cyro _____ CKC _____ TCA _____ Observation _____ other

Management option selected: _____

   Follow-up date: _____

   Note sent to Primary Care Physician:_____Yes   Date:_____   _____

                                                                Colposcopist Signature

Appendix 6-2

Colposcopy Information Sheet

What is colposcopy? It is close-up examination of the cervix using a special microscope called a colposcope.

Why do I need it? It will help identify the cause of your abnormal Papanicolaou (Pap) smear. An abnormal Pap smear may indicate cancerous and precancerous conditions, as well as some relatively harmless conditions. The Pap smear alone, however, cannot give a definitive diagnosis. The cervix must be magnified many times by the colposcope to look for the source of the abnormal cells. A small segment of these areas may be obtained for study by a pathologist. This is call a biopsy.

Is any preparation necessary? You should not douche, us any vaginal creams, or have intercourse 2 days before the examination. It is ideal to perform the colposcopy just after your period has ended. Some women find it helpful to take ibuprofen 1 to 2 hours before their appointment to reduce any cramping associated with a biopsy (do not use ibuprofen if you are allergic to it or to aspirin or if you are pregnant).

What is the examination like? It is like a regular pelvic examination, except that instead of looking at the cervix with the naked eye, the clinician will be looking through the colposcope. The entire examination takes approximately 20 to 30 minutes. If a biopsy is obtained, a slight pinching sensation may be experienced. The final step is to do a scraping of the inside of the cervix. This is called an endocervical curettage. This part of the examination lasts only about 15 seconds and is usually associated with some cramping.

What happens after the examination? You will be given a sanitary napkin to wear home. No time off from work is needed. Intercourse should be avoided until all bleeding stops. No other limitation of activities is needed. The biopsy results will be back within a specified time. Your clinician will tell you when and how you should get in touch with him/her to discuss your results and treatment plans, if necessary, as well as what follow-up is needed. Please contact your clinician if she or he has not contacted you within several weeks of your appointment. If your phone number or address changes, please inform us so that we can update your chart.

Appendix 6-3

Patient Intake Form

Referred by: _____ Your name: _____

Your address: _____ City/State: _____ Zip code: _____

Home telephone: _____ Work telephone: _____

Your age now: _____ Date of your last menstrual period: _____

Please answer the following questions. Your answers will remain strictly confidential.

Reason(s) for referral: _____ Abnormal Pap smear
_____ Vaginal discharge
_____ Vaginal bleeding
_____ DES exposure
_____ Warts
_____ For how long?_____
_____ Other_____

Any prior treatment for abnormal Pap smears? _____ Yes _____ No
If yes, please list date and type of treatment: _____

Marital status: _____ Married _____ Single _____ Divorced

Age at first intercourse: _____ (0 = not applicable)

Total number of sexual partners in your lifetime: _____

Total # of pregnancies: _____ # of Miscarriages or abortions: _____

Type of birth control currently used: _____ Birth control pill
_____ IUD
_____ Tubal ligation
_____ Norplant
_____ Vasectomy in partner
_____ Barrier method
_____ Other What?_____

Do you smoke cigarettes? _____ Yes _____ No
If yes, how many packs a day? _____ For how many years?

Have you ever been treated for any of the following?
_____ Herpes _____ Chlamydia _____ Trichomoniasis _____ Other_____ Gonorrhea _____ Syphilis _____ Warts _____ No

Has your sexual partner ever been treated for the following:
_____ Herpes _____ Chlamydia _____ Trichomoniasis _____ Other_____ Gonorrhea _____ Syphilis _____ Warts _____ No

Have you ever taken an AIDS test: _____ Yes _____ No
If yes, was the result _____ positive or _____ negative?

Do you use intravenous drug presently? _____ Yes _____ No
In the past? _____ Yes _____ No

Do you have a history of a bleeding disorder? _____ Yes _____ No

Appendix 6-4

Informed Consent fo Colposcopy with Biosy of Cervix, Endocervix, Vagina, Introitis, Perineum, or Anus

_____ or his/her assistant has explained to me the procedures and local anesthesia necessary to diagnose my condition or my dependent's condition. I understand the nature of the procedure summarized below, and I request and authorize the performance of biopsy of the cervix, endocervix, and possibly the vagina, perineum, or anus.

I have been informed and understand that the following are possible risks associated with the procedure:

_____ Light bleeding that may require a sanitary napkin

_____ Heavy bleeding (rare) that may require a stitch or hospitalization

_____ Pain during the procedure (usually mild)

_____ Infection of biopsy site or uterine lining

I have been informed of the following benefits of the procedure:

_____ Can be done in the office

_____ Helps diagnose cause of abnormal Pap smear

_____ Helps plan future therapy

I understand that the procedure to be performed will be done under the guidance of a colposcope (a special microscope). I consent to the administration of such local anesthsia as is considered necessary. I understand that video or photographic equipment may be used during my procedure for later educational purposes.

The procedure of biopsy of the cervix, endocervix, vagina, vulva, perineum, and anus has been explained to me. I have read and understand this information, and I have had all quesstions answered to my satisfaction. I consent to the procedure outlined in this form.

(Adult patient):_____

Signature:_____ Date:_____

Witness:_____ Time:_____ Date:_____

(Minor patient accompanied by parent or guardian):

I, the parent or legal guardian of the above-named minor, an unemancipated minor, do hereby consent to the procedures described above.

Signature (parent/guardian):_____Date:_____

Witness:_____ Time:_____ Date:_____

Telephone authorization for unaccompanied minors:

Parent/guardian name:_____Telephone:_____

Caller (clinician) signature:_____ Date:_____

Normal Transformation Zone

Dennis M. O'Connor

CHARACTERISTICS AND DEFINITIONS OF THE NORMAL CERVIX

Embryology of the Cervix

The cervix develops from two embryonic sites. The majority of the cervix is derived from the distally fused müllerian ducts, known as the müllerian tubercle. This area is centrally hollow and is lined by the columnar epithelium. At approximately 16 weeks' gestation, the urogenital plate expands upward to the müllerian tubercle and then undergoes cavitation, forming the rudimentary vagina. The surface of this hollow structure is lined by a stratified squamous epithelium. The point where the columnar and squamous cells meet is known as the original or native squamocolumnar junction.[1-3] The location of the original squamocolumnar junction probably varies throughout fetal life. From the late-second to the early-third trimester, the junction is located within the rudimentary endocervical canal. After 8 months of gestation, it is common to find the columnar epithelium extending out over the cervical surface.[4] At term, the columnar cells regress into the endocervical canal. In some women, however, the original squamocolumnar junction may be found extending from the cervix onto the vaginal surface.[1]

The mechanism of cellular transformation from columnar to squamous epithelium is becoming clearer. It is known that under the influence of unopposed estrogen, the surface epithelial cells will undergo proliferation and stratification. Estrogen also has the ability to regulate factors involved in the development of squamous metaplastic cells. Prolonged exposure to estrogen can delay metaplasia in the vagina and cervix, which can result in persistent columnar epithelium in the vagina, which is called adenosis. The prototype example of this effect is in-utero exposure to estrogen analogs, such as diethylstilbestrol, which results in cervical deformations, such as hoods, collars, and coxcombs.[3,5,6]

Anatomy and Topography of the Cervix

The cervix (Latin for neck) is the inferior extension of the uterus. The cervix is divided into two portions. The lower portion extends into the vagina and is the cervical surface that can be visualized using the colposcope. This region of the cervix is known as the vaginal cervix or portio. The upper cervix extends from the upper border of the vaginal fornix to the uterine isthmus and is known as the supravaginal cervix. The cervix is obliquely attached to the vagina. For this reason, the portio of the cervix is only one fourth of the total cervical length anteriorly, whereas it is one half of the total cervical length posteriorly. In the nulliparous woman, the cervix is approximately 3 cm in length and comprises approximately 50% of the total uterine volume. The normal cervix is cylindrical and measures approximately 2 cm in diameter. *The cervical surface extends from the circumferential vaginal fornix to the external cervical os; in the nulliparous woman, the os is round and measures 3 to 5 mm in diameter.* During pregnancy, the cervix enlarges owing to proliferation of the elastic and smooth muscle fibers and to vascular congestion. After vaginal delivery, the external os enlarges and takes on a linear stellate configuration as a result of scarring from cervical lacerations.[1,7]

The cervix is supported by the parametrial soft tissue, the uterosacral ligaments, and the transverse cervical or cardinal ligaments of Mackenrodt. The latter provide the major source of cervical support and are characterized by well-defined fascial ligaments that extend from the lateral cervix through the broad ligament base to the levator ani muscle. The cervical canal is approximately 3 cm in length and is fusiform in shape. The diameter of the canal varies and is approximately 8 mm at its widest point. The cervical canal contains ridges known as plicae palmatae or arbor vitae uteri. The small ridges are lost after vaginal delivery.[1,2,8]

Histology of the Normal Cervix

The majority of the portio of the cervix is covered by stratified squamous epithelium. The squamous cells have a characteristic basket-weave pattern of maturation identical to that of the squamous mucosa of the vagina. As the epithelium matures, the squamous cells enlarge and increase in overall volume, and the amount of nuclear material decreases. Maturation of squamous cells is estrogen dependent. In the premenopausal and postmenopausal states, the less mature cervical cells predominate.[1,9]

Cervical squamous cells have been arbitrarily divided into four distinct layers. The basal, or germinal, cell layer is composed of a single layer of small cuboidal cells that contain large, darkly staining nuclei. The nuclei are round to oval in shape. Mitotic figures are occasionally seen. The *parabasal or prickle cell layer* is composed of irregular polyhedral cells with large, dark, oval nuclei. Micronucleoli can be seen in these cells. On electron microscopy, tonofilaments are present, indicating a squamous differentiation. The *intermediate, or navicular cells* are flattened cells with glycogen-rich clear cytoplasm. The nuclei are small, dark, and round. The *superficial, or stratum corneum, layer* is composed of flat, elongated cells with small pyknotic nuclei. Collagen is present in the more superficial cells. Scanning electron microscopy of these squamous cells indicates numerous small ridges on the cell surface, which may indicate the presence of keratin filaments.[3] Although these four layers exist, examination of numerous cervical specimens indicates that maturation of the squamous cells varies considerably. The only two layers that can be readily identified are usually the basal and the superficial cells (Figure 7-1).[9–11]

The basement membrane lies beneath the basal cells. On electron microscopy, it usually measures 3 μm in thickness. The basement membrane is composed of the lamina densa, which borders the underlying cervix stroma, and the lamina lucida, which borders the basal cell. The basal cells possess foot processes that extend into the basement membrane.[9]

The squamous cells contain numerous cytokeratin filaments, which can be identified immunohistochemically. Cytokeratins 1, 6, 13, 14, 15, 16, 19, and 20 are found in the surface squamous cells of the ectocervix. Cytokeratin 15 predominates in the basal and parabasal cells.[12–15] The basal and parabasal cell layers also contain numerous epidermal growth factor and estrogen receptors. Epidermal growth factor stimulates cell mitotic activity and induces keratinization and squamous cell differentiation; estrogen stimulates DNA synthesis and shortens the cell cycle.[16] A relative lack of estrogen results in minimal proliferation and maturation, commonly seen in postmenopausal women who are not using hormone supplemental therapy.

The surface extending from the internal cervical os to the squamous margin is lined by a single layer of tall columnar cells. The nuclei in these cells are round to oval and basal. Most columnar cells are secretory, using apocrine and merocrine systems, but a few are ciliated and may be used for transport (Figure 7-2). Transmission electron microscopy of these cells demonstrates the presence of cilia, mucin droplets, and secretory granules of varying sizes. The endocervical columnar cells express cytokeratin 16 only.[10,14]

The endocervical cells invaginate into the cervical stroma to a depth of approximately 5 to 8 mm. This represents

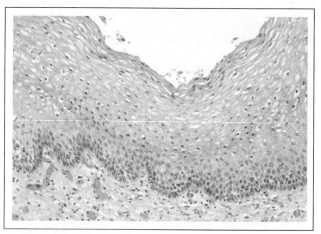

Figure 7-1 Normal ectocervical squamous epithelium. As maturation progresses, the amount of cell cytoplasm increases, and the nuclear size decreases. At the basement membrane, the basal and parabasal cells are the most closely approximated. Cytoplasmic clearing in the upper intermediate and superficial layers indicates evidence of glycogenation (hematoxylin and eosin stain, high magnification).

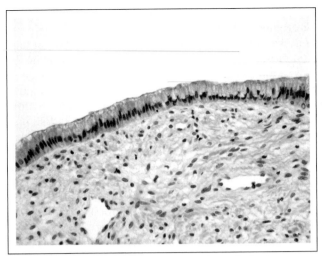

Figure 7-2 Normal endocervical cells. A single layer of tall columnar endocervical cells is shown. The nuclei are generally basal, small, dark, and round (hematoxylin and eosin stain, high magnification).

crypt formation, not true glands, because there are no ductal or acinar structures. Nevertheless the cells are called endocervical glands because of their rounded shape on cross-section.[1]

The area where the stratified squamous and columnar cells meet is known as the squamocolumnar junction. This junction is distinctive in only one third of examined specimens (Figure 7-3). The remainder has evidence of a gradual transformation from one cell type to the other (discussed later).

The cervix stroma is composed of fibrous connective tissue, with lesser amounts of smooth muscle and connective tissue fibers. In approximately 1% of cervices, small, rounded structures lined by flattened cuboidal cells can be seen laterally. These represent mesonephric or wolffian remnants.[9,14]

Cytology of the Normal Cervix

Papanicolaou (Pap) smear sampling of the cervix involves scraping of the cervical surface and a portion of the nonvisualized cervical canal using various sampling devices. Stratified squamous cells are markedly cohesive. Therefore cells removed from the ectocervix are those that have exfoliated from the surface. Under the microscope, they are seen as individual cells. The columnar cells in the cervical canal are less cohesive and can be removed in clumps. Under the microscope, they usually appear as cell groups. *In the well-estrogenized patient, the majority of the squamous cells seen under the microscope is from the superficial and intermediate layers.* As such, these cells are navicular in shape and contain abundant amounts of cytoplasm. The nuclei are usually small, centrally located, and round. When present, the columnar cells are either linear in arrangement with basal nuclei or grouped in a honeycomb pattern when seen on cross-section. In the post-menopausal patient, the exfoliated cells are mostly parabasal, with some intermediate forms. These cells are more rounded, with large, centrally located nuclei. The nuclear membranes in all cells are smooth, and the nuclear chromatin is usually granular or finely stippled (Figure 7-4).[1,11,17]

The amount of cell exfoliation varies with the menstrual cycle. During the proliferative phase, the exfoliating cells are mainly well-glycogenated superficial cells. In the secretory phase, however, the intermediate cells predominate, and there is less glycogen.[18]

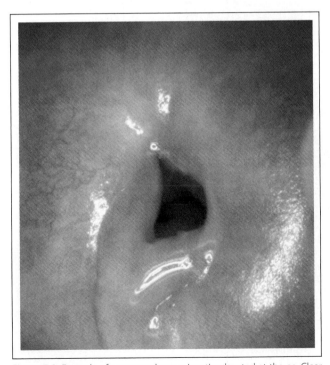

Figure 7-3 Example of squamocolumnar junction located at the os. Clear mucus is present.

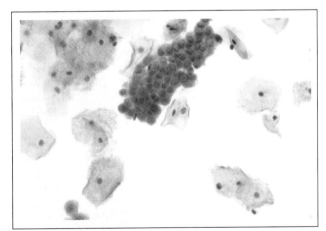

Figure 7-4 Cytology of the normal cervix. In an estrogenized woman, the squamous epithelial cells are large, with polygonal borders. The nuclei are small, round to oval, and dark. Although cell color is laboratory dependent, mature cells tend to be orange or pink. A central cluster of endocervical cells is also present. In cross-section, the cells are arranged in a honeycomb pattern. The endocervical nuclei are slightly larger, with a more open chromatin pattern and micronucleoli (thin-layer preparation, Papanicolaou stain, high magnification).

SQUAMOUS METAPLASIA

Formation of Squamous Metaplasia

Metaplasia is defined as a transformation from one mature cell type to a second mature type. This process occurs in different body sites, including the bronchi, stomach, bladder, and salivary glands. The transformation usually involves a conversion from a columnar, secretory type of cell to a stratified, squamous cell. Cervical metaplasia has always generated major interest because of its neoplastic potential.[12]

Historically, areas of cervical squamous metaplasia were originally misidentified as either early-differentiated carcinomas or folds in the upper squamous epithelium. German pathologists originally used the terms *epidermidalization* or *epidermoidalization* to describe areas of transformation from columnar to squamous cervical cells. Eventually, this process was reclassified as metaplasia, reserve cell hyperplasia, or squamocolumnar prosoplasia.[19,20]

Factors that induce squamous metaplasia in the cervix are still poorly understood, but they may include environmental conditions, mechanical irritation, chronic inflammation, pH changes, or changes in sex-steroid hormone balance. Metaplasia begins with the movement of the original squamocolumnar junction onto the portio, usually as a result of estrogen production or interval vaginal deliveries. The exposure of the delicate columnar cells to an acidic bacteria-laden vaginal environment initiates the process of inflammation and replacement with stratified squamous cells (Figure 7-5).[2,17,19]

For decades, it was unclear how this transformation took place. However, it has been more recently shown in the mouse model that the presence of p63 (a homologue of the p53 tumor suppressor gene) in the postnatal vaginal epithelium is necessary for the eventual conversion from uterine columnar to cervicovaginal squamous epithelium.[6] The mechanism of squamous metaplasia has been variously described as continued epithelialization with new squamous cells derived from previously formed squamous epithelium, proliferation of subcolumnar nests of squamous basal cells, or development from undifferentiated embryonic rests within the superficial cervix stroma.[15,23] Presently, it is felt that the process begins in the subcolumnar reserve cells. The origin of reserve cells remains obscure. Suggested parent cells include embryonal urogenital crest cells, fetal squamous cells, and stromal fibroblasts.[23] *It is believed that these reserve cells probably arise from the dedifferentiation of overlying columnar cells, and their appearance and amount may be regulated by the presence or absence of retinoids.*[12,17] The presence of various cytokeratin intermediate filaments in reserve cells (cytokeratins 5, 6, 8, 13, 14, 15, 16, 17, 18, and 19) indicates an epithelial origin of these cells. These cells also contain modulating proteins (28 kd estrogen responsive protein and p63) that initiate replication of the reserve cells and eventual transformation into squamous cells. As the reserve cells proliferate and differentiate into

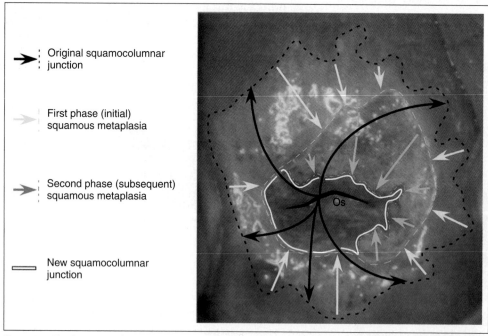

→⋮ Original squamocolumnar junction

→⋮ First phase (initial) squamous metaplasia

→⋮ Second phase (subsequent) squamous metaplasia

▭ New squamocolumnar junction

Os

Figure 7-5 The formation of squamous metaplasia. The original or native squamocolumnar junction (SCJ) migrates onto the portio as the result of changes in the hormonal milieu or of vaginal deliveries *(black arrows and dotted line)*. The conversion of the columnar surface into a mature squamous surface (squamous metaplasia) moves the SCJ toward the internal os, and eventually the endocervical canal. This can occur in phases, with the mature metaplasia *(yellow arrows and dotted line)* distal to the more recently formed immature metaplasia *(blue arrows and dotted line)*. The transformation zone is the area of squamous metaplasia between the original or native SCJ and the new SCJ *(black dotted and solid white lines)*.

squamous metaplastic cells, there is a decrease in production of cytokeratin 19 and an increase in the cytokeratins commonly seen in mature squamous cells. In contrast, cytokeratins 6 and 16 predominate in metaplastic cells that have the potential to become dysplastic.[12,14,15] Other predictors of dysplastic potential in squamous metaplasia include degree of metaplastic proliferation and rate of metaplastic change.[24,25]

Histology of Squamous Metaplasia

Sixty percent of cervices will have a gradual transformation from columnar to mature squamous epithelium. *This area of squamous metaplasia is known histopathologically as the transformation zone.* Metaplasia is most commonly seen in the lower third of the endocervical canal.[8] The first evidence of squamous metaplasia is the identification of a single layer of subcolumnar reserve cells, known histologically as reserve cell hyperplasia. The reserve cells are round to cuboidal, with large round to oval nuclei. They can be seen beneath the surface columnar cells and the columnar cells, within the endocervical glands (Figure 7-6). As the reserve cells proliferate, the resultant immature cells gain more cytoplasm, and the nuclei decrease in size. Over time, the surface columnar cells degenerate and are sloughed, and the endocervical glands solidify. The remaining stratified cells develop squamous characteristics and acquire glycogen. Eventually, these cells take on the appearance of mature squamous cells (Figure 7-7A-E).[1,7,11,26,28]

The process of metaplasia is highly variable, and it is not uncommon to see areas of well-developed metaplasia interspersed with nonmetaplastic columnar epithelium. Other areas can show a well-developed mature squamous epithelium that overlies endocervical glands with little or no metaplastic proliferation.[11]

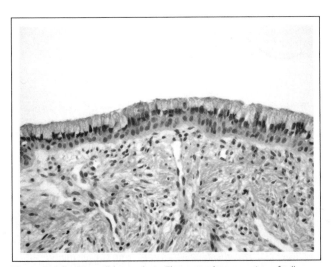

Figure 7-6 Reserve cell hyperplasia. The upper layer consists of tall columnar endocervical cells. Directly underneath is a single layer of cells with scant cytoplasm and uniform round nuclei. Although the term *hyperplasia* is used to indicate the presence of reserve cells, there is only one cell layer, and mitotic figures are absent (hematoxylin and eosin stain, high magnification).

Because metaplasia is a process brought about by irritation or inflammation, it is not uncommon to see chronic inflammatory cells. These are usually plasma cells and lymphocytes. Occasionally, acute inflammatory cells are present in the underlying stroma and the surface metaplastic cells. As the metaplasia evolves within the endocervical glands, there is squamous bridging across the lumen, resulting in smaller gland structures. In the past, this has been called adenomatous hyperplasia or mucoid degeneration.[20]

Cytology of Squamous Metaplasia

Reserve cells can be seen on a Pap smear. They are commonly found within a mucoid background in linear sheets. The cells are usually round to oval with foamy cytoplasm. The nuclei are round to degenerative in shape and are small and dark. Because of their arrangement and size, these cells must be distinguished from moderate (metaplastic cell) dysplasia (Figure 7-8).

The presence of metaplastic cells represents cytologic evidence of a transformation zone cellular sample. The cells are typically seen in small groups or sheets. They have cyanophilic cytoplasm and are smaller in size than the mature squamous epithelial cells. The nuclei are slightly larger than intermediate cell nuclei. Their membranes are smooth and round, and the chromatin is granularly to finely stippled. Micronucleoli may be present (Figure 7-9).[3]

The appearance of metaplastic cells can be cytologically similar to that of parabasal cells. For this reason, it is difficult to differentiate metaplastic cells from parabasal cells in a postmenopausal woman. Parabasal cells, however, tend to occur in larger numbers in postmenopausal women, but they are rarely seen in reproductive-age women. *Therefore the presence of small, oval cells with slightly enlarged nuclei in a background of mature squamous cells represents evidence of squamous metaplasia.*

COLPOSCOPY OF THE NORMAL TRANSFORMATION ZONE

Tissue Basis and Mechanism of Colposcopic Changes in the Normal Cervix

Colposcopy was originally developed by Hans Hinselmann in 1925 as a screening test to identify cervical neoplasia. He noted that small cervical surface abnormalities could be best identified after the application of various contrast agents. Hinselmann used cedar wood oil, iodine solution, and 3% acetic acid, noting that the acetic acid provided the best contrast, with transient development of a white surface coloration.[13] Hinselmann called this change leukoplakia, but today this coloration is known as acetowhitening of the cervix surface.

Colposcopy uses an external white light source to illuminate the cervix and distal vagina. The color changes represent the ratio of reflected to absorbed light and are related to tissue chromophores and the amount of visualized red

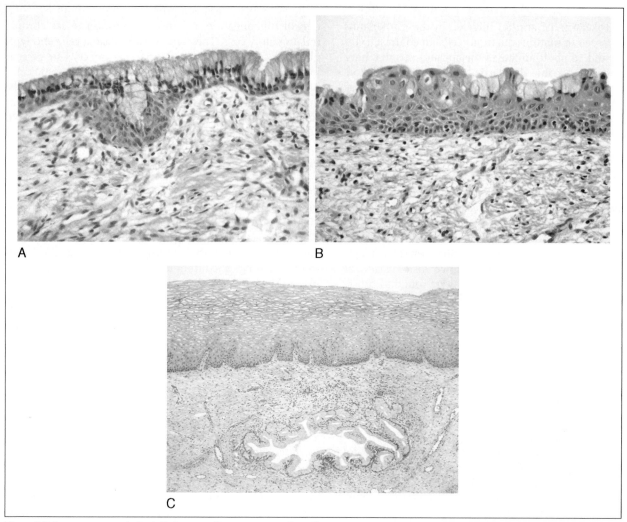

Figure 7-7 Squamous metaplasia. **A,** Early stage of immature metaplasia. The reserve cells have proliferated and created a two- to four-cell layer of uniformly round cells with scant cytoplasm and large nuclei. The endocervical cells are still present at the surface. As metaplasia progresses **(B)**, the immature squamous cells continue to proliferate. Maturation results in an increase in cytoplasmic amount, but glycogenation has not yet occurred. The remaining endocervical cells show degeneration and are difficult to recognize. A few acute and chronic inflammatory cells are also seen in the superficial stroma and at the surface. Near completion of the metaplastic process **(C)**, the metaplastic cells have matured in glycogenated squamous cells identical to the normal ectocervix. The only evidence of metaplasia is the residual endocervical glands seen under the squamous surface **(A,** hematoxylin and eosin stain, high magnification; **B,** hematoxylin and eosin stain, high magnification; **C,** hematoxylin and eosin stain, original low magnification).

(Continued)

blood cell hemoglobin. *The amount of reflected light depends on the amount of cellular material that covers a particular tissue surface.* Stratified squamous epithelium of the ectocervix has multiple cell layers that form a potential barrier between the light source and the underlying superficial cervical stromal capillaries (Figure 7-10). On the other hand, a single layer of columnar endocervical cells allows the majority of the light to be absorbed, which illuminates the underlying capillary vessels (Figure 7-11). Therefore through the colposcope, *the ectocervix has a light pink color, whereas the endocervix is more pink-red.* Occasionally, individual branching vessels that reflect capillary arcades in the superficial stroma can be identified on the ectocervix. This becomes more prominent in postmenopausal woman when there

are fewer stratified squamous cells to obstruct light absorption.[17,28]

The application of 3% to 5% acetic acid alters the cervix surface. The reasons for this are unclear. Proposed theories include agglutination of nuclear proteins; alterations in cytokeratin filaments, particularly cytokeratins 10 and 19; and cytoplasmic dehydration.[13,17] *The resultant cellular modifications produce more reflected light, and the eye discerns a surface whiteness. The effects are transient, and the acetowhite effect is lost after an interval of approximately 15 seconds to 2 minutes, depending on the number of cells, the amount of individual cell cytoplasm, and the nuclear size.*

Because squamous metaplasia has less cytoplasm and greater nuclear volume per cell, an area of metaplasia will

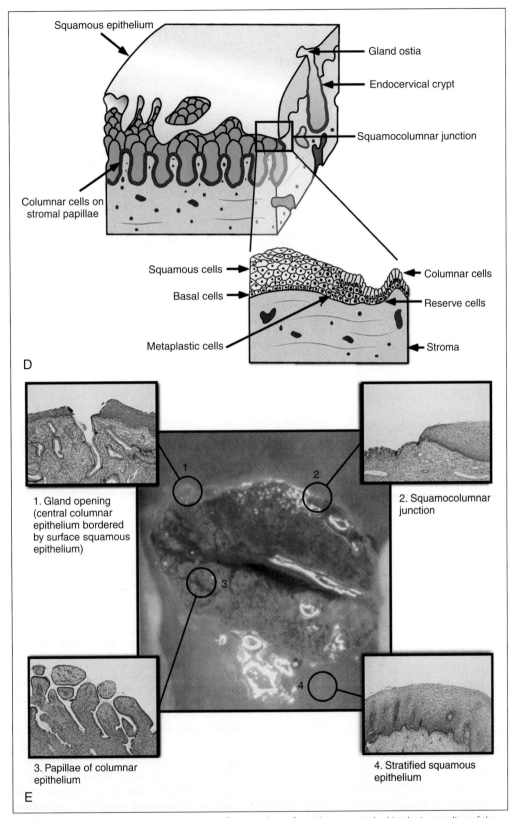

Figure 7-7—cont'd D, A graphic representation of a normal transformation zone and a histologic sampling of the squamocolumnar junction. **E,** Histologic representation of sampling the various areas of a normal cervix.

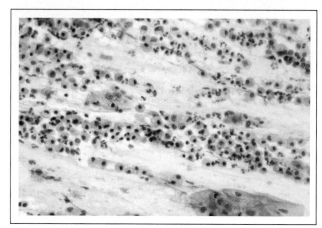

Figure 7-8 Reserve cells seen on Papanicolaou smear. The small, round cells are seen streaming across the field in a mucous background. Mature squamous epithelial cells are seen on the periphery (conventional smear, Papanicolaou stain, high magnification).

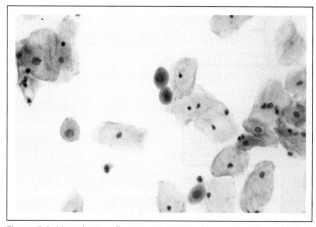

Figure 7-9 Metaplastic cells seen on Papanicolaou smear. The individual metaplastic cells are small and oval. The cytoplasm is a cyan color. The nuclei are slightly increased when compared with the nuclei of the surrounding mature squamous cells. The chromatin is fine and uniformly granular (thin-layer smear, Papanicolaou stain, high magnification).

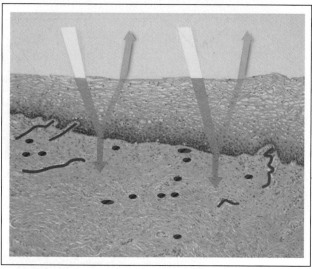

Figure 7-10 The normal ectocervix and the effects of white light exposure after dilute acetic acid application. The surface color is dependent on the amount of light absorption into the underlying stroma, which illuminates the red blood cells in the superficial capillaries (enhanced red coloration). The stratified squamous cells act as a barrier, reflecting some of the light back to the observer. The overall effect is a light pink coloration.

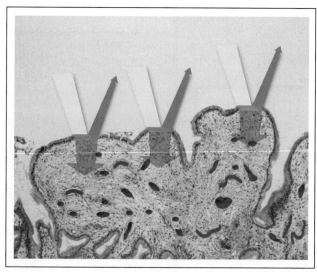

Figure 7-11 The normal endocervix and the effects of white light exposure after dilute acetic acid application. The superficial capillaries (enhanced red coloration) are directly beneath the single layer of columnar cells. Most of the light is absorbed, and little is reflected back to the observer. The overall effect is a dark pink to red coloration.

typically appear whiter than the surrounding lighter-pigmented ectocervix or darker-pigmented endocervix (Figure 7-12). Nevertheless, varying degrees of metaplastic cell maturity will require continued reapplication of 3% to 5% acetic acid to maintain this acetowhite effect.

Colposcopic Appearance of the Transformation Zone

Hinselmann described the normal cervix using the letters "O," "E," and "U." "O" represented the original mucous membrane. This area was characterized by normal squamous mucosa. "E" represented ectopy, which was the grapelike papillary topography of the endocervix. "U" represented the "umwandlung" zone. This area was felt to be an intermingling of the squamous and columnar epithelium.[20] Malcolm

Coppleson modified this terminology to incorporate the terms *native squamous epithelium, columnar epithelium, metaplastic epithelium,* and *undifferentiated metaplastic epithelium.* The fourth term was applied to areas of immature metaplasia that were difficult to distinguish from dysplasia.[28] *At the present time, we use the term transformation zone to identify an area that has the potential to transform into cervical neoplastic abnormalities.*

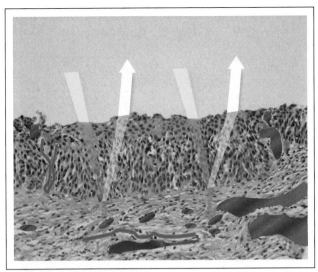

Figure 7-12 The normal transformation zone and the effects of white light exposure after dilute acetic acid application. The metaplastic squamous cells have less cytoplasm and more nuclear mass than do their mature counterparts. Most of the light is reflected back to the observer. The overall effect is a translucent to flocculent white coloration. In addition, increased vascularity (enhanced red coloration) develops from underlying inflammation, and capillary loops will grow to the surface. When seen on end, they appear as small punctate dots.

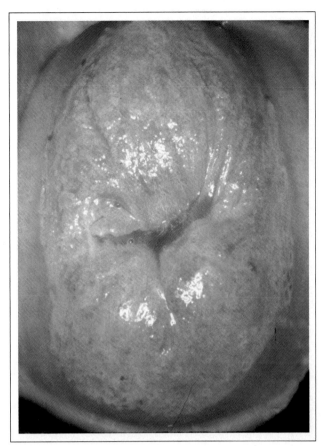

Figure 7-13 A large ectropion.

The transformation zone is defined colposcopically as the area bordered laterally by the original squamocolumnar junction and medially by the new squamocolumnar junction.[17,28,29] Whenever the term squamocolumnar junction is used, it almost always refers to the new squamocolumnar junction (Figure 7-13). The location of the (new) squamocolumnar junction is variable. During reproductive life, the squamocolumnar junction is commonly located near the external os or on the portio. In approximately 5% of women, it extends beyond the cervix onto the vagina. Twenty-five percent of women have the squamocolumnar junction within the endocervical canal. Pregnancy can cause cervical eversion and exposure of the squamocolumnar junction even if it is located within the canal. The size of the transformation zone is also altered by exposure to oral contraceptive pills, pregnancy, pH changes in the vagina, and vaginal infections. Therefore the exact size of the transformation zone varies. In children, it averages approximately 3 mm, whereas an adult's transformation zone is approximately 6 to 8 mm.[17,24,30]

The colposcopic changes that are seen with squamous metaplasia can be divided into three stages.[17] The first stage is characterized by the development of small endocervical papillae and by translucent to somewhat opaque acetowhite change (Figure 7-14). The second stage is characterized by fusion of the papillae owing to confluence of the proliferating metaplastic cells (Figure 7-15). The third stage is characterized by a smooth surface of acetowhite change (Figure 7-16). As the metaplastic cells transform into mature squamous cells, the coloration is indistinguishable from the mature ectocervix.

The interface that is easiest to identify colposcopically after the application of 3% to 5% acetic acid is the new squamocolumnar junction. This is because of the sharp contrast between the deep red, unaffected endocervix and the white, immature metaplastic area. In contrast, because the squamous cells at the original squamocolumnar junction mature gradually, *it is difficult to differentiate colposcopically where metaplasia ends and the mature squamous epithelium of the ectocervix begins. Helpful landmarks and characteristics of the transformation zone include endocervix gland openings, or gland ostia, which are characterized by a central, reddened, residual endocervix encircled by slightly raised whitened metaplasia, and nabothian cysts. The latter are cystic structures covered by a thinned surface epithelium and compressed dilated vessels that arborize normally (Figure 7-17). Because the new squamocolumnar junction represents the area of the most active immature cell proliferation, it is a site that must be completely seen by the colposcopist to accurately access areas in which high-grade dysplasia can potentially develop.*[17,29]

Although the metaplastic areas are commonly confluent, patches of metaplasia can be seen along the endocervical surface. These patches can occur above a circumferential ring of acetowhite squamous metaplasia. *The colposcopist must examine the endocervical canal carefully to identify these patches that still represent areas of the transformation zone* (Figure 7-18).

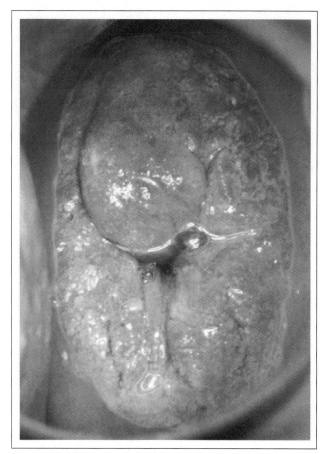

Figure 7-14 A large ectropion with the beginnings of squamous metaplasia.

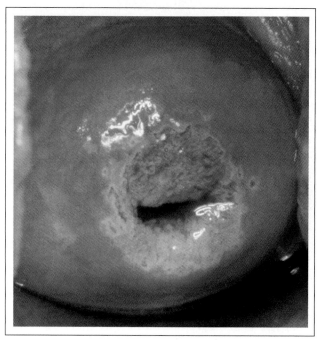

Figure 7-16 Small ectropion with a rim of metaplasia that has formed a smooth acetowhite surface.

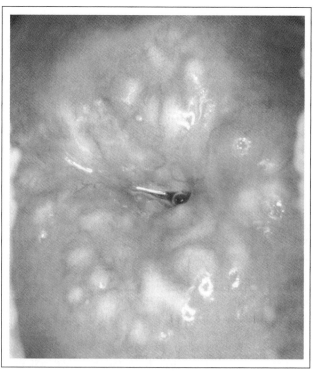

Figure 7-17 An example of multiple nabothian cysts. The most peripheral nabothian cysts mark the colposcopically visible extent of the transformation zone.

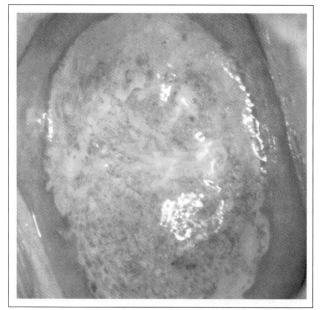

Figure 7-15 Fusion of the papillae and early formation of islands of metaplasia.

Vascular changes can be seen in areas of metaplasia. The optimal magnification to identify vascular changes is 12 to 16 times the original cervix. The vessels are usually hairpin in shape and are 50 to 250 μm apart. Capillary loops extending to the epithelial surface are seen as punctate dots.

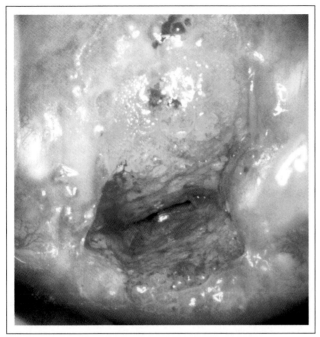

Figure 7-18 Immature metaplasia involving the endocervix.

Table 7-1 Features Suggestive of a Normal Transformation Zone:

- Nabothian cysts
- Glycogenated epithelium
- Faint acetowhite epithelium suggestive of squamous metaplasia
- Gland openings

Because the vessels that proliferate within squamous metaplasia are small, the punctation is fine, and the intracapillary distance between the dots is close. With certain vaginal infections such as trichomoniasis, the vessels will coalesce to form ecchymosis (the strawberry cervix). Mosaic tiles bordered by small-caliber capillaries are less commonly seen but can occur.[17,28,29]

A satisfactory colposcopic examination is defined by identification of the entire transformation zone. Although it is usually difficult to identify the site of the original or native squamocolumnar junction, it is felt that this site is located in an area that can usually be seen colposcopically. The area of major concern is the location of the new squamocolumnar junction. *It is commonly located at the external os or in the endocervical canal, and it has the potential to develop high-grade dysplasias or carcinoma, owing to the high rate of cell proliferation at that location. Because the new squamocolumnar junction is usually the most difficult portion of the transformation zone to visualize, a satisfactory colposcopy is often described as visualization of the entire new squamocolumnar junction.* Translucent acetowhite change that occurs on the endocervical papillae represents areas of immature metaplasia and should still be considered part of the colposcopic transformation zone. Table 7-1 summarizes the features suggestive of a normal transformation zone.

WHEN IS A BIOPSY NECESSARY?

Areas of acetowhite change and angioabnormalities represent various degrees of normal and abnormal cell proliferations that must be recognized by the colposcopist. A biopsy is necessary at any time to establish the origin of acetowhite or angiogenic change. The inexperienced colposcopist will initially biopsy multiple acetowhite sites in the transformation zone. As his or her experience increases, the colposcopist recognizes that certain surface pattern changes correlate with specific abnormalities. The number of biopsies eventually decreases as the colposcopist becomes more discriminating. Nevertheless, even areas with minimal acetowhite change or fine angiogenic proliferations may harbor a high-grade dysplasia. Although older, small series suggested that colposcopy accuracy rates approached 85% or more for high-grade dysplasias and occult carcinomas,[31] recent analysis of material from the Atypical Squamous Cells of Undetermined Significance/Low-Grade Squamous Intraepithelial Lesion Triage Study (ALTS) showed that the sensitivity of colposcopy was poor. In ALTS, the first colposcopy was able to identify only 55% of patients eventually found to have cervical intraepithelial neoplasia (CIN) 3.[32] Therefore, if any question arises, a biopsy is necessary for final diagnosis. Indeed, ALTS showed, the experience of the colposcopist notwithstanding, that *the ability to detect high-grade cervical dysplasia improves significantly when two or more biopsies are taken.*[33]

The value of endocervical curettage is highly controversial. Scraping the endocervical canal has been considered useful to evaluate areas that are not visible colposcopically. However, it has not been established whether an endocervical curettage is needed in a patient with a satisfactory colposcopic examination. Because it is assumed that squamous abnormalities occur within the transformation zone, and because glandular abnormalities are infrequent, endocervical curettage in such a patient is probably cost-ineffective. *The endocervical curettage may be valuable when the colposcopist cannot be certain that he or she saw the entire transformation zone, or in patients who have cytologic evidence of glandular abnormalities.* Evidence indicates that, in some laboratories, an endocervical brush sampling can be used as a substitute for endocervical scraping.[34]

REFERENCES

1. Hendrickson MR, Kempson RL. Uterus and fallopian tubes. In: Sternberg SS (ed). Histology for Pathologists. New York: Raven Press, 1992, pp 801–808.
2. Kurman RJ, Norris HJ, Wilkinson E. Tumors of the cervix, vagina and vulva. In: Atlas of Tumor Pathology, series 3, vol. 4. Bethesda, MD: Armed Forces Institute of Pathology, 1992, pp 1–12.

3. Robboy SJ, Bernhardt PF, Parmley T. Embryology of the female genital tract and disorders of abnormal sexual development. In: Kurman RJ (ed). Blaustein's Pathology of the Female Genital Tract, ed. 4. New York: Springer-Verlag, 1994, pp 8–10.

4. Linhartova A. Extent of columnar epithelium on the ectocervix between the ages of 1 and 13 years. Obstet Gynecol 1978;52:451–456.

5. Ciocca DR, Puy LA, Lo Castro G. Localization of an estrogen-responsive protein in the human cervix during menstrual cycle, pregnancy, and menopause and in abnormal cervical epithelia without atypia. Am J Obstet Gynecol 1986;155:1090–1096.

6. Kritia T, Mills AA, Chunha GR. Roles of p63 in the diethylstilbestrol-induced cervicovaginal adenosis. Development 2004;131:1639–1649.

7. Krantz KE. The anatomy of the human cervix, gross and microscopic. In: Blandau RJ, Moghissi K (eds). The Biology of the Cervix. Chicago: University of Chicago Press, 1973, pp 57–69.

8. Singer A. Anatomy of the cervix and physiological changes in cervical epithelium. In: Fox H, Well M (eds). Haines and Taylor Obstetrical and Gynecological Pathology. New York: Churchill Livingstone, 1995, pp 225–248.

9. Lawrence WD, Shingleton HM. Early physiologic squamous metaplasia of the cervix: Light and electron microscopic observation. Am J Obstet Gynecol 1980;137:661–671.

10. Feldman D, Romney SL, Edgcomb J, Valentine T. Ultrastructure of normal, metaplastic, and abnormal human uterine cervix: Use of montages to study the topographical relationship of epithelial cells. Am J Obstet Gynecol 1984;150:573–688.

11. Ferenczy A, Wright TC. Anatomy and histology of the cervix. In: Kurman RJ (ed). Blaustein's Pathology of the Female Genital Tract, ed 4. New York: Springer-Verlag, 1994, pp 185–199.

12. Gigi-Leitner O, Geiger B, Levy R, Czernobilsky B. Cytokeratin expression in squamous metaplasia of the human uterine cervix. Differentiation 1986;31:191–205.

13. Maddox P, Szarewski A, Dyson J, Cuzick J. Cytokeratin expression and acetowhite change in cervical epithelium. J Clin Pathol 1994;47:15–17.

14. Smedts F, Ramaekers F, Leube RE, et al. Expression of keratins 1, 6, 15, 16 and 20 in normal cervical epithelium, squamous metaplasia, cervical intraepithelial neoplasia and cervical carcinoma. Am J Pathol 1993;142:403–412.

15. Smedts F, Ramaekers F, Troyanovsky S, et al. Basal-cell keratins in cervical reserve cells and a comparison to their expression in cervical intraepithelial neoplasia. Am J Pathol 1992;140:601–612.

16. Kupryjanczyk J. Epidermal growth factor receptor expression in the normal and inflamed cervix uteri: A comparison with estrogen receptor expression. Int J Gynecol Pathol 1990;9:263–271.

17. Burke L, Antonioli DA, Ducatman BS. Colposcopy: Text and Atlas. Norwalk, CT: Appleton & Lange, 1991, pp 29–59.

18. Papanicolaou GN, Traut HF, Marchetti AA. The Epithelia of Woman's Reproductive Organs. New York: The Commonwealth Fund, 1948, pp 30–36.

19. Cullen TS. Cancer of the Uterus. New York: D Appleton, 1900, pp 180–187.

20. Fluhmann CF. The Cervix Uteri and Its Diseases. Philadelphia: WB Saunders, 1961, pp 56–78.

21. Darwiche N, Celli G, Sly L, et al. Retinoid status controls the appearance of reserve cells and keratin expression in mouse cervical epithelium. Cancer Res 1993;53:2287–99.

22. Witkiewicz AK, Hecht JL, Cviko A, et al. Microglandular hyperplasia: a model for the de novo emergence and evolution of endocervical reserve cells. Hum Pathol 2005;36:154–61.

23. Szamborski J, Liebhart M. The ultrastructure of squamous metaplasia in endocervix. Path Europ 1973;1:13–20.

24. Autier P, Coibion M, Huet F, Grivegnee AR. Transformation zone location and intraepithelial neoplasia of the cervix uteri. Br J Cancer 1996;74:488–490.

25. Moscicki AB, Burt VG, Kanowitz S, et al. The significance of squamous metaplasia in the development of low grade squamous intraepithelial lesions in young women. Cancer 1999; 85:1139–1144.

26. Gould PR, Barter RA, Papadimitriou JM. An ultrastructural, cytochemical and autoradiographic study of the mucous membrane of the human cervical canal with reference to subcolumnar basal cells. Am J Pathol 1979;95:1–16.

27. Tsutsumi K, Sun Q, Yasumoto S, et al. In vitro and in vivo analysis of cellular origin of cervical squamous metaplasia. Am J Pathol 1993;143:1150–1158.

28. Coppleson M, Pixley E, Reid B. Colposcopy. Springfield, IL: Charles C Thomas, 1971, pp 14–16, 53–110, 155–192.

29. Kolstad P, Stafl A. Atlas of Colposcopy. Baltimore: University Park Press, 1972, pp 35–56.

30. Gilmour E, Ellerbrock TV, Koulos JP, et al. Measuring cervical ectopy: Direct visual assessment of the verses computerized planimetry. Am J Obstet Gynecol 1997;176:108–111.

31. Sheshadri V, O'Connor DM. The agreement of colposcopic grading as compared to directed biopsy results. J Lower Genital Tract Dis 1999;3:150–154.

32. Jeronimo J, Schiffman M. Colposcopy at a crossroads. Am J Obstet Gynecol 2006;195:349–53.

33. Gage JC, Hanson VW, Abbey K, et al. Number of cervical biopsies and sensitivity of colposcopy. Obstet Gynecol 2006;108:264–72.

34. Anderson W, Frierson H, Barber S, et al. Sensitivity and specificity of endocervical curettage and the endocervical brush for the evaluation of the endocervical canal. Am J Obstet Gynecol 1988;159:702–707.

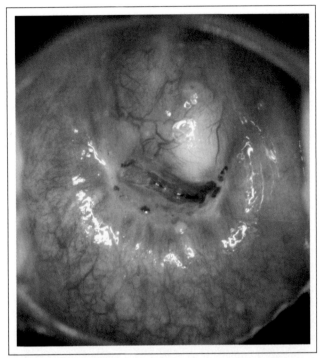

Plate 7-1 Large nabothian cyst and distinct fine normal, branching vessels of the cervical squamous epithelium.

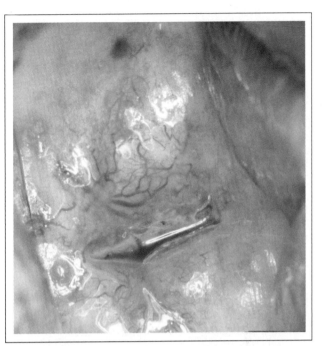

Plate 7-3 Close-up of prominent normal, arborizing vessels.

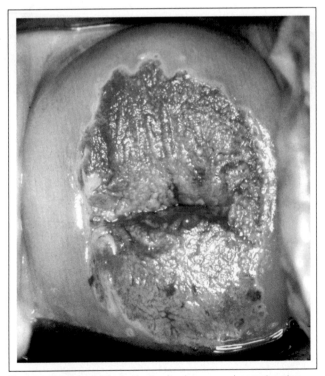

Plate 7-2 Ectropion with clearly visualized squamocolumnar junction.

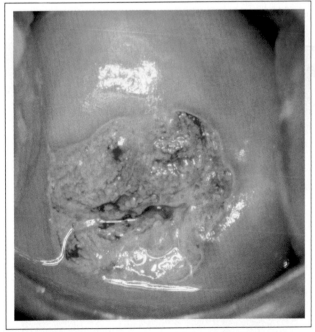

Plate 7-4 Ectropion with immature metaplasia on the anterior and posterior lips of the cervix.

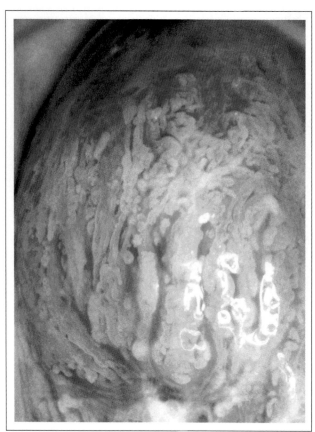

Plate 7-5 Close-up of immature metaplasia after the application of dilute acetic acid.

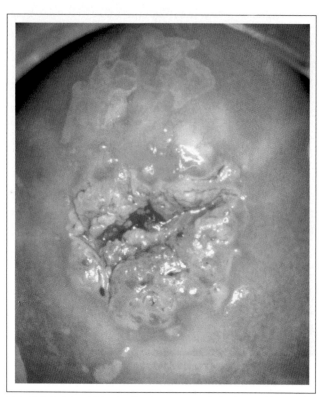

Plate 7-7 Peripheral islands of immature metaplasia along with central metaplasia.

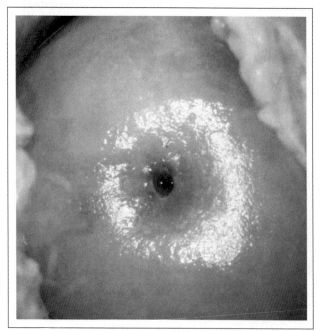

Plate 7-6 Featureless mature transformation zone with squamocolumnar junction at the narrow os.

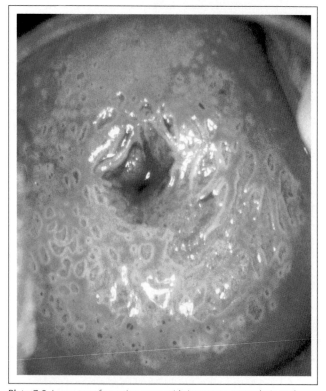

Plate 7-8 Large transformation zone with immature metaplasia and multiple islands of columnar epithelium.

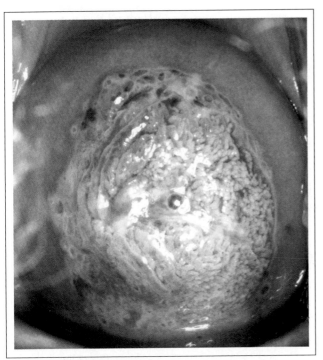

Plate 7-9 Large ectropion with very active squamous metaplasia.

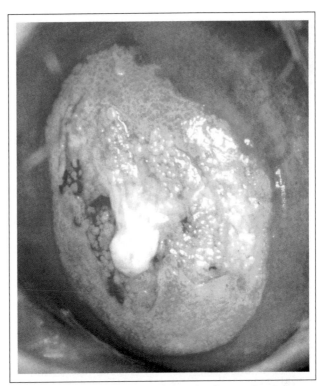

Plate 7-11 Field of immature metaplasia with a fine mosaic pattern.

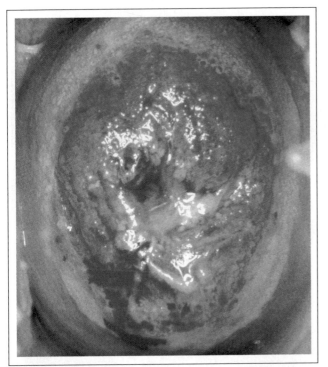

Plate 7-10 Congenitally large transformation zone with a wide rim of immature metaplasia. There is an ill-defined fine mosaic pattern present, and mucus present centrally.

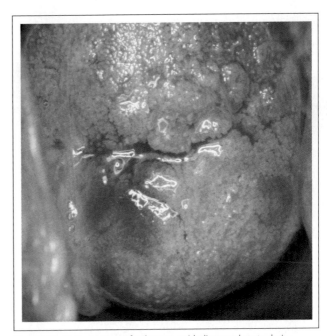

Plate 7-12 Close-up view of columnar epithelium and metaplasia.

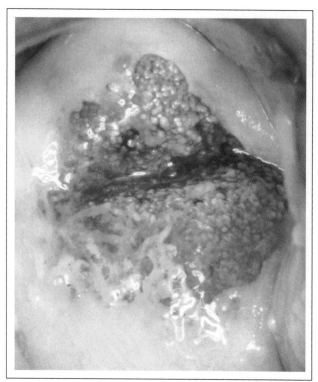

Plate 7-13 Ectropion with tongues of squamous metaplasia.

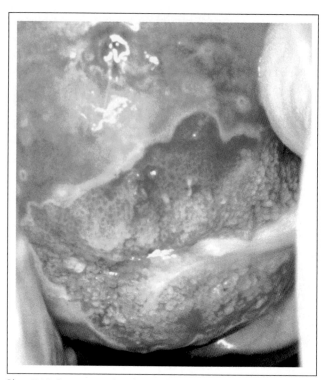

Plate 7-15 Ectropion and evidence of transformation zone remnants superiorly with several gland openings.

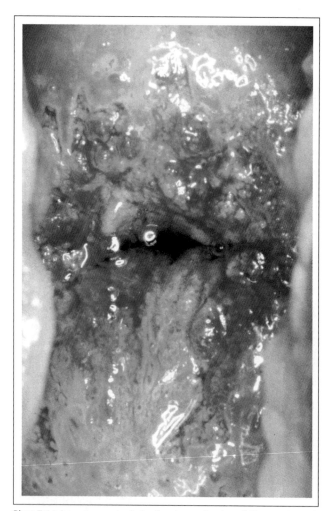

Plate 7-14 Immature metaplasia after the application of dilute acetic acid. The new squamocolumnar junction is jagged.

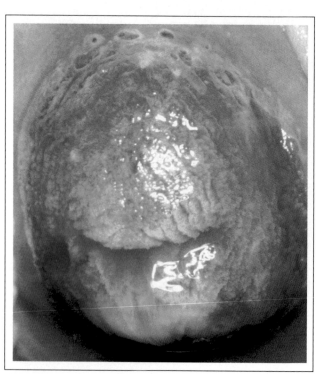

Plate 7-16 Large ectropion with islands of columnar epithelium superiorly and mucus inferiorly.

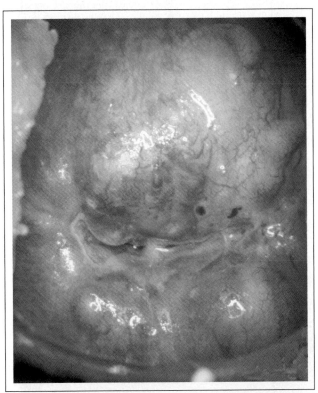

Plate 7-17 Multiple large nabothian cysts and prominent normal vessels. The squamocolumnar junction is at the os.

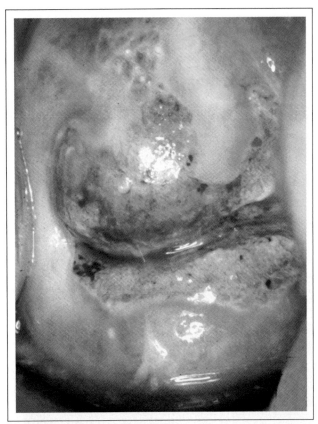

Plate 7-19 Irregular squamocolumnar junction with a maturing tongue of metaplasia on the anterior lip of the cervix.

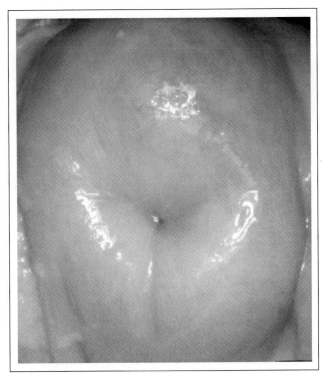

Plate 7-18 Mature transformation zone with the squamocolumnar junction recessed inside the os. There are no visible remnants of the transformation zone on the exocervix.

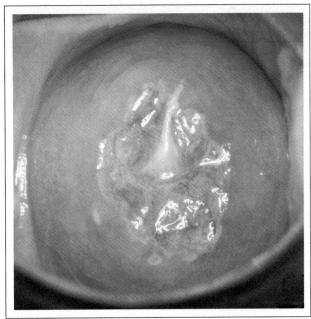

Plate 7-20 A small ectropion, squamous metaplasia, and mucus.

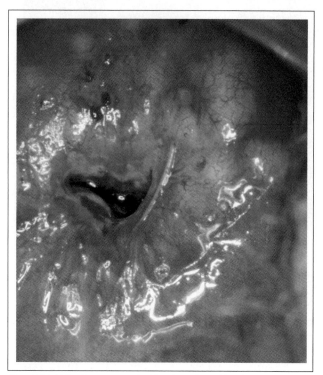

Plate 7-21 Nabothian cysts with dilated overlying blood vessels. There is a rim of metaplasia at the cervical os, and a portion has been disrupted at 6 o'clock by insertion of the speculum.

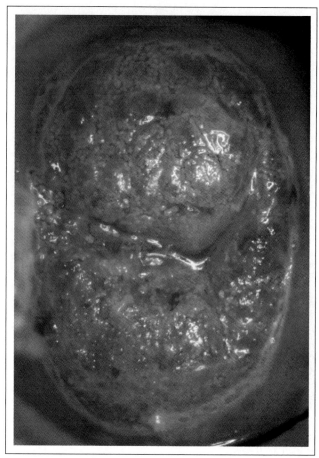

Plate 7-22 Large ectropion with a small rim of metaplasia.

CHAPTER 8

Angiogenesis of Cervical Neoplasia

Adolf Stafl

Of all the diagnostic methods for detection of cervical neoplasia, colposcopy is the only one that allows the study of the terminal vascular network of the cervix. By comparing the colposcopic, histologic, and vascular findings, it is possible to evaluate the pathogenesis of cervical neoplasia from normal cervix to invasive carcinoma.

NORMAL COLPOSCOPIC FINDINGS

In 70% of all prepubertal girls columnar epithelium everts to the ectocervix.[1,2] There are no changes in the epithelium when this congenital eversion of columnar epithelium is exposed to the alkaline vaginal environment before puberty. On colposcopic examination, the grapelike structures of columnar epithelium are visible (Figure 8-1). There is a sharp squamocolumnar junction without any metaplastic changes. The vessels below the original epithelium (columnar or squamous) are not clearly visible (Figure 8-2). Using a special photographic technique developed by Kolstad, it is possible to increase the contrast of these vessels (Figure 8-3).

However, the morphology of the vessels still cannot be sufficiently evaluated. Stafl developed a special histochemical technique for alkaline phosphatase that allows us to study the morphology of the vessels even in small cervical biopsies.[3] Using this technique, the vasculature of the original squamous epithelium is seen as a network of fine branching capillaries. *Underlying the original squamous epithelium, there is a flat capillary network on the border between the stroma and the epithelium* (Figure 8-4). In columnar epithelium, the vascular picture is completely different. *In each of the grapelike structures of columnar epithelium, there is a complicated bundle of capillaries that is separated from the observer by just one layer of columnar cells* (Figure 8-5). *This explains why the columnar epithelium looks red to the naked eye.* Although this epithelium is often described as inflamed or as an erosion, *this redness has nothing to do with inflammation or erosion but reflects the proximity of these vessels to the examiner's view.*

In puberty, because of the stimulation of estrogen, there is more glycogen in the epithelial cells. The glycogen is transformed by lactobacilli into lactic acid, and the pH of the vagina decreases. *The low pH of the vagina is the main stimulus initiating the process of squamous metaplasia.* In Figure 8-6, it is possible to recognize the grapelike structures of columnar epithelium. In between the arrows, the picture is different. Individual grapelike structures are not visible, owing to a coalescence of these structures, and a flat surface develops

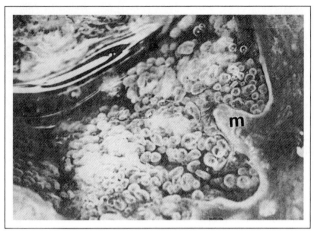

Figure 8-1 Junction between the columnar epithelium *(grapelike structures)* and the metaplastic *(m)* epithelium. (Reprinted with permission from Kolstad P, Stafl A. Atlas of Colposcopy. Oslo: Universitetsforlaget, 1982, p 55.)

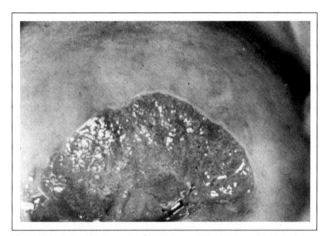

Figure 8-2 Colpophotograph of an 11-year-old prepubertal girl. A sharp squamocolumnar junction without any metaplastic changes is visible. The vessels below the original squamous epithelium and the columnar epithelium are not clearly visible.

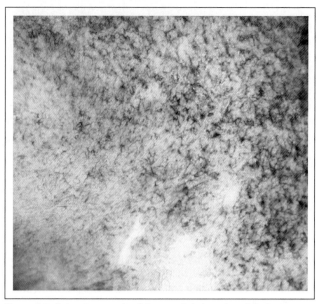

Figure 8-3 Colpophotograph of the vessels below the original squamous epithelium. A network of fine capillaries is visible.

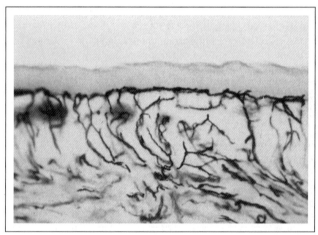

Figure 8-4 Histochemical demonstration of capillaries below the original squamous epithelium. There is a flat capillary network on the border between the squamous epithelium and stroma.

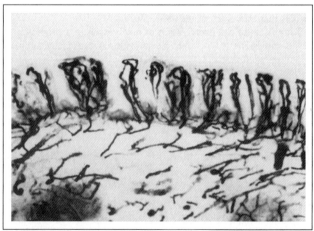

Figure 8-5 Capillaries in the grapelike structures of the columnar epithelium.

that is still covered with columnar epithelium. When squamous metaplasia begins, it starts on the top of connected papillae—a suprapapillary metaplasia. It is possible to identify the vascular structures of columnar epithelium, which are partially connected (Figure 8-7). *When the connection of the grapelike structures is not completed, two possible outcomes result. Either there is a connection with the surface or there is not. When these connections are visible, they are called* gland openings. *When the connection with the surface is lost, a retention cyst may develop. These retention cysts are called* nabothian follicles. In Figure 8-8, connected papillae are visible on the right side. Squamous metaplasia from the left side is on the top of connected papillae. The vascular pattern under a well-differentiated squamous epithelium is similar to the vascular pattern under the original squamous epithelium. There is just a flat capillary network on the border between the epithelium and its underlying stroma. Only the

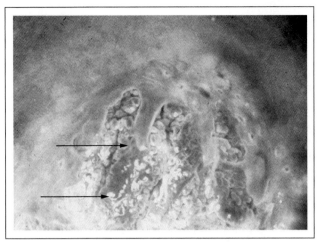

Figure 8-6 Colpophotograph of squamous metaplasia. Grapelike structures of the columnar epithelium are visible. Between the *arrows*, there is a coalescence of the papillae, and a flat surface has developed that is still covered with columnar epithelia. (Reprinted with permission from Kolstad P, Stafl A. Atlas of Colposcopy. Oslo: Universitetsforlaget, 1982, p 55.)

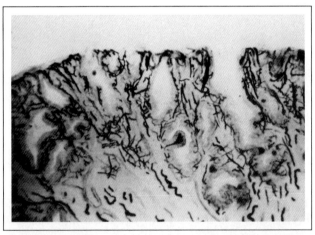

Figure 8-7 On vascular preparation, we can see the coalescence of vascular structures of the original grapelike structures of the columnar epithelium.

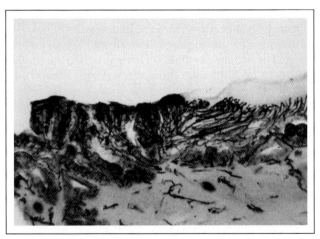

Figure 8-8 Squamous metaplasia *(right)* on the top of connected papillae.

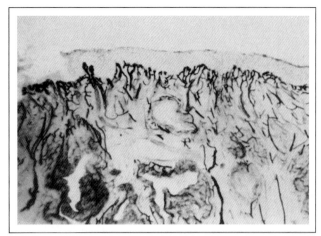

Figure 8-9 In well-differentiated metaplastic squamous epithelium, the vascular pattern is similar to that of original squamous epithelium.

remnants of columnar epithelium in the stroma signify that this is well-differentiated squamous epithelium (Figure 8-9).

VASCULAR NETWORK IN CERVICAL INTRAEPITHELIAL NEOPLASIA

In cervical intraepithelial neoplasia (CIN), vascular structures do not coalesce and metaplastic epithelium completely fills the folds and clefts of the columnar epithelium. *The original vascular structures of columnar epithelium are remodeled to vessels of either punctation or of mosaic.* Figure 8-10 shows the beginning of atypical squamous metaplasia. The vascular structures are not connected, and metaplastic epithelium completely fills the folds and clefts of the columnar epithelium. Colposcopically, we see reddish fields separated by whitish borders; this colposcopic finding is called *reverse mosaic.* In vascular preparations (Figure 8-11), vascular structures of original columnar epithelium can be recognized. They are not

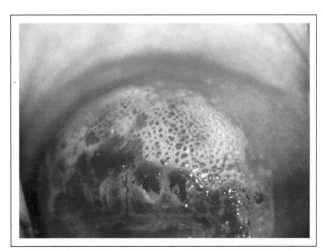

Figure 8-10 Reverse mosaic. The beginning of atypical squamous metaplasia.

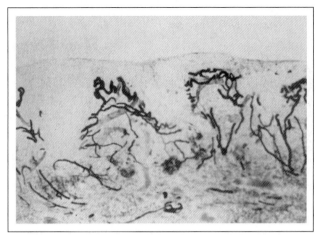

Figure 8-11 Vascular structures of the columnar epithelium are not connected, and the metaplastic epithelium completely fills the clefts of the columnar epithelium.

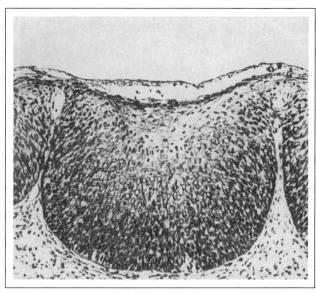

Figure 8-13 Histology in mosaic. The epithelium grows in blocks, and the vessels in the stroma papillae are compressed.

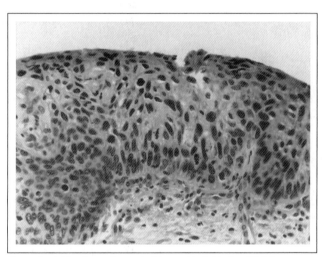

Figure 8-14 Histology of a cervical intraepithelial lesion (CIN) 3.

connected, and metaplastic epithelium fills all the clefts and folds of the columnar epithelium. By symmetrical compression of these vascular structures, punctation develops. *In the vascular preparation of punctation* (Figure 8-12), *some structures of the columnar epithelium are so compressed that they even disappear, and therefore the intercapillary distance (the distance in between the reddish points of punctation) is increased. The increased intercapillary distance relates to the degree of histopathologic changes.*

In mosaic patterns, the vessels surround blocks of pathologic epithelium in basketlike structures, and the branching of the vessels in these structures is completely irregular. The corresponding histologic picture (Figure 8-13) shows complete loss of stratification and is described as CIN 3, or carcinoma *in situ*, in older terminology. When the nuclei are observed in high magnification, their morphology is practically identical to that of invasive cancer (Figure 8-14).

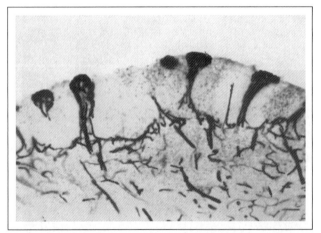

Figure 8-12 Vascular structures in an area of punctation. The original vessels of the columnar epithelium are restructured and compressed. Some are so compressed that they disappear.

Figure 8-13 shows the histologic findings of a mosaic pattern. Blocks of pathologic epithelium are visible, and they are separated by stromal papillae. There are vessels in the stromal papillae. If the epithelium proliferates, it will compress the vessels in the stromal papillae. The pathologic epithelium has high metabolic needs, but its own growth compresses the vessels that supply it. The metabolism is diminished, and a biologic equilibrium develops. The epithelium cannot further proliferate unless new vessels develop.

In summary, the capillaries in stromal papillae of a CIN 3 lesion are compressed. The metabolic supply of the epithelium is compromised. The epithelium cannot further proliferate unless new vascularization evolves. Biologic equilibrium develops, and CIN 3 can persist for years in the absence of treatment.

ANGIOGENESIS OF INVASION

In 1971 Folkman[8] wrote that tumors cannot grow beyond a few hundred thousand cells unless new capillaries develop. Tumors must send out chemical signals that induce capillaries to grow. This process is called *angiogenesis.* He demonstrated that, in mice, a small tumor could cause the proliferation of new vessels, which, in turn, supply the metabolic needs of the tumor so it can grow. Folkman suggested that this neovascularization might be caused by a hypothetical tumor angiogenesis factor.

Similar vascular findings are found in different women. In some cases of mosaic, it is possible to see new vessels growing from the top of the basketlike structure, and these vessels run parallel with the surface and are just covered with a few layers of cells (Figure 8-15). The colposcopic appearance of these vessels is termed "atypical vessels" (Figure 8-16). Based on these findings, Stafl[9] stated in 1975 that "when it will be possible to prevent angiogenesis, then it will be possible to prevent invasion."

In conclusion, what started as pure colposcopic and morphologic research of vessels during the development of cervical neoplasia could result in a new modality of treatment of cancer in the new millennium.

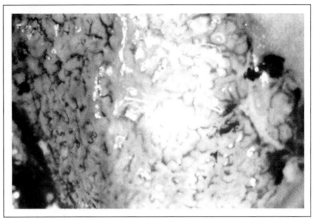

Figure 8-16 Atypical vessels in a case of microinvasive carcinoma. The vessels run parallel to the surface and are winding and small.

REFERENCES

1. Pixley E. Morphology of the fetal and prepubertal cervical vaginal epithelium. In: Jordan JA, Singer A (eds). The Cervix. Philadelphia: WB Saunders, 1976, pp 75–87.
2. Linhartova A. Congenital ectopy of the uterine cervix. Int J Gynec Obstet 1970;8:653.
3. Stafl A. Histochemical technique for visualization of capillaries of the uterine cervix. Cesk Morf 1962;10:336.
4. Petersen O. Precancerous changes of the cervical epithelium in relation to manifest cervical carcinoma. Acta Radiol 1955;127:74.
5. Lange P. Clinical and histological studies of cervical carcinoma. Acta Path Microbiol Scand 1960;143:37.
6. Green GH. Invasive potentiality of cervical carcinoma in situ. Int J Gynaec Obstet 1969;7:157.
7. Indoe WA, McLean MR, Jones RW, Mullins PR. The invasive potential of carcinoma in situ of the cervix. Obstet Gynecol 1984;64:451.
8. Folkman J. Anti-angiogenesis. Ann Surgery 1972;175:409.
9. Stafl A, Mattingly RF. Angiogenesis of cervical neoplasia. Am J Obstet Gynecol 1975;121:845.

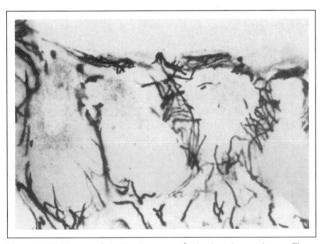

Figure 8-15 Neovascularization in a case of microinvasive carcinoma. The newly developed vessels run parallel to and just below the epithelium surface.

CHAPTER 9

Abnormal Transformation Zone

Gregory L. Brotzman • Barbara S. Apgar

KEY POINTS

- Under the influence of human papillomavirus (HPV) and oncogenic cofactors, the normal metaplastic epithelial cells are transformed to atypical metaplastic cells, and the process is initiated to convert the normal transformation zone (TZ) to an abnormal transformation zone (ATZ).
- The cellular hallmark of the ATZ is the transition to a dedifferentiated cellular state and the evolution of dedifferentiated cells, called *basaloid cells*, which are characterized by nuclear atypia and enlargement and reduction of cytoplasm.
- The ATZ is manifested as a wide spectrum of epithelial and vascular findings.
- Misinterpretation of trivial TZ changes as ATZ findings can lead to mismanagement and overtreatment of the patient.
- Leukoplakia or white plaque is visible grossly as a white, often raised, area that is not necessarily confined to the TZ.
- Epithelium that appears grossly normal but turns white after application of 3% to 5% acetic acid is called *acetowhite epithelium*.
- Any cells with an enlarged nucleus, such as metaplastic cells or cells traumatized by infection or friction, may exhibit varying degrees of acetowhiteness.
- Punctation is a colposcopic finding reflecting the capillaries in the stromal papillae that are seen end-on and penetrate the epithelium.
- If the punctation or mosaic is not located in a field of acetowhite epithelium, it is unlikely to be associated with cervical intraepithelial neoplasia (CIN).
- Although atypical vessels are the hallmark of invasion, they can be associated with other conditions such as inflammation, postradiation effect, condyloma, or normal epithelium.
- When a breach of the epithelium occurs, the underlying stromal vessels are revealed, leading to a reddish appearance of the epithelium.

The normal transformation zone (TZ) contains mature stratified squamous epithelium, squamous metaplasia, nabothian cysts, gland openings, and normal arborizing or fine reticular blood vessels. Normal squamous cells are well glycogenated and contain very little protein.[1] *Under the influence of human papillomavirus (HPV) and oncogenic cofactors, the normal metaplastic epithelial cells are transformed to atypical metaplastic cells, and the process is initiated to convert the normal TZ to an abnormal transformation zone (ATZ).*

The ATZ occurs as a result of one or more oncogenic factors that stimulate metaplastic cells to become atypical metaplastic cells, thus developing into blocks of epithelium that exhibit pleomorphism, nuclear atypia, and disorganization rather than the normal pattern of stratification of the squamous epithelial cells. These abnormal cells stimulate the capillary endothelial cells of adjacent capillaries, thus initiating an alteration of the vascular network. The blood vessels become compressed and tortuous and extend up to the surface of the epithelium, where they can be recognized by their characteristic colposcopic appearance. The abnormal cells expand centripetally by mechanically displacing and eventually replacing the normal squamous and columnar epithelium.[2] *The cellular hallmark of the ATZ is the transition to a dedifferentiated cellular state and the evolution of dedifferentiated cells, called* basaloid cells, *which are characterized by nuclear atypia and enlargement and reduction of cytoplasm (increased nuclear:cytoplasmic ratio).* On an ultrastructural level, the abnormal epithelial cells exhibit decreased glycogen and disruption of desmosomes (cellular bridges).[3,4]

The primary responsibility of the colposcopist is to rule out the presence of invasive cancer in each ATZ. Because invasive cervical cancer is rare compared with cervical intraepithelial neoplasia (CIN), the colposcopist must look for signs of invasive disease each time the ATZ is examined. The early warning signs of cervical cancer may not be obvious to the colposcopist unless a high index of suspicion is present. Each patient must be presumed to have invasive carcinoma until the absence of an invasive lesion is verified colposcopically. Accurate identification of the entire TZ and appropriate recognition of the colposcopic signs of CIN and invasive cancer are essential steps in the colposcopic examination. Understanding the development of the normal TZ will lead to an appreciation of why CIN and invasion occur within the confines of the TZ in the vast majority of cases.

The colposcopic patterns of the ATZ reflect disorganization or derangement of the normal epithelial and stromal architecture. The visual expression of abnormal cellular changes in the squamous and columnar epithelium is the hallmark of the abnormal TZ. These changes may be manifested colposcopically as a wide spectrum of epithelial and vascular findings that are discussed in more detail in chapters 10, 12–15, 19, 21, and 22. It appears that in the majority of cases, cervical neoplasia progresses through various stages of CIN to invasion over an extended period of time.[5] Colposcopically, the cellular transformation from metaplasia to atypia, then to intraepithelial neoplasia and invasion, results in characteristic features of the ATZ including leukoplakia, acetowhite epithelium, abnormal blood vessels (mosaic and punctation), atypical blood vessels, and ulcerations (Figures 9-1 and 9-2). The colposcopically visible epithelial and vascular abnormalities of the ATZ may vary in appearance from one examination to the next. The ATZ may appear normal to the naked eye, but characteristic abnormal findings may become evident on colposcopic examination.

The hallmark features of the ATZ associated with preinvasive disease include acetowhite epithelium and the presence of vascular abnormalities referred to as *mosaic* and *punctation*. In more advanced lesions, particularly invasion, atypical blood vessels may be present and the full extent of the ATZ may not be visible. At times, normal epithelial and vessel variations that occur with estrogen deficiency and pregnancy can produce an abnormal-appearing TZ. Distinguishing physiologic changes associated with pregnancy, such as decidualization and squamous metaplasia, from CIN can prove to be a formidable challenge to the colposcopist. Colposcopists should biopsy multiple areas of acetowhite epithelium to differentiate the normal TZ from ATZ findings. *Misinterpretation of trivial TZ changes as ATZ findings can lead*

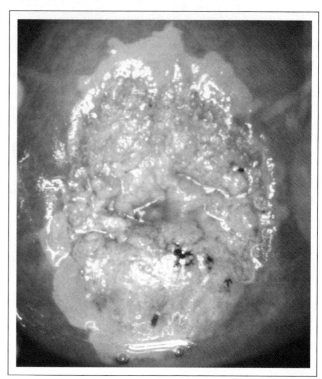

Figure 9-2 Abnormal, large transformation zone with shiny acetowhite epithelium with geographic margins, consistent with a low grade lesion.

to mismanagement and overtreatment of the patient. The goals of the colposcopist should be to develop accurate skills for recognition of the ATZ, including warning signs of cervical cancer, and to appropriately identify the spectrum of normal colposcopic findings, including variations that have no clinical significance.

Because recognition of the findings of the ATZ is of critical importance, various techniques are used to highlight the abnormal epithelial and vascular components and to allow the colposcopist to perform appropriate biopsies. Features that can help distinguish the ATZ from a normal TZ are discussed more specifically in chapters 10, 12 to 15, 19, 21, and 22. They include the following general guidelines[6]:

- Color of the lesion before and after the application of 3% to 5% acetic acid
- Sharpness of the margins separating the lesion from the surrounding normal epithelium
- Presence and characteristics of blood vessels
- Uptake or rejection of iodine solution

LEUKOPLAKIA

Leukoplakia (white plaque) is visible grossly as a white, often raised, area that is not necessarily confined to the TZ. Because leukoplakia appears white before the application of 3% to 5% acetic acid, it is differentiated from epithelium that appears white only after the application of acetic acid

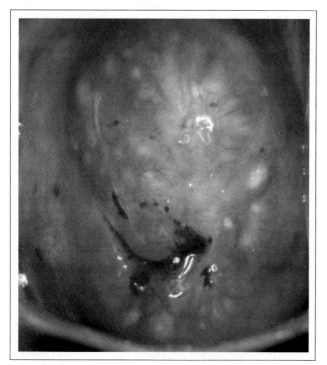

Figure 9-1 Normal, large transformation zone with multiple nabothian cysts present.

(acetowhite epithelium) (Figure 9-3). Cytologically, leukoplakia is represented by hyperkeratosis (squamous cells without the presence of nuclei) or parakeratosis (squamous cells with pyknotic or degenerating nuclei). Histologically, leukoplakia may be represented as thickened, keratinized squamous epithelium. Normal glycogen-producing squamous epithelium of the cervix does not exhibit keratin. When the epithelium is keratinized and light cannot effectively pass thorough the epithelial layers, the light rays are reflected back, giving the tissue a whitish appearance (Figure 9-4). Depending on its adherence to the underlying epithelium, leukoplakia may be dislodged during cytologic sampling or after wiping the cervix with a cotton swab.

Leukoplakia usually occurs as a result of irritation to the epithelium, such as trauma, chronic infection, or neoplasia. Leukoplakia can result from diaphragm or cervical cap use; from developmental variants, such as benign acanthotic non-glycogenated epithelium; and, less often, from CIN or invasive carcinoma.[7] Leukoplakia is often a benign finding, but histologic sampling must be performed to distinguish between benign hyperkeratosis and neoplasia.[2,8] Growth of a significant lesion, such as keratinizing carcinoma, may produce a dense, irregular surface contour, but the most apparent colposcopic finding may be leukoplakia. Biopsy is necessary to distinguish between normal and abnormal epithelium.

ACETOWHITE EPITHELIUM

In contrast to leukoplakia, *epithelium that appears grossly normal but turns white after the application of 3% to 5% acetic acid is referred to as* acetowhite epithelium. The exact mechanism of the acetowhite reaction change is not completely understood. One explanation is that the application of dilute acetic acid leads to a temporary dehydration of the epithelium. When dilute acetic acid is applied to normal, mature squamous epithelium, it has no effect. The light is absorbed by the epithelium, and it will appear pink. Abnormal epithelial cells contain an increased amount of protein, and application of dilute acetic acid results in overlapping of the enlarged nuclei. Light is not able to pass through the epithelium and is reflected back at the colposcopist, appearing white (Figure 9-5). There can be varying degrees of acetowhiteness, depending on epitheial thickness and degree of nuclear enlargement and density.

Colposcopists evaluate the color and density of the acetowhite reaction to assess the severity of the lesion. Abnormal acetowhite epithelium varies from a faint or a bright white (low-grade changes) (Figure 9-6) to a dense gray-white (high-grade lesions) (Figure 9-7). Unlike metaplastic cells that progress from immature to well-differentiated, the ATZ cells remain immature or dedifferentiated to varying degrees,

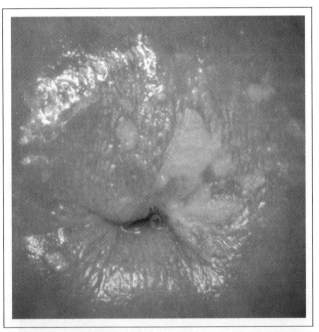

Figure 9-3 Example of leukoplakia extending from the 12- to the 4-o'clock position.

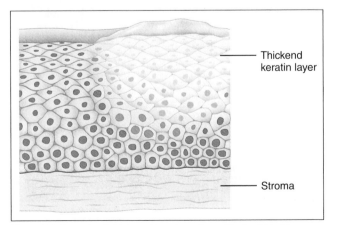

Thickend keratin layer

Stroma

Figure 9-4 Example of thickened keratin surface of leukoplakia. The epithelium is white before the application of dilute acetic acid.

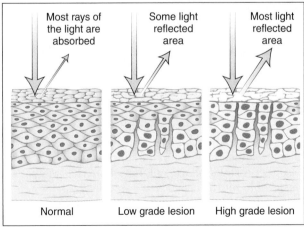

Most rays of the light are absorbed

Some light reflected area

Most light reflected area

Normal   Low grade lesion   High grade lesion

Figure 9-5 Example of how light is reflected when abnormal epithelium is present.

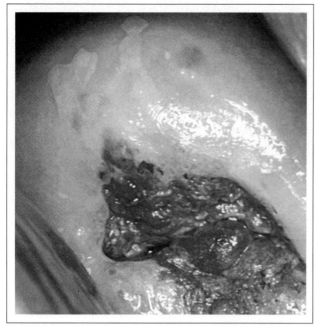

Figure 9-6 Peripheral, mild acetowhite epithelium of a low-grade lesion.

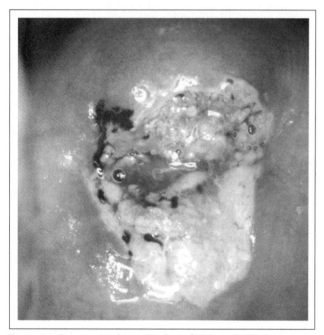

Figure 9-7 Dense acetowhite epithelium of high-grade CIN on the posterior lip of the cervix.

depending on the severity of the abnormality, and undergo an acetowhite reaction.[5]

Not all epithelium that turns acetowhite is abnormal. *Any cell with an enlarged nucleus, such as metaplastic cells or cells traumatized by infection or friction, may exhibit varying degrees of acetowhiteness.* For this reason, further colposcopic assessment of acetowhite epithelium is important. Gross visual inspection of the cervix after 3% to 5% acetic acid application without magnification and illumination has limitations. The

magnified, illuminated examination can help differentiate abnormal epithelium from normal variants such as immature metaplasia and reparative changes. At times, it may be impossible to differentiate between benign and neoplastic findings, and biopsy is the only solution.

It is possible to have varying degrees of acetowhiteness within the same lesion, with peripheral faint acetowhite change accompanied by a central dense acetowhite reaction. This finding is known as an *internal margin*, and it may be associated with significant high-grade lesions (Figures 9-8 and 9-9). Histologically, an internal border is represented by a sharp demarcation between the two intraepithelial grades of severity. It is important to recognize an internal margin. If the colposcopist performs a biopsy of only the peripheral component of the acetowhite lesion, the histology will not be reflective of the true severity of the lesion because the most abnormal area is often adjacent to the squamocolumnar junction. It is therefore important to sample the central lesion because the central and peripheral lesions likely represent two significantly different pathologic processes in the same lesion.

It is important to determine whether the acetowhite reaction is present on the squamous or columnar epithelium. If the columnar epithelium exhibits an acetowhite reaction, it may represent metaplastic epithelium or a glandular epithelial abnormality. If there is cytologic evidence of a glandular lesion, the columnar epithelium should be carefully visualized (Figure 9-10). If intraepithelial neoplasia is present at

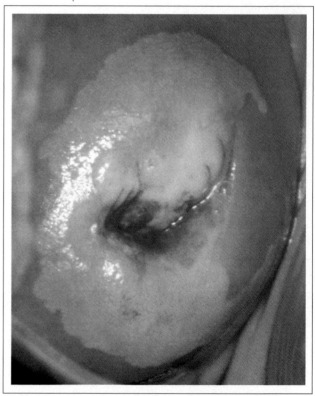

Figure 9-8 Peripheral low-grade lesion and a central denser acetowhite epithelium of a high-grade lesion at 12 o'clock, with an internal margin noted.

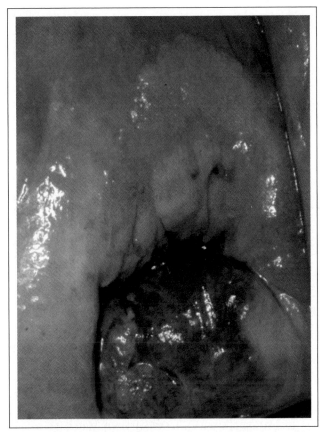

Figure 9-9 Peripheral low-grade lesion and a central denser acetowhite epithelium of a high-grade lesion. The internal margin is noted at 12 o'clock. Some background blood is present at 2 o'clock.

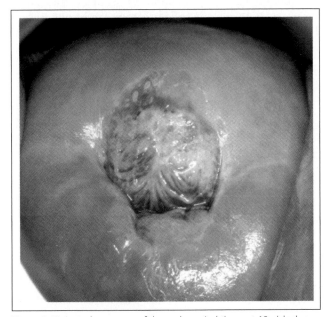

Figure 9-10 Irregular contour of the endocervical tissue at 12 o'clock may represent a glandular lesion.

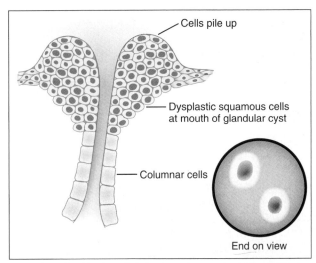

Figure 9-11 Graphic of a cuffed gland opening seen in a high-grade lesion.

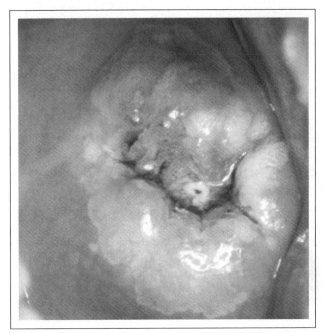

Figure 9-12 Large lesion, with peripheral low grade and central high grade, and a cuffed gland at 12 o'clock.

the mouth of a glandular crypt, it may appear as a white-cuffed gland opening (Figures 9-11 and 9-12). These cuffed gland openings should be easily distinguished from the faint rim of metaplastic epithelium surrounding normal gland openings.

UPTAKE OR REJECTION OF IODINE

In addition to the use of dilute acetic acid to define the ATZ, dilute Lugol's solution is used to more precisely define the lesion tissue. Normal squamous epithelium is well glycogenated, and when a dilute iodine solution is applied, a mahogany-brown stain of the epithelium is produced

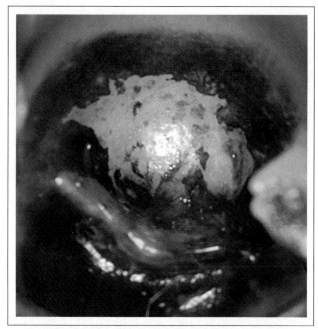

Figure 9-13 Example of rejection of iodine with CIN.

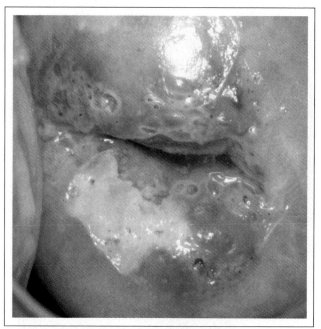

Figure 9-14 Example of a high-grade lesion with dense acetowhite epithelium on the posterior lip of the cervix and no abnormal vessels present.

(Figure 9-13). Normal columnar epithelium, condylomata acuminata, high-grade lesions, and many low-grade lesions do not contain glycogen and will "reject" iodine when it is applied. Either a mustard-yellow or a variegate uptake pattern is produced, indicating the lack of cellular glycogen.

PUNCTATION AND MOSAIC

The arrangement of the terminal vessels in the stroma underlying the squamous epithelium leads to the colposcopic vascular findings, which can be normal, arborizing vessels or abnormal vessels called *punctation* or *mosaic*.[5] If the abnormal epithelium does not contain any stromal papillae, it will appear white only after the application of 3% to 5% acetic acid and will lack colposcopically apparent vessels

(Figure 9-14).[4] *Punctation is a colposcopic finding reflecting the capillaries in the stromal papillae that are seen end-on and penetrate the epithelium* (Figures 9-15 and 9-16). When the stroma and accompanying capillaries are "pressed" between islands of squamous epithelium in a continuous fashion, a cobblestone or chicken-wire pattern called *mosaic* is produced (Figures 9-17 and 9-18).[4,9]

Punctation and mosaic can be seen in both normal and abnormal cervical epithelium. Abnormal vessels can be visualized with a red-free (green-filtered) light. Examples of non-neoplastic epithelium exhibiting punctation, mosaic, or both include inflammatory conditions such as trichomoniasis (Figure 9-19), gonorrhea, or chlamydial infection or very active immature squamous metaplasia.

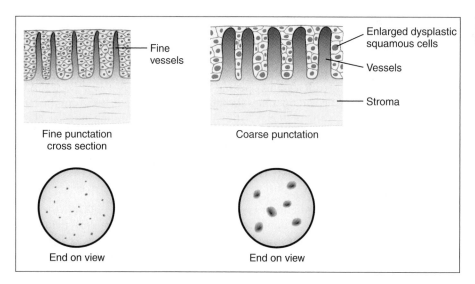

Fine vessels

Fine punctation cross section

End on view

Enlarged dysplastic squamous cells

Vessels

Stroma

Coarse punctation

End on view

Figure 9-15 Perpendicular and cross-sectional graphic of punctation.

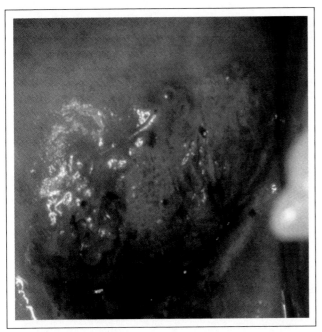

Figure 9-16 High-power view of a coarse punctation vessel pattern.

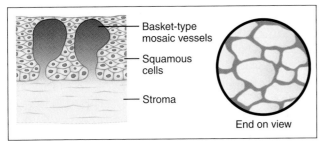

Figure 9-17 Perpendicular and cross-sectional graphic of mosaic.

Basket-type mosaic vessels

Squamous cells

Stroma

End on view

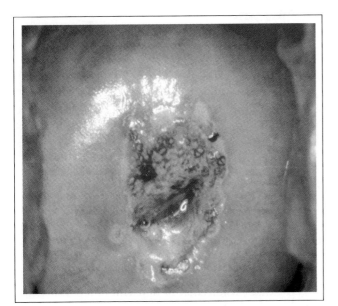

Figure 9-18 Example of cobblestone appearance of mosaic in a high-grade lesion.

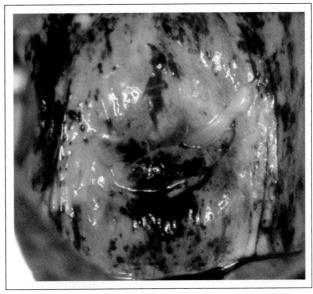

Figure 9-19 Inflammed cervix with bleeding, scattered subepithelial hemorrhages, and punctations.

If the punctation or mosaic is not located in a field of acetowhite epithelium, it is unlikely to be associated with CIN. The punctation or mosaic pattern is described as fine or coarse. If the vessels are fine in caliber, regular, and located close together, it is more likely that the patterns represents a benign process or low-grade CIN (Figures 9-20 and 9-21). If the intercapillary distance of the vessels is increased and they are coarser in appearance, the grade of the lesion is usually more severe, and it is unlikely that a benign process is present (Figures 9-22 and 9-23). It should be emphasized that many preinvasive lesions lack abnormal vessels and are identified only by the presence of acetowhite epithelium.

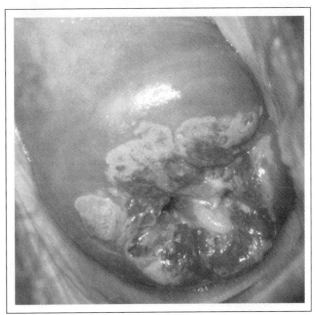

Figure 9-20 Low-grade lesion with fine punctation at 12 o'clock and mosaic at 9 o'clock.

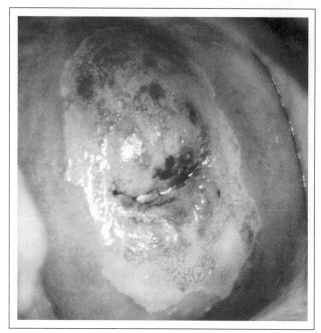

Figure 9-21 Peripheral, fine mosaic in a large, low-grade lesion.

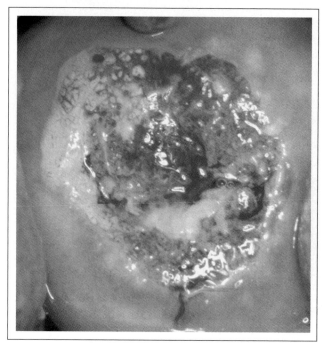

Figure 9-23 Coarse mosaic in a field of acetowhite epithelium at the 10- to 12-o'clock position.

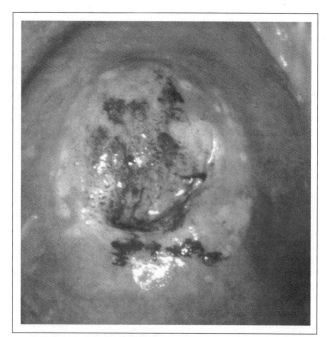

Figure 9-22 Coarse punctation at the 9-o'clock position.

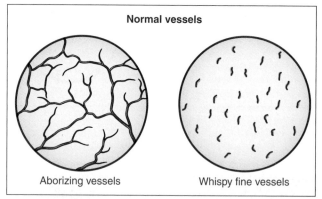

Figure 9-24 Graphic of normal blood vessels.

ATYPICAL VESSELS

When an intraepithelial lesion progresses to a microinvasive or frankly invasive lesion, there may be release of tumor angiogenic factor, leading to the development of aberrant vessels, known as *atypical vessels*.[5] These vessels do not display the normal arborizing vessel patterns (Figures 9-24 and 9-25). Rather, they are described as nonarborizing, atypical vessels with corkscrew, comma, or hairpin patterns (Figures 9-26 to 9-28). *Atypical vessels are a hallmark sign of microinvasive or frankly invasive cervical cancer. They may also be seen in other conditions where there may be aberrant vessel growth, such as healing granulation tissue, postradiation changes, inflammatory conditions, and exophytic condylomata acuminata* (Figures 9-29 and 9-30).

ULCERATIONS

In addition to acetowhite epithelium, red areas such as ulcerations and erosions may be apparent in the ATZ. *When the overlying squamous epithelium is interrupted for some reason and there is a breach of the epithelium, the underlying stromal*

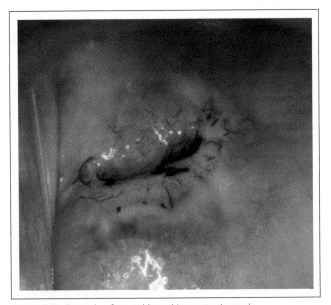

Figure 9-25 Example of several branching normal vessels.

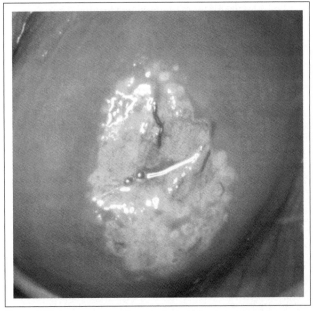

Figure 9-28 Large, sausage-shaped, atypical blood vessel.

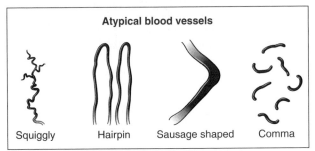

Atypical blood vessels

Squiggly   Hairpin   Sausage shaped   Comma

Figure 9-26 Graphic demonstrating atypical blood vessel pattern.

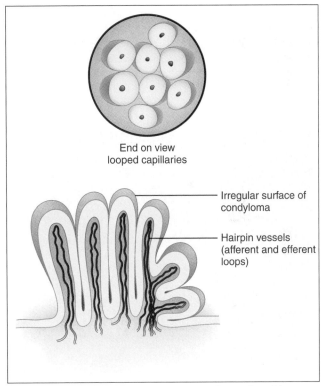

End on view
looped capillaries

Irregular surface of
condyloma

Hairpin vessels
(afferent and efferent
loops)

Figure 9-29 Graphic of hairpin vessels seen in the fronds of condyloma.

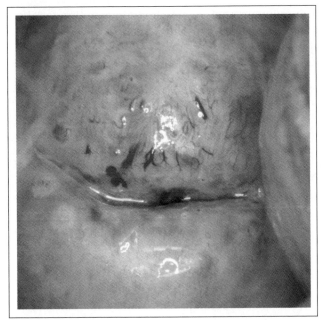

Figure 9-27 Atypical vessels on the anterior aspect of the cervix.

vessels are revealed, leading to a reddish appearance of the epithelium (Figure 9-31). Although these red areas may be traumatic in origin and not portend any neoplastic process, careful colposcopic evaluation and directed biopsy are essential. Ulcerations can also result from infections such as herpes simplex virus. Benign ulcerations can occur as a result of speculum or tampon trauma or pessary use.

The cellular debris present in the ulcer imparts a whitish or gray appearance to the ulcer base. Whenever an ulcer associated with a neoplastic process is suspected, it should be biopsied. Even when the suspicion of neoplasia is low, any ulcer that has not resolved over a period of a few weeks

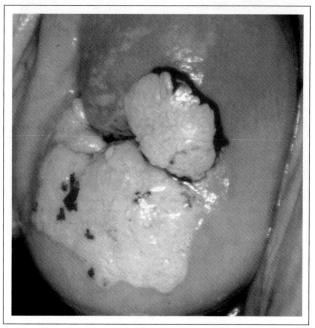

Figure 9-30 The tips of looped capillaries are noted throughout this cervical condyloma.

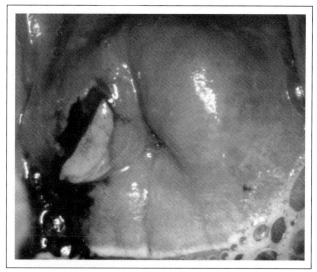

Figure 9-31 Traumatic erosion from a speculum at the 9-o'clock position.

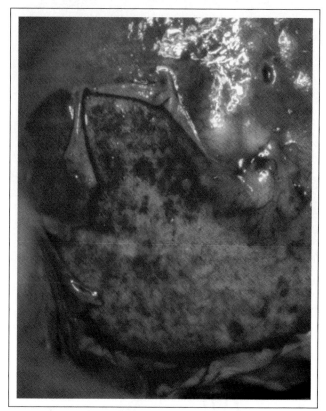

Figure 9-32 Example of how epithelial edges can roll up when detached from the underlying basement membrane.

should be biopsied. Scrutiny of the ulcer margins can help distinguish a true ulcer from a traumatic epithelial lesion. Following a traumatic event, the edges of the ulcer are usually normal in appearance.[5] With high-grade CIN, a decreased number of desmosomes is present, thus accounting for the finding of peeling edges and true erosions.[10] The epithelium is actually peeling off the underlying basement membrane, producing an erosion or rolled lesion margin (Figure 9-32).

INFECTION

If an infection is present, the colposcopic features of the ATZ can be altered, especially with trichomoniasis (Figure 9-33). A classic although infrequent manifestation of a trichomonal infection are "strawberry spots" (Figure 9-34). These red blotches are the result of the sloughing of the superficial epithelium and exposure of the dilated and inflamed stromal vessels. Because infection can cause sloughing of cells, the typical features noted during a colposcopic exam can be

Figure 9-33 Graphic of epithelial denudation that occurs with certain infections.

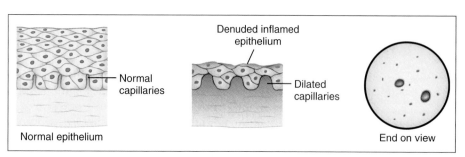

Normal epithelium

Normal capillaries

Denuded inflamed epithelium

Dilated capillaries

End on view

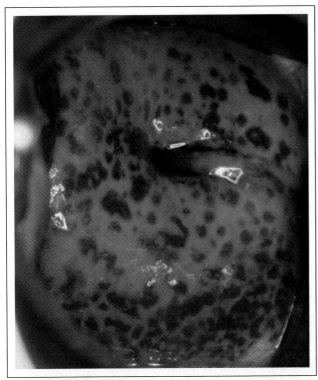

Figure 9-34 Example of colpitis due to trichomoniasis. "Strawberry spots" are evident.

to absent or patchy update or the so-called leopard-skin appearance. If infection is noted, the colposcopist may need to reschedule the examination until after the infection has been treated.

REFERENCES

1. Cartier R. Dysplasias of squamous epithelium. In: Practical Colposcopy. Paris: Laboratorie Cartier, 1984, pp 21–23.
2. Ferency A, Wright T. Anatomy and histology of the cervix. In: Kurman R (ed). Blaustein's Pathology of the Female Genital Tract, ed 4. New York: Springer-Verlag, 1994.
3. Feldman D, Romney S, Edgcomb J, et al. Ultrastructure of normal, metaplastic, and abnormal human uterine cervix: use of montages to study the topographical relationship of epithelial cells. Am J Obstet Gynecol 1984;150:573–688.
4. Coppleson M, Pixley E, Reid B. Colposcopy. A Scientific and Practical Approach to the Cervix, Vagina and Vulva in Health and Disease, ed 3. Springfield, IL: Charles C Thomas, 1987.
5. Coppleson M, Dalrymple J, Atkinson K. Colposcopic differentiation of abnormalities arising in the transformation zone. Obstet Gynecol Clin North Am 1993;20:83–110.
6. Burghardt E, Pickel H, Girardi F (eds). Colposcopy Cervical Pathology Textbook and Atlas, ed 3. New York: Thieme, 1998.
7. Wespi H. Colposcopic-histologic correlations in the benign acanthotic nonglycogenated squamous epithelium of the uterine cervix. Colp Gynecol Laser Surg 1986;2:147–158.
8. Gray LA. Colposcopy. In: Gray LA, ed. Dysplasia, Carcinoma-in-Situ and Microinvasive Cancer of the Cervix Uteri. Springfield, IL: Charles C Thomas, 1964, pp 246–249.
9. Burghardt E. Premalignant conditions of the cervix. Clin Obstet Gynaecol 1976;3:257–294.
10. Richart R. Cervical intraepithelial neoplasia. Pathol Ann 1973;8:301–328.

altered. The white epithelium may not be as obvious due to the thinness of the skin, and the tissue is more easily traumatized and often bleeds. The basal layers of epithelium are not very well glycogenated, so the application of iodine will lead

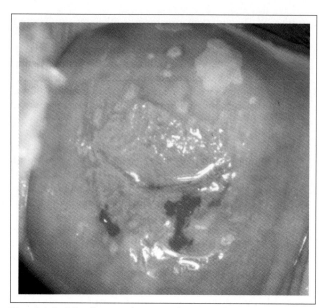

Plate 9-1 Peripheral geographic acetowhite epithelium of a low-grade cervical intraepithelial lesion.

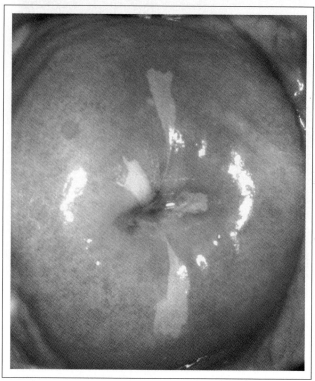

Plate 9-3 Low-grade lesion with mild acetowhite epithelium in geographic patterns.

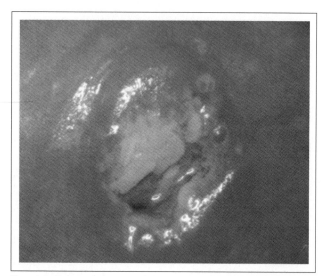

Plate 9-2 High-grade lesion with dense acetowhite epithelium on the anterior lip of the cervix.

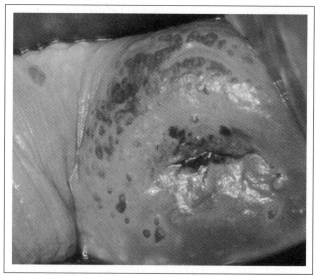

Plate 9-4 Abnormal transformation zone with blotchy areas of erythema (so-called strawberry spots) from *Trichomonas vaginalis*.

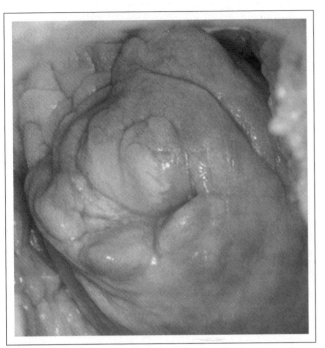

Plate 9-5 Cervix distorted from prior treatment, exhibiting leukoplakia from 9 to 12 o'clock.

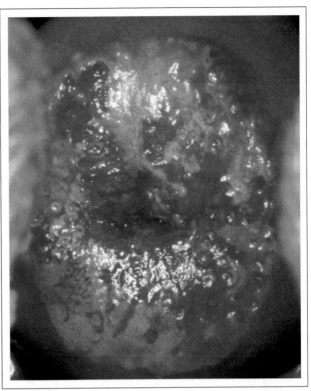

Plate 9-7 High-grade lesion with diffuse acetowhite epithelium and coarse mosaic.

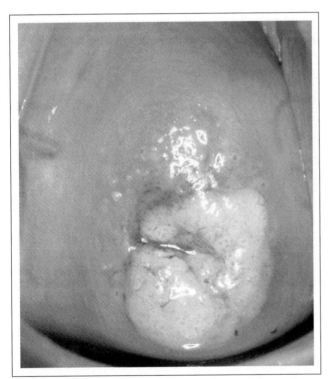

Plate 9-6 High-grade lesion with dense acetowhite epithelium and an irregular surface contour.

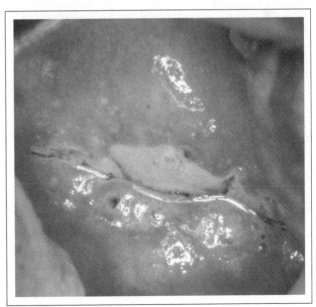

Plate 9-8 Acetowhite epithelium on the anterior lip of cervix with inadequate view of squamocolumnar junction.

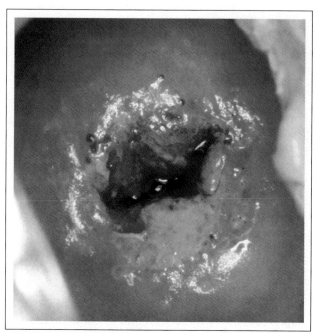

Plate 9-9 Low-grade lesion with mild acetowhite epithelium on the posterior lip of the cervix.

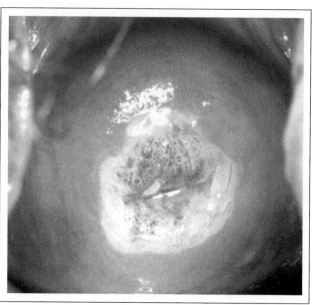

Plate 9-11 High-grade lesion with coarse punctation on the anterior lip of the cervix.

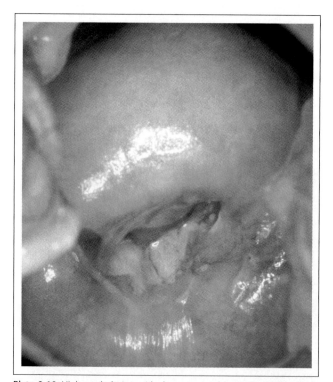

Plate 9-10 High-grade lesion with dense acetowhite epithelium on the posterior lip of the cervix near the os.

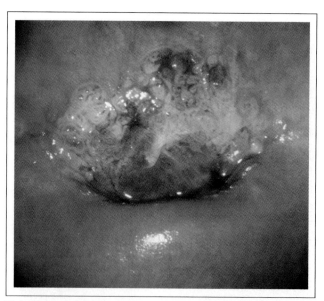

Plate 9-12 Acetowhite epithelium with mosaic that was determined to be high-grade cervical intraepithelial lesion on biopsy.

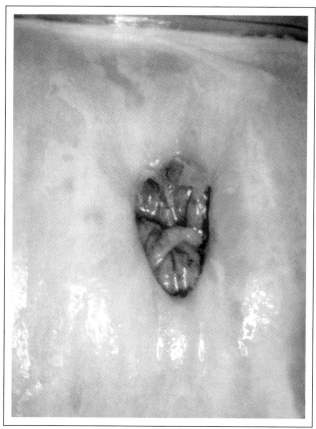

Plate 9-13 Low-grade lesion with mild acetowhite epithelium on the anterior lip of the cervix.

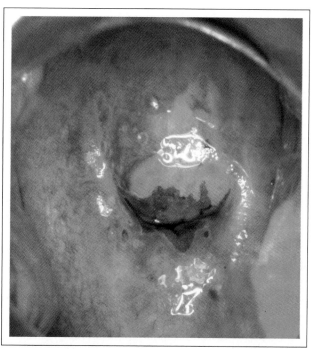

Plate 9-15 Low-grade lesion on the anterior lip of the cervix with a shiny, almost translucent appearance.

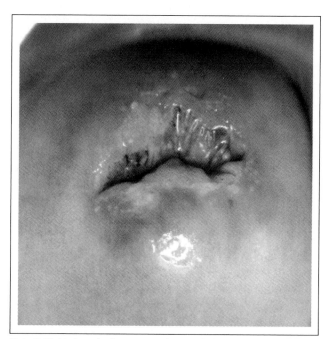

Plate 9-14 Moderately dense acetowhite epithelium on the posterior lip and a fainter white lesion on the anterior lip.

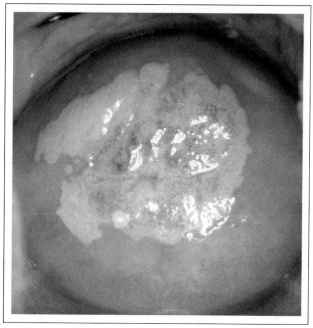

Plate 9-16 Acetowhite, low-grade lesion with geographic borders, as well as punctation and mosaic more centrally on the anterior lip. This may indicate that a higher-grade lesion is present centrally.

CHAPTER 10

Colposcopic Assessment Systems

10.1: Rubin and Barbo Colposcopic Assessment System

Mary M. Rubin • Dorothy M. Barbo

KEY POINTS

» The purpose of a thorough and systematic colposcopic assessment is to direct the colposcopist to the most abnormal lesions to biopsy in order to exclude the presence of invasive disease.

» The task of selecting the most appropriate site for biopsy can be challenging if the lesion is complex and occupies the large portions of the transformation zone.

» The Rubin and Barbo assessment method includes some of the common descriptors of abnormal colposcopic findings and also includes descriptors for normal cervical findings.

» The Rubin and Barbo assessment method not only measures the intensity of the acetowhite epithelial changes but also addresses other color-tone changes, such as red, yellow, and dull gray, that suggest the presence of invasive cancer.

» In milder degrees of dysplasia, there may be no apparent vessel pattern, or only a fine mosaic and punctation may be present. As the vascular network becomes more disorganized as a result of increasing disease severity and neovascularization, the caliber, shape, and arrangement of the vessels produce the bizarre patterns of atypical vessels.

» The borders of low-grade lesions are indistinct or feathered, whereas the borders of high-grade lesions are sharply demarcated and may even exhibit peeling or separation from the underlying stroma.

» The surface epithelium can range from the relatively flat or micropapillary surface of low-grade lesions to the markedly raised or even exophytic lesions of invasive disease.

COLPOSCOPIC GRADING HISTORY

The purpose of a colposcopic assessment system is to assist the colposcopist in selecting the most abnormal lesions to biopsy and to rule out the presence of invasive cancer. Using a systematic approach to colposcopic assessment is not a new exercise. In the early days of colposcopic evaluation, pioneers of the art and science of colposcopy, such as Burghardt, Coppelson, and Kolstadt and Stafl, defined certain colposcopic criteria that were thought to be associated with histologic abnormalities, especially higher-grade lesions.[1-3] These abnormal findings included leukoplakia, acetowhite epithelium, punctation, mosaic, and atypical vessels. Squamous metaplasia, gland openings, islands of columnar epithelium, and nabothian cysts were considered normal findings. More recently, others have used modifications of these same colposcopic descriptors and have developed grading systems to help distinguish between normal and abnormal findings.[4]

The presence of any abnormal findings during colposcopic examination usually initiates performance of a colposcopically directed biopsy. When a focal lesion is present or when several similar lesions are observed, the choice of a biopsy site is relatively clear. However, when complex squamous lesions are present that occupy large portions of the transformation zone, *the task of selecting the biopsy sites that best represent the most abnormal lesion can be challenging, especially for the novice colposcopist.* Attempts to clarify the abnormal findings by adding descriptors to these entities and by creating a quantifiable grading system are described later in this chapter.[5] Clinician educators such as Wright and Burke and their colleagues have also developed modified versions of a quantifiable system.[6,7]

In an attempt to provide the colposcopist with an organized framework for critically assessing the health of the cervix, *Rubin and Barbo[8] developed an assessment method that retains the best descriptors of some of the previous colposcopic grading systems but eliminates the numbers, which can be confusing. In addition, this system includes descriptors for normal findings.* More importantly, it includes descriptors that focus the clinician's pattern-recognition process on the possibility of microinvasive or frankly invasive disease. The Rubin and Barbo colposcopic assessment method evolved from the authors' many years of experience performing colposcopic examinations and from their collaborative colposcopic teaching efforts. The system was initially tested on new learners of colposcopy and subsequent revisions were made. All clinicians (physicians and advanced practice professionals alike) can benefit from a systematic method that points out the key features of the normal and abnormal transformation zones and assists in selecting the most severe findings for biopsy.

The Rubin and Barbo colposcopic assessment system is a systematic review of the chief features of the transformation zone: color, vessel, border, and surface. It helps the novice or occasional colposcopist develop colposcopic skills and locate small, early, and most severe changes in the atypical transformation zone for directed biopsies. This methodology is most applicable to squamous lesions, although adenocarcinoma or adenosquamous lesions will show some of these features, especially surface and vascular changes.

No assessment system is perfect, as squamous lesions do not always fit neatly into one line of descriptors. However, this system assists the colposcopist in a more thoughtful assessment of the epithelial and vascular features of a lesion, resulting in more precise biopsy site selection.

The pathologist thus receives the most representative tissue specimen. This process enables the clinician to make accurate treatment and management decisions. Ultimately, both the colposcopist and the patient benefit from this reasoned approach to colposcopic evaluation.

RUBIN AND BARBO COLPOSCOPIC ASSESSMENT CONCEPTS

The key concepts of the system include the dimensions of color, vessel, border, and surface pattern. Descriptors of cervical findings in each category (normal, preinvasive disease, and invasive disease) are presented in a grid format summarized in Table 10.1-1. Appropriate application of the descriptors in each category enables the colposcopist to accurately determine the most severe lesion for colposcopic biopsy.

Color

The color of normal cervical epithelium ranges from the pink hue of normal mature squamous epithelium (Figure 10.1-1)

Table 10.1-1 Colposcopic Abnormality: Rubin and Barbo Colposcopic Assessment System

Grade	Color	Vessels	Border	Surface
Normal	Pink	Fine	Normal transformation zone	Flat
	Translucent	Lacy		
		Normal branching		
Grade 1	White	None	Diffuse	Flat
HPV/mild dysplasia	Shiny white	Fine punctation	Feathery	Micropapillary
CIN 1	Snow white	Fine mosaic	Flocculated	Macropapillary
LSIL			Geographic	
Grade 2	Whiter	None	Demarcated	Flat
Moderate dysplasia	Shiny gray	Punctation		Slightly raised
CIN 2	White	Mosaic		
HSIL				
Grade 3	Whitest	None	Sharp	Raised
Severe dysplasia/CIS	Dull white	Coarse punctation	Demarcated	
CIN 3	Oyster white	Coarse mosaic	Straight	
HSIL		Dilated	Internal border	
		↑ Intercapillary distance		
Microinvasion	Red	Atypical	Clearly demarcated	Nodular
Frank invasion	Yellow	Irregular	Peeling	Ulcerated
	Dull gray	Bizarre	Rolled edges	Necrotic
				Exophytic

HPV, Human papilloma virus; *CIN*, cervical intraepithelial neoplasia; *LSIL*, low-grade squamous intraepithelial lesion; *HSIL*, high-grade squamous intraepithelial lesion; *CIS*, carcinoma *in situ*.

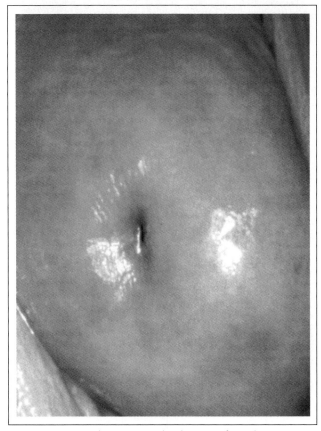

Figure 10.1-1 Normal cervix covered with mature, featureless squamous epithelium.

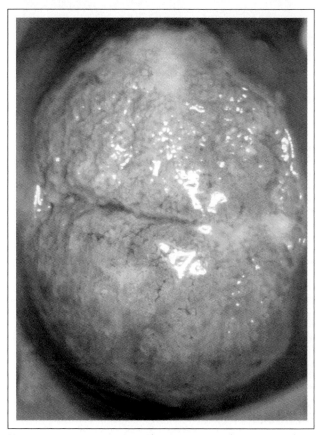

Figure 10.1-2 Large ectropion with immature metaplasia.

to the translucent appearance of squamous metaplasia (Figure 10.1-2). As abnormal epithelium evolves, it initially takes on an acetowhite characteristic, sometimes appearing shiny white (Figure 10.1-3) or snow white (Figure 10.1-4). *As the nuclear:cytoplasmic ratio of the cells increases, the intensity of the acetowhiteness also increases. In cervical intraepithelial neoplasia (CIN) grade 2 (CIN 2), this results in a whiter color or in a gray-white tone* (Figure 10.1-5). *When the cellular abnormality progresses to CIN 3, the acetowhiteness becomes very intense, the whitest of any category.* The epithelium can also appear dull, opaque, or pearly oyster-white in this grade of abnormality (Figure 10.1-6). *With microinvasion or frank invasion, the color tone becomes a dull yellow or red, consistent with the increased vascularity.* As ulceration of the epithelium occurs, a yellow tone appears first, followed by a dull gray tone indicating cell death and necrosis (Figures 10.1-7 and 10.1-8). *It is important to observe not only the intensity of the color tone changes but also the speed at which acetowhite changes occur, as well as their duration and the rate of disappearance. This often correlates with the severity of the histopathology.*

Vessel

Experts in the field of colposcopy, such as Kolstadt and Stafl, provide in-depth explanations for the progression of vascular abnormalities (see Chapter 8).[3] *Vascular patterns associated with normal mature or maturing squamous epithelium can range from a lacy network of fine vessels* (Figure 10.1-9) *to a dilated but branching configuration that*

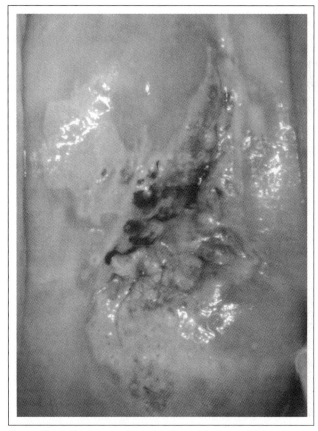

Figure 10.1-3 Shiny acetowhite epithelium with geographic borders typical of low-grade lesions.

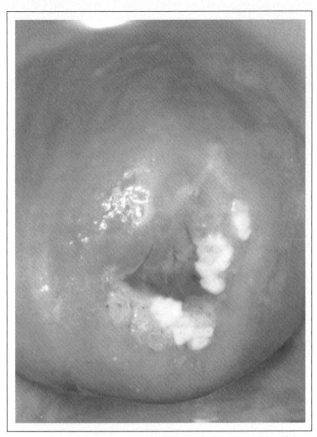

Figure 10.1-4 Bright snow-white epithelium on the posterior lip of the cervix associated with condyloma. There is also some faint white epithelium from 6 o'clock to 9 o'clock, associated with cervical intraepithelial neoplasia, grade 1.

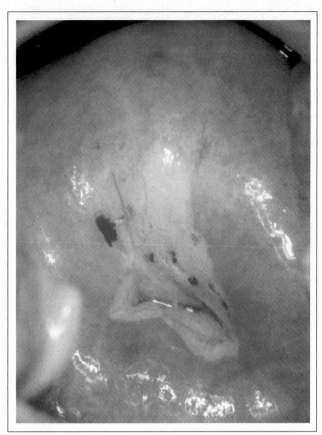

Figure 10.1-6 Dull, acetowhite, high-grade lesion. The squamocolumnar junction is not visible.

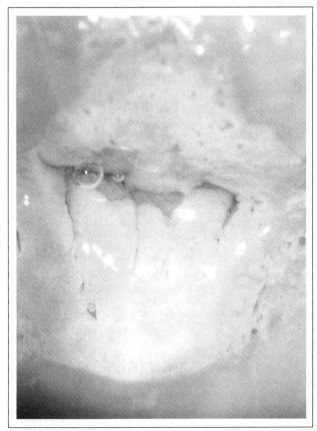

Figure 10.1-5 High-grade lesion with dense acetowhite epithelium on the posterior lip of the cervix.

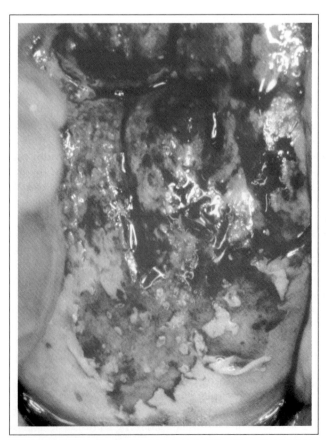

Figure 10.1-7 Example of an invasive cancer with yellow color, peeling epithelium, resultant ulcerations, and bleeding.

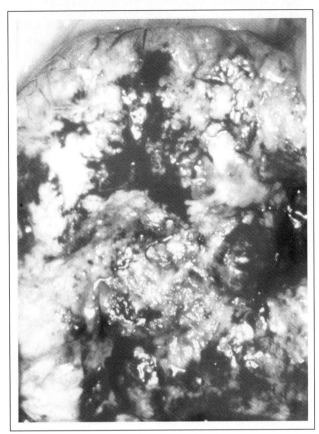

Figure 10.1-8 Large cancer with necrotic yellow base and raised surface contour.

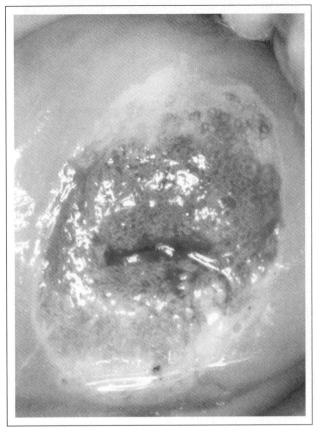

Figure 10.1-9 Ectropion with a rim of metaplasia and a fine, irregular mosaic pattern anteriorly.

overlies nabothian cysts (Figure 10.1-10). In milder degrees of dysplasia, there may be no apparent vessels, or only very fine mosaic and punctation may be present (Figure 10.1-11). *As epithelial change progresses to CIN 2, finer vascular changes disappear, leaving either no vessels or the abnormal vessels of punctation or mosaic* (Figure 10.1-12). When preinvasive cellular change reaches the CIN 3 category, the neovascular proliferation may not have kept pace with the cellular growth, and many lesions may be devoid of vessel patterns. However, if vascular changes are present, *the punctation and mosaic patterns usually appear coarse or dilated, with an increasing intercapillary distance.* The vessel patterns may exhibit variation in size (Figure 10.1-13). As the neoplastic cells breach the basement membrane and become microinvasive or frankly invasive disease, the vascular network becomes disorganized in its attempt to nourish the rapidly proliferating cellular growth. *Changes in vessel size, caliber, shape, and mutual arrangement produce the bizarre atypical vessels often viewed as "hockey sticks," "commas," or "corkscrews"* (Figure 10.1-14). As the cancer advances, the thin-walled, dilated vessels can break through the epithelial surface,

creating lakes and pools easily seen on colposcopic examination (Figure 10.1-15). Atypical vessels are best viewed with a red-free (green) filter before application of dilute acetic acid. This increases the contrast between the vessels and the rest of the epithelium, making abnormal vessels such as punctation and mosaic more pronounced.

Border

Mature squamous epithelium does not have sharp identifiable borders. Immature squamous metaplasia often has a border that represents the outer limits of the transformation zone (see Figure 10.1-2).

The borders of low-grade disease may often be indistinct or have a flocculated, feathered appearance (Figure 10.1-16). As the grade of dysplasia advances to CIN 2, the borders become more well demarcated and occasionally geographic (Figure 10.1-17). *The characteristics of CIN 3 lesions include sharply demarcated, smoother, straighter borders* (Figure 10.1-18). High-grade lesions are often closest to the squamocolumnar junction, where the cells are the most immature and have the greatest mitotic activity.

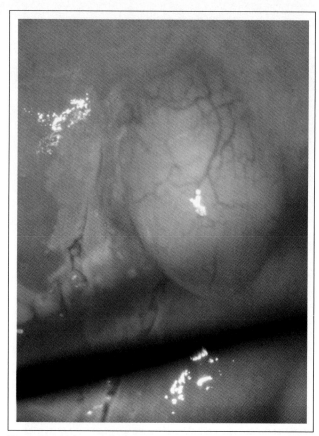

Figure 10.1-10 Large nabothian cyst with prominent, normal-branching blood vessels.

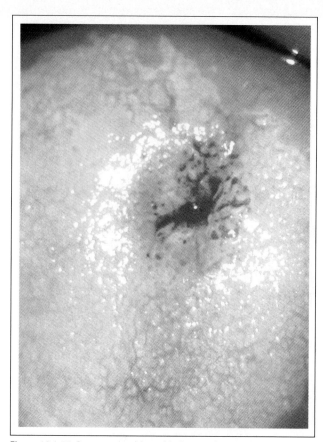

Figure 10.1-12 Dense acetowhite epithelium with coarse mosaic pattern.

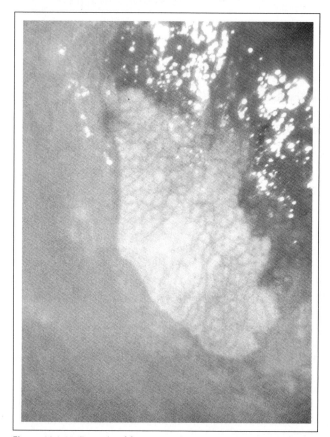

Figure 10.1-11 Example of fine mosaic and punctation on the lateral aspect of the cervix.

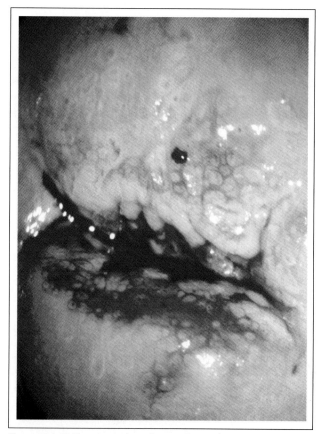

Figure 10.1-13 Very coarse, irregular mosaic vessels.

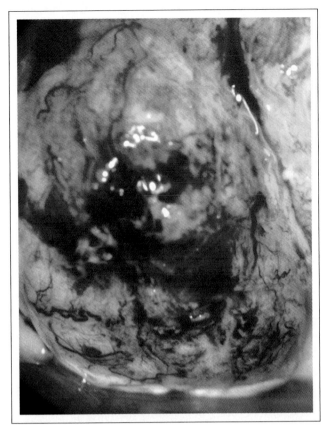

Figure 10.1-14 Example of atypical vessels with irregular, nonbranching patterns.

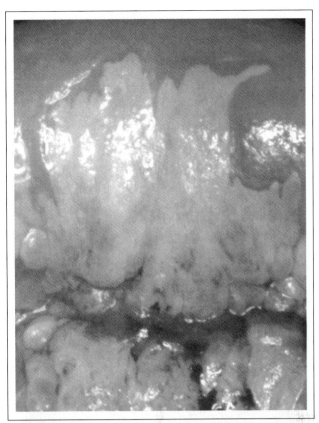

Figure 10.1-16 Example of irregular geographic border of a low-grade lesion.

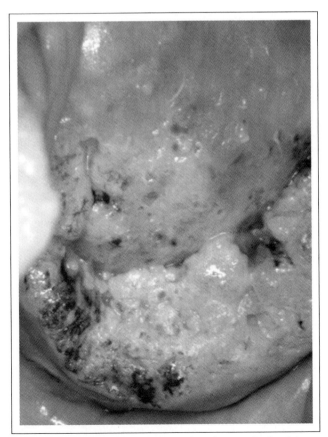

Figure 10.1-15 Example of a vascular pool on the posterior lip of the cervix in a patient with invasive cancer.

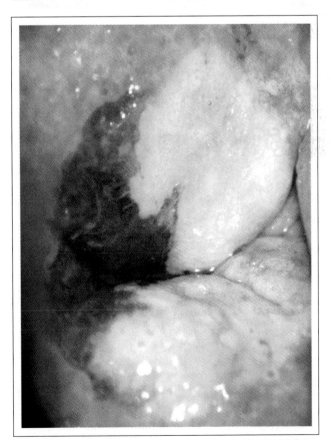

Figure 10.1-17 Example of a high-grade lesion (cervical intraepithelial lesion, grade 3) at 12 o'clock, with sharper borders compared with a low-grade lesion. A CIN 2 lesion is present on the posterior lip.

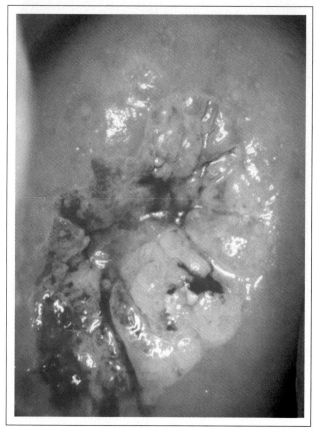

Figure 10.1-18 Example of a high-grade cervical intraepithelial lesion with dense acetowhite epithelium and sharp margins in the lower left quadrant of the cervix.

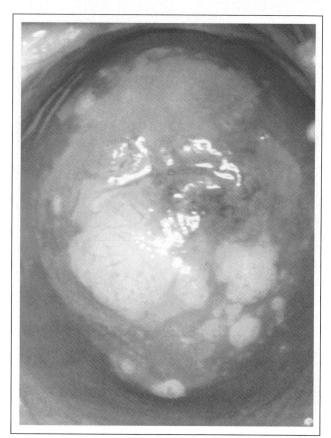

Figure 10.1-19 Large, low-grade lesion with central, denser, acetowhite, high-grade lesion.

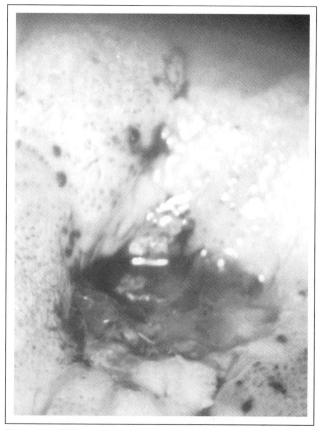

Figure 10.1-20 Dense acetowhite epithelium with very coarse mosaic and peeling edges at 5 o'clock and 12 o'clock.

A lesion within a lesion, as first discussed by Reid, creates an internal border outlining the greater abnormality (Figure 10.1-19). *As the lesion advances and becomes microinvasive or frankly invasive, the borders are often seen to be peeling or rolled* (Figure 10.1-20).

Surface

Normal epithelium is usually flat (Figure 10.1-21). The epithelium of minor-grade dysplastic change is also relatively flat (see Figure 10.1-11). However, integration of *human papillomavirus (HPV) can produce a micropapillary or a macropapillary (exophytic, condylomatous) surface* (Figure 10.1-22). As preinvasive disease progresses to CIN 2, the lesions sometimes become slightly raised but most are still relatively flat (Figure 10.1-23). CIN 3 lesions are most likely to be raised. This further intensifies the demarcation of the borders (Figure 10.1-24). Microinvasive and frankly invasive lesions can appear ulcerated. *As tumor diathesis occurs, lesions may present as ulcerated, nodular, or exophytic growths* (see Figures 10.1-8 and 10.1-15).

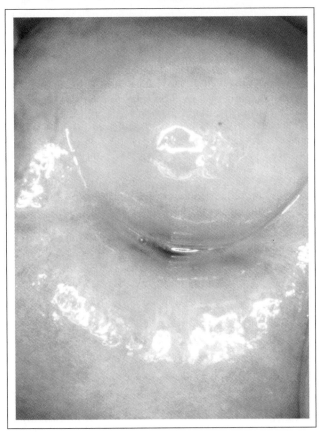

Figure 10.1-21 Example of flat, featureless, normal squamous epithelium.

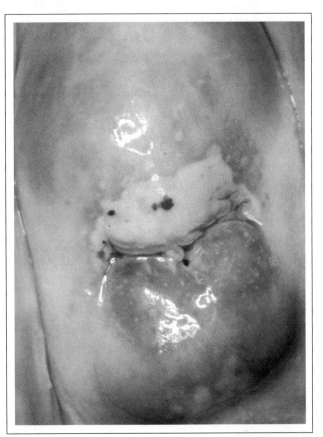

Figure 10.1-23 High-grade lesion with acetowhite epithelium and a relatively flat surface contour.

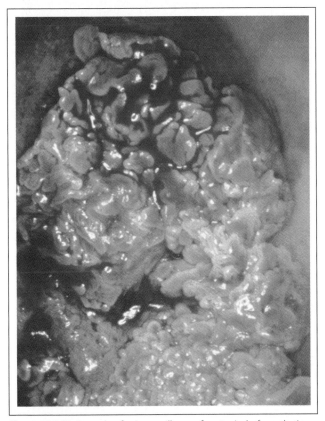

Figure 10.1-22 Example of micropapillary surface typical of exophytic condyloma.

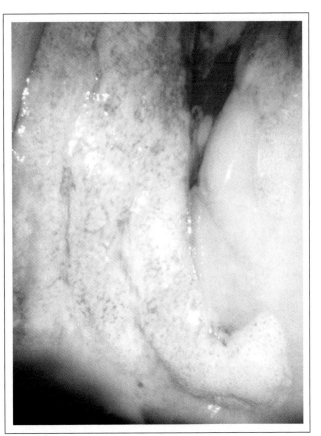

Figure 10.1-24 High-grade lesion with thick, raised, acetowhite epithelium, a sharp border, and coarse punctation.

REFERENCES

1. Burghardt E. Histopathologic basis of colposcopy. In: Burghardt E, ed. Colposcopy-Cervical Pathology Textbook and Atlas, ed 2. New York: Georg Thieme Verlag, 1991, pp. 61–98.
2. Coppleson M, Pixley E, Reid B. The tissue basis of colposcopic appearances. In: Coppleson M, Pixley E, Reid B, eds. Colposcopy: A Scientific and Practical Approach to the Cervix, Vagina, and Vulva in Heath and Disease, ed 3. Springfield, IL: Charles C Thomas, 1986, p 114.
3. Kolstadt P, Stafl A. Diagnostic criteria. In: Kolstadt P, Stafl A, eds. Atlas of Colposcopy, ed 2. Baltimore: University Park Press, 1977, p 23.
4. Anderson M, Jordan J, Morse A, et al. Colposcopic appearances of cervical intraepithelial neoplasia. In: Anderson MC, Jordan JA, Morse AR, Sharp F, Stafl A, eds. A Text and Atlas of Integrated Colposcopy, ed 2. London: Chapman & Hall Medical, 1996, p 87.
5. Campion M, Ferris D, diPaola F, et al. The abnormal cervix. In: Campion MJ, Ferris DG, Di Paolo F, Reid R, Miller MD, eds. Modern Colposcopy: A Practical Approach. Augusta, GA: Educational Systems, 1991, pp 7-17–7-27.
6. Wright C, Lickrish G, Shier, M. The abnormal transformation zone. In: Wright VC, Lickrish GM, Shier MS, eds. Basic and Advanced Colposcopy, ed 2. Komoka, Ontario: Biomedical Communications, 1995, pp 9–12.
7. Burke L, Antonioli D, Ducatman B. Atypical transformation zone. In: Burke L, Antonioli D, Ducatman B, eds. Colposcopy Text and Atlas. Norwalk, CT: Appleton & Lange, 1991, p 61.
8. Rubin M. Follow-up of an abnormal Pap test and colposcopy. In: Wallis LA (ed). Textbook of Women's Health. New York: Little, Brown, 1997, p 901.

10.2: Reid's Colposcopic Index

Richard I. Reid

KEY POINTS

▪ The Reid's Colposcopic Index (RCI) uses four colposcopic criteria (acetowhite reaction, color, margins, and vessels) to formulate a colposcopic impression and to aid in the selection of the most appropriate sites for colposcopically directed biopsy.

▪ The use of acetowhite change and abnormal vessels alone as descriptors of preinvasive lesions may lead to an inaccurate impression of the histologic severity.

▪ Because prominent areas of colposcopic change do not necessarily coincide with areas of greatest histologic severity, large areas of minor-grade lesions or squamous metaplasia are often overinterpreted, and subtle areas of high-grade lesions are easily overlooked.

▪ Although the final diagnosis is ultimately determined by the histologic interpretation, the colposcopic impression is a necessary safeguard against inaccurate or confusing histologic diagnoses.

▪ Margins are scored based on whether they are feathered, straight, or peeling.

▪ Color is determined by the degree of acetowhite change obtained following the application of copious amounts of 3% to 5% acetic acid. In practice, most lesions are scored in the intermediate category based on color (score 1).

▪ Vessels are scored based on how prominent (coarse) they are, but most high-grade lesions lack visible vessels.

▪ Iodine staining is graded by the epithelial uptake of dilute Lugol's solution and may range from partial uptake to total rejection of iodine. Normal columnar epithelium and epithelial-altering conditions such as vaginitis or atrophy are not scored in this category.

▪ Each of the four categories is assigned a score. The calculation of the scoring is cumulative; therefore the numerator fluctuates and the denominator is fixed at 8.

▪ A lesion that scores 5 or higher is typically high grade, whereas a score of 2 or lower usually indicates low-grade disease.

An effective colposcopic grading scheme will improve diagnostic reliability, reduce interobserver variability, speed colposcopic teaching, and simplify computerized data collection. However, *attempting to grade lesion severity solely based on the prominence of the acetowhite reaction or by the mere presence of aberrant vessels is unreliable.* This chapter describes four colposcopic criteria, all of which are correlated with histologic severity. Each colposcopic sign (margins, color, vascular patterns, and iodine staining) is graded into three semi-objective categories and scored as 0, 1, or 2 points. Scores for the four individual criteria are then added together to produce the Reid's Colposcopic Index (RCI). If used in strict accordance with the stated criteria, an accuracy of ≈90% can be achieved. However, departures from the validated criteria (e.g., by not adhering to the exact definitions or by omitting the iodine staining) quickly erode this performance standard.

WHAT IS REQUIRED OF A COLPOSCOPIC EXAMINATION?

Predicting histology from the colposcopic impression has never been a formal requirement of the triage process. Some believe that it is unnecessary and that rigid adherence to the triage rules will protect the clinician from error. Unfortunately, *the most prominent areas of colposcopic change do not necessarily coincide with the areas of greatest histologic severity. Large, minor-grade lesions or squamous metaplasia are often overinterpreted, and subtle avascular patches of cervical intraepithelial neoplasia, grade 3 (CIN 3) are easily overlooked.* These difficulties can easily lead to the clinician missing the correct diagnosis, even when multiple samples are obtained. Also, clinicians who depend on a mechanical approach to colposcopy will not develop that clinical sixth sense that often keeps them from errors. Hence, to compensate for a myriad or often misleading colposcopic features, robust grading systems have been developed over the past 50 years. The RCI is a guide to expected histologic severity and neoplastic potential.

Colposcopic triage is done with several purposes in mind, as follows:

- The most immediate objective is to determine whether a colposcopic explanation can be found for the abnormal cytology and whether any such lesion was seen in its entirety. If so, colposcopy is used to identify the most severe areas of any lesion and to take a directed biopsy under colposcopic control. This process breaks down if the clinician is unable to differentiate among normal, minimally abnormal, and significantly abnormal colposcopic patterns.
- The next practical issue is to establish where the treatment margins will be set. Establishing topography with certainty again depends upon the colposcopist's grading ability. Those who cannot differentiate subtle CIN 2,3 from immature metaplasia will never be truly sure whether some of their examinations were satisfactory or unsatisfactory.
- As important as these practical matters are, it should be not be forgotten that the primary goal of a colposcopic examination is to ensure that invasive disease is not missed and thus mistakenly undertreated.

Unless one is a skilled colposcopist, it is often difficult to be sure that these requirements have been fulfilled.

Colposcopists who do not use a grading system are merely using the colposcope as a visual aid to finding various acetowhite areas for biopsy, with the therapeutic response being largely decided by the pathologist.

HOW AND WHY DOES THE REID'S COLPOSCOPIC INDEX WORK?

Squamous metaplasia, CIN, and cervical cancers can all exhibit a degree of acetowhite change, with or without abnormal vessel patterns. Learning to differentiate benign changes from low-grade or high-grade CIN is a challenge. Although similarities exceed differences, there are some relatively objective criteria that do allow a skilled colposcopist to differentiate one end of the morphologic spectrum from the other. The strength of the RCI is that it relies on critical analysis (rather than on pattern recall) to ensure that serious disease is not missed and that trivial findings are not overinterpreted. By minimizing dependence on pattern recall, use of this grading system may simplify the teaching of colposcopy. In converting qualitative colposcopic data into a derived numeric score, the RCI has been used in software programs for computerized patient follow-up.

The criteria in the original RCI were distilled from a list of colposcopic characteristics shown in a series of pilot studies to define the colposcopic morphology of CIN 1–3 lesions. This list was later reduced to just four criteria by a prospective computer analysis. Each individual criterion was chosen because it was statistically independent (by factor analysis) from the other potentially usable colposcopic signs on that list and because it could be consistently graded into three semi-objective categories. These four criteria, as a group, were studied in a population of women attending an urban gynecology oncology clinic for colposcopic triage of abnormal cytology (i.e., a single high-grade or =3 low-grade cytologies). The criteria were shown to be predictive of the eventual histologic diagnosis.

The acetowhite reaction seems to occur through different mechanisms at different points in the neoplastic spectrum. High-grade lesions become acetowhite through osmotic dehydration of the abnormal chromatin within the undifferentiated basal cells. Hence, foci of CIN 3 turn optically dense for a couple of minutes, such that the normal red hue of the underlying stromal vessels can no longer be seen from the epithelial surface. Acetowhitening of minor lesions, on the other hand, is thought to be due to a transient reaction between dilute acetic acid and abnormal keratins within human papillomavirus (HPV)-infected keratinocytes of the upper layers. The acetowhite change of intermediate-grade lesions appears to reflect a combination of osmotic dehydration of the abnormal chromatin in the undifferentiated basal layers and the distorted keratins within the cell membranes of HPV-infected (but differentiating) surface cells.

DEFINITIONS OF COLPOSCOPIC CRITERIA

Abnormal colposcopic signs have been grouped into four categories, as follows:

- Sharpness of the margins
- Epithelial color
- Vascular patterns
- Iodine staining

The predictive accuracy of the RCI is maximized only when these individual colposcopic criteria are grouped into an aggregate score.

For each criterion:

- A category was correlated with the typical appearances of high-grade intraepithelial change (CIN 2,3, moderate to severe dysplasia, high-grade squamous intraepithelial lesion [HSIL]). This was scored 2 points.
- Another category fell short of being highly abnormal but was still beyond what would be regarded as merely nonspecific change. This category was scored 1 point and was shown to be reasonably predictive of low-grade intraepithelial changes (HPV/CIN 1, mild dysplasia, low-grade squamous intraepithelial lesion [LSIL]).
- Other, less defined patterns of acetowhitening or vascular atypia were scored as 0 points because they had a low predictive value for bona fide CIN.

Precise definitions of these gradations follow and are summarized in Table 10.2-1.

With respect to the examination sequence, the first three colposcopic signs are scored after the application of a generous amount of 3% to 5% acetic acid (vinegar). If an area of acetowhite change appears, the lesion is assessed and then scored. It is important to note that this grading scheme was based on studies that correlated the findings in a target biopsy taken from a specific site[1-3]; hence, when multiple colposcopic patterns coexist, the RCI must be separately derived for each disease focus. Diluted Lugol's iodine is then applied sparingly with a soaked cotton ball so that the iodine staining reaction can be assessed and scored.

COLPOSCOPIC SIGNS

Sharpness of Peripheral Margins

The following types of lesions indicate a score of 0:

- Lesions with feathered, finely scalloped margins (resembling "beat to beat" variation on an electronic fetal heart rate monitoring tracing) (Figure 10.2-1)
- Angular, irregularly shaped, or geographic (map-like) lesions (even if a portion of the lesion has a relatively straight course, because the lesion itself would have been assessed as a minor one based on its shape) (Figure 10.2-2)
- Flat lesions with indistinct borders (Figure 10.2-3)

Table 10.2-1 Reid's Colposcopic Index

Colposcopic Sign	0 Points	1 Point	2 Points
Margin	Condylomatous or micropapillary contour	Regular lesions with smooth, straight outlines	Rolled, peeling edges
	Indistinct borders	Sharp peripheral margins	Internal borders between areas of differing appearance
	Flocculated or feathered margins		
	Jagged, angular lesions		
	Satellite lesions, acetowhite change that extends beyond the transformation zone		
Color	Shiny, snow-white color	Shiny, gray-white	Dull, oyster-gray
	Indistinct acetowhite change, semitransparent rather than completely opaque	Intermediate white	
Vessels	Uniform, fine caliber	Absence of surface vessels	Definite punctation or mosaic
	Randomly arranged patterns		Individual vessels dilated, arranged in sharply demarcated, well-defined patterns
	Nondilated capillary loops		
	Ill-defined areas of fine punctation or mosaic		
Iodine staining	Positive iodine uptake, producing a mahogany-brown color	Partial iodine uptake (variegated and tortoiseshell)	Yellow staining of a lesion, which is scored 3/6
	Yellow staining by an area that is recognizable as a low-grade lesion by above criteria (<2/6)		Mustard-yellow appearance
Colposcopic score	0–2 = HPV or CIN 1 (low-grade disease)	3–4 = CIN 1 or CIN 2 (intermediate-grade disease)	5–8 = CIN 2 or CIN 3 (high-grade disease)

HPV, Human papilloma virus; *CIN*, cervical intraepithelial neoplasia.

- *Satellite* lesions, not contiguous with the new squamocolumnar junction (SCJ)
- Any lesion showing an irregular surface contour that appears condylomatous, micropapilliferous, or microconvoluted (Figures 10.2-4 and 10.2-5)

The following type of lesions indicates a score of 1:

- Ovoid, symmetrically shaped lesions with smooth, relatively straight margins (Figure 10.2-6)

The following types of lesions indicate a score of 2:

- Lesions in which cell-to-cell cohesiveness is so fragile that the epithelial edges tend to detach from the underlying stroma and curl back on themselves. Such microtrauma may be caused by inadvertently "scraping" the tissue while inserting and opening the speculum, or it may be deliberately evoked by the colposcopist gently pushing on the lesion surface with a cotton swab. Rolling or peeling edges are found almost exclusively at the new SCJ, and such lesions are scored 2, regardless of the appearance of their peripheral margins (Figure 10.2-7).

- An internal demarcation (internal margin) between two different colposcopic patterns, within the same part of an abnormal transformation zone (ATZ). With *two-in-one lesions*, the peripheral area may be more visually prominent but will nonetheless be found to reflect a minor-grade change. Conversely, the central area is often very subtle but will invariably represent a focus of high-grade dysplasia at the advancing edge of the new squamocolumnar junction (NSCJ) (Figure 10.2-8).

Finding a small focus of emerging CIN 3 within a complex ATZ can be like *finding a needle in a haystack*. Detection of an internal margin can be of great assistance in this difficult task. However, it is important to remember that the colposcopic sign of a *two-in-one lesion* is only valid if a definite internal demarcation can be seen between the central and

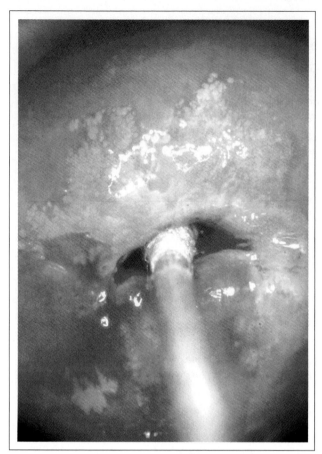

Figure 10.2-1 The acetowhite lesion found on the anterior cervix has peripheral margins that are irregular and feathered. This is a biopsy-proven CIN 1 (low-grade squamous intraepithelial lesion), and the colposcopy was unsatisfactory.

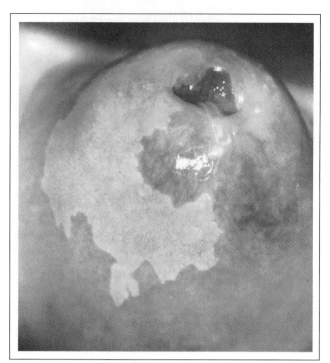

Figure 10.2-2 This lesion represents a geographic map-like, low-grade dysplasia. The lesion itself is irregular, and it extends to the posterior cervical portio.

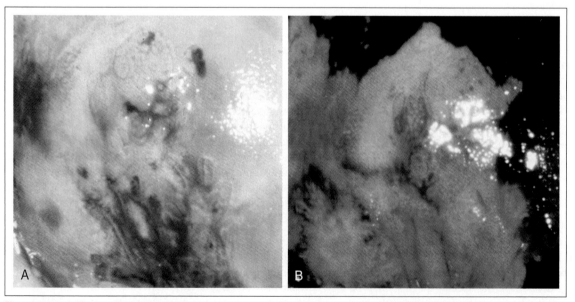

Figure 10.2-3 A, This is a CIN 3 lesion. The peripheral margin is indistinct at 12 o'clock. B, Peripheral margin becomes distinct only after the application of dilute Lugol's iodine.

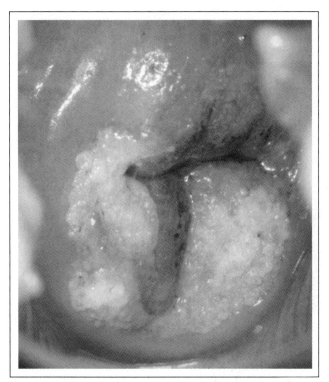

Figure 10.2-4 Example of a non-exophytic condylomatous lesion, micropapilliferous in appearance.

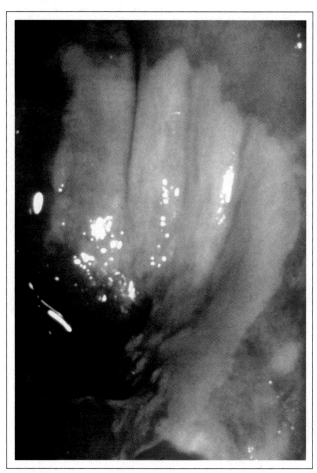

Figure 10.2-6 A small, focal CIN 3 at 12 o'clock demonstrates the biologically regular lesion. These thickened and smooth types of lesions that do not have surface blood vessels are commonly high grade.

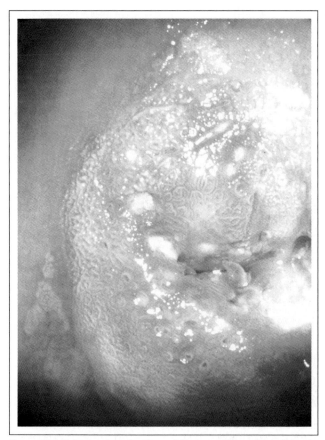

Figure 10.2-5 A microconvoluted, condylomatous lesion with an irregular and inconsistent surface contour.

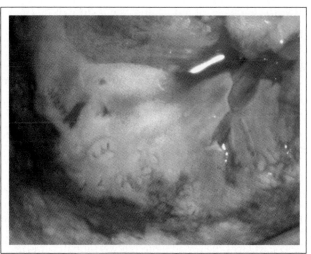

Figure 10.2-7 This high-grade CIN demonstrates a rolled, peeling margin at 6 o'clock. The epithelium that is peeling is a result of a lack of desmosomes that adhere the surface epithelium to the underlying stroma.

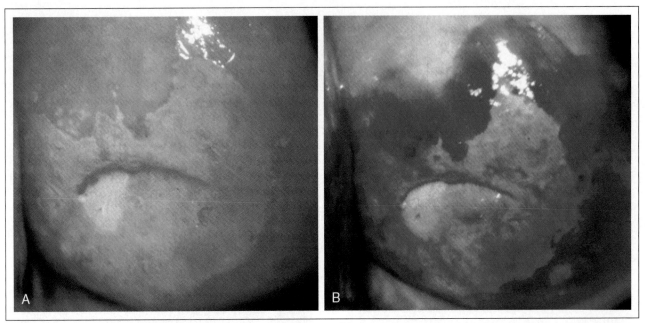

Figure 10.2-8 **A,** Example of two lesions in one, in which the central lesion is of higher grade than the peripheral one. An internal margin is evident during colposcopist inspection, moving from the periphery toward the center on any radius. **B,** Demonstrates the value of iodine in further identifying different lesions.

peripheral parts of a the same lesion. This internal demarcation must be visible as inspection moves centrally along any given radius, starting at the original SCJ and moving inward to the colposcopically visible SCJ. *When two different colposcopic patterns are seen on a single radius, the central lesion will invariably be of higher grade than the peripheral lesion and hence should be the site of target biopsy.*

Iodine staining is particularly useful in assisting in the identification of subtle CIN that is easily missed when assessment is performed with 3% to 5% acetic acid alone.

Epithelial Color

The following types of lesions indicate a score of 0:

* Less intense degrees of acetowhite change, seen as semitransparent (rather than completely opaque) (Figure 10.2-9)
* Lesions that show a pure, snow-white color (typical of an exophytic condyloma) or those that demonstrate a very intense surface shine (Figure 10.2-10)

Minor-grade lesions are often quite transient in that they appear and disappear quickly.

The following type of lesions indicates a score of 1:

* Lesions with a somewhat nondescript gray-white color. It is believed that this intermediate color category represents a fusion of two differing influences. The grayish discoloration reflects light absorption by atypical nuclei within the basal layers, whereas the surface reflectivity is probably due to continuing keratin formation within areas of cellular maturation in the upper layers (Figure 10.2-11).

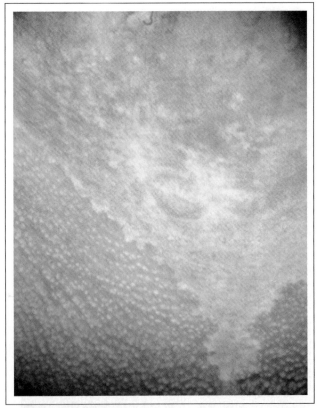

Figure 10.2-9 The color in this example is indistinct, and the lesion is semitransparent. This type of surface acetowhitening is indicative of CIN 1 or physiologic metaplasia.

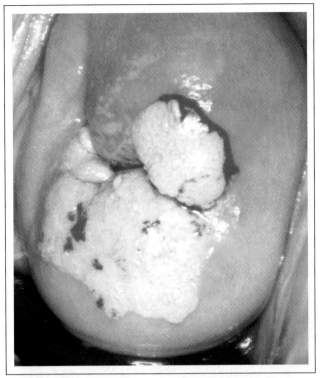

Figure 10.2-10 This exophytic condyloma exhibits a shiny, snow-white color, whereas condylomatous-looking invasive cancers are typically dull yellowish-white lesions.

In practice, most lesions will be scored within the intermediate category.

The following type of lesions indicates a score of 2:

- Thick patches of dull, oystershell-white epithelium. The matte, nonreflective quality is due to the paucity of cytoplasm within the neoplastic basal cells throughout

the entire thickness of the epithelium in high-grade lesions. In the absence of surface keratin, light passes down to the basal layers, where it is absorbed by the dense chromatin deposits in the abnormal nuclei, thus imparting a dull, oystershell hue (Figure 10.2-12).

Major-grade lesions may take longer to appear after dilute acetic acid application; when they do appear, however, they usually remain visible longer than minor-grade lesions.

Vascular Patterns

The following type of lesions indicates a score of 0:

- Areas of fine punctation or fine mosaic, ill-defined, yet prominent vessels formed by loose aggregations of nondilated capillaries of uniform caliber. These vessels represent normal intraepithelial looped capillaries that have been exaggerated because of a proliferative effect due to HPV infection (Figure 10.2-13).

Prominent vascular changes in minor-grade lesions closely resemble the surface vessels seen in congenital metaplasia. Hence, it can be quite difficult to distinguish between congenital metaplasia and a low-grade lesion (Figure 10.2-14).

The following type of lesions indicates a score of 1:

- *Most CIN 2,3 lesions do not display abnormal surface vascular patterns when dilute acetic acid is applied.* Conversely, when the colposcopic examination is performed with saline, these same high-grade lesions have abundant epithelial vessels. This disparity suggests that the application of dilute acetic acid soaking to a high-grade, nuclear-dense lesion causes enough epithelial swelling to transiently compress most intraepithelial looped capillaries, preventing them from being visualized (Figure 10.2-15).

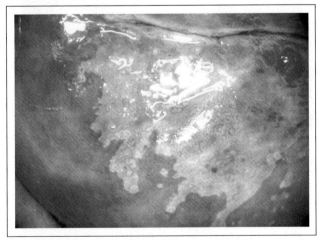

Figure 10.2-11 This CIN 1 lesion is typical in that it exhibits an irregular margin and a shiny gray color, with a fine mosaic pattern. Most low-grade lesions are gray-white in color.

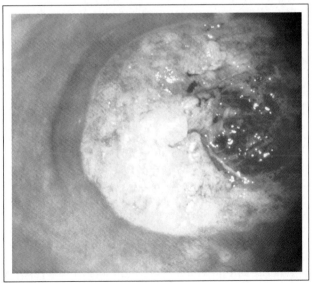

Figure 10.2-12 Most high-grade lesions are dull oystershell-white in color. This lesion has smooth and regular margins and is devoid of surface vessels.

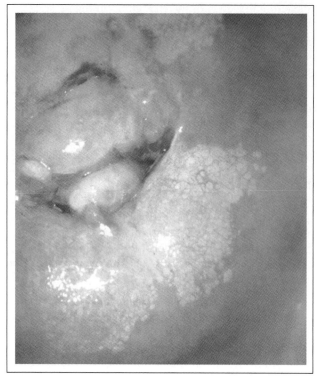

Figure 10.2-13 Low-grade lesions often exhibit a fine mosaic and punctation pattern. This example reveals loose arcades of haphazardly oriented surface vessels that represent an exaggeration of the normal looped cervical capillaries.

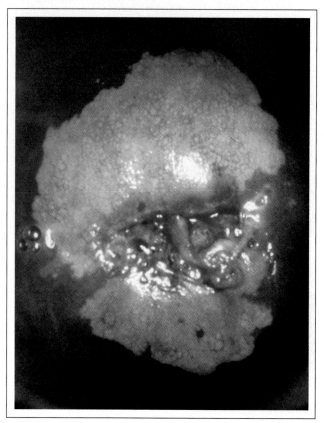

Figure 10.2-14 Although the vessels in this example are prominent, they are nondilated and irregular.

The following type of lesions indicates a score of 2:

- Coarse, dilated punctation or significant mosaic vascular patterns. These vessels are confined to significant plaques of acetowhite change, dilated, and arranged in sharply demarcated, well-defined patterns.

These vessels are formed because of angiogenesis (e.g., new vessels feeding a neoplasia), as distinct from the vessels found in low-grade disease (Figure 10.2-16).

Iodine-Staining Reaction

The following types of lesions indicate a score of 0:

- Uniform iodine uptake (positive staining) by intracellular glycogen deposits within well-differentiated vaginal epithelium. The chemical reaction between glycogen and iodine produces a deep mahogany-brown color (Figure 10.2-17).
- An area of epithelium that was recognizable as a minor-grade lesion on the three acetic acid criteria (because it scored <3 points) but failed to stain mahogany brown. Histologically, most such lesions represent areas of parakeratosis, without the rich intracellular glycogen stores normally found in benign vaginal mucosa. Despite the absence of intracellular glycogen, the surface keratin deposits in such lesions do retain enough iodine to stain a mustard-yellow color (Figure 10.2-18). This pattern is termed *negative iodine staining.*

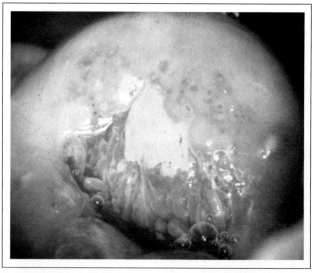

Figure 10.2-15 This CIN 3 does not exhibit surface blood vessels because of the thickened epithelium. Most CIN 2,3 lesions do not have visible surface vessels.

The following type of lesions indicates a score of 1:

- An irregular mixture of iodine uptake and iodine rejection, imparting a variegated, *tortoise-shell* appearance (Figure 10.2-19). This pattern, termed *partial iodine staining,* is typical of low-grade dysplasia.

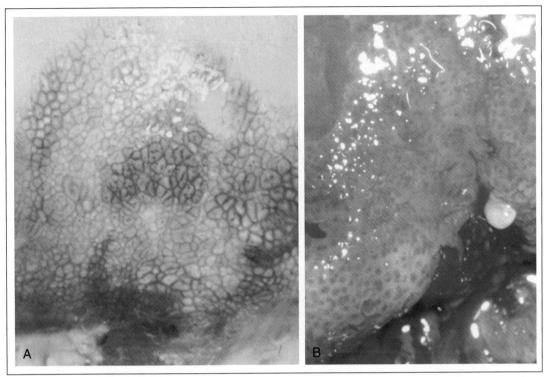

Figure 10.2-16 The vessels depicted in **A** here and in B represent neovascularization or an angiogenic response to a significant neoplasia. **A** reveals a classic mosaic pattern typical of late-stage lesions on the verge of malignant transformation. **B,** Dilated, coarse punctation is evident.

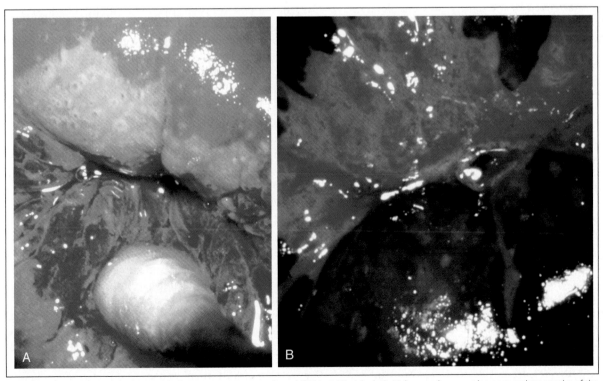

Figure 10.2-17 A, The acetowhite epithelium represents an equivocal CIN 1 at 12 o'clock. **B,** Mahogany brown color or complete uptake of the iodine is consistent with normal epithelium.

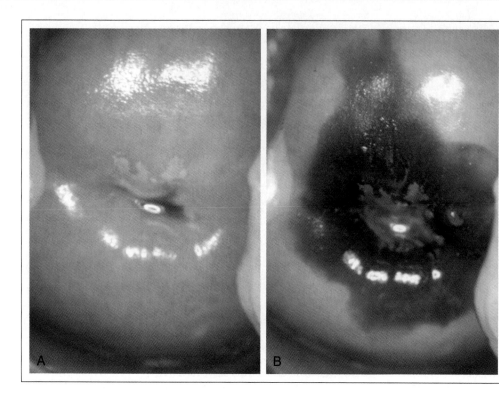

Figure 10.2-18 A, Example of a minor-grade lesion with respect to the margins, color, and vessels. **B,** Lesion is mustard yellow when iodine is applied.

The following type of lesions indicates a score of 2:

- Mustard-yellow staining in an area that was already recognized as being high grade by the three dilute acetic acid criteria. It is important to understand that the negative iodine staining seen in both trivial and major lesions is characterized by the same yellow discoloration. Hence, determining whether a focus of negative iodine stain attracts 0 or 2 points depends on the application of other colposcopic features, not on the shade of the iodine reaction (Figure 10.2-20).

The following are important considerations:

- Normal columnar epithelium, biopsy sites, and other epithelial altering conditions (e.g., vaginitis, atrophy) may result in yellowish discoloration as well. However, because these areas are not acetowhite lesions, they are not to be scored.
- The Lugol's iodine parameter helps in two important ways, and colposcopists should consider it an important part of the index. First, Lugol's iodine staining improves sensitivity by reducing the number of false-negative exams caused by overlooking thin, high-grade lesions that are still in the process of emerging within an actively metaplasing transformation zone. Second, Lugol's iodine staining also improves specificity by helping to downgrade false-positive calls that are often evoked by areas of benign, acanthotic, non-neoplastic epithelia laid down by a metaplastic process occurring during intrauterine life. Many such congenital transformation zones present florid acetowhite and vascular change but are usually easily recognized as

non-neoplastic by their pattern of iodine uptake (see later discussion).

Applying the Reid's Colposcopic Index Scoring System

Overall, the positive predictive value of any individual colposcopic criterion in the RCI is around 80%. This is noteworthy but not robust enough for genuine clinical utility. Hence, an aggregate score is calculated by adding the points assigned for the four categories. The numerator of the RCI fluctuates according to colposcopic appearance, but the denominator remains fixed at 8.

- Lesions that score 5 points are likely to predict high-grade histology.
- Lesions that score 2 points are likely to predict low-grade histology.
- Lesions that score 3 or 4 points usually represent low- to moderate-grade histology.

Most commonly, high-grade lesions are characterized by distinctly definable margins, absent vessels, dull-white color, and a confirmatory iodine yellow staining. Small, subtle, high-grade lesions sometimes closely resemble immature physiologic metaplasia. Both appear as areas of acetowhite reaction with absent vessels. However, the color of immature metaplasia is generally semi-transparent and margins are indistinct and confluent (Figures 10.2-21 and 10.2-22). Additionally, the acetowhite change of normal metaplastic epithelium often occupies most of the circumference of the transformation zone and is always contiguous with the SCJ.

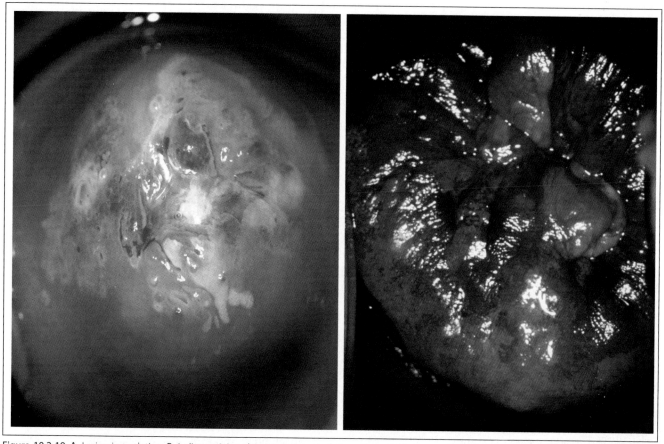

Figure 10.2-19 A, Lesion in evolution. **B,** Iodine staining shows a tortoiseshell-like pattern, in that areas of both mustard yellow and mahogany brown are present.

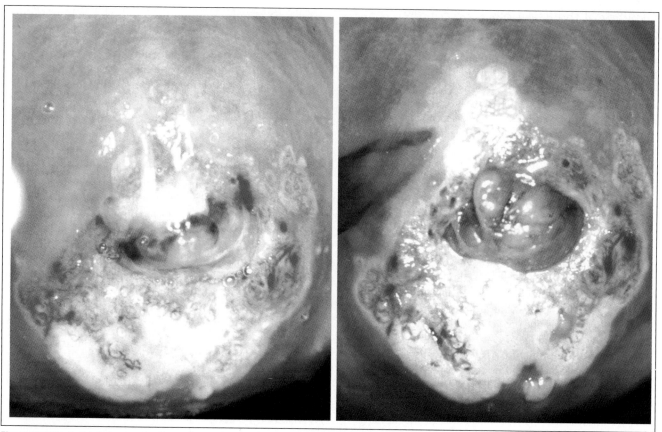

Figure 10.2-20 A, This lesion has significant abnormalities, including atypical blood vessels and dense acetowhite epithelium with sharp borders. **B,** This image shows how the lesion rejects the iodine, giving a mustard-yellow appearance to the areas of acetowhite epithelium.

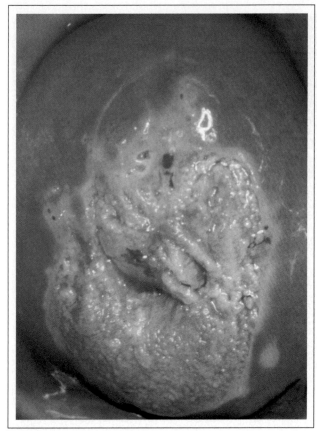

Figure 10.2-21 Example of metaplasia with a semitransparent acetowhiteness.

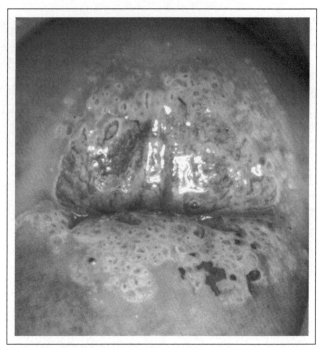

Figure 10.2-22 Metaplasia with mild acetowhiteness and several islands of columnar epithelium present.

Accuracy of the Reid Colposcopic Index Grading Scheme

The original RCI was based on correlations seen in two tertiary referral clinics, where patients tended to manifest well-developed, often quite florid lesions sited within mature abnormal transformation zones. In this setting, the RCI is robust and highly reproducible. However, in some situations it is more difficult to obtain the same degree of excellence, as follows:

- *When the RCI is used in the work-up of women with very mild or non-representative cytology* (e.g., in the triage of very young women with smear abnormalities and immature transformation zones), *specificity can weaken,* especially if the colposcopist is less experienced. The main difficulty is the large number of women with normal cytology who harbor patches of unusually acanthotic (but physiologic) epithelium that is laid down by fetal metaplasia during intrauterine development. Such *congenital transformation zones* present florid acetowhite and vascular change that will result in a false-positive prediction of high-grade histology.
- Conversely, in triaging women with lesions that are still emerging within immature ATZs, any focus of HSIL will usually be both subtle and nonrepresentative, resulting in a false-negative prediction with respect to high-grade histology.

- Another source of apparent inaccuracy lies in the reduced correlation that can exist at the lower end of the morphologic spectrum. For good reason, histology is universally accepted as the *gold standard* for diagnosing invasive cervical cancer and CIN 3. However, histology, cytology, and colposcopy can all be subjective. Moreover, for HPV infection and even CIN 1, histologic change typically lags behind the development of cytologic or colposcopic change. This phenomenon has been well described in studies showing high levels of interobserver and intraobserver differences for selected material.

SUMMARY

It is easy to derive the four proven colposcopic criteria that can be quickly compiled into an index (the RCI) that helps the clinician recognize lesion severity at the time of colposcopy. However, using the colposcopic index to infer approximate histologic findings does not eliminate the importance of biopsy. Clinicians should always follow the triage rules conscientiously, including the need to carefully perform selected colposcopically directed biopsy specimens. The value of these individual colposcopic signs is maximized by combining them into a weighted scoring system. The overall predictive accuracy of the combined colposcopic index is greater than 95%.[1-3]

The formal calculation of this colposcopic index produces a meaningful clinical assessment of lesion severity, against which the clinician can reconcile the cytologic and histologic findings.

REFERENCES

1. Reid R, Stanttope CR, Herschman BR, et al. Genital warts and cervical cancer. IV. A colposcopic index for differentiating subclinical papillomaviral infection from cervical intraepithelial neoplasia. Am J Obstet Gynecol 1984;149:815–823.

2. Reid R, Herschman BR, Crum CP, et al. Genital warts and cervical cancer. V. The tissue basis of colposcopic change. Am J Obstet Gynecol 1984;149:293–303.

3. Reid R, Scalzi P. Genital warts and cervical cancer. VI. An improved colposcopic index for differentiating benign papillomaviral infections from high-grade cervical intraepithelial neoplasia. Am J Obstet Gynecol 1985;153:611–618.

CHAPTER 11

The Management of Women with Atypical Squamous Cells

Thomas C. Wright, Jr.

KEY POINTS

- The pooled prevalence of biopsy-confirmed cervical intraepithelial neoplasia, grades 2 and 3 (CIN 2,3) or cancer in women in atypical squamous cells of undetermined significance (ASC-US) is 9.7%.
- Almost half of women with ASC-H cytology will have biopsy-confirmed CIN 2,3 identified at colposcopy.
- The most appropriate threshold for referring women to colposcopy is a repeat cytology result of ASC or greater.
- The sensitivity of a single repeat cytology for identifying women with CIN 2,3 at an ASC-US threshold was 82%. At this threshold 51% of all women would be referred to colposcopy. When a threshold of LSIL or greater is used, the sensitivity drops to only 46%.
- Testing for HPV should only be for high-risk types of HPV. Testing for low-risk types of HPV only increases costs without providing clinical benefit.
- The sensitivity of HC 2 for detecting CIN 2,3 is 93%, and would refer 42% of the patients to colposcopy.
- In the ASC-US/LSIL Triage Study (ALTS) clinical trial, risk for CIN 3 was identical in HPV DNA–positive women with ASC-US and women with LSIL; therefore HPV–DNA positive women with ASC-US should receive the same evaluation and follow-up as women with LSIL.
- Women with ASC-US who are HPV DNA negative have a very low risk of having CIN 3
- "Reflex" HPV DNA testing is the preferred approach to managing women with ASC-US whenever liquid-based cytology is used.
- The use of HPV testing to manage adolescents with ASC-US would refer the vast majority to colposcopy, even though they are at very low risk for having cancer.
- The 2006 Consensus Guidelines recommend against performing HPV DNA testing in adolescents for any reason.
- The 2006 Consensus Guidelines discourage performing colposcopy in adolescents for the initial management of ASC-US or LSIL.
- A woman with ASC-H has a 2 to 5 times greater risk of having CIN 2,3 than does a woman with ASC-US.
- In ALTS only 40% of women with ASC-H 35 years and older were HPV DNA positive. This suggests that HPV DNA testing might potentially be useful in this subset of women with ASC-H.

When the Bethesda System terminology for reporting cervical cytology was first introduced in 1988, it was recognized that because of the subjective nature of cytology, cytopathologists needed an equivocal category. This equivocal category would alert the clinician and patient as to the possibility that a high-grade cervical cancer precursor, referred to as *cervical intraepithelial neoplasia grades 2 and 3* (CIN 2,3), was present in cases in which equivocal cytologic changes were too severe to fit into the category of reactive or reparative changes but insufficient to allow a cytologic diagnosis of a squamous intraepithelial lesion (SIL). In the 1988 Bethesda System classification, this category was termed *atypical squamous cells of undetermined significance* (ASC-US).[1] When ASC-US was originally introduced, cytopathologists were encouraged to subcategorize ASC-US results by stating whether they thought the changes were suggestive of a reactive/reparative process, suggestive of neoplastic process, or even suggestive of invasive cervical cancer.

By 1993, shortly after the introduction of ASC-US, the median ASC-US rate of laboratories responding to the College of American Pathologists (CAP) laboratory questionnaire was 2.8%.[2] However, by 1996 the median ASC-US rate in a repeat CAP survey had increased to 4.4%.[3] This represented a significant increase from the rate reported in 1993 and occurred despite the fact that at this point most laboratories were still using conventional glass Papanicolaou (Pap) tests.[3] The reasons why such a large increase took place are unclear, but undoubtedly concerns about potential litigation played an important role. During the 1990s the number of malpractice cases against laboratories and cytopathologists for "failure to diagnose" cervical cancers skyrocketed. Such cases are often quite difficult to defend because even with expert cytologists, the diagnosis of ASC-US is poorly reproducible.[4–6]

In 2001, when the Bethesda System underwent revision to improve usability and to reflect our increased knowledge of role of human papillomavirus (HPV) in the pathogenesis of cervical cancer, it was recognized that ASC-US was one area where change was needed. Not only had *the ASC-*

US rate increased dramatically, but several studies showed that *modifiers such as "suggestive of a reactive/reparative process" were misleading.* This is because the *interpretation of minor cytologic changes is so subjective that cytopathologists could not reproducibly distinguish between those ASC-US changes associated with neoplasia and those associated with inflammation.* At the conference at which the 2001 Bethesda System was developed, a number of individuals recommended that the ASC-US category be eliminated and that cervical cytology specimens be classified as either normal or as SIL. However, the majority of the conference participants believed that retaining category of ASC-US was useful because a considerable proportion CIN 2,3 cases detected in any given clinical practice are identified during the evaluation of women with ASC-US. For example, in the Kaiser Permanente Northern California experience, 39% of all CIN 2,3 lesions were diagnosed in women undergoing colposcopy for ASC-US.[7] The potential impact of eliminating the ASC-US category was also documented by a study in which the referral cytology specimens of 100 women referred for colposcopy because of an ASC-US diagnosis were blindly re-evaluated by a panel of pathologists who were instructed to classify the specimens as either normal or SIL.[8] In 10 of 17 (59%) cases of CIN 2,3, the ASC-US referral cytology was reclassified as normal when the ASC-US category was eliminated. Therefore the 2001 Bethesda System retained a borderline or equivocal cytologic category but changed the name as well as the criteria for diagnosing ASC-US. The use of modifiers was also discouraged. *The 2001 Bethesda System defined atypical squamous cells (ASC) as cytologic changes suggestive of SIL that are quantitatively or qualitatively insufficient for a definitive interpretation.*[9]

The 2001 Bethesda System also formally subdivided ASC into two categories. One is considered to be a relatively low-risk category that is quite commonly encountered and in which a minority of women will have CIN 2,3. This low-risk category ASC is called *atypical squamous cells of undetermined significance* (ASC-US) (Figure 11-1). The other category is relatively uncommon but is associated with a much higher risk of having associated CIN 2,3 lesions. This category is termed *atypical squamous cells; cannot exclude high-grade squamous intraepithelial lesion* (ASC-H) and should essentially be considered to be an equivocal high-grade squamous intraepithelial lesion (HSIL). *ASC-H is used when cytologic features suggestive of HSIL are present but definite evidence is lacking.* Typically this means that either only a few HSIL cells are present or the HSIL cells seen on the slide do not have all of the cytologic features of HSIL (Figure 11-2). It is important for clinicians managing women with abnormal cervical cytology results to recognize that *the diagnosis of ASC is poorly reproducible.*[4-6] For example, in the recent National Cancer Institute's ASC-US/LSIL Triage Study (ALTS) clinical trial, only 55% of the cytology specimens originally diagnosed as ASC were subsequently given a diagnosis of ASC by the pathology quality control group.[6] Thirty-one percent of the cases were downgraded to within normal limits and 14% upgraded to a SIL.[10]

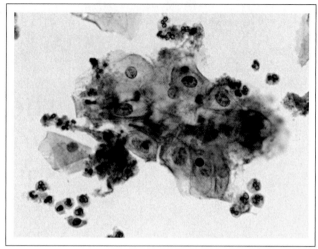

Figure 11-1 ASC-US: The cells shown here have some features of LSIL. The nuclei are somewhat enlarged and hyperchromatic. However, the cells do not show sufficient cytologic alterations to be classified as diagnostic of LSIL. Moreover, there is a considerable amount of inflammation present that may be contributing to the cytologic changes. Therefore the laboratory classified this case as ASC-US.

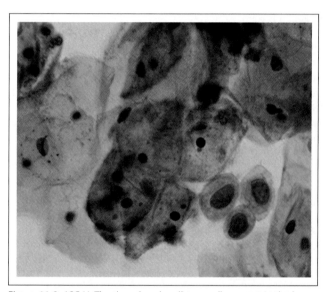

Figure 11-2 ASC-H: The three "parabasal" type cells present in the lower-right corner of the photograph have a number of the cytologic features usually associated with HSIL. The nuclei are hyperchromatic and also are somewhat enlarged, resulting in an increased nuclear:cytoplasmic ratio. The nuclear outlines are also somewhat irregular, which is another feature of HSIL. In this case there were only three atypical cells present on the slide, and the cytopathologist was uncomfortable making a definitive diagnosis of HSIL and instead classified the case as ASC-H.

RATE OF REPORTING OF ATYPICAL SQUAMOUS CELLS IN U.S. LABORATORIES

Our best data on the rate of reporting of ASC come from laboratory questionnaires that are collected by CAP every several years. The most recent CAP survey covered the period from 2002 to early 2003 and collected data for conventional cervical cytology separately from liquid-based cytology. Reporting rates for the different cytologic abnormalities are shown in Table 11-1.[11] *For conventional cytology the mean reporting rate for ASC-US was 3.8%, and for liquid-based cytology it was 4.8%. What is striking about the laboratory reporting rates is the huge variation observed between laboratories.* The reporting rate for ASC-US in the bottom 5% of the reporting range (1 of 20 laboratories) is less than 1%, whereas the reporting rate in laboratories in the upper 5% of the reporting range is 11%. Although the mean reporting rate of ASC-H is similar for both liquid-based cytology and conventional cytology, about 0.5%, there also are striking differences in reporting rates for ASC-H between laboratories. Almost one fourth of U.S. laboratories rarely if ever make a cytologic diagnosis of ASC-H (see Table 11-1). This means that *it is very important for clinicians to know how their laboratories diagnose ASC.*

CLINICAL SIGNIFICANCE OF AN ATYPICAL SQUAMOUS CELL DIAGNOSIS

The clinical significance of ASC is directly proportional to the underlying prevalence of CIN 2,3. *A woman with a cytologic diagnosis of ASC-US on a routine screening cervical cytology has a 5% to 16% chance of having biopsy-confirmed CIN 2,3 identified at colposcopy* (Table 11-2). A recent meta-analysis including 20 studies found that the pooled prevalence of biopsy-confirmed CIN 2,3 or cancer in women with ASC-US is 9.7%.[12] The underlying rate of CIN 2,3 in women with ASC-US is considered high enough that most experts and professional societies, both in the United States and in other countries, recommend some form of additional workup or follow-up for these women. In contrast, the prevalence of CIN 2,3 in women with ASC-H is much higher than the prevalence in women with ASC-US (Table 11-3).

Table 11-2 Prevalence of Biopsy-Confirmed CIN 2,3 in Women with ASC-US

		Number (%)	
Author	**Country**	**ASC-US**	**CIN 2,3**
Manos, 1999	United States: Kaiser	956	63 (7%)
Bergeron, 2000	France	111	12 (11%)
Morin, 2001	Canada	359	19 (5%)
Solomon, 2001	United States: multisite	2313	267 (12%)
Lonky, 2003	United States: Kaiser	278	33 (12%)
Carozzi, 2005	Italy	199	35 (35%)
Srodon, 2006	United States: Johns Hopkins	351	32 (9%)
Alvarez, 2007	United States: multisite	794	97 (12%)

Modified from references 34, 36–42.
CIN, Cervical intraepithelial neoplasia; *ASC-US*, atypical squamous cells of undetermined significance.

Table 11-1 Cytologic Abnormality Rates Reported in U.S. Laboratories, 2002–2003

			Percentile Reporting Rate				
Category	**N***	**Mean**	**5th**	**25th**	**50th**	**75th**	**95th**
Conventional Smears							
LSIL	243	2.06	0.3	0.8	1.4	2.1	5.6
HSIL+	233	0.7	0.1	0.2	0.4	0.7	2.2
ASC-US	237	3.81	0.5	1.6	3.1	4.8	9.7
ASC-H	148	0.48	0.0	0.0	0.1	0.3	2.1
Liquid-Based Cytology Specimens							
LSIL	232	2.92	0.8	1.6	2.4	3.6	6.9
HSIL+	224	0.84	0.1	0.4	0.5	0.9	2.0
ASC-US	222	4.76	0.9	2.6	4.1	5.9	11.0
ASC-H	142	0.55	0.0	0.1	0.2	0.4	1.5

Data modified from Davey DD, Neal MH, Wilbur DC, et al. Bethesda 2001 implementation and reporting rates: 2003 practices of participants in the College of American Pathologists Interlaboratory Comparison Program in Cervicovaginal Cytology. Arch Pathol Lab Med 2004;128:1224–1229.
LSIL, Low-grade squamous intraepithelial lesion; *HSIL*, high-grade squamous intraepithelial lesion; *ASC-US*, atypical squamous cells of undetermined significance; *ASC-H*, atypical squamous cells: cannot exclude HSIL.
*Number of reporting laboratories in the United States.

Table 11-3 Prevalence of Biopsy-Confirmed CIN 2,3 in Women with ASC-H

| Author | Country | Number (%) | |
		ASC-H	CIN 2,3
Duncan, 2005	United States: reference lab	99	40 (40%)
Liman, 2005	United States: University of Rochester	48	22 (46%)
Srodon, 2005	United States: Johns Hopkins	96	19 (20%)
Sherman, 2006	United States: multisite	101	50 (50%)

Modified from references 33–35, 43.

CIN, Cervical intraepithelial neoplasia; ASC-H, atypical squamous cells: cannot exclude high-grade squamous intraepithelial neoplasia.

In most studies *almost half of women with ASC-H will have biopsy-confirmed CIN 2,3 identified at colposcopy.* Because of the high underlying prevalence of CIN 2,3, women with ASC-H need to be managed in a more aggressive manner than women with ASC-US.

MANAGEMENT OF WOMEN WITH ATYPICAL SQUAMOUS CELLS OF UNDETERMINED SIGNIFICANCE

Repeat Cervical Cytology

Repeat cytology has traditionally been used for managing women with equivocal cytologic findings. The concept for this approach is simple: If a significant cervical lesion is present, it should be detected the next time the cytology exam is repeated. However, it is well recognized that the sensitivity of cytology is relatively low. In recent, well-controlled clinical trials the sensitivity of a single cervical cytology for identifying women with CIN 2,3 in a screening setting has ranged from 0.4 to 0.76.[13-15] To compensate for this, clinicians have frequently repeated the cytology examination several times prior to returning the patient to routine screening. *Based on several studies, the most appropriate threshold for referring women to colposcopy is a repeat cytology result of ASC or greater.*[16,17] Using higher referral thresholds, such as low-grade squamous intraepithelial lesion (LSIL) or HSIL, as the basis for referral to colposcopy results in too many women with CIN 2,3 being missed. Table 11-4 presents a number of studies in which women with ASC underwent a colposcopic examination and either a repeat cytology or HPV deoxyribonucleic acid (DNA) testing. In these studies

Table 11-4 Performance of Repeat Cytology or HPV Testing for Identifying CIN 2,3 Lesions in Women with ASC Cytology

| Author | Repeat Cytology* | | HPV DNA Testing | |
	Sensitivity	% Referred	Sensitivity	% Referred
Goff, 1993	0.60	46%	NA	NA
Slawson, 1994	0.67	37%	NA	NA
Cox, 1995	0.73	NA	NA	NA
Wright, 1995	0.73	49%	NA	NA
Ferris, 1998	0.70	56%	0.89	43%
Manos, 1999	0.76	38%	0.89	40%
Bergeron, 2000	0.67	32%	0.83	43%
Lin, 2000	NA	NA	1.00	52%
Shlay, 2000	NA	NA	0.93	31%
Morin, 2001	NA	NA	0.90	29%
Solomon, 2001	0.85	59%	0.96	57%
Kulasingam, 2002	NA	NA	0.89	35%
Pretorius, 2002	NA	NA	0.89	32%
Guyot, 2003	NA	NA	1.00	52%
Lonky, 2003	NA	NA	0.81	30%
Dalla Palma, 2005	NA	NA	0.94	70%

Modified from references 36–40, 44–54.

HPV, Human papillomavirus; CIN, cervical intraepithelial neoplasia; ASC, atypical squamous cells; DNA, deoxyribonucleic acid; NA, not applicable.

*Using an ASC-US (atypical squamous cells of undetermined significance) cutoff for referral to colposcopy.

the sensitivity for identifying women with CIN 2,3 of a single repeat cervical cytology at an ASC-US cut-off ranged from 0.60 to 0.85. In these studies a repeat single cytology would have referred 32% to 59% of the women to colposcopy. A meta-analysis of the effectiveness of repeat cytology in women with ASC-US identified 9 studies that provided sufficient information to allow sensitivity to be evaluated.[18] There was considerable heterogeneity in results among the studies in both sensitivity and the proportion of women referred to colposcopy with repeat cytology. *The pooled estimate of the sensitivity of a single repeat cytology for identifying women with CIN 2,3 at an ASC-US threshold was 82%. At this threshold, 51% of all women would be referred to colposcopy. When a threshold of LSIL or greater is used as the basis for referral to colposcopy, sensitivity drops to only 46%.*

These studies focus on the results achieved with a single repeat cytologic examination. Relatively few clinical studies have evaluated the effectiveness of a program of repeat cytology for women with ASC, and evidence is missing regarding the best interval to repeat the cytology, as well as the number of repeats that are necessary. *In a heavily screened population such as in the United States, more than two repeat cytology tests would be expected to provide minimal benefit.* The best data that we have on the effectiveness of a program of repeat cervical cytology come from the ALTS trial, as women in this trial were followed prospectively for 2 years.[16] In ALTS, a single repeat cytology examination with referral for an ASC-US or greater result on the repeat cytology would have identified 83% of the women with CIN 3 lesions and referred 58% of the women to colposcopy. Repeating cytology twice increased sensitivity to 95% but also increased the referral rate to 67%. A third repeat cytology resulted in a minimal increase in sensitivity (to 97%) and a slight increase in referrals (to 73%). A program of two repeat cytology examinations using an LSIL result as the basis for referral to colposcopy had a sensitivity of 74% and a referral rate of 32%. *The approach of repeating cervical cytology has some disadvantages compared with other potential management options. It can significantly delay the diagnosis of CIN 2,3 or cervical cancer, and even in populations with good access to healthcare, adherence to recommendations becomes a significant problem when multiple visits are required.*

Testing for High-Risk Human Papillomavirus Types

A number of the studies have used the only Food and Drug Administration (FDA)-approved molecular HPV DNA test (Hybrid capture 2 [HC 2] Digene, a Qiagen Company, Gaithersburg, MD to evaluate women with ASC (see Table 11-4). *It is important to stress that although this test can test for both low-risk and high-risk types of HPV, testing should only be for high-risk types of HPV. Testing for low-risk types of HPV only increases costs, without providing clinical benefit.* Not all of the studies shown in Table 11-4 separated women with ASC-US from those with ASC-H, and only a few have directly compared HPV testing with repeat cytology. The sensitivity of HPV DNA testing in these studies for identifying women

with CIN 2,3 ranges from 0.81 to 1.00. A recent meta-analysis of the performance of HPV DNA testing in women with ASC-US reported that *the pooled sensitivity of HC 2 for detecting CIN 2,3 is 93%.*[12] An important finding of the meta-analysis was that the sensitivity of HPV testing was similar in the different studies and the pooled estimate of sensitivity was quite stable. In contrast, there was considerable heterogeneity among the different studies in the reported prevalence of high-risk HPV DNA positivity in women with ASC-US. *The pooled estimate for the proportion that would be referred to colposcopy if HPV DNA testing were performed is 42%.* The meta-analysis concluded that evidence exists for improved sensitivity of HPV DNA testing compared with repeat cervical cytology for the management of women with ASC-US. It also concluded that the specificity of both cytology and HPV DNA testing was low.

Requiring women to return to the office so that a sample for HPV DNA testing can be collected increases both cost and inconvenience. "Reflex" HPV DNA testing is an approach in which the original liquid-based cytology specimen is tested for HPV DNA if an ASC-US result is obtained.[19] *Reflex HPV DNA testing offers significant advantages because women do not need an additional clinical examination for specimen collection and 40% to 60% of women will be spared a colposcopic examination.* Moreover, HPV DNA–negative women can be rapidly assured that that they do not have a significant lesion. Several cost-effectiveness analyses have evaluated the use of reflex HPV DNA testing to manage women with ASC-US.[20,21] These studies have shown that HPV DNA testing is a very attractive option compared with either immediate colposcopy or repeat cytology. *Because the prevalence of HPV decreases with age, this approach becomes more specific in older women, and thus it is more attractive from a cost-effectiveness standpoint.*

When considering how to manage women with ASC-US who are high-risk HPV DNA positive, it is useful to remember that *in the ALTS clinical trial, risk for CIN 3 was identical in HPV DNA–positive women with ASC-US and women with LSIL.*[22] The overall risk for CIN 3 in women with ASC-US, irrespective of HPV status, was 9%. If a woman with ASC-US was high-risk HPV DNA positive, her risk for CIN 3 increased to 15%. This is exactly the same as the risk for CIN 3 for women with LSIL enrolled in ALTS.[23] Therefore *HPV DNA–positive women with ASC-US should receive the same evaluation and follow-up as women with LSIL.* This is generally accepted to be a colposcopic examination. In contrast, *women with ASC-US who are HPV DNA negative have a very low risk of having CIN 3. In ALTS, only 22 of 1559 (1.4%) of the HPV-negative women with ASC-US had CIN 3 identified during the 2-year study.*[16]

POST-COLPOSCOPY MANAGEMENT OF WOMEN WITH ATYPICAL SQUAMOUS CELLS OF UNDETERMINED SIGNIFICANCE

It is important to recognize that a single colposcopic examination is not as sensitive as previously thought. *In ALTS, approximately 36% of the CIN 2,3 lesions appear to have been missed when women with ASC-US underwent immediate colposcopy.*[16] The sensitivity of colposcopy improved somewhat when only HPV-positive women were referred to colposcopy, *but initial colposcopy still missed 30% of CIN 2,3 lesions.* This means that *women with ASC-US who are referred for a colposcopic examination and found not to have CIN require some form of additional follow-up.* ALTS evaluated several different follow-up approaches and concluded that HPV-positive women in whom no CIN lesion is identified at colposcopy could be followed-up using *one of two approaches.*[24] These approaches are either repeat cervical cytology at 6 and 12 months with referral to colposcopy if either repeat Pap test is diagnosed as ASC-US or greater, or HPV DNA testing at 12 months with referral to colposcopy if the woman is found to be persistently high-risk HPV DNA positive. In ALTS, repeating cervical cytology twice would have detected 88% of CIN 2,3 lesions missed at initial colposcopy and referred 64% of the women for a second colposcopy (Table 11-5).[24] For comparison, HPV DNA testing at 12 months would have detected 92% of the missed CIN 2,3 lesions and referred 55% of all the women for a second colposcopy. Women with ASC-US who are of unknown HPV status are at slightly lower risk for having a missed CIN 2,3 lesion after a negative colposcopy than are women who are high-risk HPV DNA positive. Risk of a missed CIN 2,3 lesion after a negative colposcopy is 6% in women whose HPV status is unknown versus 8% for those who are high-risk HPV positive. Although the risk is only minimally different in these two groups of women, the 2006 Consensus Guidelines recommend that women of unknown HPV status undergo repeat cytology at 12 months after a negative colposcopy.[25] Performing both HPV DNA testing and cytology at the 12-month follow-up visit provides a very minimal increase in sensitivity but results in a greater number of women being referred to colposcopy (see Table 11-5). Therefore the 2006 Consensus Guidelines do not recommend performing both tests at the 12-month follow-up visit. However, in the United States it is unlikely that many clinicians will perform HPV testing without also performing cytology.

2006 CONSENSUS GUIDELINES FOR WOMEN WITH ATYPICAL SQUAMOUS CELLS OF UNDETERMINED SIGNIFICANCE

In 2001 the American Society for Colposcopy and Cervical Pathology (ASCCP) held a consensus conference in Bethesda, Maryland at the National Institutes of Health (NIH), together with 29 other professional societies and national and international healthcare agencies, to develop comprehensive guidelines for managing women with cytologic abnormalities.[17] These guidelines were updated in 2006.[25] *The 2006 Consensus Guidelines identify three approaches that are safe and effective for managing women with ASC-US* (Table 11-6, Figure 11-3). *These are: (1) performing repeat cytology twice at 6 and 12 months and referring women with a repeat abnormal cytology of ASC-US or greater on either of the two repeats to colposcopy; (2) performing an immediate colposcopic examination in all women; and (3) testing for high-risk types of HPV with referral to colposcopy for women who are high-risk HPV positive. Because of the convenience of HPV DNA testing to patients and its attractiveness in cost-effectiveness*

Table 11-5 Strategies for Post-Colposcopy Follow-Up

Strategy	Sensitivity	Percent Referred for Colposcopy
Repeat cytology at 6 and 12 months	88.0%	63.6%
HPV alone at 12 months	92.2%	55.0%
HPV and cytology at 12 months	94.8%	64.1%

Modified from Ref. 24.

Table 11-6 Recommended Management of Women with ASC-US

General Management Approaches

A program of DNA testing for high-risk (oncogenic) types of HPV, repeat cervical cytological testing, or colposcopy are all acceptable methods for managing women older than 20 years with ASC-US. (**AI**) When liquid based cytology is used, or when co-collection for HPV DNA testing can be done, reflex HPV DNA testing is the preferred approach. (**AI**) Women with ASC-US who are HPV DNA negative can be followed up with repeat cytological testing at 12 months. (**BII**) Women who are HPV DNA positive should be managed in the same fashion as women with LSIL and be referred for colposcopic evaluation. (**AII**) Endocervical sampling is preferred for women in whom no lesions are identified (**BII**) and those with an unsatisfactory colposcopy (**AII**) but is acceptable for women with a satisfactory colposcopy and a lesion identified in the transformation zone. (**CII**) Acceptable postcolposcopy management options of women with ASC-US who are HPV positive but in whom CIN is not identified are HPV DNA testing at 12 months and repeat cytological testing at 6 and 12 months. (**BII**) It is recommended that HPV DNA testing not be performed at intervals less than 12 months. (**EIII**) When a program of repeat cytological testing is used for managing women with ASC-US, it is recommended that cytological testing be performed at 6-month intervals until 2 consecutive "negative for intraepithelial lesion or malignancy" results are obtained. (**AII**) Colposcopy is recommended for women with ASC-US or greater cytological abnormality on a repeat test. (**AII**) After 2 repeat "negative for intraepithelial lesion or malignancy" results are obtained, women can return to routine cytological screening. (**AII**) When colposcopy is used to manage women with ASC-US, repeat cytological testing at 12 months is recommended for women in whom CIN is not identified. (**BIII**) Women found to have CIN should be managed according to the 2006 Consensus Guidelines for the Management of Cervical Intraepithelial Neoplasia. Because of the potential for overtreatment, the routine use of diagnostic excisional procedures such as the loop electrosurgical excision is unacceptable for women with an initial ASC-US in the absence of histologically diagnosed CIN 2,3. (**EII**)

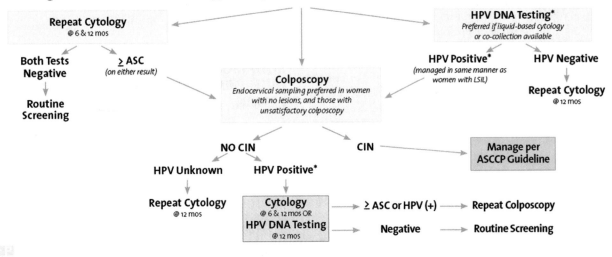

Test only for high-risk (oncogenic) types of HPV

Figure 11-3 Reprinted from *The Journal of Lower Genital Tract Disease* Vol. 11 Issue 4, with the permission of ASCCP © American Society for Colposcopy and Cervical Pathology 2007. No copies of the algorithms may be made without the prior consent of ASCCP.

modeling, reflex HPV DNA testing is considered the preferred approach to managing women with ASC-US whenever liquid-based cytology is used. When repeat cytology is used, women who are negative on both repeat tests can return to routine cytologic screening. This is because two repeat cytology examinations had a sensitivity in ALTS of 95.4%.[16] When HPV DNA testing is used to manage women with ASC-US, women found to be high-risk HPV DNA negative should have a repeat cervical cytology at 12 months. This is because their risk for having CIN 2,3 is low—only 3% in ALTS.[16]

Because of the risk that a CIN lesion was missed at initial colposcopy, *HPV-positive women with ASC-US who are not found to have CIN at initial colposcopy should be followed using one of two approaches (see Figure 11-3). These are either repeat cervical cytology at 6 and 12 months with referral to colposcopy if either repeat Pap test is diagnosed as ASC-US or greater, or HPV DNA testing at 12 months with referral to colposcopy if the woman is found to be persistently high-risk HPV DNA positive.*

ADOLESCENTS WITH ATYPICAL SQUAMOUS CELLS OF UNDETERMINED SIGNIFICANCE

Adolescents, who are defined as women 13 to 20 years of age (prior to their 21st birthday) in the 2006 Consensus Guidelines, are at very low risk for having an invasive cervical cancer. Our best estimate of the number of cases of invasive cervical cancer in the United States comes from the Surveillance Epidemiology and End Results (SEER) program, which is a national tumor database run by the NIH. *According to the SEER data, there were only 12 cases of invasive cervical cancer in females 10 to 19 years of age in the United States in 2002.[26]* In females 20 to 24 years of age, the age-specific incidence of invasive cervical cancer is only 1.5 per 100,000.[26] For comparison, the incidence of invasive cervical cancer is 11.4 per 100,000 for females 30 to 34 years of age. *Despite their low risk*

for cancer, mild cytologic abnormalities are extremely common in adolescent women. This is due to the high prevalence of HPV infections in this population.[27] Approximately 20% to 25% of sexually active women younger than 21 years will be HPV DNA positive at any single point in time, and within several years of initiating sexual activity the majority of adolescents will become HPV DNA positive.[27]

HPV DNA positivity is particularly high in adolescents with ASC-US. In ALTS, 72% of the women 18 to 20 years of age with ASC-US were HPV positive.[28] Similar results have been reported from another study of adolescents with ASC-US, in which 77% were found to be high-risk HPV positive.[29] This means that *using HPV testing to manage adolescents with ASC-US would refer the vast majority to colposcopy, even though they are at very low risk for having cancer.* It is also important to note that *many adolescents experience multiple sequential HPV infections.[30]* As a result, *finding a repetitively positive HPV test in this age group could mean either that the adolescent has a persistent high-risk HPV infection or that they have repeated transient infections with different types of HPV. Because of these considerations, the 2006 Consensus Guidelines recommend against performing HPV DNA testing in adolescents for any reason (see Chapter 22).[25]*

HPV infections are often associated with minor cytologic abnormalities, the vast majority of which spontaneously disappear without any intervention within a couple of years as the HPV infection clears.[31] *Because of the transient nature of the associated HPV infection, most cytologic abnormalities are of little long-term clinical significance in adolescents, and the 2006 Consensus Guidelines discourage performing colposcopy in adolescents for either ASC-US or LSIL.[25]* All that colposcopy achieves in this age group is to identify large numbers of cervical lesions that have minimal long-term oncogenic significance. Moreover, *identifying cervical lesions in this age group can lead to unnecessary treatment than can have a negative impact on future pregnancies (see Chapter 22).[32]*

Because of these considerations, the 2006 ASCCP Consensus Guidelines recommend that *adolescent women with ASC-US undergo a repeat cervical cytology in 12 months* (Table 11-7, Figure 11-4). *If the repeat result is anything other than HSIL, cytology should be repeated again in another 12 months. If a result of ASC-US or greater is diagnosed on the second repeat taken 24 months after the initial ASC-US, the adolescent can then be referred to colposcopy. Adolescents with an HSIL result on the 12-month repeat should be referred to colposcopy.* This conservative approach provides time for minor-grade lesions and HPV infections to spontaneously resolve. *If HPV testing is inadvertently performed, the HPV status should not influence management.*

Table 11-7 ASC-US in Special Populations

ADOLESCENT WOMEN

In adolescents with ASC-US, follow-up with annual cytological testing is recommended (Figure 11-4). (**BII**) At the 12-month follow-up, only adolescents with HSIL or greater on the repeat cytology should be referred to colposcopy. At the 24-month follow-up, those with an ASC-US or greater result should be referred to colposcopy. (**AII**) HPV DNA testing and colposcopy are unacceptable for adolescents with ASC-US. (**EII**) If HPV testing is inadvertently performed, the results should not influence management.

IMMUNOSUPPRESSED AND POSTMENOPAUSAL WOMEN

HIV infected, other immunosuppressed women, and postmenopausal women with ASC-US should be managed in the same manner as women in the general population. (**BII**)

PREGNANT WOMEN

Management options for pregnant women older than 20 years with ASC-US are identical to those described for nonpregnant women, with the exception that is acceptable to defer colposcopy until at least 6 weeks postpartum. (**CIII**) Endocervical curettage is unacceptable in pregnant women. (**EIII**)

MANAGEMENT OF WOMEN WITH ATYPICAL SQUAMOUS CELLS: CANNOT EXCLUDE HIGH-GRADE SQUAMOUS INTRAEPITHELIAL LESION

As mentioned previously in this chapter, a diagnosis of ASC-H should be considered as an equivocal HSIL. This is because women with ASC-H have a 20% to 50% risk of having a CIN 2,3 lesion (see Table 11-3). Thus *a woman with ASC-H has a 2 to 5 times greater risk of having CIN 2,3 than does a woman with ASC-US. This makes intermediate triage much less attractive than in women with ASC-US because the risk that a CIN 2,3 lesion would be missed is significantly higher.* In addition, the majority of women with ASC-H are high-risk HPV DNA positive. Rates of HPV DNA positivity in women with ASC-H have ranged from 84% in ALTS to 79% in the series of Liman et al. to 67% in the experience of Srodon et al.[33-35] The combination of a high rate of underlying CIN 2,3 combined with a relatively high rate of HPV DNA positivity means that HPV DNA testing is not an attractive option for managing women with ASC-H. It should be noted, however, that *in ALTS the prevalence of HPV DNA positivity in women with ASC-H dropped significantly with increasing age.[35] Eighty-nine percent of women with ASC-H younger than age 35 were HPV DNA positive, but only 40% of those 35 years and older were HPV DNA positive. This suggests that HPV DNA testing could potentially be useful in the subset of older women with ASC-H.* This was not recommended

Management of Adolescent Women with Either Atypical Squamous Cells of Undetermined Significance (ASC-US) or Low-grade Squamous Intraepithelial Lesion (LSIL)

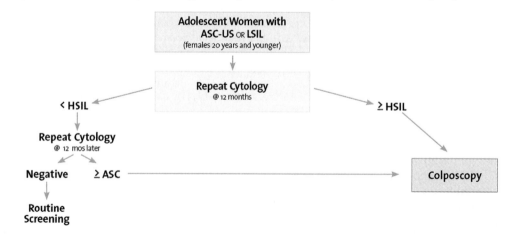

Figure 11-4 Reprinted from *The Journal of Lower Genital Tract Disease* Vol. 11 Issue 4, with the permission of ASCCP © American Society for Colposcopy and Cervical Pathology 2007. No copies of the algorithms may be made without the prior consent of ASCCP.

in the 2006 Consensus Guidelines because the published experience with ASC-H in older women remains quite small, and it was decided that the safety of using HPV DNA testing for triage in this population is not yet established.

2006 CONSENSUS GUIDELINES FOR WOMEN WITH ATYPICAL SQUAMOUS CELLS: CANNOT EXCLUDE HIGH-GRADE SQUAMOUS INTRAEPITHELIAL LESION

The 2006 Consensus Guidelines recommend that all women with ASC-H be referred for colposcopy (Table 11-8, Figure 11-5). *If CIN 2,3 is not identified at colposcopy, the women should be followed similar to high-risk HPV DNA–positive women with ASC-US, using either cytology performed at 6 and 12 months or HPV DNA testing performed at 12 months.* Women with an ASC-US or greater result on repeat cytology at either 6- or 12-month follow-up and those found to be HPV DNA positive at the 12-month follow-up should be referred for another colposcopy. Those who are HPV DNA negative or

Table 11-8 Recommended Management of Women with ASC-H

The recommended management of women with ASC-H is referral for colposcopic evaluation (Figure 11-5). **(AII)** In women in whom CIN 2,3 is not indentified, follow-up with HPV DNA testing at 12 months or cytological testing at 6 and 12 months is acceptable. **(CIII)** Referral to colposcopy is recommended for women who subsequently test positive for HPV DNA or who are found to have ASC-US or greater on their repeat cytological tests. **(BII)** If the HPV DNA test is negative or if 2 consecutive repeat cytological tests are "negative for intraepithelial lesion or malignancy," return to routine cytological screening is recommended. **(AI)**

who have two "within normal limits" cytology results can be returned to routine screening.

MANAGEMENT SCENARIOS

Scenario 1

Sentinel Pap: ASC-US
Colposcopic findings or histologic cell type if a biopsy was done:
   No colposcopy done
HPV testing for high-risk (oncogenic) HPV types: Negative
Satisfactory colposcopy: Not applicable (NA)
Fertility desires: N/A

The results of the ALTS indicated that the negative predictive value of HPV testing for high-risk (oncogenic) HPV types is 99% in women with ASC-US smears. These women are extremely unlikely to have high-grade disease, and their risk for occult, unrecognized cancer is virtually nil. These women can be reassured that their cytologic abnormality is not clinically significant, and they may be returned to annual screening protocols.

Scenario 2

Sentinel Pap: ASC-US
Colposcopic findings or histologic cell type if a biopsy was done:
   No SIL found
HPV testing for high-risk (oncogenic) HPV types: Positive
Satisfactory colposcopy: Yes or no
Fertility desires: N/A

The risk of high-grade CIN in a patient with ASC-US cytology who tests positive for oncogenic HPV types is comparable to that in a woman with LSIL cytology. This case

Management of Women with Atypical Squamous Cells: Cannot Exclude High-grade SIL (ASC - H)

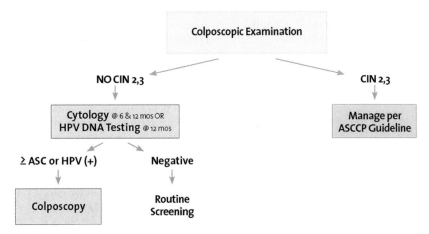

Figure 11-5 Reprinted from *The Journal of Lower Genital Tract Disease* Vol. 11 Issue 4, with the permission of ASCCP © American Society for Colposcopy and Cervical Pathology 2007. No copies of the algorithms may be made without the prior consent of ASCCP.

represents either a woman with latent HPV infection without any clinical lesion, a woman with a lesion at the time of the Pap smear that has now regressed, a woman who was evaluated with colposcopy when a very small and possibly growing lesion (early in its natural history) was present that may have been missed on examination, or a woman with a lesion that should have been detected on colposcopy but was not. Alternatively, the cytologic abnormality may be due to a vaginal or vulvar lesion that was missed on colposcopic assessment, or it may represent cytologic overcall. Endocervical sampling is preferred if no lesion is identified (unless the patient is pregnant). This woman should be re-evaluated in 12 months with HPV DNA testing or in 6 and 12 months with cytology, with referral for colposcopy if ASC-US or a more severe abnormality is reported on the repeat Pap smear or if HPV DNA testing is positive. An excisional procedure is *not* an acceptable treatment alternative in this setting.

Scenario 3

Sentinel Pap: ASC-US in a patient ≤20 yrs old
Colposcopic findings or histologic cell type if a biopsy was done:
    Colposcopy not done
HPV testing for high-risk (oncogenic) HPV types: Not done
Satisfactory colposcopy: N/A
Fertility desires: N/A

HPV DNA testing is unacceptable for evaluation of adolescents with ASC-US, and colposcopy is unacceptable in the initial evaluation of ASC-US in adolescents but is instead reserved for adolescents whose ASC-US cytology has persisted for at least 24 months. Most of the disease detected in this population is trivial, and aggressive evaluation may lead to overtreatment. Instead of reflex HPV testing or colposcopy, the recommended evaluation of an adolescent with ASC-US is to repeat cytology in 12 months. If HSIL is detected, colposcopy should be performed. If less than HSIL, repeat cytology is done in another 12 months. If the cytology still shows ASC-US or worse, the patient should be referred to colposcopy.

COUNSELING

When faced with abnormal cytology, women often feel vulnerable and concerned about the implications of an ASC-US smear in regard to their gynecologic health. Patients should be reassured that ASC-US is a very common cytologic diagnosis and infrequently associated with invasive cancer. This can provide some degree of reassurance to the patient. Our goal as clinicians is to adequately evaluate ASC-US while preventing overdiagnosis and overtreatment of trivial disease. The current 2006 ASCCP guidelines provide a rational, evidence-based approach to ASC-US. Application of these guidelines to our daily practices will necessarily require many clinicians to change ingrained practices in the evaluation of ASC-US cytology, especially in the adolescent population.

It will also require diligence on the part of clinicians to be sure they check the appropriate boxes when submitting their cytology specimens to prevent inadvertent performance of reflex HPV DNA testing and subsequently having to deal with a positive HPV test that the current guidelines recommend essentially ignoring. It may also be a challenge to persuade patients presenting with ASC-US cytology that they do not need a colposcopic evaluation. Education of patients as to the evaluation plan (and the reasons for it) can assist patients in better understanding the meaning of an ASC-US Pap.

REFERENCES

1. Luff RD. The Bethesda System for reporting cervical/vaginal cytologic diagnoses: report of the 1991 Bethesda workshop. The Bethesda System Editorial Committee. Hum Pathol 1992;23:719–721.
2. Davey DD, Naryshkin S, Nielsen ML, et al. Atypical squamous cells of undetermined significance: interlaboratory comparison and quality assurance monitors. Diagn Cytopathol 1994;11: 390–396.
3. Jones BA, Davey DD. Quality management in gynecologic cytology using interlaboratory comparison. Arch Pathol Lab Med 2000;124:672–681.
4. Robb JA. The "ASCUS" swamp. Diag Cytopathol 1994;11: 319–320.
5. Sherman ME, Schiffman MH, Lorincz AT, et al. Toward objective quality assurance in cervical cytopathology. Correlation of cytopathologic diagnoses with detection of high-risk human papillomavirus types. Am J Clin Pathol 1994;102: 182–187.
6. Stoler MH, Schiffman M. Interobserver reproducibility of cervical cytologic and histologic interpretations: realistic estimates from the ASCUS-LSIL Triage Study. J Am Med Assoc 2001; 285:1500–1505.
7. Kinney WK, Manos MM, Hurley LB, et al. Where's the high-grade cervical neoplasia? The importance of minimally abnormal Papanicolaou diagnoses. Obstet Gynecol 1998;91: 973–976.
8. Pitman MB, Cibas ES, Powers CN, et al. Reducing or eliminating use of the category of atypical squamous cells of undetermined significance decreases the diagnostic accuracy of the Papanicolaou smear. Cancer 2002;96:128–134.
9. Solomon D, Davey D, Kurman R, et al. The 2001 Bethesda System: terminology for reporting results of cervical cytology. J Am Med Assoc 2002;287:2114–2119.
10. Solomon D, Schiffman M, Tarrone R. Comparison of three management strategies for patients with atypical squamous cells of undetermined significance: baseline results from a randomized trial. J Natl Cancer Instit 2001;93:293–299.
11. Davey DD, Neal MH, Wilbur DC, et al. Bethesda 2001 implementation and reporting rates: 2003 practices of participants in the College of American Pathologists Interlaboratory Comparison Program in Cervicovaginal Cytology. Arch Pathol Lab Med 2004;128:1224–1229.
12. Arbyn M, Sasieni P, Meijer CJ, et al. Chapter 9: Clinical applications of HPV testing: a summary of meta-analyses. Vaccine 2006;24(Suppl 3):S78–S89.
13. Petry KU, Menton S, Menton M, et al. Inclusion of HPV testing in routine cervical cancer screening for women above 29 years in Germany: results for 8466 patients. Br J Cancer 2003; 88:1570–1577.

14. Taylor S, Kuhn L, Dupree W, et al. Direct comparison of liquid-based and conventional cytology in a South African screening trial. Int J Cancer 2006;118(4):957-962.

15. Cuzick J, Clavel C, Petry KU, et al. Overview of the European and North American studies on HPV testing in primary cervical cancer screening. Int J Cancer 2006;119:1095–1101.

16. ASCUS-LSIL Triage Study (ALTS) Group. Results of a randomized trial on the management of cytology interpretations of atypical squamous cells of undetermined significance. Am J Obstet Gynecol 2003;188:1383–1392.

17. Wright TC Jr, Cox JT, Massad LS, et al. 2001 consensus guidelines for the management of women with cervical cytological abnormalities. J Am Med Assoc 2002;287:2120–2129.

18. Arbyn M, Buntinx F, Van Ranst M, et al. Virologic versus cytologic triage of women with equivocal Pap smears: a meta-analysis of the accuracy to detect high-grade intraepithelial neoplasia. J Natl Cancer Inst 2004;96:280–293.

19. Wright TC Jr, Lorincz A, Ferris DG, et al. Reflex human papillomavirus deoxyribonucleic acid testing in women with abnormal Papanicolaou smears. Am J Obstet Gynecol 1998; 178:962–966.

20. Kim JJ, Wright TC, Goldie SJ. Cost-effectiveness of alternative triage strategies for atypical squamous cells of undetermined significance. J Am Med Assoc 2002;287:2382–2390.

21. Kim JJ, Wright TC, Goldie SJ. Cost-effectiveness of human papillomavirus DNA testing in the United Kingdom, The Netherlands, France, and Italy. J Natl Cancer Inst 2005;97: 888–895.

22. Cox JT, Schiffman M, Solomon D. Prospective follow-up suggests similar risk of subsequent cervical intraepithelial neoplasia grade 2 or 3 among women with cervical intraepithelial neoplasia grade 1 or negative colposcopy and directed biopsy. Am J Obstet Gynecol 2003;188:1406–1412.

23. ASCUS-LSIL Triage Study (ALTS) Group. A randomized trial on the management of low-grade squamous intraepithelial lesion cytology interpretations. Am J Obstet Gynecol 2003;188:1393–1400.

24. Guido R, Schiffman M, Solomon D, et al. Postcolposcopy management strategies for women referred with low-grade squamous intraepithelial lesions or human papillomavirus DNA-positive atypical squamous cells of undetermined significance: a two-year prospective study. Am J Obstet Gynecol 2003;188:1401–1405.

25. Wright TC Jr, Massad LS, Dunton CJ, Spitzer M, Wilkinson EJ, Solomon D; for the 2006 ASCCP-Sponsored Consensus Conference. 2006 consensus guidelines for the management of women with abnormal cervical screening tests. J Low Genit Tract Dis. 2007 Oct;11(4):201–222.

26. SEER Cancer Statistics Review 1975-2003. Accessed December 1, 2005, at *www.seer.cancer.gov/cgi-bin/csr/1975_2003/search.pl#results*.

27. Burchell AN, Winer RL, de Sanjose S, et al. Chapter 6: Epidemiology and transmission dynamics of genital HPV infection. Vaccine 2006;24(Suppl 3):S52–S61.

28. Sherman ME, Schiffman M, Cox JT, et al. Effects of age and HPV load on colposcopic triage: data from the ASCUS LSIL Triage Study (ALTS). J Natl Cancer Inst 2002;94:102–107.

29. Boardman LA, Stanko C, Weitzen S, et al. Atypical squamous cells of undetermined significance: human papillomavirus testing in adolescents. Obstet Gynecol 2005;105:741–746.

30. Brown DR, Shew ML, Qadadri B, et al. A longitudinal study of genital human papillomavirus infection in a cohort of closely followed adolescent women. J Infect Dis 2005;191: 182–192.

31. Moscicki AB, Schiffman M, Kjaer S, et al. Chapter 5: Updating the natural history of HPV and anogenital cancer. Vaccine 2006;24(Suppl 3):S42–S51.

32. Kyrgiou M, Koliopoulos G, Martin-Hirsch P, et al. Obstetric outcomes after conservative treatment for intraepithelial or early invasive cervical lesions: systematic review and meta-analysis. Lancet 2006;367:489–498.

33. Liman AK, Giampoli EJ, Bonfiglio TA. Should women with atypical squamous cells, cannot exclude high-grade squamous intraepithelial lesion, receive reflex human papillomavirus-DNA testing? Cancer 2005;105:457–460.

34. Srodon M, Parry Dilworth H, Ronnett BM. Atypical squamous cells, cannot exclude high-grade squamous intraepithelial lesion: diagnostic performance, human papillomavirus testing, and follow-up results. Cancer 2006;108:32–38.

35. Sherman ME, Castle PE, Solomon D. Cervical cytology of atypical squamous cells-cannot exclude high-grade squamous intraepithelial lesion (ASC-H): characteristics and histologic outcomes. Cancer Cytopathology 2006;108:298–305.

36. Manos MM, Kinney WK, Hurley LB, et al. Identifying women with cervical neoplasia: using human papillomavirus DNA testing for equivocal Papanicolaou results. J Am Med Assoc 1999;281:1605–1610.

37. Bergeron C, Jeannel D, Poveda J, et al. Human papillomavirus testing in women with mild cytologic atypia. Obstet Gynecol 2000;95:821–827.

38. Morin C, Bairati I, Bouchard C, et al. Managing atypical squamous cells of undetermined significance in Papanicolaou smears. J Reprod Med 2001;46:799–805.

39. Solomon D. ALTS results. Personal communication, 2001.

40. Lonky NM, Felix JC, Naidu YM, et al. Triage of atypical squamous cells of undetermined significance with hybrid capture II: colposcopy and histologic human papillomavirus correlation. Obstet Gynecol 2003;101:481–489.

41. Carozzi FM, Del Mistro A, Confortini M, et al. Reproducibility of HPV DNA testing by Hybrid Capture 2 in a screening setting. Am J Clin Pathol 2005;124:716–721.

42. Alvarez RD, Wright TC. Effective cervical neoplasia detection with a novel optical detection system: a randomized trial. Gynecol Oncol 2007;104:281–289.

43. Duncan LD, Jacob SV. Atypical squamous cells, cannot exclude a high-grade squamous intraepithelial lesion: the practice experience of a hospital-based reference laboratory with this new Bethesda system diagnostic category. Diagn Cytopathol 2005;32:243–246.

44. Goff BA, Muntz HG, Bell DA, et al. Human papillomavirus typing in patients with Papanicolaou smears showing squamous atypia. Gynecol Oncol 1993;48:384–388.

45. Slawson DC, Bennett JH, Simon LJ, et al. Should all women with cervical atypia be referred for colposcopy: a HARNET study. Harrisburgh Area Research Network. J Fam Pract 1994;38: 387–392.

46. Cox T, Lorincz AT, Schiffman MH, Sherman ME, et al. Human papillomavirus testing by hybrid capture appears to be useful in triaging women with a cytologic diagnosis of atypical squamous cells of undetermined significance. Am J Obstet Gynecol 1995;172:946–954.

47. Wright TC, Sun XW, Koulos J. Comparison of management algorithms for the evaluation of women with low-grade cytologic abnormalities. Obstet Gynecol 1995;85:202–210.

48. Ferris DG, Wright TC Jr, Litaker MS, et al. Triage of women with ASCUS and LSIL on Pap smear reports: management by

repeat Pap smear, HPV DNA testing, or colposcopy? J Fam Pract 1998;46:125–134.

49. Lin CT, Tseng CJ, Lai CH, et al. High-risk HPV DNA detection by Hybrid Capture II. An adjunctive test for mildly abnormal cytologic smears in women > or = 50 years of age. J Reprod Med 2000;45:345–350.

50. Shlay JC, Dunn T, Byers T, et al. Prediction of cervical intraepithelial neoplasia grade 2–3 using risk assessment and human papillomavirus testing in women with atypia on Papanicolaou smears. Obstet Gynecol 2000;96:410–416.

51. Kulasingam SL, Hughes JP, Kiviat NB, et al. Evaluation of human papillomavirus testing in primary screening for cervical abnormalities: comparison of sensitivity, specificity, and frequency of referral. J Am Med Assoc 2002;288:1749–1757.

52. Pretorius RG, Peterson P, Novak S, et al. Comparison of two signal-amplification DNA tests for high-risk HPV as an aid to colposcopy. J Reprod Med 2002;47:290–296.

53. Guyot A, Karim S, Kyi MS, et al. Evaluation of adjunctive HPV testing by Hybrid Capture II in women with minor cytological abnormalities for the diagnosis of CIN 2/3 and cost comparison with colposcopy. BMC Infect Dis 2003;3:23.

54. Dalla Palma P, Pojer A, Girlando S. HPV triage of women with atypical squamous cells of undetermined significance: a 3-year experience in an Italian organized programme. Cytopathology 2005;16:22–26.

CHAPTER 12

Low-Grade Squamous Intraepithelial Lesions

Alan G. Waxman

KEY POINTS

- The great majority of low-grade squamous intraepithelial lesion (LSIL) cases are associated with high-risk human papillomavirus (HPV) types, most commonly HPV 16.
- The majority of women with LSIL harbor more than one HPV type.
- Most LSIL cytology will spontaneously revert to normal or remain unchanged over time. Progression to cancer is rare.
- As much as 91% of LSIL cytology in young women will spontaneously revert to normal over 3 years.
- Cervical intraepithelial neoplasia (CIN), grade 1 (CIN 1) is most often a manifestation of a productive viral infection and has a very low premalignant potential. Therefore CIN 1 rarely requires treatment.
- The risk of CIN 2 or worse in women with LSIL and HPV-positive atypical squamous cells of undetermined significance (ASC-US) is identical. As many as 28% will have CIN 2 or 3 on colposcopic-directed biopsy if followed for 2 years. Therefore adult women with LSIL cytology must undergo further evaluation to rule out high-grade dysplasia.
- Although cytologic diagnosis is not highly reproducible in general, LSIL is the most reproducible diagnosis among the cytologic abnormalities.
- Colposcopic findings of low-grade lesions are variable. An accurate colposcopic diagnosis of low-grade lesions is less precise and less reproducible than high-grade lesions.
- The cytologic and colposcopic diagnoses of LSIL are less reliable in older than in younger women.
- On colposcopy, it may be hard to distinguish LSIL from squamous metaplasia.

Low-grade squamous intraepithelial lesions (LSILs) are non-neoplastic manifestations of infection with human papillomavirus (HPV) and include both flat acetowhite lesions and raised condyloma acuminata. The terminology *low-grade squamous intraepithelial lesion* is included in the Bethesda System of nomenclature for cervical cytology devised in 1988 in part to distinguish these benign cervical lesions from high-grade squamous intraepithelial lesions (HSILs) that have true premalignant potential. Accordingly, the term *intraepithelial lesion* replaced *intraepithelial neoplasia* in cytologic diagnosis. The terminology for histologic lesions is not governed by the Bethesda nomenclature, and thus these lesions are still called *cervical intraepithelial neoplasia* (CIN). The term *low-grade squamous intraepithelial lesion* includes cytologic lesions previously called "mild dysplasia," cervical intraepithelial neoplasia, grade 1 (CIN 1), and HPV changes or cellular changes consistent with koilocytosis.[1]

In this chapter, the virology, natural history, cytology, and histology of low-grade lesions and colposcopic findings that characterize them will be discussed. These colposcopic findings will be distinguished from benign changes such as squamous metaplasia or repair following treatment. The colposcopist will need to consider how the behavior and significance of LSIL cytology may vary at various stages in the life cycle including adolescence, pregnancy, and after menopause. Finally, the guidelines for managing women with LSIL cytology or CIN 1 biopsy will be presented.

RISK FACTORS AND EPIDEMIOLOGY

LSIL and CIN 1 reflect the benign cytologic and pathologic effects of infection with HPV. Although more than 100 HPV viral types have been identified, 30 to 40 are known to infect the lower anogenital tract. HPV has been divided into low-risk and high-risk types based on their association with high-grade lesions and invasive cervical cancer. Fifteen high-risk types have been identified.[2,3] Although several of the low-risk types (most commonly types 6 and 11) are commonly found in LSIL, high-risk types including types 16, 18, 45, 56, 31, 33, and 35 are also commonly associated with LSIL.[4,5] *Investigators in the ASC-US (atypical squamous cells of undetermined significance)/LSIL Triage Study (ALTS) found high-risk HPV types in as many as 86.1% of cases of LSIL.*[6] HPV type 16, the most prevalent of the high-risk types, was found in 24.8%. This large multicenter trial was designed in part to determine whether the presence of high-risk HPV types could predict which low-grade lesions had true malignant potential. However, the LSIL arm of the study was prematurely discontinued because of the high frequency at which high-risk HPV types were found in these low-grade lesions. These findings were confirmed in other studies from around the world. Clifford et al. performed a meta-analysis of 53 studies from five continents that included 8308 low-grade lesions; 64% were cytologic LSIL, and 36% were histologic CIN 1. HPV diagnosis was based on PCR.[7] Seventy-one percent of women with LSIL (range 29–100%) were HPV positive. In all continents represented, HPV 16 was the most common HPV type, present in 26.3% of all women who had HPV-positive LSIL. The prevalence of other HPV types present in LSIL varied from region to region, the second most common being HPV 31 in Europe, HPV 51 in North America, HPV 33 in South and Central America, and HPV 58 in Africa and Asia. Of note, the prevalence of HPV 16 and HPV 18 increased dramatically when the authors evaluated the data on HSIL and invasive cancer, respectively. In this study, HPV 16 and/or HPV 18 were present in 35% of LSIL but in 70% of cervical cancers worldwide. The prevalence of almost all other HPV types in cancer decreases dramatically when their prevalence is compared with LSIL.[8,9]

Young women become infected with HPV very quickly after initiating sexually activity.[10,11] *Numerous studies have shown a high prevalence of high-risk HPV types in women younger than 30 years of age that declines substantially with age.* The prevalence of these infections among women in their 20s is 22% to 24%.[12–14] Not surprisingly, high-risk HPV types are also more common in younger women with LSIL. In ALTS, 87% of women younger than 29 years with LSIL were positive for high-risk HPV types compared with 75% of older women.[15] Evans et al., using more sensitive polymerase chain reaction (PCR) analysis for HPV deoxyribonucleic acid (DNA) testing, reported a similar trend. In their study, 60% of women aged 30 and younger with LSIL were high-risk HPV DNA-positive compared with 46% of older women.[16]

In contrast to HSIL, in which most women are infected with a single HPV type, most women with LSIL lesions are infected with multiple HPV types.[4,17] In ALTS, more than one HPV type was found in 58.9% of women with LSIL.[17]

DO HUMAN PAPILLOMAVIRUS–NEGATIVE LOW-GRADE SQUAMOUS INTRAEPITHELIAL LESIONS EXIST?

Cellular processes such as metaplasia, inflammation, repair, and atrophy can produce cytologic changes in the cervical epithelium that may be misinterpreted as LSIL. However, *with rigorous cytologic interpretation and the use of sensitive HPV detection methodology, high- or low-risk types of HPV can be found in virtually all cases of LSIL.* Evans et al. performed PCR analysis on 200 thin-layer cytology specimens diagnosed as LSIL. HPV was diagnosed in 97.5%, of which 55.5% were high-risk types and 42% were "other" HPV types.[16] Zuna et al., reporting for the ALTS group, found that most HPV-negative LSIL cytology reflected either overreading of the cytology or a false-negative HPV DNA test. Of 401 liquid-based specimens with a diagnosis of LSIL made by a consensus of four independent pathologists, only 7 (2%) were HPV DNA negative by both the Hybrid Capture 2 (HC 2) test of 13 high-risk types and PCR for 27 high- and low-risk HPV types. Of the 7 found to be HPV negative, all but 2 became positive within 2 years.[18]

Although virtually all women with LSIL are infected with HPV, only a minority of women who test positive for HPV will develop an actual lesion. LSIL has been reported in 1.1% to 7% of adolescents and young women.[19] Risk factors associated with the development of LSIL include young age, infection with high-risk HPV, duration of infection, and daily cigarette smoking. Both the incidence of HPV infection and the development of LSIL peak in the late teens and early 20s and decline thereafter. *HPV infection parallels the onset of sexual activity in women with an immature transformation zone, whereas HPV clearance correlates with cell-mediated immune response and a decline in number of new partners.*[5] Because infection with HPV is the primary risk factor for development of LSIL, the risk factors for acquiring HPV and LSIL coincide. In a study of adolescents aged 13 to 21 years, Moscicki et al. found the number of new sexual partners per month, history of herpes simplex virus, and history of vulvar warts were all risk factors for acquisition of HPV infection. However, in their multivariate analysis, only duration of HPV infection and daily cigarette smoking were risks for LSIL.[19]

NATURAL HISTORY

The mechanism of HPV infection has been well studied in recent years. The virus enters the cervical epithelium through microlacerations occurring most commonly during intercourse. On the cervix, the relatively thin metaplastic tissue is more susceptible to viral infection than the thicker, more mature squamous epithelium. HPV infects the basal cells, sheds its capsid, and exists in the host nucleus separate from the host genome in an episomal state. Initially it replicates only locally and infects neighboring basal cells. It may remain in this latent form for months to years with no greater proliferation or morphologic expression. This latent period is a time of steady-state viral density. The episomal material replicates each time the cell divides but does not further proliferate. When as yet poorly identified co-factors are present and in the absence of successful suppression by the host's cell-mediated immune system, viral replication and proliferation beyond the basal layer may be stimulated. As the epithelial cells mature, they migrate away from the basement membrane toward the surface. On reaching the intermediate layer, viral genetic material begins to become encapsulated, replicate, and proliferate within the cell. In this form, LSIL is a productive viral infection. Intermediate and superficial cells will have many virions per cell. Morphologically, the cells will develop koilocytes (enlarged, irregular nucleus with a perinuclear halo), the cytopathic effects of the virus. Colposcopically a lesion will have the gross appearance of a flat acetowhite lesion or an exophytic condyloma.[4,20,21] *For most low-grade lesions, this is the ultimate expression of the HPV infection and the cytopathic effects will never convert to a truly invasive process.*

An alternative developmental pathway has been proposed for those lesions destined to become high grade.

The HPV DNA is thought to leave its episomal state and become integrated into the DNA of the host cells at the basal layer of the epithelium. As these cells mature, they move progressively toward the surface of the epithelium, retaining the dysplastic characteristics of an enlarged irregular nucleus and relatively reduced cytoplasmic volume. Integration of the HPV DNA has been found in the majority of squamous cell cervical cancers but much less so in CIN.[4] *Some suggest that lesions destined to become high grade may not arise from LSIL but from a separate population of cells.*[5] The concept of a large but transient low-grade lesion clinically masking an initially small but growing high-grade lesion within its borders has biological plausibility. High-grade lesions are not infrequently seen within the borders of larger low-grade lesions. Moreover, different HPV types have been found in adjacent CIN 1 and CIN 3 lesions.[22]

Moscicki et al. proposed that the rate at which the cervix undergoes squamous metaplasia over time is a key factor in the development of LSIL. Young college women were monitored with periodic colpophotographs, and changes were documented in the area of immature metaplasia prior to development of LSIL. They demonstrated that the development of LSIL correlated with the rate of recent metaplasia, but not with the area of cervical ectopy per se.[20]

The proportion of women with LSIL whose lesions regress or progress has not been fully elucidated. This is due in part to methodologic difficulties inherent to natural history studies. Without performing colposcopy and directed biopsies on all study patients with normal and abnormal findings, it is impossible to accurately classify which cervix is truly normal and which harbors some degree of dysplasia. Because of the inaccuracy of a single colposcopy in predicting histologic change and in identifying the highest-grade lesion, even colposcopy with directed biopsy may not identify high-grade disease. Furthermore, the effect of biopsy on the natural history of the lesion may further confound the ideal study design by accelerating regression.

As many as 28% of women with cytologic LSIL will harbor CIN 2 or 3.[23] Moreover, the poor reliability of the diagnosis of LSIL assures some degree of misclassification in studies of natural history based on cytology alone. Kinney et al., reporting on colposcopically directed biopsies in 46,009 women, found CIN 2,3 or cancer in 15.2% of women with only LSIL cytology.[24]

It is important to recognize these methodologic limitations when evaluating cross-sectional studies that suggest 70% to 80% of low-grade lesions remain unchanged over time or resolve spontaneously without treatment. *Resolution is especially the rule in younger women, but in a small but significant number, a higher-grade lesion will develop.* Nasiell et al. followed 555 women with cytologic evidence of LSIL. They treated only those who progressed to CIN 3. Over the course of the study, 62% returned to normal, and 16% progressed to CIN 3 and were then treated. Two women who dropped out of the study were found to have invasive cancer 2 and 6 years later.[25] Melnikow et al. performed a meta-analysis of studies that followed women with

abnormal Papanicolaou (Pap) tests over time without treatment. Although 47.4% of those with LSIL returned to normal within 2 years, 20.8% progressed to CIN 2,3 and 0.15% progressed to cancer.[26]

Schlecht et al. followed 118 women with LSIL for a mean duration of 53.3 months and found that 88.1% regressed to ASC-US or negative, whereas 9.2% progressed to HSIL. The mean time to regression was 10.5 months (median 6.0 months). Not unexpectedly, the mean time to regression for those testing positive for oncogenic HPV types by PCR was almost twice as long (13.8 months) as for those with only non-oncogenic HPV DNA types (7.8 months) or those who were HPV negative (7.6 months). The differences in median times were not significantly different (6.1, 5.3, and 6.0 months, respectively). Women who progressed to HSIL took considerably longer, with a mean of 85.7 months. Those positive for oncogenic HPV DNA types who progressed did so more rapidly, within an average of 67.0 months.[27]

The transient nature of HPV infection in young women, even with high-risk types, has been well documented.[10,28,29] Ho et al. followed a cohort of college women for 3 years and found 43% of those who were HPV negative on entering the study acquired the infection during the study period. The median duration of these incident infections was 8 months. Seventy percent of those who became HPV positive during the study reverted to negative after 12 months, and 91% tested negative after 24 months. Only 5.1% of women who were HPV positive during the 3-year period developed a squamous intraepithelial lesion (SIL). Of these, 93% had low-grade lesions. This included women who were HPV positive at the start of the study as well as those who developed the infection during the study period. Factors related to the development of SIL included infection with a high-risk HPV DNA type and persistence of infection for at least 6 months.[10] Young women are infected with HPV at a very high rate and, not unexpectedly, develop SIL, especially LSIL. Moscicki et al.[28] followed 187 young women with LSIL for an average of 61 months. The mean age was 19.1 years (range 13–22 years). Sixty-one percent spontaneously returned to negative cytology in the first year of follow-up. By 36 months, 91% had regressed. Regression was defined as the first of at least three negative cervical cytology examinations. Of those whose cytology remained LSIL at 12 months of follow-up, 51% regressed in the next 12 months. Of those who still had LSIL at 24 months, another 60% regressed in the following year. Only 3% of these young women progressed to HSIL.

SCREENING

Cervical cytology (the Pap test) is the most widely used cancer screening test in most industrialized countries. It is the first step in the diagnosis of early invasive cervical cancer and cervical cancer precursors (i.e., high-grade squamous or glandular intraepithelial lesions). The finding of LSIL is essentially an intermediate step in the quest for HSIL and heralds the presence of CIN 2 or greater in as many as 28% of cases. Of note, *in ALTS, the rates of immediate and delayed diagnosis of CIN 2 or greater were identical in women with LSIL and HPV-positive ASC-US (i.e., 17.8% and 17.9% for immediate diagnosis, and 27.6% and 26.7% over a 2-year follow-up, respectively).*[23]

Liquid-based and conventional cytology allow the inspection of cells exfoliated predominantly from the superficial and intermediate layers. An exception is epithelial atrophy in postmenopausal and lactating women. In estrogen-deprived vaginal and cervical epithelium, the most superficial layer is the parabasal layer. The characteristics of LSIL are most prominent in the cells exfoliated from the uppermost superficial cell layer. Cytologically, LSIL is characterized by nuclear enlargement to at least three times the size of a normal intermediate cell nucleus. This increases the nuclear:cytoplasmic ratio. There is also moderate variation in nuclear size and shape, sometimes including bi- and multi-nucleation. When irregularities are present in the nuclear contour, they are usually mild. Chromatin density may be variable and range from granular to smudged or opaque. Conventional cytology may demonstrate nuclear hyperchromasia, but this feature is frequently absent in liquid-based preparations.[1] *Cellular cytoplasm is pushed to the periphery of the cell, creating a perinuclear halo. This feature when accompanied by nuclear atypia results in a cellular change called koilocytosis.* However, LSIL may be present without manifesting koilocytosis (Figure 12-1).

Rigorous attention to these nuclear abnormalities is essential to prevent cytologic misclassification of minor cellular changes into the category of LSIL. *To make the diagnosis of LSIL, nuclear enlargement with atypia is necessary* (Figure 12-2). A frequent source of false-positive LSIL cytology is the diagnosis of koilocytosis based on the presence of a perinuclear halo with nuclear enlargement but without the requisite nuclear irregularity and hyperchromasia. In more than two thirds of such patients, HPV DNA will be absent.[1]

Age plays a role in the histologic confirmation of LSIL detected on Pap testing. Wright et al. found that CIN was confirmed histologically more often in women with LSIL who are younger than 29 years than in those older than 29 years. On the other hand, among those with HSIL cytology, histologically confirmed CIN was found equally among younger and older women.[30]

The inclusion of HPV-associated koilocytosis in LSIL remains controversial. Lonky et al., studying a previously well-screened population, compared colposcopic-directed biopsy results of women whose LSIL Paps were based on HPV with koilocytosis versus those whose LSIL Paps lacked the viral cytopathic effect. LSIL changes with HPV effect were more than twice as likely to be negative for dysplastic lesions on colposcopy or CIN on biopsy. In addition, those whose Paps showed LSIL without HPV cytopathic features were significantly more likely to harbor high-grade histologic lesions.[31] Kurman et al. justified the inclusion of cytologic findings of CIN 1 and HPV effect into LSIL based on the behavior and virology of the two component lesions. They noted studies showing a 16% rate of progression to

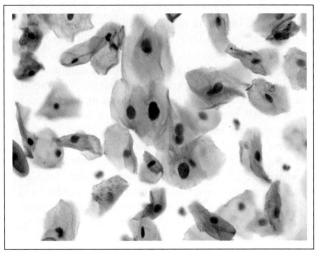

Figure 12-1 Liquid-based cytology classified as epithelial cell abnormality, low-grade squamous intraepithelial lesion. Note particularly the cells in the center. They have enlarged nuclei compared with those in the cells to the left and below. This feature is required for a diagnosis of LSIL. The nuclear contours are irregular. One cell to the right of center is binucleated, a common feature in LSIL. (Cytology image courtesy of Nancy Joste, MD.)

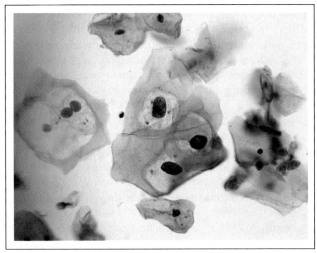

Figure 12-2 Epithelial cell abnormality, low-grade squamous intraepithelial lesion. This liquid-based cytology shows changes characteristic of HPV effect or koilocytosis. Nuclear enlargement is present with some irregularity of the borders. Perinuclear halos are prominent, the distinctive feature of HPV effect. Compare the size of the dysplastic nuclei with the nuclei in the adjacent normal superficial and intermediate squamous cells. (Cytology image courtesy of Nancy Joste, MD.)

CIN 3 among women with CIN 1 without HPV changes, compared with 14% among those with HPV cytopathic changes. Furthermore, they noted that both CIN 1 and HPV changes are associated with a heterogeneous complement of high-risk and low-risk HPV DNA types.[32]

Although rigorous criteria have been established for the cytologic and histologic diagnoses of low-grade lesions, the subjective nature of microscopic interpretation leads to variation in interpretation. Woodhouse et al. found an

83% rate of correct diagnoses of LSIL on validated cytology slides that were examined by more than 17,000 pathologists. The majority of those that were misdiagnosed were overcalled as HSIL (12%).[33] Stoler et al. showed similar variability in data from ALTS. A total of 4948 liquid-based cytology tests and 2237 colposcopic biopsies were subjected to quality control review after initial diagnoses were made by ALTS clinical center pathologists. Agreement on diagnosis between clinical center and quality control pathologists was highest with a diagnosis of "negative for intraepithelial lesion or malignancy." *Among cytologic abnormalities, LSIL had the highest degree of concurrence with agreement in 68% of cases.* Twenty-six percent of slides originally called LSIL were downgraded to ASC-US or negative by the quality control pathologists, and 6% were upgraded to HSIL.[34]

COLPOSCOPIC FINDINGS

The degree of acetowhite change seen colposcopically in LSIL is variable (Table 12-1). Acetowhite epithelium appears pale translucent pink-white or a dense snowy white, depending on whether overt condylomatous changes are present. Dysplastic epithelium appears acetowhite when light directed from the colposcope is reflected off the different layers of cervical epithelium and away from the underlying network of basal capillaries at the stromal-epithelial junction. In cases of increased nuclear:cytoplasmic ratio, less light penetrates to the stroma and more is reflected back from the epithelial layers. In LSIL, this results from the relative enlargement of the nucleus. However in HSIL, the nuclear enlargement is less pronounced but the cytoplasm is contracted.

With the exception of overt condylomas, low-grade lesions appear as pale, relatively translucent pink-white or shiny, snowy white lesions (Figure 12-3). *The acetowhite effect is more gradual in onset and more transient in duration than the acetowhite reaction seen in higher-grade dysplasia.* In addition, *the dilute acetic acid needs to be reapplied frequently for optimal visualization of the lesion.* These lesions arise in areas of squamous metaplasia and abut the squamocolumnar junction (SCJ).

Condylomatous changes brought about by certain types of HPV, most notably types 6 and 11, may present on the cervix as exophytic condylomata acuminata or as flat to slightly raised *satellite lesions* (Figure 12-4). These may or may not be contiguous with the SCJ and may be found beyond the transformation zone. They may appear as multiple small, well-circumscribed acetowhite lesions on the portio vaginalis of the cervix and may extend onto the vagina as well (Figure 12-5). Histologically, condylomatous lesions are often characterized by surface keratinization resulting from hyperkeratosis or parakeratosis. *Colposcopically, these lesions will have a dense snowy-white appearance after the application of dilute acetic acid because most of the light projected from the colposcope will reflect off the surface keratin with very little reaching the red subepithelial capillaries. This surface keratin may even appear white*

Table 12-1 Colposcopic Findings Suggestive of Low-Grade Squamous Intraepithelial Lesion

| Acetowhite: |
| Pale, translucent white |
| Snow white |
| Margins: |
| Indistinct |
| Geographic |
| Flocculated |
| Contours: |
| Flat |
| Raised and irregular in condylomata |
| Vessels: |
| Absent |
| If present, fine mosaic and/or punctation |

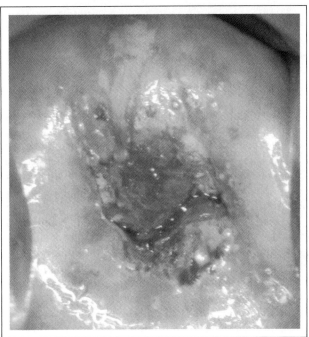

Figure 12-3 A low-grade lesion is demonstrated at 12 o'clock on this cervix. Note the pale acetowhite color and indistinct borders. Repeated applications of dilute acetic acid would be required to maintain visibility of this lesion.

without the application of dilute acetic acid (leukoplakia). It will poorly take up Lugol's solution, appearing white to pale yellow.[35]

Condylomatous lesions may vary in surface contour, from flat acetowhite lesions to slightly raised areas with regular fine papilla to florid exophytic condylomata acuminata. Flat acetowhite macular lesions are sometimes referred to as flat condylomata.[35]

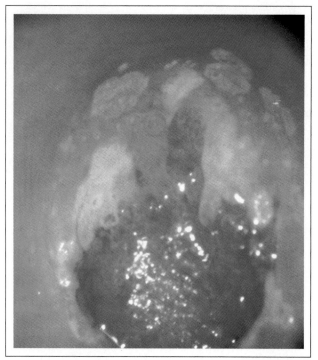

Figure 12-4 Multiple pale and denser white lesions are seen above the cervical os. Note that several of these lesions appear as discrete islands, not connected to the SCJ. They are slightly raised and condylomatous in appearance. Such "satellite" lesions are almost always low grade.

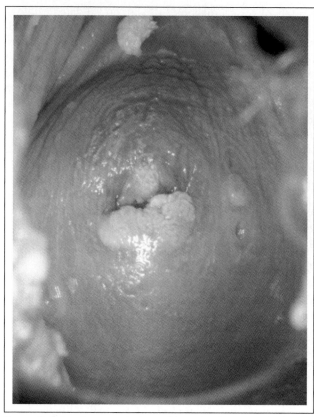

Figure 12-5 Prominent exophytic condyloma in a woman with LSIL on cytology. Note the dense acetowhite color. This may represent surface keratin. Note the presence of a condyloma on the anterior vagina as well as on the cervix.

Each papilla in an exophytic condyloma acuminata has a central capillary loop that may be most easily seen after the dilute acetic acid has begun to fade. Early condylomata may be difficult to distinguish from high-grade lesions because they may have only a minimally raised surface with shallow projections. The central capillary loops may appear as punctation.[35]

Alternatively, immature condylomata with papillae but lacking keratin may be mistaken for the papillae of endocervical columnar epithelium that also have a central capillary, although the papillae of the endocervix have more blunt, rounded tips (Figure 12-6). The distinction between condylomata acuminata and invasive cancer may also be challenging. However, unlike the exophytic lesion of invasive cancer, condylomata have no atypical vessels or areas of necrosis. However, contact bleeding may be present, especially in the presence of an accompanying bacterial infection (Figure 12-7).

In non-condylomatous, low-grade intraepithelial lesions, the surface contours are flat. The margins may be indistinct, with the acetowhite changes noted at the SCJ fading into the background color of the mature squamous epithelium. The margins may also appear irregular in contrast to the sharp, straight margins of high-grade lesions. Numerous terms are used to describe the margins of low-grade lesions, including *flocculated* (like gathered cloth or cumulus clouds) and *geographic* (with the map-like appearance of bays and peninsulas) (Figures 12-8 to 12-10). Low-grade squamous lesions may exhibit vascular changes including punctation and mosaic. However, unlike high-grade lesions, the

vascular patterns in low-grade lesions tend to be fine, of small caliber, regular in their distribution, and of normal intercapillary distance (50–250 μm). Atypical vessels are exceedingly rare in low-grade lesions (Figure 12-11).[36]

The colposcopic findings of low-grade lesions are variable. Hellberg and Nilsson reported the colposcopic appearance of 165 women with histologically documented CIN 1. They found acetowhite epithelium in 52.1%, punctation in 22.4%, mosaic pattern in 18.2%, and atypical vessels in 2.4%.[37] Other smaller series have reported higher rates for punctation, mosaic vascular changes, and especially acetowhite epithelium, which was reported as almost universally present.[38]

Correctly predicting LSIL based on the colposcopic impression is in many ways more challenging than diagnosing a high-grade lesion. *The colposcopic impression of low-grade lesions is less precise and less reproducible than the colposcopic impression of higher-grade lesions.*[38–40] Hopman et al. reviewed eight studies that reported colposcopic impression and histologic correlates in patients with satisfactory colposcopy examinations. They found a colposcopic impression of CIN 1 correctly predicted the histologic diagnosis only 42.8 % of the time (range 20.0–60.0%) compared with rates of 61.6%, 59.0%, and 78.3% for no CIN, CIN 2, and CIN 3, respectively.[38] The same group found intraobserver agreement of 66.7% when 23 expert colposcopists reviewed slide

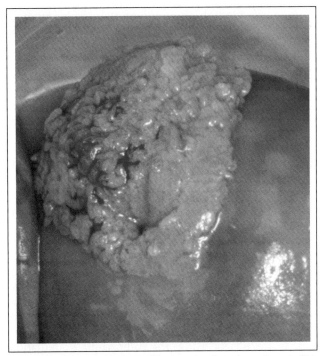

Figure 12-6 Large exophytic condyloma arising from the endocervix. This could easily be mistaken for a prominent ectropion (i.e., everted endocervical epithelium).

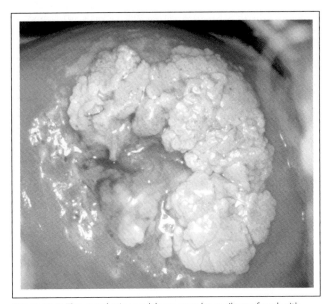

Figure 12-7 This exophytic condyloma may be easily confused with cancer. The absence of atypical vessels and lack of surface bleeding makes cancer less likely. When in doubt, biopsy!

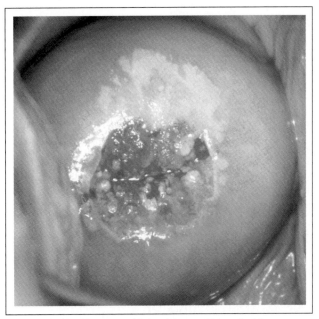

Figure 12-8 Map-like geographic borders are apparent in this low-grade lesion. Note also the pale acetowhite color and small satellite lesions.

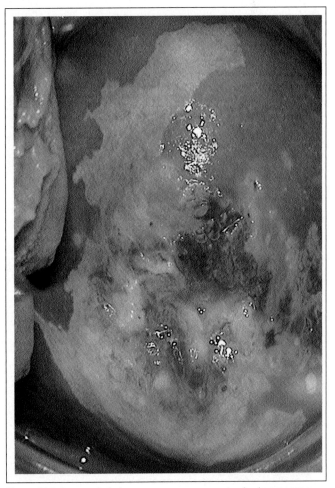

Figure 12-9 Low-grade lesions may appear more extensive in pregnancy. This patient is 13 weeks pregnant. Note the pale acetowhite color and geographic borders of this lesion.

colpophotographs of varying degrees of dysplasia during two study sessions 2 to 3 months apart. The interobserver agreement for the two readings was only 52.4% and 51.0%, respectively. *They found both inter- and intraobserver concordance to be worse with CIN 1 and CIN 2 than with the categories of no CIN and CIN 3.*[40]

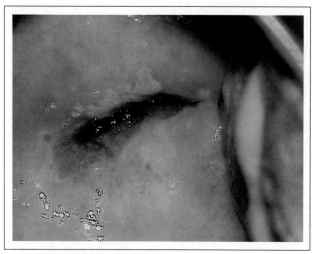

Figure 12-10 This low-grade lesion has flocculated borders and a pale white color. Also note the presence of a faint, fine mosaic pattern.

COLPOSCOPIC MIMICS OF LOW-GRADE LESIONS

With the exception of findings characteristic of condylomata acuminata, the colposcopic findings of LSIL differ only by degree from those seen with immature squamous metaplasia. In immature squamous metaplasia, multiple layers of reserve cells underlie immature non-glycogenated squamous cells and the last remnants of the columnar epithelium. After application of dilute acetic acid, this nuclear-dense tissue will frequently appear a pale acetowhite color (although less dense and more translucent than in low-grade lesions). The borders are irregular and may be indistinct from those of low-grade SIL. Fine regular mosaic and punctate vascular patterns may also be seen. These acetowhite changes are especially prominent around gland openings and the new SCJ (Figures 12-12 and 12-13).

The colposcopic findings of repair are similar to those of squamous metaplasia. Such findings may be seen after treatment for CIN. Pale acetowhite changes and even fine mosaic or punctation patterns may be present within the first 4 to 6 months after treatment with cryotherapy or loop excision procedures (Figures 12-14 and 12-15).

Caution must be in exercised when making the colposcopic diagnosis of low-grade lesions in older women. This is especially true in postmenopausal women in whom atrophy limits the epithelial strata to basal and parabasal layers. Zahm et al. found the acetowhite response, irregular surface contours, and distinct borders of high-grade lesions were more likely to be blunted in women aged 35 or older. It was observed that the colposcopic examination in older women is less sensitive than in younger women, even when the older women are premenopausal. Obvious trivial findings had a higher frequency of harboring significant CIN (Figure 12-16).[41]

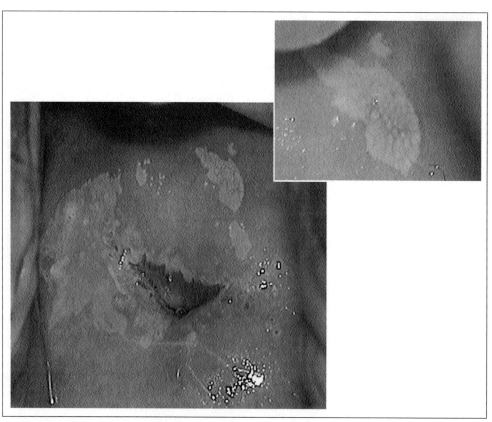

Figure 12-11 This low-grade lesion has an obvious flat satellite lesion. A fine mosaic vascular pattern in the satellite lesion is apparent in the higher-power inset.

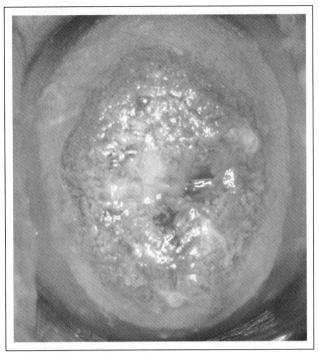

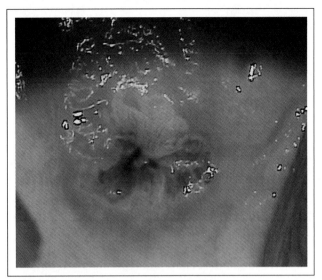

Figure 12-14 Six months after a loop electrosurgical excision procedure (LEEP), this cervix has a pale acetowhite lesion with geographic borders (i.e., characteristic LSIL changes). Biopsy showed only squamous metaplasia.

Figure 12-12 Surrounding the SCJ in this cervix is a band of pale acetowhite epithelium. Biopsy shows squamous metaplasia. This could easily be mistaken for LSIL. Biopsy is needed to make the distinction.

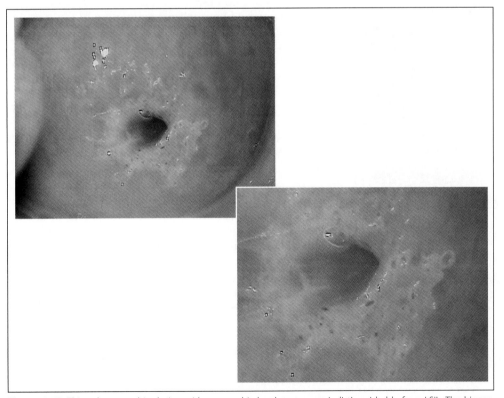

Figure 12-13 This pale acetowhite lesion with geographic borders appears indistinguishable from LSIL. The biopsy showed only squamous metaplasia.

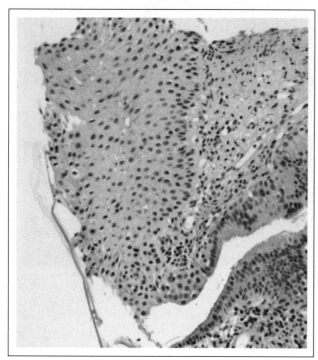

Figure 12-15 Histology of lesion in Figure 12-14. Note widely spaced nuclei with homogeneity of shape and size and lack of crowding. The metaplastic squamous epithelium can be seen starting to move down the neck of the endocervical gland at the bottom of the picture. (Histology image courtesy of Nancy Joste, MD.)

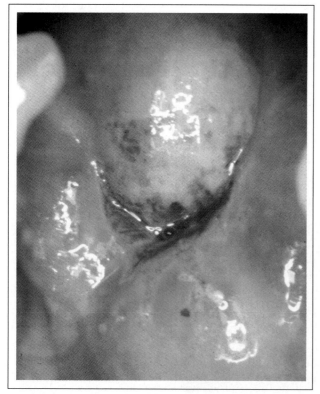

Figure 12-16 This is the cervix of a 50-year-old woman. The lesion is pale acetowhite with ill-defined borders. Although the colposcopic impression was LSIL, the biopsy showed CIN 3.

The acetowhite reaction may also become blunted in pregnancy as the cervix becomes increasingly edematous and congested. Economos et al. reported substantial under-diagnosis on colposcopic examination of pregnant women.[42] Fourteen percent of women with a colposcopic impression of low-grade lesions actually had CIN 3 on biopsy. On the other hand, the estrogen-mediated eversion of the endocervix common in pregnancy may cause normal physiologic changes to be overdiagnosed as low-grade dysplasia. Eversion permits the extension of squamous meta-plasia centrally and creates the appearance of low-grade acetowhitening. The newly proliferated endocervical papil-lae will also often have an acetowhite response at their tips. In pregnant women, low-grade lesions more commonly have mosaic patterns or punctation than in the non-pregnant state. This is due to a physiologic neovascular-ization in pregnancy (Figure 12-17). *The interpretation of low-grade lesions in pregnancy challenges even the most experienced colposcopist.*

HISTOLOGY

Although increasing numbers of pathologists are adapting a dichotomous terminology to histologic diagnoses (low grade and high grade), most still use the *cervical intraepithe-lial neoplasia* or *dysplasia* terminology. Low-grade lesions therefore will be diagnosed as CIN 1 or mild dysplasia. Exo-phytic condylomatous lesions will usually be diagnosed as condyloma acuminata.

Histologic findings of low-grade intraepithelial lesions are characterized by a delayed maturation of the stratified squamous epithelium of the cervix. This is manifested by a loss of the normal progressive cellular differentiation in the bottom third of the epithelial layer, although there is some progressive maturation with more horizontal orien-tation and successive decrease in nuclear size in the upper two thirds of the epithelium. Instead of having a narrow band of basal cells, with their enlarged nuclei and high nuclear:cytoplasmic ratio, low-grade lesions exhibit a widened band of basal-like dysplastic cells. Frequently mitoses are present above the basal layer but are confined to the lower third of the epithelium. The cells in the upper two thirds of the epithelium may appear normal but more often continue to have some degree of nuclear enlargement and morphologic atypia (Figures 12-18 and 12-19). Condylomatous lesions are characterized by acanthosis of the basal layers with cellular changes con-sistent with CIN 1. Frequently disorders of keratin pro-duction such as parakeratosis and hyperkeratosis are present on the surface. Koilocytosis is the hallmark. In contrast to CIN 1, histologic CIN 2 and 3 have loss of cel-lular maturation extending to encompass the upper two thirds of the epithelial layer. Mitotic activity may also per-sist into the upper strata of the epithelium.

Similar to the cytologic diagnosis of LSIL, the histologic diagnosis of CIN 1 is subject to some variability. In the pathology review of ALTS, quality review pathologists

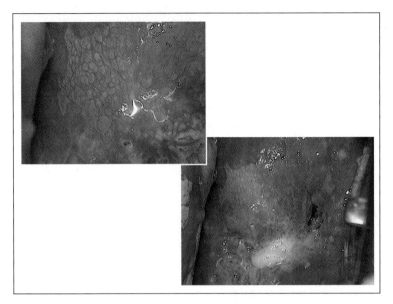

Figure 12-17 Prominent mosaic patterns and (less commonly) punctation may be seen in low-grade lesions in pregnancy due to the neovascularization common to the pregnant state. This cervix at 23 weeks' gestation shows a pale acetowhite lesion with geographic borders. The higher-power inset shows a prominent mosaic pattern with a wide, variable intercapillary distance. In a non-pregnant patient, this would be expected to herald a higher-grade lesion.

reexamined biopsy specimens initially diagnosed by community pathologists. Among colposcopic-directed biopsy specimens, concordance was greatest when a diagnosis was made of HSIL/cancer with 77% agreement. Fewer than half (43%) of the biopsies originally diagnosed as LSIL were also called LSIL by the quality review pathologist. Forty-one percent were read as negative for dysplasia; 4% were called ASC-US and 13% HSIL or greater. This lack of precision makes natural history studies difficult to interpret. *However, from a clinical standpoint, sufficient safeguards are built into the recommended management guidelines that patient care will rarely be adversely affected by the inherent variation in histologic diagnosis.*

MANAGEMENT GUIDELINES

Rationale

Although cytologic LSIL is thought to reflect the cytopathic effects of HPV infection rather than a true premalignant lesion, the imprecision of the diagnosis mandates further evaluation. LSIL diagnosed by one pathologist may be called HSIL by another as often as 12% of the time.[33] Furthermore, in ALTS, women with LSIL were found to have CIN 2 or 3 on directed biopsies in 17.8% of cases, and another 9.8% were found to have CIN 2 or 3 on close follow-up over the next 2 years.[23] It is therefore recommended that *the first step in*

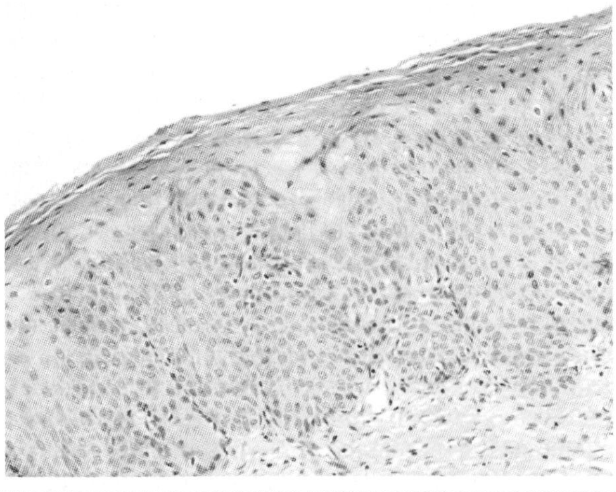

Figure 12-18 CIN 1. Note the delayed maturation of the nuclei. There is little change in the nuclear appearance throughout the lower third of the epithelium. In the upper layers, the nuclei become smaller and are oriented more horizontally. No mitoses are seen in this section. There is surface parakeratosis and keratin production with residual nuclei. This lesion lacks obvious koilocytes. (Histology image courtesy of Nancy Joste, MD.)

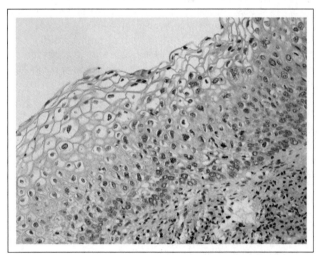

Figure 12-19 This biopsy of CIN 1 has obvious koilocytosis. Note again the lack of maturation in the lower third of the epithelium. In this biopsy, however, as maturation does occur the cells begin to take on glycogen, which is seen as cytoplasmic clearing with tiny nuclei or no visible nuclei. Contrast this normal maturation with the HPV-infected koilocytes. The koilocytes have enlarged, more central nuclei, and the clear space surrounding the nuclei is a virus-laden vacuole, not glycogen. (Cytology image courtesy of Nancy Joste, MD.)

the management of most women with LSIL on cytology is colposcopy with biopsies as indicated (Table 12-2).

Sampling of the endocervical canal, either with endocervical curettage or brushing, should be part of the evaluation if the colposcopy exam is unsatisfactory or if no lesion is seen. Endocervical curettage in the presence of a satisfactory colposcopy examination is justified by findings of a recent study by Pretorius et al. These authors, working in Shanxi Province in China, found CIN 2 or worse in the endocervical curetting of 29.2% of 364 women with a satisfactory colposcopy, including 13 of 88 women who had LSIL on cytology. It is unclear how many of these 13 women had no lesion visible on their ectocervix, but in the overall study population of women with satisfactory colposcopy exams, CIN 2 or worse was diagnosed on endocervical curettage (ECC) alone in 20 (5.5%)[43] (see Table 12-2).

Adolescence, Menopause, and Pregnancy

Although colposcopy is the appropriate first step in the management of most women with LSIL, more conservative follow-up may be appropriate for women at the extremes of the life cycle and in pregnancy.[44]

Adolescence

The incidence of invasive cervical cancer is exceedingly low in women younger than age 21.[45] Moreover, although sexually active adolescents readily acquire HPV infections,[10-14] they are equally efficient at clearing HPV spontaneously.[10,46]

Table 12.2 ASCCP Guidelines for the Management of Women with LSIL

Colposcopy is recommended for managing women with LSIL, except in special populations (see Table 12.3). **(AII)** Endocervical sampling is preferred for non-pregnant women in whom no lesions are identified **(BII)** and those with an unsatisfactory colposcopy **(AII)** but is acceptable for those with a satisfactory colposcopy and a lesion identified in the transformation zone. **(CII)** Acceptable post-colposcopy management options for women with LSIL cytology in whom CIN 2,3 is not identified are testing for high-risk (oncogenic) types of HPV at 12 months or repeat cervical cytological testing at 6 and 12 months. **(BII)** If the HPV DNA test is negative or if two consecutive repeat cytological tests are "negative for intraepithelial lesion or malignancy," return to routine cytological screening is recommended. **(AI)** If either the HPV DNA test is positive or if repeat cytology is reported as ASC-US or greater, colposcopy is recommended. **(AI)** Women found to have CIN should be managed according to the appropriate 2006 Consensus Guidelines on the Management of Cervical Intraepithelial Neoplasia. In the absence of CIN identified histologically, diagnostic excisional or ablative procedures are unacceptable for the initial management of patients with LSIL. **(EII)**

LSIL, Low-grade squamous intraepithelial lesion; *CIN,* cervical intraepithelial lesion; *HPV,* human papillomavirus; *DNA,* deoxyribonucleic acid; *ASC-US,* atypical squamous cells of undetermined significance.
From Ref. 44.

Although a relatively small proportion will develop high-grade dysplastic lesions (3% in a recent study of college students from the state of Washington),[11] *the very long latent period required for the development of invasive disease permits the safe use of cytology for surveillance of low-grade lesions in adolescents.* In adolescents and young women, 61% of LSIL lesions will spontaneously regress in 1 year of follow-up, with another 20% regressing in the second year.[46] Colposcopy, biopsy, and the fear of cancer may be especially traumatic to adolescents. *It therefore seems safe and prudent to delay colposcopy in women of this age group with LSIL unless HSIL is found on follow-up cytology or the LSIL fails to resolve over a 2-year observation period.* This rationale supports the recommended management for LSIL in women younger than 21 years of the American Society for Colposcopy and Cervical Pathology (ASCCP). These young women should be followed with a Pap test 12 months after the initial LSIL result with referral to colposcopy for a result of HSIL or worse. If the first follow-up cytology shows LSIL, atypical squamous cells cannot exclude a high grade lesion (ASC-H), ASC-US, or negative, a second repeat cytology is recommended 12 months later with referral to colposcopy if this Pap test shows ASC-US or greater[44] (Table 12-3). In a young woman with LSIL who is judged to be unlikely to present for recommended follow-up, colposcopy is a reasonable option. Because of the high prevalence of HPV in adolescents, triage with HPV DNA testing is not recommended and the results should be ignored if HPV testing is done inadvertently (see Table 12-3).

Postmenopausal Women

Well-screened, previously negative postmenopausal women are likewise at low-risk for invasive cervical cancer.[47] Furthermore, *the physiologic changes in the postmenopausal cervical and vaginal epithelium may present a false-positive Pap result.* This is a consequence of the interrupted maturation inherent in the atrophic epithelium and inflammation that frequently accompanies atrophy. Without estrogen stimulation, the epithelial strata are limited to basal and parabasal layers with minimal development of intermediate and superficial cells. The cells that are exfoliated are likely to have enlarged nuclei with hyperchromasia and a slight increase in the nuclear:cytoplasmic ratio. This effect is less common in liquid-based than conventional cytology.[1] Schiffman et al. showed a decreased association between LSIL and HPV in older women, although the upper age stratum in their study was 40 years and older.[48] The physiologic changes associated with atrophy explain the overinterpretation of LSIL in older women.

Postmenopausal women with LSIL on cytology may be triaged directly to colposcopy. Other acceptable options include *reflex* HPV DNA testing, reserving colposcopy for those who test positive for high-risk HPV DNA types. In women with previously negative Pap tests, another acceptable alternative to immediate colposcopy is follow-up with repeat cytology at 6-month intervals for 1 year, with referral to colposcopy should either Pap test show ASC-US or

Table 12.3 ASCCP Guidelines for the Management of LSIL in Special Populations

Adolescents

In adolescents with LSIL, follow-up with annual cytologic testing is recommended. **(AII)** At the 12-month follow-up, only adolescents with HSIL or greater on the repeat cytology should be referred to colposcopy. At the 24 month follow-up, those with an ASC-US or greater result should be referred to colposcopy. **(AII)** HPV DNA testing is unacceptable for adolescents with LSIL. **(EII)** If HPV DNA testing is inadvertently performed, the results should not influence management.

Postmenopausal Women

Acceptable options for the management of postmenopausal women with LSIL include reflex HPV DNA testing, repeat cytologic testing at 6 and 12 months, and colposcopy. **(CIII)** If the HPV DNA test is negative or CIN is not identified at colposcopy, repeat cytology in 12 months is recommended. If either the HPV DNA test is positive or the repeat cytology is ASC-US or greater, colposcopy is recommended. **(AII)** If two consecutive repeat cytological tests are "negative for intraepithelial lesion or malignancy," return to routine cytologic screening is recommended.

Pregnant Women

Colposcopy is preferred for pregnant, non-adolescent women with LSIL cytology. **(BII)** Endocervical curettage is unacceptable in pregnant women. **(EIII)** Deferring the initial colposcopy until at least 6 weeks postpartum is acceptable. **(BIII)** In pregnant women who have no cytologic, histologic, or colposcopically suspected CIN 2,3 or cancer at the initial colposcopy, postpartum follow-up is recommended. **(BIII)** Additional colposcopic and cytologic examinations during pregnancy are unacceptable for these women. **(DIII)**

LSIL, Low-grade squamous intraepithelial lesion; *HSIL*, high-grade squamous intraepithelial lesion; *ASC-US*, atypical squamous cells of undetermined significance; *HPV*, human papillomavirus; *DNA*, deoxyribonucleic acid; *CIN*, cervical intraepithelial lesion.
From Ref. 44.

greater.[44] After two consecutive negative Paps, the patient can return to routine screening (see Table 12-3).

Pregnancy

Management of LSIL during pregnancy should be the same as in the non-pregnant state. The management of pregnant adolescents should follow the guidelines for adolescents. Nonadolescent pregnant women with LSIL should be referred for colposcopy, although this may be deferred until after delivery. *If colposcopy is performed for LSIL, additional colposcopy examinations are not indicated during pregnancy unless a high-grade lesion is diagnosed.* If no evidence of CIN 2 or greater is found, a postpartum examination is indicated. The regimen recommended for follow-up of LSIL in the non-pregnant women will be satisfactory in most pregnant women with LSIL. *Biopsy in pregnancy should be reserved for lesions suspicious for HSIL or cancer* (see Table 12-3).

Follow-Up after Colposcopy

Findings at colposcopy will dictate subsequent management. *The objective of colposcopy in women with LSIL is to detect the <27% who have high-grade CIN.* The majority of the HSIL (17%) will be found on initial biopsy. With close follow-up over the next year, most of the remaining 10% will be diagnosed. The ALTS investigators explored three strategies to determine the optimal follow-up strategy when colposcopy failed to detect CIN 2 or worse in a woman with LSIL or HPV + ASC-US on cytology. A strategy of follow-up with two liquid-based Pap tests 6 months apart and referral to colposcopy if either is found to be ASC-US or greater identified 88.0% of the women with CIN 2+ while referring 63.6% of those followed to repeat colposcopy. Ninety-two percent of the residual high-grade lesions were identified by a strategy that employed a single HPV DNA test (HC 2) performed 12 months after the initial colposcopy with repeat colposcopy if the test was positive for high-risk HPV DNA types. This approach referred 55.0% of women to colposcopy. The combination of cytology and HPV DNA testing resulted in a nonsignificant improvement in sensitivity (94.8% of the high-grade lesions found) but with the highest rate of colposcopy referral (64.1%).[49] The first two strategies are equally acceptable in the 2006 ASCCP guidelines.[44] *Because of the additional cost and lack of increased sensitivity, the combined cytology plus HPV strategy was discouraged* (see Table 12-2; Figure 12-20). Again, because of the high prevalence of HPV in adolescents and the likelihood that a positive test may represent a new incident infection rather than a persistent infection, women younger than 21 years should be followed with cytology and not HPV DNA testing. *If an HPV DNA test is inadvertently ordered, the results should not be considered in the subsequent management of an adolescent* (see Table 12-3; Figure 12-21).

When the initial colposcopy is unsatisfactory and the histologic findings are CIN 1 or less (in a patient whose referral cytology showed LSIL or less), post-colposcopy management remains controversial. In one of the few studies to examine such patients Spiezer et al. 43 women reported on a group of 43 women managed with excision for LSIL on cytology or biopsy and unsatisfactory colposcopy. CIN 2 or 3 was uncovered in 4 (9.3%). No cancers were found.[50] Although these numbers are small, they give support to conservative management with cytology or HPV DNA testing in these women. *Diagnostic excision in this situation is unnecessary given its morbidity and the low risk of cancer* (Table 12-4).[51]

Cervical Intraepithelial Neoplasia 1 Preceded by Cytology Showing Atypical Squamous Cells or a Low-Grade Squamous Intraepithelial Lesion

Because of the low likelihood of cancer when colposcopy reveals only CIN 1, treatment with excision or ablation is unacceptable for initial management. CIN 1 is not considered a precancerous lesion and is likely to resolve spontaneously or

Management of Women with Low-grade Squamous Intraepithelial Lesion (LSIL) *

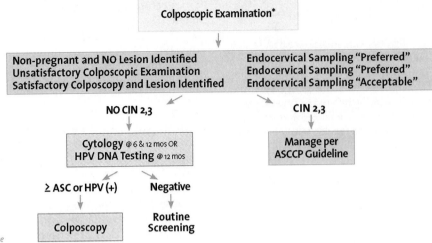

Management options may vary if the woman is pregnant, postmenopausal, or an adolescent - (see text)

Figure 12-20 Reprinted from *The Journal of Lower Genital Tract Disease* Vol. 11 Issue 4, with the permission of ASCCP © American Society for Colposcopy and Cervical Pathology 2007. No copies of the algorithms may be made without the prior consent of ASCCP.

Management of Women with a Histological Diagnosis of Cervical Intraepithelial Neoplasia Grade 1 (CIN 1) Preceded by ASC-US, ASC-H or LSIL Cytology

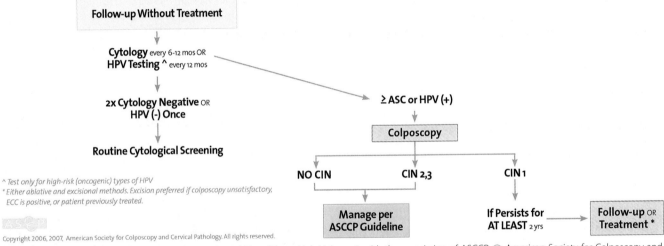

^ Test only for high-risk (oncogenic) types of HPV
* Either ablative and excisional methods. Excision preferred if colposcopy unsatisfactory, ECC is positive, or patient previously treated.

Figure 12-21 Reprinted from *The Journal of Lower Genital Tract Disease* Vol. 11 Issue 4, with the permission of ASCCP © American Society for Colposcopy and Cervical Pathology 2007. No copies of the algorithms may be made without the prior consent of ASCCP.

persist unchanged during a 2-year follow-up period. Among women enrolled in ALTS who presented with LSIL or HPV-positive ASC-US on initial cytology and were found to have CIN 1 on initial colposcopy, 13% were subsequently found to have CIN 2 or 3 (8.9% CIN 3) and none had cancer during the 24-month follow-up period. This rate of high-grade dysplasia on follow-up was similar to women whose colposcopy was completely negative, had no biopsy performed (11.3%), and whose biopsy was negative for CIN (11.7%).[23] Conservative management allows adequate time to identify cases that are likely to have been initially misclassified or to progress to higher-grade lesions with minimal risk of developing cancer.

The rationale for avoiding treatment in favor of more conservative follow-up is related to the cost, discomfort, and potential morbidity of commonly used treatment modalities. Cryotherapy is associated with a profuse discharge and, although significant stenosis is uncommon,[51] lesser degrees of narrowing of the os and migration of the SCJ can make follow-up colposcopy difficult. *Recent studies have shown a significant risk of premature delivery and preterm premature rupture of membranes in pregnant women previously treated with loop electrosurgical excision procedure (LEEP).*[53–55] This is especially significant in young women with CIN 1, a group for whom future pregnancy complications are a concern and a group very likely to have spontaneous regression.[46]

How long may CIN 1 be safely followed without treatment? Although persistence of CIN 1 is associated with a higher risk of high-grade dysplasia and the likelihood of regression decreases the longer dysplasia persists, cancer can be effectively prevented with continued follow-up. *Hence, it is safe to follow a compliant patient with semi-annual cytology exams or annual HPV DNA testing with colposcopy as indicated for women with positive high-risk HPV DNA or cytology of ASC-US or greater.* Because some women will have anxiety with prolonged conservative management of a condition that does not resolve, eventual treatment is acceptable. *Conservative management should be followed for at least 2 years.* If CIN 1 has not resolved after 2 years, treatment is acceptable with excision or ablation if the colposcopy remains satisfactory[55] (see Table 12-4). *There are no data, however, to preclude continued follow-up beyond 2 years.*

Cervical Intraepithelial Neoplasia 1 Preceded by Cytology Showing Atypical Squamous Cells or a low-Grade Squamous Intraepithelial Lesion

Under the old guidelines, this scenario would have resulted in review of the cytology and histology and a diagnostic excisional procedure if the diagnosis were confirmed. However, the 2006 guidelines changed in two ways. First, because experience has shown that most pathologists are unlikely to downgrade their own or another pathologist's diagnosis of HSIL, the necessity for a review of the cytology and histology was made optional. Furthermore, for women with a satisfactory colposcopy and a negative ECC, in addition to the option of a diagnostic excisional procedure, the option to follow with colposcopy and cytology at 6-month intervals for 1 year was added. In women with a repeat HSIL diagnosis or an unsatisfactory colposcopy, a diagnostic excisional procedure is recommended. Those with two consecutive negative cytology results can return to routine screening[44] (Table 12-4, Figure 12-22).

Cervical Intraepithelial Neoplasia 1 Preceded by Cytology Showing Atypical Squamous Cells or a Low-Grade Squamous Intraepithelial Lesion

Adolescent Women. The management of adolescents with CIN 1 is the same as adolescents with LSIL (see Table 12-5, Figure 12-23).

Pregnant Women. The recommended management of pregnant women with a histological diagnosis of CIN 1 is follow-up without treatment. Treatment of pregnant women for CIN 1 is unacceptable (see Table 12-5).

MANAGEMENT SCENARIOS

Scenario 1

Sentinel Pap: LSIL
Colposcopic findings or histologic cell type if a biopsy was done:
No SIL found

Table 12.4 ASCCP Guidelines for the Management of Women with CIN 1

CIN 1 Preceded by ASC-US, ASC-H, or LSIL Cytology
The recommended management of women with a histologic diagnosis of CIN 1 preceded by an ASC-US, ASC-H or LSIL cytology is follow-up with either HPV DNA testing every 12 months or repeat cervical cytology every 6 to 12 months. **(BII)** If the HPV DNA test is positive or if repeat cytology is reported as ASC-US or greater, colposcopy is recommended. If the HPV test is negative or two consecutive repeat cytology tests are "negative for intraepithelial lesion or malignancy," return to routine cytological screening is recommended. **(AII)**

  If CIN 1 persists for at least 2 years, either continued follow-up or treatment is acceptable. **(CII)** If treatment is selected and the colposcopic examination is satisfactory, either excision or ablation is acceptable. **(AI)** A diagnostic excisional procedure is recommended if the colposcopic examination is unsatisfactory, the endocervical sampling contains CIN, or the patient has been previously treated. **(AIII)** Treatment modality should be determined by the judgment of the clinician and should be guided by experience, resources, and clinical value for the specific patient. **(AI)** In patients with CIN 1 and an unsatisfactory colposcopic examination, ablative procedures are unacceptable. **(EI)** Podophyllin or podophyllin-related products are unacceptable for use in the vagina or on the cervix. **(EII)** Hysterectomy as the primary and principal treatment for histologically diagnosed CIN 1 is unacceptable. **(EII)**

CIN 1 Preceded by HSIL or AGC-NOS (atypical glandular cells not otherwise specified) Cytology
Either a diagnostic excisional procedure or observation with colposcopy and cytology at 6-month intervals for 1 year is acceptable for women with a histologic diagnosis of CIN 1 preceded by a HSIL or AGC-NOS cytology, provided in the latter case that the colposcopic examination is satisfactory and endocervical sampling is negative. **(BIII)** In this circumstance it is also acceptable to review the cytologic, histologic, and colposcopic findings; if the review yields a revised interpretation, management should follow guidelines for the revised interpretation. **(BII)**

  If observation with cytology and colposcopy is elected, a diagnostic excisional procedure is recommended for women with repeat HSIL cytological results at either the 6- or 12-month visit. **(CIII)** After 1 year of observation, women with two consecutive "negative for intraepithelial lesion or malignancy" results can return to routine cytologic screening. A diagnostic excisional procedure is recommended for women with CIN 1 preceded by a HSIL or AGC-NOS cytology in whom the colposcopic examination is unsatisfactory, except in special populations (e.g., pregnant women). **(BII)**

*CIN, cervical intraepithelial neoplasia; ASC-US, atypical squamous cells of undetermined significance; ASC-H, ***; LSIL, low-grade squamous intraepithelial lesion; HPV, human papillomavirus; DNA, deoxyribonucleic acid.*
From Ref. 51.

Management of Women with a Histological Diagnosis of Cervical Intraepithelial Neoplasia - Grade 1 (CIN 1) Preceded by HSIL or AGC-NOS Cytology

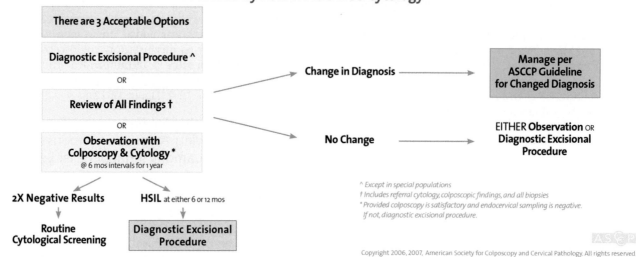

Figure 12-22 Reprinted from *The Journal of Lower Genital Tract Disease* Vol. 11 Issue 4, with the permission of ASCCP © American Society for Colposcopy and Cervical Pathology 2007. No copies of the algorithms may be made without the prior consent of ASCCP.

Table 12.5 ASCCP Guidelines for the Management of Women with CIN 1 in Special Populations

Adolescents

Follow-up with annual cytologic assessment is recommended for adolescents with CIN 1. **(AII)** At the 12-month follow-up, only adolescents with HSIL or greater on the repeat cytology should be referred to colposcopy. At the 24-month follow-up, those with an ASC-US or greater result should be referred to colposcopy. **(AII)** Follow-up with HPV DNA testing is unacceptable. **(EII)**

Pregnant Women

The recommended management of pregnant women with a histologic diagnosis of CIN 1 is follow-up without treatment. **(BII)** Treatment of pregnant women for CIN 1 is unacceptable. **(EII)**

CIN, cervical intraepithelial neoplasia; ASC-US, atypical squamous cells of undetermined significance; HPV, human papillomavirus; DNA, deoxyribonucleic acid. From Ref. 51.

HPV testing for high-risk (oncogenic) HPV types: Positive (This test is relevant only in postmenopausal women and should only be done in that age group. In adults it is cost-inefficient, and in adolescents the results should be ignored.)
Satisfactory colposcopy: Yes
Fertility desires: N/A

If the colposcopic findings are negative and no biopsy is performed, a reasonable search for dysplasia is prudent in sites other than the ectocervix. This was a satisfactory colposcopy, meaning the entire SCJ was well visualized. Findings of high-grade dysplasia on ECC have been reported in the presence of a satisfactory exam with no visible ectocervical lesion, but such findings are rare.[43] In addition to sampling the endocervical canal with an ECC or cytobrush, careful examination of the vagina and vulva will occasionally reveal an explanation for the abnormal Pap.

ALTS found high-grade CIN in 17.8% of women with LSIL cytology who underwent immediate colposcopy. The cumulative incidence of high-grade dysplasia was 27.6% in women followed for 2 years. This suggests that this patient has an almost 10% risk of being diagnosed with high-grade dysplasia if followed appropriately.[23] The ALTS investigators proposed that most of these high-grade lesions were already present but were clinically undetectable at the time of initial colposcopy. In ALTS, two follow-up options were available: two Pap tests 6 months apart and referral to colposcopy for cytology reported as ASC-US or greater, or a single HC 2 HPV DNA test in 1 year and colposcopy if it was positive for high-risk HPV types. Cytology follow-up had a sensitivity of 88.0% in uncovering those residual high-grade lesions, whereas 63.6% of the women undergoing cytology follow-up were referred to colposcopy. Follow-up with HPV DNA testing resulted in referral of 55.0% of the women to colposcopy while detecting 92.2% of high-grade lesions. Of note, follow-up with the combination of cytology plus HPV testing was not significantly more sensitive (94.8%) but sent more women to colposcopy (64.1%).[49]

Diagnostic excision is not appropriate at this time.

Scenario 2

Sentinel Pap: LSIL
Colposcopic findings or histologic cell type if a biopsy was done: No SIL found
HPV testing for high-risk (oncogenic) HPV types: Positive (This test is relevant only in postmenopausal women and should only be done in that age group. In adults it is cost-inefficient, and in adolescents the results should be ignored.)
Satisfactory colposcopy: No
Fertility desires: N/A

Management of Adolescent Women (20 Years and Younger) with a Histological Diagnosis of Cervical Intraepithelial Neoplasia - Grade 1 (CIN 1)

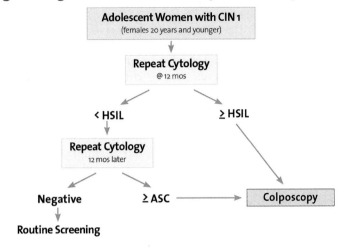

Figure 12-23 Reprinted from *The Journal of Lower Genital Tract Disease* Vol. 11 Issue 4, with the permission of ASCCP © American Society for Colposcopy and Cervical Pathology 2007. No copies of the algorithms may be made without the prior consent of ASCCP.

This scenario raises the question of whether diagnostic excision (LEEP or cold-knife conization) is indicated because of the unsatisfactory colposcopy. Most high-grade dysplastic lesions begin at the SCJ. With an unsatisfactory colposcopy, the SCJ is not visible, and thus a lesion, if present, may not be apparent. In this case, *endocervical sampling with curettage or brush is recommended* and may find such a hidden lesion. *If the endocervical sampling is negative, a continued search for a possible high-grade lesion using a diagnostic excision with LEEP or cold-knife cone seems logical, but its value is not supported by the evidence.* Given its cost and potential for morbidity, excision is not recommended in this case scenario. The limited available data suggest a low rate of high-grade dysplasia and a negligible rate of cancer in this situation. Spitzer et al. found only a 9.4% rate of high-grade CIN on conization in women with unsatisfactory colposcopy and LSIL on Pap or colposcopic biopsy. They found no cancers.[50] This patient should be followed-up in a similar manner as recommended in Scenario 1.

Scenario 3

Sentinel Pap: LSIL
Colposcopic findings or histologic cell type if a biopsy was done: CIN 1
HPV testing for high-risk (oncogenic) HPV types: Positive or not done (This test is relevant only in postmenopausal women and should only be done in that age group. In adults it is cost-inefficient, and in adolescents the results should be ignored.)
Satisfactory colposcopy: Yes or No
Fertility desires: N/A

From the 1970s through most of the 1990s, biopsy-proven CIN 1 was treated with cryosurgery. It had a high apparent cure rate.[52] Subsequent studies have shown that *much of the resolution of CIN 1 that was attributed to cryosurgery especially in young women would have occurred without any treatment.*[46] Those lesions destined to progress to CIN 2 or 3 generally have a sufficiently long latent period to permit timely treatment. *The patient in this scenario can safely be followed with Pap tests at 6-month intervals with colposcopy referral for ASC-US or greater, or with HPV DNA tests annually with referral to colposcopy for high-risk HPV DNA results.* Although the risk of progression increases with duration of persistence of CIN 1, so does the chance of spontaneous regression. Treatment after 24 months of persistent CIN 1 is a reasonable option if the patient prefers not to continue with conservative management.

Scenario 4

Sentinel Pap: LSIL
Colposcopic findings or histologic cell type if a biopsy was done: CIN 1
HPV testing for high-risk (oncogenic) HPV types: Positive or not done (This test is relevant only in postmenopausal women and should only be done in that age group. In adults it is cost-inefficient, and in adolescents the results should be ignored.)
Satisfactory colposcopy: Yes or No
Fertility desires: Actively trying to get pregnant

This patient should be managed identically to the woman in Scenario 3. She should not be discouraged from trying to conceive during the follow-up period. *If CIN 2 or 3 is diagnosed during follow-up, it can be safely followed without treatment during a pregnancy. If CIN 2 or 3 is diagnosed during pregnancy,* colposcopy with a limited number of biopsies is appropriate. Treatment should be delayed until the postpartum period.

If CIN 1 persists through the 2-year follow-up period and the patient desires to conceive at that point, continued follow-up should be encouraged rather than treatment, as treatment with excisional procedures has been shown to increase the risk of preterm delivery.[52–55] Unfortunately, there is only scanty and contradictory evidence dealing with the risk of prematurity after cryosurgery. *It should not be assumed that cryosurgery results in lower complication rate than LEEP.*

Scenario 5

Sentinel Pap: LSIL in an adolescent
Colposcopic findings or histologic cell type if a biopsy was done: Colposcopy should not be done
HPV testing for high-risk (oncogenic) HPV types: Not done (or if done, the results should be ignored)
Satisfactory colposcopy: N/A
Fertility desires: N/A

This patient is younger than 21 years of age and has LSIL cytology. Her risk of CIN 2 or 3 is very small,[23] and her risk of invasive cancer is almost zero.[45] Because 91% CIN 1 in adolescents is expected to regress spontaneously over 36 months, *the recommended management for adolescents with biopsy-proven CIN 1 is observation.*[46]*Because of the high rate of spontaneous regression of CIN 2 in the adolescent, low progression rate, and pregnancy-related complications associated with treatment, the recommended management for adolescents with biopsy-proven CIN 2 is also observation.*[55]*Because most CIN 2,3 in adolescents is actually CIN 2, if the pathologist is unable to differentiate CIN 2 from CIN 3 in an adolescent, the lesion should be assumed to be CIN 2 and managed with observation* (see Chapter 22). This leads to the recommendation to defer colposcopy in this patient pending the results of repeated cytology at 12-month intervals. A Pap result of HSIL 12 months after the initial LSIL suggests progression and warrants colposcopy. If that first repeat Pap shows only LSIL or less, this implies persistence or regression of the lesion and allows continued conservative follow-up with another Pap test 12 months later. If the cytology has not reverted to negative by 24 months after the initial LSIL result (i.e., it is ASC-US or greater), a colposcopy exam with biopsies as indicated is appropriate. This conservative approach requires a compliant patient and a good follow-up system on the part of the colposcopist.

COUNSELING SCENARIOS

The critical element in counseling women with LSIL and CIN 1 is to make clear to them that the reason for concern about their condition is because of the almost 30% risk that they have a precancerous condition (CIN 2,3) and not because LSIL and CIN 1 are themselves precancerous. This is sometimes a difficult concept for patients to grasp and is sometimes even difficult for the healthcare provider to accept because they may be afraid of missing a precancerous condition. *Because patients are incredibly perceptive, they will pick up on the healthcare provider's body language hints of discomfort with the recommendation to follow LSIL or CIN 1 without treatment and will insist on treatment, putting even more pressure on the provider.* The patient's fear and the provider's insecurity merge into a self-fulfilling prophecy. The way to overcome this slippery slope is to confidently counsel the patient that LSIL and CIN 1 are simple viral infections that do not require treatment. The patient needs to be evaluated for the possibility that she has CIN 2,3, but the intuitive notion that if we catch the condition early (as CIN 1) we can improve the cure rate is simply not true. The cure rate for CIN 1 and CIN 2,3 are all the same. Because most CIN 1 will regress spontaneously, treating it is unnecessary in most women and potentially harmful in all of them. *The healthcare provider needs to tell this to the patient in a confident and reassuring manner.*

REFERENCES

1. Solomon D, Nayar R (eds). The Bethesda System for Reporting Cervical/Vaginal Cytologic Diagnoses: Definitions, Criteria, and Explanatory Notes, ed 2. New York: Springer-Verlag, 2004.
2. Lorincz AT, Reid R, Jenson AB, et al. Human papillomavirus infection of the cervix: relative risk associations of 15 common anogenital types. Obstet Gynecol 1992;79:328–337.
3. Muñoz N, Bosch FX, de Sanjosé S, et al. Epidemiologic classification of human papillomavirus types associated with cervical cancer. N Engl J Med 2003;348:518–527.
4. Park T, Fujiwara H, Wright TC. Molecular biology of cervical cancer and its precursors. Cancer 1995;76:1902–1913.
5. Schiffman MH, Brinton LA. The epidemiology of cervical carcinogenesis. Cancer 1995;76:1888–1901.
6. ASCUS-LSIL Triage Study (ALTS) Group. A randomized trial on the management of low-grade squamous intraepithelial lesion cytology interpretations. Am J Obstet Gynecol 2003; 188:1393–1400.
7. Clifford GM, Smith JS, Aguado T, et al. Comparison of HPV type distribution in high-grade cervical lesions and cervical cancer: a meta-analysis. Br J Cancer 2003;89:101–105.
8. Clifford GM, Rana RK, Franceschi S, et al. Human papillomavirus genotype distribution in low-grade cervical lesions: comparison by geographic region and with cervical cancer. Cancer Epidemiol Biomarkers Prev 2005;14:1157–1164.
9. Clifford GM, Franceschi S, Diaz M, et al. Chapter 3: HPV type-distribution in women with and without cervical neoplastic diseases. Vaccine 2006;24s3:S3/26–S3/34.
10. Ho GYF, Bierman R, Beardsley L, et al. Natural history of cervicovaginal papillomavirus infection in young women. N Engl J Med 1998;338:423–428.
11. Winer RL, Lee S, Hughes JP, et al. Genital human papillomavirus infection: incidence and risk factors in a cohort of female university students. Am J Epidemiol 2003;157:218–226.
12. Clavel C, Masure M, Bory JP, et al. Human papillomavirus testing in primary screening for the detection of high-grade cervical lesions: a study of 7932 women. Br J Cancer 2001;84:1616–1623.

13. Sellors JW, Mahony JB, Kaczorowiski J, et al, and the Survey of HPV in Ontario Women (SHOW) Group. Prevalence and predictors of human papillomavirus infection in women in Ontario, Canada. CMAJ 2000;163:503–508.

14. Kulasingam SL, Hughes JP, Kiviat NB, et al. Evaluation of human papillomavirus testing in primary screening for cervical abnormalities comparison of sensitivity, specificity, and frequency of referral. J Am Med Assoc 2002;288:1749–1757.

15. Sherman ME, Schiffman M, Cox JT; Atypical Squamous Cells of Undetermined Significance/Low-Grade Squamous Intraepithelial Lesion Triage Study Group. Effects of age and human papilloma viral load on colposcopy triage: data from the randomized Atypical Squamous Cells of Undetermined Significance/Low-Grade Squamous Intraepithelial Lesion Triage Study (ALTS). J Natl Cancer Inst 2002;94:102–107.

16. Evans MF, Adamson CS, Papillo JL, et al. Distribution of human papillomavirus types in ThinPrep Papanicolaou tests classified according to the Bethesda 2001 terminology and correlations with patient age and biopsy outcomes. Cancer 2006;106:1054–1064.

17. The Atypical Squamous Cells of Undetermined Significance/Low-Grade Squamous Intraepithelial Lesions Triage Study (ALTS) Group. Human papillomavirus testing for triage of women with cytologic evidence of low-grade squamous intraepithelial lesions: baseline data from a randomized trial. J Natl Cancer Inst 2000;92:397–402.

18. Zuna RE, Wang SS, Rosenthal DL, et al. Determinants of human papillomavirus-negative, low-grade squamous intrepeithelial lesions in the atypical squamous cells of undetermined significance/low-grade squamous intraepithelial lesions triage study (ALTS). Cancer (Cancer Cytopathol) 2005;105:253–262.

19. Mosiscki AB, Hills N, Shiboski S, et al. Risks for incident human papillomavirus infection and low-grade squamous intraepithelial lesion development in young females. J Am Med Assoc 2001;285:2995–3002.

20. Moscicki AB, Burt VG, Kanowitz S, et al. The significance of squamous metaplasia in the development of low-grade squamous intraepithelial lesions in young women. Cancer 1999;85:1139–1144.

21. Reid R, Campion MJ. HPV-associated lesions of the cervix: biology and colposcopic features. Clin Obstet Gynecol 1989;32:157–179.

22. Park J, Sun D, Genest DR, et al. Coexistence of low and high-grade squamous intraepithelial lesions of the cervix: morphologic progression or multiple papillomaviruses? Gynecol Oncol 1998;70:368–391.

23. Cox JT, Schiffman M, Solomon D. Prospective follow-up suggests similar risk of subsequent cervical intraepithelial neoplasia grade 2 or 3 among women with cervical intraepithelial neoplasia grade 1 or negative colposcopy and directed biopsy. Am J Obstet Gynecol 2003;188:1406–1412.

24. Kinney WK, Manos MM, Hurley LB, et al. Where's the high-grade cervical neoplasia? The importance of minimally abnormal Papanicolaou diagnoses. Obstet Gynecol 1998;91:973–976.

25. Nasiell K, Roger V, Nasiell M. Behavior of mild cervical dysplasia during long-term follow-up. Obstet Gynecol 1986;67:665–669.

26. Melnikow J, Nuovo J, Willan AR, et al. Natural history of cervical squamous intraepithelial lesions: a meta-analysis. Obstet Gynecol 1998;92:727–735.

27. Schlecht NF, Platt RW, Duarte-Franco E, et al. Human papillomavirus infection and time to progression and regression of cervical intraepithelial neoplasia. J Natl Cancer Inst 2003;95:1336–1343.

28. Moscicki AB, Shiboski S, Broering J, et al. The natural history of human papillomavirus infection as measured by repeated DNA testing in adolescent and young women. J Pediatr 1998;132:277–284.

29. Burk RD, Kelly P, Feldman F, et al. Declining prevalence of cervicovaginal human papillomavirus infection with age is independent of other risk factors. Sex Transm Dis 1996;23:333–341.

30. Wright TC, Xiao WS, Koulos J. Comparison of management algorithms for the evaluation of women with low-grade cytologic abnormalities. Obstet Gynecol 1995;85:202–210.

31. Lonky NM, Navarre GL, Saunders S, et al. Low-grade Papanicolaou smears and the Bethesda system: a prospective cytohistopathologic analysis. Obstet Gynecol 1995;85:716–720.

32. Kurman RJ, Malkasian GD, Sedlis A, et al. From Papanicolaou to Bethesda: the rationale for a new cervical cytology classification. Obstet Gynecol 1991;77:779–781.

33. Woodhouse SL, Stastny JF, Styer PE, et al. Interobserver variability in subclassification of squamous intraepithelial lesions: results of the College of American Pathologists Interlaboratory Comparison Program in Cervicovaginal Cytology. Arch Pathol Lab Med 1999;123:1079–1084.

34. Stoler MH, Schiffman M, for the ALTS Group. Interobserver reproducibility of cervical cytologic and histologic interpretations: realistic estimates from the ASCUS-LSIL Triage Study. J Am Med Assoc 2001;285:1500–1505.

35. Meisells A, Fortin R, Roy M. Condylomatous lesions of the cervix II. Cytologic, colposcopic, and histopathologic study. Acta Cytol 1977;21:379–390.

36. Kolstad P. The development of the vascular bed in tumors as seen in squamous cell carcinoma of the cervix uteri. Br J Radiol 1965;38:216.

37. Hellberg D, Nilsson S. 20-year experience of follow-up of the abnormal smear with colposcopy and histology and treatment by conization or cryosurgery. Gynecol Oncol 1990;8:166–169.

38. Hopman EH, Kenemans P, Helmerhorst TJM. Positive predictive rate of colposcopic examination of the cervix uteri: an overview of literature. Obstet Gynecol Surv 1998;53:97–106.

39. Ismail SM, Colclough AB, Dinnen JS, et al. Observer variation in histopathological diagnosis and grading of cervical intraepithelial neoplasia. Br Med J 1989;298:707–710.

40. Hopman EH, Voorhorst FJ, Kenemans P, et al. Observer agreement on interpreting colposcopic images of CIN. Gynecol Oncol 1995;48:206–209.

41. Zahm DM, Ninkl I, Greinke C, et al. Colposcopic appearance of cervical intraepithelial neoplasia is age dependent. Am J Obstet Gynecol 1998;179:1298–1304.

42. Economos K, Veridiano NP, Delke I, et al. Abnormal cervical cytology in pregnancy: a 17-year experience. Obstet Gynecol 1993;81:915–918.

43. Pretorius RG, Zhang W, Belinson JL, et al. Colposcopically directed biopsy, random cervical biopsy, and endocervical curettage in the diagnosis of cervical intraepithelial neoplasia II or worse. Am J Obstet Gynecol 2004;191:430–434.

44. Wright TC Jr, Massad LS, Dunton CJ, Spitzer M, Wilkinson EJ, Solomon D; for the 2006 ASCCP-Sponsored Consensus Conference. 2006 consensus guidelines for the management of women with abnormal cervical screening tests. J Low Genit Dis 2007;11(4):201–222.

45. Reis LAG, Eisner MP, Kosary CL et al. SEER Cancer Statistics Review 1975–2001. National Cancer Institute. Available at: *seer.cancer.gov/cst/1975_/*. Accessed June 20, 2004.

46. Moscicki AB, Shiboski S, Hills N, et al. Regression of low-grade squamous intra-epithelial lesions in young women. Lancet 2004;364:1678–1683.

47. Sawaya GF. Should routine screening Papanicolaou smears be done for women older than 65 years? Arch Intern Med 2004;164:243–245.

48. Schiffman MH, Manos MM, Sherman ME et al. Human papillomavirus and cervical intraepithelial neoplasia (response). J Natl Cancer Inst 1993;85:1868–1880.

49. Guido R, Schiffman M, Solomon D, et al. Postcolposcopy management strategies for women referred with low-grade squamous intraepithelial lesions or human papillomavirus DNA-positive atypical squamous cells of undetermined significance: a two-year prospective study. Am J Obstet Gynecol 2003;188:1401–1405.

50. Spitzer M, Chernys AE, Shifrin A, et al. Indications for cone biopsy: pathologic correlations. Am J Obstet Gynecol 1998;178:74–79.

51. Wright TC Jr, Massad LS, Dunton CJ, Spitzer M, Wilkinson EJ, Solomon D; 2006 American Society for Colposcopy and Cervical Pathology-sponsored Consensus Conference. 2006 consensus guidelines for the management of women with cervical intraepithelial neoplasia or adenocarcinoma in-situ. J Low Genit Tract Dis 2007;11(4):223–39.

52. Mitchell MF, Tortorlero-Luna G, Cook E, et al. A randomized clinical trial of cryotherapy, laser vaporization, and loop electrosurgical excision for treatment of squamous intraepithelial lesions of the cervix. Obstet Gynecol 1998; 92:737–744.

53. Crane JMG. Pregnancy outcome after loop electrosurgical excision procedure: a systematic review. Obstet Gynecol 2003;102: 1058–1061.

54. Samson SA, Bentley JR, Fahey TJ, et al. The effect of loop electrosurgical excision procedure on future pregnancy outcome. Obstet Gynecol 2005;105:325–332.

55. Sadler L, Saftlas A, Wang W, et al. Treatment for cervical intraepithelial neoplasia and risk of preterm delivery. J Am Med Assoc 2004;291:2100–2106.

56. Wright TC Jr, Massad LS, Dunton CJ, Spitzer M, Wilkinson EJ, Solomon D; 2006 consensus guidelines for the management of women with cervical intraepithelial neoplasia or adenocarcinoma in situ. Am J Obstet Gynecol 2007;197:340–345.

CASE STUDY 1 QUESTIONS

HISTORY

A 19-year-old gravida 0, para 0 is referred to you with an abnormal Pap smear. She has been sexually active since age 16 years with four partners. She is a smoker.

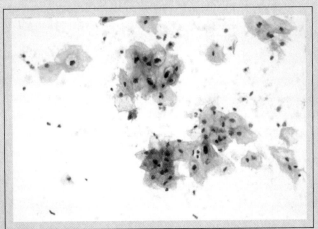

Figure 12-24 This is her Pap smear.

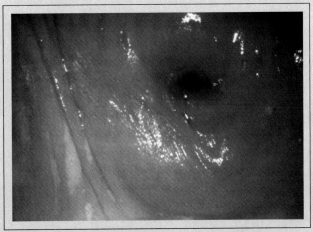

Figure 12-26 This is a colpophotograph of the right vaginal fornix.

- What is the cytologic diagnosis?
- Is the transformation zone fully visualized?
- Describe what you see.
- What is the next step in this patient's evaluation?
- What do you see?

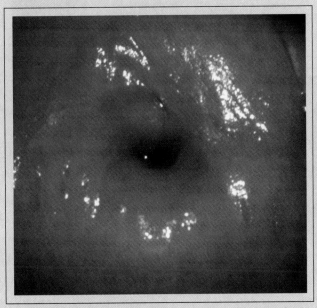

Figure 12-25 This is a colpophotograph of her cervix after the application of 5% acetic acid.

CASE STUDY 1 ANSWERS

FIGURE 12-24

Several cells are seen with enlarged hyperchromatic nuclei, irregular nuclear borders, and sharply punched-out perinuclear halos. These are koilocytes indicative of HPV infection.

FIGURE 12-25

The transformation zone is not fully visualized. Only normal squamous epithelium is seen.
There is no indication for an ectocervical biopsy. The ectocervical epithelium is normal. Because the transformation zone is in the endocervical canal and was not fully visualized, ECC is indicated. It is also necessary to evaluate the vagina for possible disease.

FIGURE 12-26

There are islands of acetowhite epithelium consistent with HPV change in the vagina. Biopsy confirmed the colposcopic impression.

CASE STUDY 2 QUESTIONS

HISTORY

A 28-year-old gravida 1, para 1 is sent to you for evaluation of a Pap smear suggestive of LSIL.

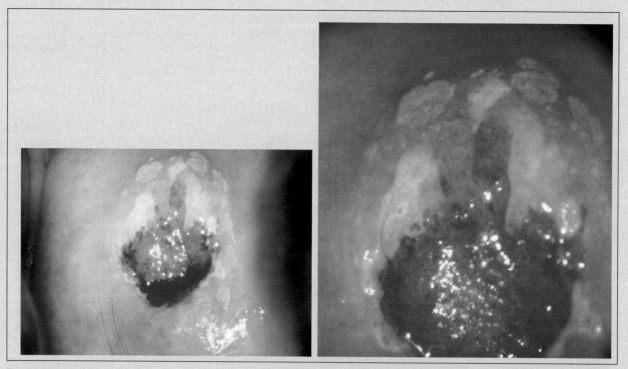

Figures 12-27 and 12-28 These are colpophotographs after the application of 5% acetic acid.

- Is the transformation zone fully visualized?
- Describe any colposcopic findings.
- What is your pathologic diagnosis?
- What are the management options in this patient?

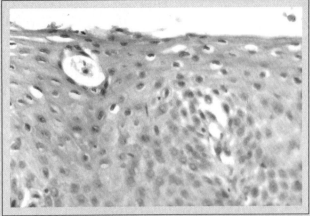

Figure 12-29 The histology of the most severe colposcopic lesion is shown.

CASE STUDY 2 ANSWERS

FIGURES 12-27 AND 12-28

The SCJ is seen along the posterior lip of the cervix, but in Figure 1, bleeding in the endocervical canal obscures the SCJ anteriorly. In Figure 2, it is not possible to see the SCJ despite removal of the blood, but by careful manipulation it was visible (not seen in these views).

There is bright acetowhite epithelium with a sharp geographic border seen adjacent to the SCJ on the posterior lip of the cervix, with some other islands of grayer acetowhite epithelium distally.

FIGURE 12-29

Biopsy at the 6-o'clock position showed bland, well-spaced nuclei without hyperchromasia and only a few scattered perinuclear halos and "raisinoid" nuclei. This is metaplastic epithelium with some suggestion of HPV changes.

There is no reason to treat this patient. Her cervical cytology, colposcopy, and biopsy did not show any evidence of high-grade disease, and even definitive low-grade disease could not be confirmed by biopsy. She is best followed with repeat cytology at 6 and 12 months or HPV testing at 12 months. If these tests are normal, she may return to cytological screening.

CASE STUDY 3 QUESTIONS

HISTORY

A 43-year-old gravida 3, para 3 is seen in your office. She is a smoker (one pack of cigarettes a day) with a history of genital warts 15 years ago. Her Pap smear is depicted in Figure 30.

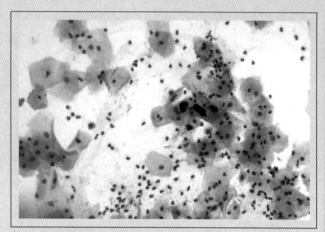

Figure 12-30

- What do you see?
- What is your diagnosis?
- Is the transformation zone fully visualized?
- Describe your findings.
- What is your colposcopic impression of the grade of the lesion?
- What is your diagnosis?
- What should be the next step in this patient's management?

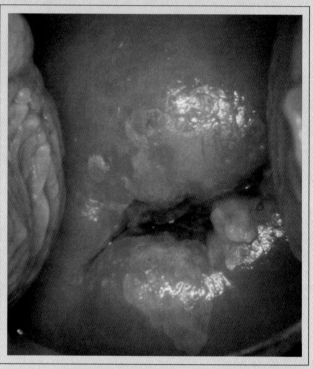

Figure 12-31 This is a photograph of her cervix after the application of 5% acetic acid.

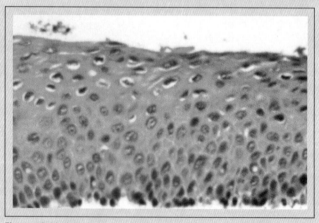

Figure 12-32 A representative colposcopically directed biopsy was taken.

CASE STUDY 3 ANSWERS

FIGURE 12-30

Several cells are seen with large, hyperchromatic nuclei but with abundant cytoplasm. This is consistent with a low-grade lesion.

FIGURE 12-31

The transformation zone is not fully visualized. Although the SCJ is seen from 6 o'clock to 10 o'clock, there is acetowhite epithelium extending into the endocervical canal along the rest of the cervix. However, with some manipulation, the SCJ was seen in its entirety (not shown). There is a gray-white lesion on both the anterior and the posterior lips of the cervix, although some of the lesion is a bit more translucent. The border is geographic. There are no vascular changes.

This appears to be a low-grade lesion.

FIGURE 12-32

There is nuclear crowding about one third to one half of the way to the epithelium with irregular, hyperchromatic nuclei and perinuclear halos seen on the surface. This is consistent with a CIN 1 to CIN 2 lesion with HPV changes.

The recommended follow-up is repeat cytology at 6 and 12 months or an HPV test in 12 months. If cytology shows ASC-US or worse or if the HPV test is positive, repeat colposcopy is recommended. Should the CIN 1 persist for at least 2 years, continued observation or treatment are appropriate options. Excision or ablative treatment is acceptable assuming the colposcopic exam remains satisfactory.

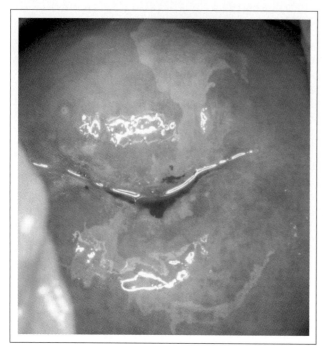

Plate 12-1 Pale acetowhite lesion with jagged "geographic" borders. Classic findings in a low-grade lesion.

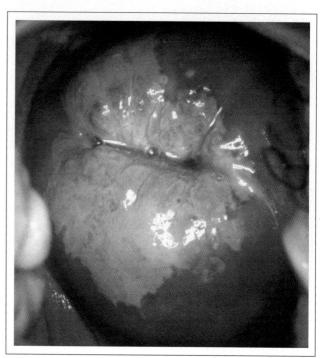

Plate 12-3 This low-grade lesion is more snowy white than the previous two. The geographic borders suggest that this is low grade. This is a satisfactory examination. The SCJ can be easily outlined. There is a suggestion of an internal border at the 5-o'clock position. Observing the lesion over time as the acetic acid effect fades would provide clarification.

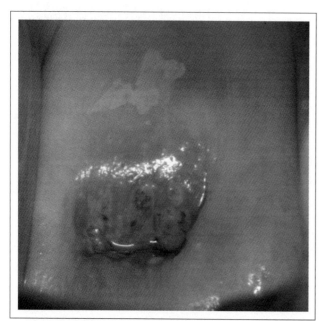

Plate 12-2 The irregular SCJ is outlined with a thin rim of acetowhite epithelium. This is typical of squamous metaplasia. A pale white satellite lesion is visible on the anterior lip. It is called a "satellite" as it is not contiguous with the SCJ. Satellite lesions are usually low-grade lesions or metaplasia.

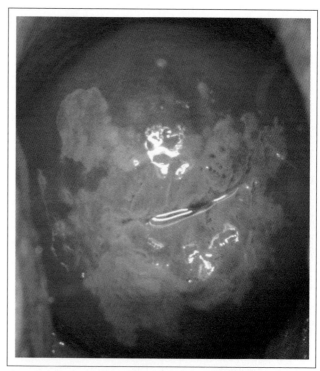

Plate 12-4 There is an extensive pale acetowhite area punctuated by numerous gland openings. Patchy areas of seemingly dense white do not represent true internal borders, as the latter tend to be adjacent to the SCJ. This is a low-grade lesion.

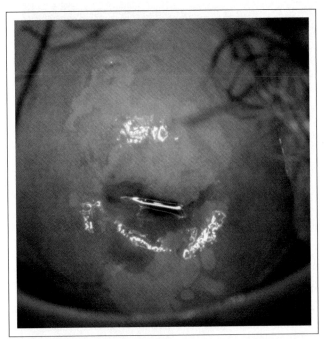

Plate 12-5 The lesion on the anterior lip is pale white with faint "flocculated" borders, more rounded than the usual geographic border. Unlike the lesion on the posterior lip, which although large is a satellite, the anterior lesion begins at the SCJ. Both have features of low-grade lesions.

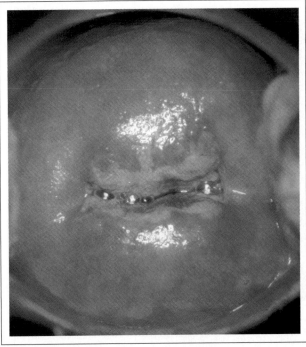

Plate 12-7 A pale acetowhite lesion surrounds the external os. The exam is not satisfactory, as the entire SCJ cannot be outlined. The colposcopist could possibly make the exam satisfactory with a little manipulation of the cervix. Biopsy showed CIN 1.

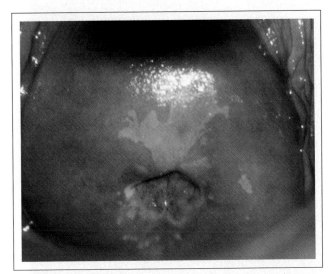

Plate 12-6 The green filter is used on this image. A pale white lesion arises from the SCJ on the anterior lip. Satellite lesions are also visible. These are low-grade lesions. A denser white lesion is barely visible at 9 o'clock. This may represent a small, coincident high-grade lesion.

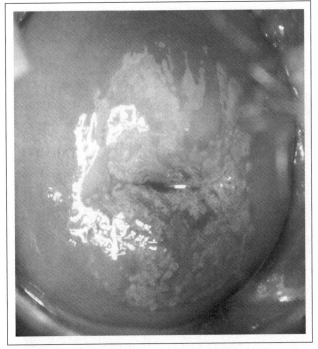

Plate 12-8 A pale acetowhite lesion with jagged "geographic" margins and satellite lesions is noted on the anterior lip. This is a low-grade lesion. Posteriorly, columnar epithelium and squamous metaplasia are noted.

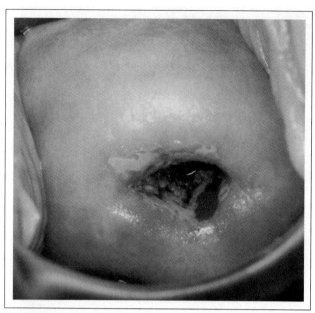

Plate 12-9 A small, pale, low-grade lesion with geographic borders is seen on the anterior lip of the cervix. Vessels are absent.

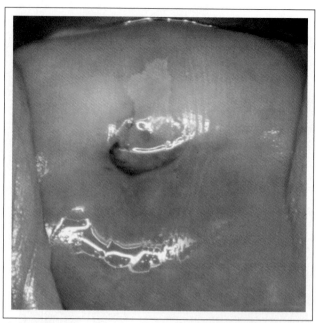

Plate 12-11 Pale acetowhite lesion arising on the anterior lip of the cervix. No vessels are visible. Findings are typical of low-grade squamous intraepithelial lesions.

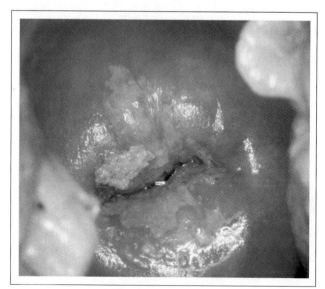

Plate 12-10 Flat low-grade lesions seen on the anterior and posterior lips of the cervix. An exophytic condyloma is seen at 11 o'clock. This is another manifestation of low-grade lesions and may represent infection with a different HPV type than the flat lesion.

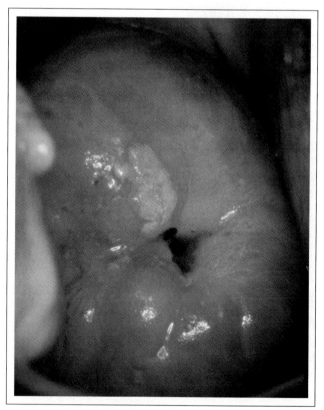

Plate 12-12 Raised condylomatous lesion on the anterior lip of the cervix.

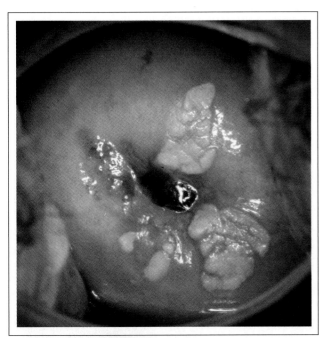

Plate 12-13 Prominent plaques characterized by hyperkeratosis and irregular surface features. This most likely represents condyloma accuminata. As the appearance is somewhat unusual, biopsies would be indicated.

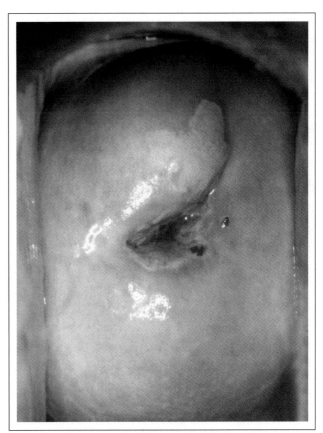

Plate 12-15 Low-grade lesion presenting as a pale acetowhite lesion with geographic borders arising from the anterior lip of the cervix.

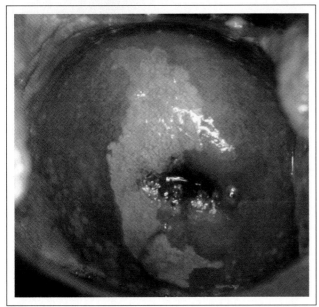

Plate 12-14 This large acetowhite lesion is characterized by geographic borders and a fine mosaic vascular pattern. A biopsy of CIN 1 would be expected. The large acetowhite area in the right lateral portio vaginalis should also be evaluated.

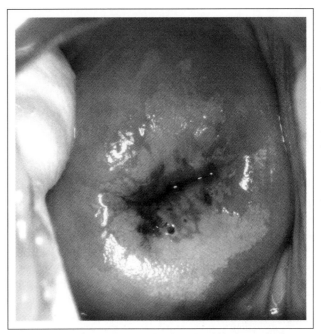

Plate 12-16 This low-grade lesion has flocculated borders and a fine mosaic vascular pattern barely visible on the pale acetowhite background.

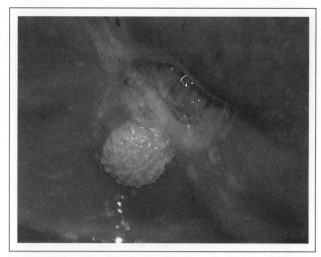
Plate 12-17 Small condyloma arising from margin of previous LEEP

CHAPTER 13

High-Grade Squamous Intraepithelial Lesions

L. Stuart Massad

KEY POINTS

- A cytologic finding of a high-grade squamous intraepithelial lesion (HSIL) accounts for only about 0.5% of all Papanicolaou (Pap) tests.
- Approximately 70% to 75% of women with HSIL will have underlying cervical intraepithelial neoplasia, grade 2 or 3 (CIN 2,3), and about 1% to 4% will have invasive cancer.
- Distinguishing moderate dysplasia (CIN 2) from severe dysplasia (CIN 3) is not highly reproducible but may be useful in managing individual women, especially in cases of discordance between cytologic and colposcopy results.
- Intensive screening leads to earlier diagnosis of CIN 2,3. This means that lesions are smaller and colposcopically more subtle than in classic descriptions. These smaller lesions also may have a longer latency period before the development of invasive cancer and may regress more often than previously reported.
- High-grade lesions found after HSIL cytology may be larger, and colposcopy may be more sensitive in women with HSIL.
- Two options are acceptable in managing women with an HSIL cytology result: either immediate loop excision or colposcopy with colposcopic-directed biopsy.
- Women with HSIL cytology remain at significant risk for CIN even if their colposcopy or biopsy does not show high-grade CIN.
- In women with HSIL, careful examination of the vagina using both 3% to 5% acetic acid and Lugol's solution may reveal a high-grade vaginal lesion not previously appreciated.
- When discordant colposcopic or biopsy findings follow HSIL cytology, two options are available: either proceeding with treatment or following women until either regression is documented or treatment is prompted by persistently abnormal cytology or the appearance of new lesions. Ablative treatments such as cryotherapy or laser ablation are inappropriate.
- Women with an unsatisfactory colposcopic examination and those with CIN of any grade on endocervical assessment may have occult endocervical cancers and are not candidates for ablative treatments. They must undergo excisional therapy. If they are to be treated, the treatment must be excisional.
- Most women with CIN 2,3 have prior borderline cytology. CIN 3 lesions identified after atypical squamous cells of undetermined significance (ASC-US) or low-grade squamous intraepithelial lesion (LSIL) cytology tend to be small, and their short-term cancer risk may be lower than for women diagnosed after HSIL, who may have large lesions that are more easily discernible. However, management guidelines do not differ by antecedent Pap result, and all women with CIN 2,3 should be considered at risk for cancer.
- Acetowhitening is a dynamic process, peaking in intensity some 60 to 90 seconds after application of 3% to 5% acetic acid. High-grade lesions will retain acetowhiteness longer, whereas less serious lesions often fade quickly.

SIGNIFICANCE

A cytologic finding of a high-grade squamous intraepithelial lesion (HSIL) is uncommon, accounting for only about 0.5% of all Papanicolaou (Pap) tests.[1] The risk for HSIL varies by age and is highest among women 25 to 29 years of age.[2] Given the large number of women who have Pap tests each year, approximately 100,000 cases of HSIL will be reported annually in the United States. These women are at substantial risk for cervical cancer, but not all of these women have true preinvasive disease. The critical skill for colposcopists managing women with HSIL is to distinguish women with preinvasive lesions who require treatment from those who do not. Failure to treat women with premalignant lesions can result in progression to cancer, with devastating consequences. On the other hand, treating women with self-limited HPV infections wastes limited resources, creates anxiety and stigmatization, and increases the risk for subsequent pregnancy-related complications. The colposcopist evaluating a woman with HSIL must exclude invasive cancer and define the area of the cervical transformation zone (TZ) appropriate for either immediate treatment or directed biopsy.

High-grade cervical intraepithelial neoplasia (CIN) and cancer are common in women with cytology interpreted as HSIL. *Approximately 70% to 75% of women with HSIL will have underlying cervical intraepithelial neoplasia, grade 2 or 3 (CIN 2,3), and about 1% to 4% will have invasive cancer.*[3,4] The significance of HSIL cytology relates to the underlying cervical disease. A College of American Pathologists (CAP) study found that 7% of women with an HSIL result had no lesion identified, whereas 16% had low-grade changes; 75% had CIN 2,3; and 0.5% had cancer.[3] In a more recent single-institution study, 12% of women with HSIL had no lesions identified at colposcopy and 7% still had no lesion despite months of subsequent follow-up, whereas an additional 18% had only low-grade changes; 71% had CIN 2,3; and 4% had cancer.[4] Negative results may be most confusing in postmenopausal women, in whom atrophy is associated with high nuclear:cytoplasmic ratios and repair after atrophy can result in significant cytologic atypia. Both of these studies suggested that the likelihood of finding no abnormality was greater when colposcopy was delayed. Unfortunately, many of these women had unsatisfactory colposcopy, and cancer usually cannot be excluded without conization.

CYTOLOGY

Under the Bethesda System 2001 for squamous intraepithelial lesions, HSIL encompasses moderate dysplasia (CIN 2) and severe dysplasia, carcinoma *in situ* (CIN 3).[5] *The two-tiered low-grade squamous intraepithelial lesion (LSIL)/HSIL terminology remains unchanged from the 1988 Bethesda System. It is understood that subdividing HSIL into moderate and severe dysplasia or CIN 2 and CIN 3 is not very reproducible. However, LSIL versus HSIL is a fairly reproducible diagnostic breakout. As in previous versions of the Bethesda System, CIN or dysplasia terminology can be used either as a substitute for SIL or as an additional descriptor.*[5,6]

The cells of HSIL are characterized by progressive dedifferentiation, smaller cell size, marked nuclear atypia, and decreased amounts of cytoplasm. As the grade of squamous intraepithelial lesion (SIL) becomes more severe, the cell size becomes smaller. In HSIL, the overall cell size is as small or smaller than normal basal or parabasal cells. In contrast, the cells of a low-grade lesion are larger and approximate in size to a normal intermediate cell. *Although the HSIL nuclei are about the same size as those of LSIL, the nuclei appear larger because of the decrease in the cytoplasmic volume.*

Compared with lower-grade lesions, a marked increase in the nuclear:cytoplasmic ratio occurs in HSIL. Unlike LSIL, HSIL is characterized by lack of human papillomavirus (HPV)-related cytopathic effects, such as perinuclear halos[6] (Figure 13-1). *The absence of koilocytosis in HSIL reflects the absence of a productive HPV infection.* Abnormal mitotic figures frequently observed in histologic sections of HSIL are not commonly seen in cytologic smears.

Only a small rim of cytoplasm may remain around the nucleus *(naked nuclei)*, making the nuclei appear more

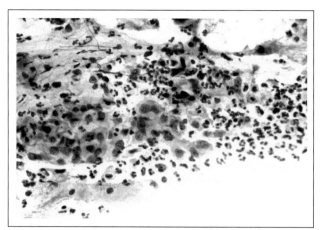

Figure 13-1 Cervical Pap smear: epithelial cell abnormality, HSIL. Dysplastic epithelial cells are seen mixed with acute inflammatory cells. The epithelial cells show moderate nuclear pleomorphism with coarse nuclear chromatin and irregular nuclear outlines. The background is otherwise clean.

prominent. The nuclear outlines become more irregular as the dysplastic process evolves. Hyperchromasia is usually prominent, and the chromatin may be finely or coarsely granular and may appear clumped. Nucleoli are usually absent. The cells may occur singly, in poorly defined sheets, or in syncytial aggregates with poorly defined cytoplasmic borders.

IMPACT OF CERVICAL DISEASE TREATMENTS ON FUTURE PREGNANCY OUTCOME

Before a discussion of triage and management of HSIL, the following data that may affect treatment decisions should be considered. *Several studies published in recent years have documented that treatment for cervical disease results in roughly a doubling of the risk of preterm delivery and other pregnancy-related complications.*[7–9] Treatments responsible for this effect include knife conization, loop excision, and possibly even laser ablation, as well as cryotherapy. These studies are retrospective, and results may be biased if treatment for CIN is linked to other risk factors for preterm delivery. In fact, women with cervical lesions are at increased risk for preterm birth, and treatment may be a marker for other risk factors, including drug use, prior spontaneous or induced pregnancy loss, and medical comorbidity.[10] However, the observation makes sense biologically because all cervical treatments destroy cervical stroma in order to treat CIN buried within endocervical glands. Loss of cervical stroma may remove a margin of safety that might allow otherwise marginal pregnancies to proceed to term. *Some but not all studies of excisional therapy have shown that the depth of cervical destruction is correlated with the risk of preterm delivery, which suggests that for women who need treatment, efforts to minimize the depth of treatment to the shallowest depth that will still result in an effective cure may mitigate future pregnancy risk.*

INITIAL MANAGEMENT

Traditionally, the management of HSIL cytology has relied on the colposcopic identification of high-grade CIN, followed by treatment when lesions are found.[11] This strategy has proven highly successful in reducing cervical cancer rates in developed countries. Most impressive results have come from Scandinavian countries, where national health programs result in near-universal screening. Screening has reduced the incidence of squamous carcinomas but not adenocarcinomas.[12] It has also resulted in the diagnosis of cervical cancers that do develop at earlier stages, with improvements in survival.[12,13] Screening has also reduced the incidence of CIN.[14] *Regrettably, most cervical cancers are now found in women who have defaulted from standard cervical cancer screening protocols.*[15–17] In addition, *intensive screening leads to earlier diagnosis of CIN 2,3. This means that lesions are smaller and colposcopically more subtle than in classic descriptions. These smaller lesions also may have a longer latency period before the development of invasive cancer and may regress more often than previously reported.*

Recently, several concerns have arisen regarding the traditional approach to HSIL cytology results. First, two to three visits are required: one for colposcopy, a second for counseling about results, and if therapy cannot be done that day, a third visit for treatment. Compliance with follow-up is frequently a problem for women with abnormal cytology, especially among less-educated women of lower socioeconomic status—precisely the women at highest risk for later developing cervical cancer. This has made a single-visit strategy attractive to those working with highest-risk women. The introduction of loop excision in the 1990s made immediate treatment feasible. In this strategy, women with HSIL cytology undergo excision of the TZ in the office under local anesthesia at the time of counseling about Pap test results. This strategy has been shown to be feasible and cost-effective.[18–21]

More fundamentally, however, concerns have arisen about the sensitivity of colposcopy in the identification of CIN 2,3. In the ASC-US (Atypical Squamous Cells of Undetermined Significance)/LSIL Triage Study, the sensitivity of colposcopy for identification of CIN 3 was only 54%.[22] *High-grade lesions found after HSIL cytology may be larger, and colposcopy may be more sensitive in women with HSIL cytology results. Studies of immediate loop excision have found CIN 2 in some 35% of women with HSIL and CIN 3 in 45%.*[18,19] Conversely, women have had CIN 1 or no lesion in 15% to 25% of cases. Women with negative colposcopy after abnormal cytology have substantial rates of subsequent disease, which suggests that lesions were missed.[23,24] Indeed, *diligent biopsy of small lesions improves the sensitivity of colposcopy. Colposcopic sensitivity does not appear to improve with experience or training.*[25,26] In fact, random biopsy may be useful in women with HSIL.[27]

According to the 2006 Consensus Conference on Management of Abnormal Cervical Cytology and CIN, organized by the American Society for Colposcopy and Cervical Pathology (ASCCP), *two options are acceptable in managing the woman with an HSIL cytology result: either immediate loop excision or colposcopy with directed biopsy.*[28] Which management is elected depends on several factors. Immediate loop excision may be more appropriate for the older woman, the woman who has missed prior appointments and may default from subsequent follow-up, or the woman who has completed childbearing. Older women are at higher risk for CIN 2 or CIN 3 and are less likely to experience disease regression. Conversely, women considering future pregnancy who have a history of complying with prior appointments are good candidates for colposcopy with directed biopsy (with subsequent management based on the results of the colposcopy and biopsy). In selected cases, immediate excision may be more appropriate for women with large colposcopic lesions, especially those with prominent high-grade features, whereas women with small lesions that have a lower colposcopic grade may be managed with colposcopy and biopsy, with treatment reserved for those with high-grade biopsy results. However, *because of the limited accuracy of colposcopy generally and of colposcopic grading in particular, colposcopic assessment is no longer required before immediate excision.* Nevertheless, prudence would suggest that colposcopy is needed to tailor the excision to the size of the lesion and the limits of the TZ.

Some management strategies are unsuitable for women with HSIL. *Because of the high prevalence of carcinogenic HPV infection in women with HSIL and because of the high rate of underlying high-grade CIN, triage using repeat cytology or HPV testing is unfounded.* A positive test adds nothing to management, and a negative test may be falsely negative, inhibiting the aggressive pursuit of precursors that may progress to cancer during a period of unwarranted observation. Similarly, only immediate excision is acceptable; cervical ablation for HSIL cytology without colposcopy may result in the destruction of occult cancer, with potentially fatal results.

MANAGEMENT OF WOMEN WITH HIGH-GRADE SQUAMOUS INTRAEPITHELIAL LESION BUT NO CERVICAL INTRAEPITHELIAL LESION, GRADE 2 OR 3, AT COLPOSCOPY

When colposcopy with directed biopsy is elected as management of an HSIL cytology result, women with CIN 2 or CIN 3 should be managed according to guidelines for those results (Table 13-1; Figure 13-2). However, discordant results (a negative colposcopy or an exam with abnormalities but biopsies read either as CIN 1 or no lesion) present a dilemma. As noted above, the sensitivity of colposcopy is limited, and these women may harbor an unsuspected high-grade lesion. A British study found that 44% of women with negative evaluations after moderate or severe dyskaryosis had CIN found during follow-up[23] while a Swedish study found 22% of women with HSIL cytology were found to have CIN during follow-up after negative colposcopy.[24] *Women with HSIL cytology remain at significant risk for CIN even if their colposcopy or biopsy does not show high-grade CIN.* However, their immediate risk for cancer appears to be quite low. Furthermore, as noted in the opening of this chapter, the predictive value of an HSIL cytology result is limited, and some women with HSIL have CIN 1, subclinical HPV infections without colposcopically visible lesions, or even no disease. Finally, *cytologic interpretation is subjective, and women with HSIL diagnoses may not have HSIL.* In a study of the reproducibility of cervical cytology, 27% of women with HSIL were found to have LSIL on review of their slides, whereas 23% had ASC-US and 3% had negative results.[29] For women with CIN 1 at colposcopic biopsy, the likelihood of CIN 2,3 at loop excision ranges from 18% to 55%, regardless of prior cytology.[30] Rates are likely to be higher after HSIL.

Before deciding that colposcopy is negative after HSIL cytology, some precautions may be in order. *Careful examination of the vagina using both 3% to 5% acetic acid and Lugol's solution may reveal a high-grade vaginal lesion.* In such a case, although the cervix in fact has no lesion(s), the cytology is correctly positive, and the patient's disease can be cleared with appropriate therapy. *Application of Lugol's solution to the cervix may also identify high-grade lesions not previously appreciated.* For clinicians practicing outside centers of excellence, review of material by an expert gynecologic pathologist may lead to an altered diagnosis, either downgrading of the HSIL cytology or upgrading of biopsy material. If the diagnosis changes, then the course of management should follow the

Table 13-1 2006 ASCCP Management Guidelines for Women with HSIL

- An immediate loop electrosurgical excision or colposcopy with endocervical assessment is an acceptable method for managing women with HSIL, except in special populations (see below). **(BII)**
- When CIN 2,3 is not identified histologically, either a diagnostic excisional procedure or observation with colposcopy and cytology at 6-month intervals for 1 year is acceptable, provided in the latter case that the colposcopic examination is satisfactory and endocervical sampling is negative. **(BIII)**
  - In this circumstance it is also acceptable to review the cytological histological and colposcopic findings; if the review yields a revised interpretation, management should follow guidelines for the revised interpretation. **(BII)**
  - If observation with cytology and colposcopy is elected, a diagnostic excisional procedure is recommended for women with repeat HSIL cytologic results at either the 6- or 12-month visit. **(CIII)**
  - After 1 year of observation, women with two consecutive "negative for intraepithelial lesion or malignancy" results can return to routine cytologic screening.
- A diagnostic excisional procedure is recommended for women with HSIL in whom the colposcopic examination is unsatisfactory, except in special populations (e.g., pregnant women). **(BII)**
- Women with CIN 2,3 should be managed according to the appropriate 2006 Consensus Guideline for the Management of Women with Cervical Intraepithelial Neoplasia. Ablation is unacceptable in the following circumstances: colposcopy has not been performed; CIN 2,3 is not identified histologically; or the endocervical assessment identifies CIN of any grade. **(EII)**
- Triage using either a program of only repeat cytology or HPV DNA testing is unacceptable. **(EII)**

ASCCP, American Society for Colposcopy and Cervical Pathology; *HSIL*, high-grade squamous intraepithelial lesion; *CIN*, cervical intraepithelial neoplasia; *HPV*, human papillomavirus; *DNA*, deoxyribonucleic acid.
From Ref. 28.

Management of Women with High-grade Squamous Intraepithelial Lesion (HSIL) *

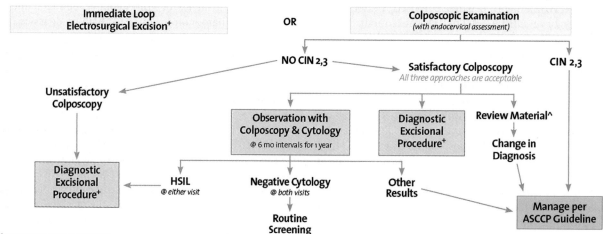

+ Not if patient is pregnant or an adolescent
^ Includes referral cytology, colposcopic findings, and all biopsies
* Management options may vary if the woman is pregnant, postmenopausal, or an adolescent

Figure 13-2 Reprinted from *The Journal of Lower Genital Tract Disease* Vol. 11 Issue 4, with the permission of ASCCP © American Society for Colposcopy and Cervical Pathology 2007. No copies of the algorithms may be made without the prior consent of ASCCP.

new diagnosis. Finally, referral to an expert colposcopist may be in order to obtain additional opinion of the case.

These considerations were weighed during deliberations preceding publication of the 2006 ASCCP Guidelines on Management of Cervical Cytology.[28] *When discordant colposcopic or biopsy findings follow HSIL cytology, clinicians and the women they counsel have two options: either proceeding with treatment or following women until either regression is documented or treatment is prompted by persistently abnormal cytology or the appearance of new lesions* (see Table 13-1 and Figure 13-2). The considerations are similar to those applied at initial management. Concern about occult preinvasive disease is weighed against impact on future childbearing. Cancer must be excluded, and

women with unsatisfactory colposcopic examinations and those with positive endocervical sampling must be treated with excisional therapies. Older women, those with a history of noncompliance, and those who have completed childbearing are optimal candidates for immediate treatment. On the other hand, younger women, especially those contemplating future childbearing, may be more likely to accept the risk of occult high-grade disease and are very unlikely to progress to cancer in the short term.

According to ASCCP guidelines, observation requires both repeat cytology and colposcopy at 6-month intervals until both are negative twice (see Table 13-1 and Figure 13-2). Cytology alone or a single repeat combination examination may be insufficiently sensitive for identifying CIN 2 or CIN 3.

However, once two combination tests are negative, routine screening can be resumed. *If HSIL cytology persists at either of the two follow-up visits, diagnostic excision is required.* If any of the examinations result in atypical squamous cells (ASC) or LSIL cytology or a CIN 1 biopsy, then management should follow the recommendations for those abnormalities (see relevant chapters). However, truncating the observation period at any time by proceeding to treatment may be reasonable because treatment will shorten time to regression and reduce the inconvenience, anxiety, and cost associated with repeated colposcopy and cytology.

In a woman with HSIL cytology in whom no lesion is found, ablative treatments such as cryotherapy or laser ablation are inappropriate because cancer has not been excluded. An occult invasive focus may lie within the endocervical canal beyond the limits of colposcopic detection or may have been missed colposcopically. Such a focus may be destroyed by ablation, leaving behind colposcopically undetectable, deeply infiltrating cancer. The opportunity to detect the need for radical cancer therapy may be missed, which places that patient at risk for later recurrence and death. Furthermore, *women with an unsatisfactory colposcopic examination and those with CIN of any grade on endocervical assessment* (endocervical curettage [ECC], endocervical brushing, or endocervical colposcopic visualization) *may have occult endocervical cancers and thus are not candidates for ablative treatments.* In fact, cancers have been reported after cryotherapy when endocervical assessment was omitted or ignored when positive.[31,32] Instead, such women should undergo excisional treatments, such as loop excision, knife conization, or laser conization.

Most women with HSIL have high-risk HPV deoxyribonucleic acid (DNA). A positive test does not alter management, and testing increases costs without changing outcomes. On the other hand, negative HPV tests in women with HSIL may be falsely negative. A negative test may lead to reassurance and suboptimal surveillance and thus may allow undetected lesions to progress to cancer. *There is no role for HPV testing to guide the management of women with HSIL.* Similarly, the sensitivity of cytology in the identification of CIN 2,3 may be as low as 50%.[33] Repeat cytology may miss a progressive lesion, and cancer may not be identified cytologically until advanced. However, exceptions to this principle exist. The risk of invasive cancer is low before the age of 21 years, and some high-grade lesions regress, especially in younger women. High-grade lesions also rarely progress to invasive cancer during the few months of pregnancy. For these reasons, observation of adolescents, young women, and pregnant women with HSIL appears to be a safe and reasonable approach (Table 13-2).

Management in Adolescents and Young Women with HSIL

The 2006 ASCCP Consensus Conference developed special guidelines for managing adolescents and young women with HSIL.[28] The guidelines defined adolescents as those before their 21st birthday. As noted in chapter 22, many of these women have newly acquired HPV infections that will regress if observed over time. Although their lifetime risk

for developing invasive cervical cancer may be substantial, the likelihood of cancer before their 21st birthday is quite small. The window of opportunity for identifying persistent high-grade cancer precursors is consequently longer, and the urgency of immediate intervention is absent. Thus *immediate excision is inappropriate, and colposcopy with biopsy of visible lesions is the recommended initial management for all adolescents and young women with HSIL cytology* (see Table 13-2; Figure 13-3).

The ASCCP Consensus Conference developed guidelines for the management of adolescents and young women when colposcopy reveals CIN 2 and CIN 3 (see later discussion). However, when colposcopy shows no lesion or when biopsies show either CIN 1 or no neoplasia, the likelihood of cervical cancer being occult or developing during short-term observation is extremely low. Unsatisfactory colposcopy is unusual in adolescents. However if the colposcopy is unsatisfactory or when endocervical sampling yields CIN, diagnostic excision is indicated. In the author's opinion, an exception to this not covered in the 2006 ASCCP Consensus Guidelines would be the younger adolescent with unsatisfactory colposcopy either because of a small, tight nulliparous cervix or because a typical condyloma confirmed by biopsy obscures the endocervical canal. *Except in very unusual circumstances, observation appears prudent for adolescents and young women with satisfactory colposcopy and negative endocervical sampling.* An example of an exception might be the woman approaching 21 years of age with multiple prior abnormal Pap tests and missed clinic appointments who now presents with HSIL cytology. For others, serial Pap testing and colposcopy at 6-month intervals for as long as 2 years is advised. If both Pap testing and colposcopy are negative at two consecutive visits, then routine annual assessment can resume.

If a high-grade colposcopic lesion appears during follow-up, biopsy is indicated. If HSIL cytology persists for 1 year, repeat biopsy of a lesion previously identified as CIN 1 or non-neoplastic changes is recommended (see Table 13-2 and Figure 13-3). Random biopsy may be helpful, and *if HSIL cytology persists for 1 year, random biopsy is recommended even in the face of normal, satisfactory colposcopy.* If CIN 2 or CIN 3 is found in one of these repeat biopsies, then management should follow guidelines for those diagnoses (see later discussion). Similarly, if colposcopy remains negative but cytology is reported as ASC or LSIL, or if CIN 1 is found at repeat biopsy, then management should follow the guidelines for those diagnoses (see chapters 11 and 12). However, *if HSIL cytology persists for 2 years, then a diagnostic excision procedure is required.*

Management in Pregnant Women with HSIL

The goal of cytology and colposcopy during pregnancy is to identify invasive cancer that requires treatment at or before the time of delivery. CIN harms neither the mother nor the fetus, whereas cervical treatments designed to eradicate CIN can result in fetal loss, preterm delivery, and maternal hemorrhage. Similarly, ECC may result in laceration of the soft cervix with consequent hemorrhage, and it may also lead to perforation of amniotic membranes with fetal loss. *ECC is*

Table 13-2 2006 ASCCP Management Guidelines for Special Populations of Women with HSIL

Adolescent Women

- In adolescents with HSIL, colposcopy is recommended. Immediate LEEP (i.e., "see and treat") is unacceptable in adolescent women. **(AII)**
  - When CIN 2,3 is not identified histologically, observation for as long as 24 months using both colposcopy and cytology at 6-month intervals is preferred, provided the colposcopic examination is satisfactory and endocervical sampling is negative. **(BIII)**
  - In exceptional circumstances, a diagnostic excisional procedure is acceptable. **(BIII)**
  - If during follow-up a high-grade colposcopic lesion is identified or HSIL cytology persists for 1 year, biopsy is recommended. **(BIII)**
  - If CIN 2,3 is identified histologically, management should follow the 2006 Consensus Guideline for the Management of Women with Cervical Intraepithelial Neoplasia. **(BIII)**
  - If HSIL persists for 24 months without identification of CIN 2,3, a diagnostic excisional procedure is recommended. **(BIII)**
  - After two consecutive "negative for intraepithelial lesion or malignancy" results, adolescents and young women without a high-grade colposcopic abnormality can return to routine cytologic screening. **(BIII)**
- A diagnostic excisional procedure is recommended for adolescents and young women with HSIL when colposcopy is unsatisfactory or CIN of any grade is identified on endocervical assessment. **(BII)**

Pregnant Women

- Colposcopy is recommended for pregnant women with HSIL. **(AII)**
  - It is preferred that the colposcopic evaluation of pregnant women with HSIL be conducted by clinicians who are experienced in the evaluation of colposcopic changes induced by pregnancy. **(BIII)**
  - Biopsy of lesions suspicious for CIN 2,3 or cancer is preferred; biopsy of other lesions is acceptable. **(BIII)**
- Endocervical curettage is unacceptable in pregnant women. **(EIII)**
- Diagnostic excision is unacceptable unless invasive cancer is suspected based on the referral cytology, colposcopic appearance, or cervical biopsy. **(EII)**
- Re-evaluation with cytology and colposcopy is recommended no sooner than 6 weeks postpartum for pregnant women with HSIL in whom CIN 2,3 is not diagnosed. **(CIII)**

ASCCP, American Society for Colposcopy and Cervical Pathology; *HSIL*, high-grade squamous intraepithelial lesion; *CIN*, cervical intraepithelial neoplasia.
From Ref. 28.

Management of Adolescent Women (20 Years and Younger) with High-grade Squamous Intraepithelial Lesion (HSIL)

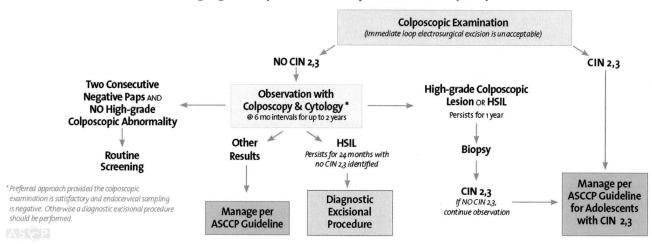

Figure 13-3 Reprinted from *The Journal of Lower Genital Tract Disease* Vol. 11 Issue 4, with the permission of ASCCP © American Society for Colposcopy and Cervical Pathology 2007. No copies of the algorithms may be made without the prior consent of ASCCP.

almost always contraindicated during pregnancy. For these reasons, *immediate excision for HSIL is contraindicated during pregnancy.* All women with HSIL should undergo colposcopy. A strong theoretical case could be made for allowing pregnant adolescents with HSIL to defer colposcopy until after pregnancy, especially if the young woman is within 3 years of sexual debut, but this was not included in recent consensus guidelines.

Colposcopy during pregnancy can be difficult because of increasing eversion (especially in primigravid women), expanding metaplasia, cervical hyperemia, the development of prominent normal epithelial changes that mimic preinvasive disease colposcopically, obscuring mucus, contact bleeding, prolapsing vaginal walls, and bleeding following biopsy (see chapter 21).[34] Colposcopy during pregnancy is best left to experienced examiners. Biopsy during pregnancy has not been linked to fetal loss or preterm delivery. Failure to perform biopsies during pregnancy has been linked to missed invasive cancer.[35-37] Biopsy is especially important if the colposcopic impression is high grade, especially in the older gravida at higher risk for invasive cancer. Although some experts recommend limiting biopsy only to pregnant women with colposcopic findings suspicious for invasive cancer,[36-38] these recommendations came from institutions with high-volume colposcopy clinics. These recommendations probably cannot be generalized to most colposcopy practitioners who rarely see invasive cancer.

Once cancer has been excluded, cervical therapy can be deferred until postpartum. *CIN may regress during the interval between antenatal cytology and a postpartum examination,* either because time elapses, allowing maternal immunity to clear the lesion, or because cervical trauma at the time of delivery destroys superficial lesions. In women with biopsy-proven CIN 2 during pregnancy, the risk of microinvasive cancer at the postpartum visit is negligible, whereas the risk after CIN 3 is substantially less than 10% and deeply invasive cancers are rare.[39,40] For this reason, reassessment after delivery is important in tailoring therapy, whereas re-evaluation during pregnancy may prompt needless intervention that may jeopardize current and future pregnancies.

Colposcopic reassessment can be deferred until at least 6 weeks postpartum if no CIN 2 or CIN 3 is found after HSIL cytology during pregnancy. This avoids potential bleeding that may follow biopsy later in pregnancy. Diagnostic excision for discordance between HSIL cytology and lesser abnormalities on colposcopy or biopsy is unacceptable during pregnancy. Diagnostic excision should only be attempted when invasive cervical cancer is suspected based on cytology, biopsy, or colposcopic appearance. In that case, knife conization should be undertaken in the controlled environment of an operating room after placement of a hemostatic circumferential suture. Office loop excision could be catastrophic for the patient, fetus, and operator.

For all women with HSIL during pregnancy (except those already treated for invasive cancer), colposcopy should be undertaken at least 6 weeks postpartum. This allows for uterine involution and minimizing of blood loss that might otherwise occur from a hypervascular cervix. High-grade lesions may persist, resolve, or progress to invasive cancer during the postpartum period,[41,42] so ablation or excision of the TZ without confirmation of persistent disease is inappropriate.

CERVICAL INTRAEPITHELIAL NEOPLASIA, GRADES 2 AND 3

Background

Through the early and middle years of the last century, the premalignant nature of high-grade CIN was debated. This was because such CIN was often associated with frank cervical cancers and, prior to the development of colposcopy, it was difficult to exclude occult carcinoma adjacent to biopsy sites.

Cytologic screening became increasingly popular through the 1940s and 1950s but required conization to confirm the underlying histology. Because of this, minor grades of abnormality were often followed without intervention. In the 1960s and 1970s, with the popularization of colposcopy in the English-speaking world, clinicians were able to identify precancerous lesions, and their premalignant nature became apparent. Richart devised the current three-tier classification system for CIN[43] although he later described a two-tier system combining CIN 2 and CIN 3 that has been adopted by many pathologists.[44] The development of cryotherapy allowed for office-based therapy. This was followed by the development of laser procedures in the 1980s and loop excision in the 1990s, leading to current standards of practice.

Histology

As HPV-infected cells accumulate mutations, the histologic appearance of the resulting lesions becomes increasingly atypical. Once basal atypia extends into the middle third of the cervical squamous epithelium, CIN 2 is diagnosed. CIN 3 is reported when atypia extends into the upper third of the epithelium. In all grades of CIN, the basement membrane remains intact, and there is no extrusion of basaloid cells into the underlying stroma (Figure 13-4).

As the dysplastic process advances, the basaloid cells exhibit less glycogen and lose the ability to adhere to one another. On an ultrastructural level, the cells begin to lose the surface microridges and develop the presence of abundant microvilli. *The desmosomes and junctional units are lost. The desmosomes no longer effectively attach the epithelium to the basement membrane. Clinically, this process is reflected in the peeling edges of high-grade lesions.*

As CIN progresses, advancing layers exhibit less cytoplasmic maturation, and the cytoplasmic borders become less distinct. In a full-thickness intraepithelial neoplasia, it may not be possible to distinguish the characteristic basal, intermediate, and superficial cell layers. The higher grades of

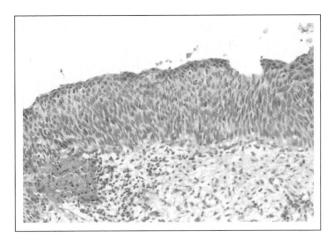

Figure 13-4 CIN 3 biopsy. The epithelium has complete loss of maturation of keratinocytes with marked crowding and vertical orientation of the nuclei. There is virtually no maturation of the squamous epithelial cells from the basal to the superficial layer. Within the submucosa is mild, superficial, chronic inflammation.

CIN tend to be characterized by more mitotic activity in the upper layers. As the mitotic activity increases, basaloid cells replace normal cells in the superficial layers.

Normal cells are diploid, and condyloma acuminatum is often polyploid, but high-grade CIN and invasive cancers are generally aneuploid. As aneuploidy develops, cellular mitotic activity commences throughout all layers of the epithelium. This evidence of a derangement in DNA replication may result in multiple mutations in the genetic structure and result in the progression of the neoplastic process. Cervical lesions with diploid or polyploid DNA contents generally retain polarity of the basal cell layer and lack abnormal mitotic figures. On the other hand, aneuploid lesions have more marked nuclear atypia and more cellular disorganization, and abnormal mitotic figures are present. The best histologic correlate of aneuploidy is abnormal mitotic figures, usually present in the superficial layers of the epithelium. Although an epithelial lesion exhibiting abnormal mitotic figures should be classified as high-grade CIN, high-grade CIN lacking abnormal mitotic figures should still be classified as CIN 2 or CIN 3 if other well-known features of high-grade CIN are present. Although koilocytosis is a characteristic of low-grade lesions, some high-grade cervical intraepithelial lesions will exhibit koilocytosis in the superficial layers but should still be classified as high-grade CIN if they meet the high-grade criteria (Figures 13-5 and 13-6).

Etiology and Natural History

CIN 2,3 arises after infection with specific types of HPV. As noted in Chapter 2, a consensus has emerged that essentially all cervical cancers arise as a result of persistent infection with types of HPV in which the E6 and E7 gene products have high affinity for the tumor-suppressor proteins p53 and pRb.[45] These high-risk carcinogenic types include 16, 18, 31, 33, 35, 39, 45, 51, 52, 56, 58, 59, 68, and 73. Binding of the protein product of the HPV E6 gene

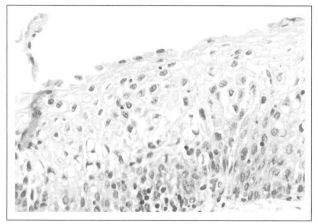

Figure 13-5 CIN 2 with HPV. Nuclear crowding is present in the parabasal area, and the cells within the epithelium lack some degree of maturation, although maturation is present in the upper half of the epithelium. Some of the cells near the surface show some distinct perinuclear halos with binucleation and features of koilocytosis.

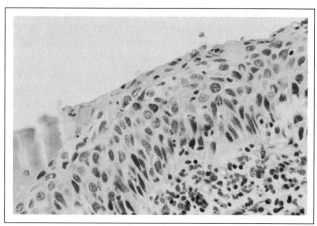

Figure 13-6 CIN 3. There is crowding and irregularity of the cells along the basal layer with lack of maturation involving the lower two thirds of the epithelium. Nuclear pleomorphism within the epithelial cells is very evident here. Inflammatory cells and blood are noted within the superficial stroma. No evidence of HPV is apparent in this biopsy specimen.

leads to inactivation of p53. p53 inactivation in turn leads to multiple effects (impairment of DNA repair and loss of control of mutant cell growth through induced apoptosis). Tetraploidy, chromosome loss, and aneuploidy follow. Degradation of pRb after E7 binding also results in multiple effects, including loss of cell cycle checkpoint controls on cell proliferation. Persistent HPV infection with long-term expression of E6 and E7 leads to clonal proliferations of mutated cervical epithelial cells that grow into lesions visible on colposcopy. Cells in these lesions may acquire constitutive telomerase activation, which in turn leads to immortalization. Over time, lesions enlarge. In order to nourish and oxygenate themselves, these large and metabolically active lesions must stimulate angiogenesis, or the ingrowth of new blood vessels. These vessels are visible colposcopically as mosaic and punctation patterns.

Although rapid progression to invasive cancer has been reported, especially in immunocompromised young women,[46] *in most cases the transition from HPV infection to cancer takes years.* The modal interval from HPV infection to CIN 3 is 7–15 years, with the prevalence of CIN 3 peaking between 25 and 30 years of age, and progression to cancer takes at least a decade longer.[47] Studies of progression are limited by methodology: *Biopsy may induce disease regression, and studies that omit or limit biopsies may miss high-grade disease initially, so later positive biopsies may actually represent persistent disease rather than newly evolved lesions.* Whether CIN 3 and cancer are preceded by stepwise progression from HPV infection to CIN 1 to CIN 2 or whether HPV infection may persist for a long time without detectable lower-grade CIN is controversial.[47] The relatively long latency period between HPV infection and cancer, combined with a high although age-dependent rate of regression, means that some women with CIN 2,3 can be followed without treatment, at least initially.

CIN 3 is generally considered to be a cancer precursor although not all CIN 3 lesions will progress to cancer. The risk of progression of CIN 3 is unclear because most consider the risk too high to justify observation. A biopsy diagnosis of CIN 3 may miss occult invasive cancer, and apparent progression after a colposcopic biopsy diagnosis may reflect missed prevalent cancers. The risk of progression appears to be high but is not absolute. One review found that the likelihood of CIN 3 progressing to invasion was 12%, with 33% regressing and the remainder having stable disease.[48] Studies of topical or oral therapies for CIN have shown somewhat higher regression rates although many of these concluded with excision, and thus the durability of regression in these cases remain in doubt.[49,50] Smaller lesions with more minor colposcopic features are more likely to regress, whereas larger lesions with coarse vascular changes are less likely to regress.[49] CIN 2,3 lesions associated with HPV 16 are less likely to regress, as are those in women with the HLA*201 phenotype.[50] In perhaps the only prospective study, cervical or vaginal cancer developed in 22% of women with carcinoma *in situ* of the cervix who were observed without treatment over an observation interval of 5 to 28 years.[51] Latency periods before progression to cancer extend over many years, allowing for diagnosis and intervention. This may be because most cancers arise in large CIN 3 lesions,[52] and the clonal proliferation of premalignant lesions occurs over extended time periods. Even though the sensitivity of a single Pap test is suboptimal, serial testing over decades according to current guidelines decreases cervical cancer risk by 92%.[53]

For many years, clinicians considered cervical carcinogenesis to be a stepwise process, beginning with CIN 1 and progressing to CIN 2, then to CIN 3, and finally to invasive cancer.[54] Current understanding is more nuanced.[55] Carcinogenesis begins with infection with a carcinogenic HPV, even before development of CIN 1. *It appears that for some HPV types, rapid transition to CIN 3 may occur without an intervening low-grade lesion although the further progression to cancer still requires several years.*[55] *For other women, low-grade disease regresses, HPV is cleared through cell-mediated immunity, and cancer never develops. For yet others, the classical pathway of progression from CIN 1 through CIN 3 and on to cancer still appears valid.*

The significance of CIN 2 is unclear. The risk of progression to CIN 3 and cancer appears greater than for women with CIN 1. However, many women with CIN 2 will have regression of their lesions without therapy. In one review, CIN 2 progressed to cancer in 5% and to CIN 3 in 20%, persisted in 40%, and regressed in 40%.[48] Many CIN 2 lesions are polyclonal, whereas cancers appear to arise from monoclonal proliferations.[56] No accepted tests are available to distinguish CIN 2 that reflects an exuberant HPV infection from that with true malignant potential. *The cutoff between CIN 1 and CIN 2 on the one hand and between CIN 2 and CIN 3 on the other is arbitrary. The reproducibility of a diagnosis of CIN 2 is poor, and many women will have either CIN 1 or CIN 3.*[57] Many pathologists do not attempt to distinguish between CIN 2 and CIN 3, instead reporting a composite diagnosis: *CIN 2,3*. The 2006 ASCCP Consensus Guidelines reflect this evolution in reporting.

The decision among leaders in colposcopy and cervical cancer prevention in the United States has been to consider CIN 2 the threshold for treatment for most U.S. women.

This provides a margin of safety and ensures that, despite the risk of underdiagnosis, significant numbers of women with CIN 3 are unlikely to progress to cancer while being observed for regression. However, newer data show that cervical therapies may have adverse effects on pregnancy, including preterm delivery and low birth weight.[8,9] These findings have led many experts to advocate observation of CIN 2, especially among younger women.

Although the likelihood of CIN 2,3 after HSIL is much greater than that after ASC-US or LSIL, the higher prevalence of these lesser cytologic results means that *most women with CIN 2,3 present with borderline cytology.*[58] *CIN 3 lesions identified after ASC-US or LSIL cytology tend to be small, and their short-term cancer risk may be lower than for women diagnosed after HSIL, who may have large lesions that are more easily discernible.*[59] *However, management guidelines do not differ by antecedent Pap result, and all women with CIN 2,3 should be considered at risk for cancer.*

Colposcopy

Traditionally, grading systems have been employed to help define the likelihood that a colposcopic lesion reflects underlying CIN 2,3. The most commonly taught of these systems is the Reid Colposcopic Index (RCI) (see chapter 10.2).[60] The RCI involves scoring lesions according to acetowhitening, contour, vascular changes, and color change in response to application of 5% acetic acid and Lugol's iodine. Caution should be exercised in interpreting these features. *Acetowhitening is a dynamic process, peaking in intensity some 60 to 90 seconds after application of 3% to 5% acetic acid.*[61] *High-grade lesions will retain dense whiteness, whereas lesser lesions often fade quickly.* Vascular changes may be more prominent using the green filter. More severe lesions tend to be associated with coarse mosaic and punctation in response to neovascularizing stimuli from increasingly dedifferentiated premalignant cells. However, variations in the coarseness of vascular changes are continuous and designation of vascular changes as coarse is subjective.

The colposcopic features suggestive of high-grade disease have been defined by the International Federation for Cervical Pathology and Colposcopy.[62] These include the following:

- A generally smooth surface with a sharp outer border
- Dense acetowhite change that appears early, is slow to resolve and is often oyster white in color
- Coarse punctation and wide irregular mosaics of differing size
- Iodine negativity, with a yellow appearance in an area that was densely white after application of acetic acid

In addition, classic high-grade colposcopic lesions are commonly large, multiquadrant lesions. *The coarse vascular changes in high-grade colposcopic lesions may be either mosaic, or punctation, or both.* Contact bleeding may obscure the most pronounced vascular changes, and *some high-grade lesions have no vascular changes. The margins of a high-grade lesion are usually smooth, in contrast to the irregular, geographic, or flocculated margins of lower-grade lesions. The edges of a high-grade* lesion may peel, a reflection of aberrant expression of intercellular and matrix binding proteins as cells become more atypical. High-grade lesions often are present inside an internal margin near the squamocolumnar junction (SCJ), associated with a larger low-grade lesion with more translucent acetowhite epithelium and fine punctate or mosaic vascularity. Identifying internal margins within large and prominent low-grade lesions is critical to correct colposcopic diagnosis, as biopsy of the more impressive lesion may result in underdiagnosis and failure to treat a preinvasive lesion.

It is easier to distinguish high-grade lesions of the cervix from low-grade lesions than it is to distinguish low-grade lesions from normal findings or from an inflammatory process. The high sensitivity and low specificity of colposcopy are most likely due to "overcalling" of low-grade lesions. The specificity of colposcopy improves when the threshold is set to distinguish high-grade lesions and cancer from less severe abnormalities.

Treatment is based on the highest grade of CIN present, regardless of the other grades of CIN that may be present. High-grade cervical lesions may be found anywhere in the TZ, but most are seen close to the SCJ. It has been suggested that CIN 2 or CIN 3 begins as a small focus of highly dysplastic epithelium near the SCJ, probably in an area of immature squamous metaplasia, and eventually expands peripherally. Areas of high-grade CIN can also form at the proximal edge of the field of a preexisting low-grade lesion. The detection of an internal line of demarcation (internal margin) that separates a central area of significant colposcopic atypia from a larger field of lower-grade acetowhite epithelium is a reliable sign of high-grade cervical disease (Figure 13-7). This observation highlights the centripetal structure of CIN, with the less-differentiated, higher-grade component being more centrally located and the better-differentiated portion residing at the periphery. In general, the most abnormal area of a lesion will be contiguous with the SCJ. This is an important point because a large lesion may have

rather spectacular (but low-grade) geographic change at its peripheral margin but centrally harbor a more ominous high-grade lesion. If the colposcopist fails to note the less obvious but more severe central lesion, as demonstrated by a lesion with an internal margin, the colposcopic biopsy may be misdirected, and the patient may subsequently be undertreated.

The size of the TZ and of the lesion, the intensity of the color, the distinctiveness of the margins, the pattern of the vessels, and the presence of micropapillae are all highly and independently correlated with the histologic grade. The likelihood of finding a higher histologic grade was estimated as an odds ratio (OR). Variation in the acetowhite color was the most important finding with an OR of 16 (95% confidence interval [CI], 10–26). Coarse vessels versus no vessels had an OR of 10 (95% CI, 3.2–34). Fine vessels versus no vessels had an OR of 1.6 (CI, 1.1–2.5). Large and medium-sized lesions showed ORs of 3.6 and 2, respectively.

When viewed with a red-free (green) filter before the application of 3% to 5% acetic acid, high-grade lesions may exhibit abnormal vessel patterns such as mosaic and punctation (Figure 13-8). These patterns may disappear after the application of 3% to 5% acetic acid owing to the constriction of narrow vessels by the intense swelling of the dysplastic epithelium. Not all high-grade lesions exhibit abnormal vessel patterns; therefore the absence of vessels does not imply that the lesion lacks significance. In fact, punctation and mosaic patterns are seen more often in low-grade CIN.

As the metabolic rate increases within HSIL, vascular dilation resists the constrictive effects of epithelial swelling, thus resulting in persistence of the mosaic and punctation patterns after the application of 3% to 5% acetic acid. However, the presence or absence of a vascular pattern is not diagnostic of either a high-grade lesion or a low-grade lesion. As the intercapillary distance of the vessels increases, the vessel patterns appear coarser, and the vessels can achieve significant dilation (Figures 13-9 and 13-10). As lesion severity progresses, the abnormal vessels may transition to atypical vessels as the vessels begin to run horizontally across the epithelium.

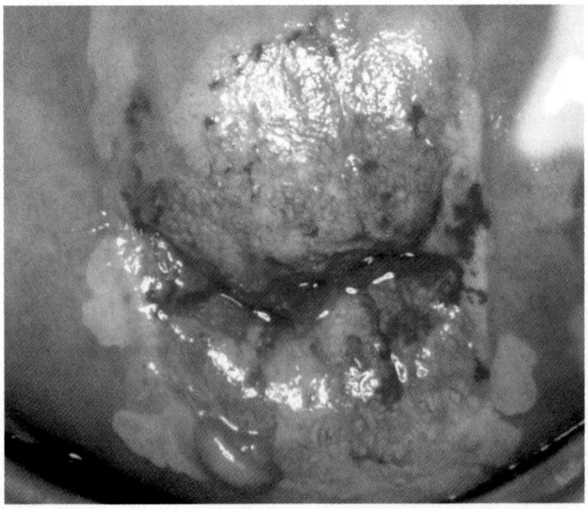

Figure 13-7 A large, high-grade lesion with an internal border on the anterior lip of the cervix. Note how the geographic peripheral color changes abruptly toward the os, taking on a denser, whitish color. A coarse mosaic is also present. Disease is present on the posterior lip of the cervix as well. Multiple punch biopsies revealed CIN 3.

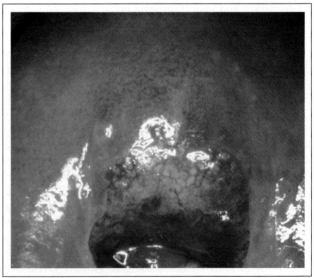

Figure 13-8 Example of green filter examination showing accentuation of mosaic.

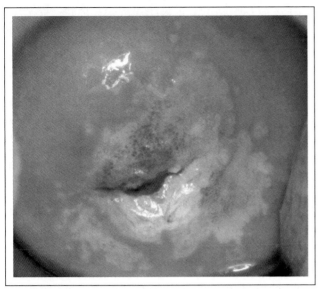

Figure 13-9 Peripheral low-grade squamous intraepithelial lesion, with irregular margins and central HSIL with coarse punctation anteriorly and with dense acetowhite epithelium and internal margin at 3 to 5 o'clock. Biopsy revealed CIN 2.

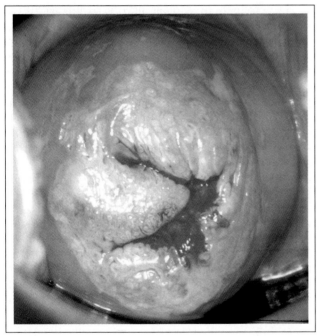

Figure 13-10 Large HSIL with coarse mosaic at 10 to 11 o'clock.

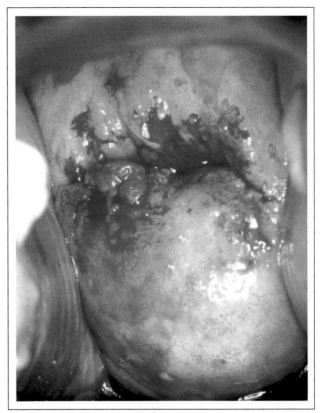

Figure 13-11 HSIL with dense acetowhite epithelium on the anterior lip that is peeling off after being touched with a cotton-tipped applicator.

It has been demonstrated that patients younger than 35 years with documented CIN 2 or CIN 3 may present with trivial colposcopic findings of doubtful significance. However, women older than 35 years with CIN 2 or CIN 3 are much more likely to present with trivial findings.

Care must be taken when examining a high-grade lesion to avoid detaching the surface epithelium by abrasion. As cervical lesions become more abnormal, the desmosomal anchors loosen, allowing the overlying diseased epithelium to more easily detach from the basement membrane. Colposcopically, this epithelial detachment is exhibited as a rolled or peeling margin (Figure 13-11). Care must be taken when examining a high-grade lesion to avoid detaching the surface epithelium by abrasion. Sometimes manipulation with a cotton-tipped applicator alone for the purposes of better visualization of the cervix is enough to detach the epithelium. If the cervical biopsy specimen is submitted to pathology unattached to the basement membrane and underlying stroma, it is impossible to determine the grade of the lesion or whether the lesion is invasive, often yielding the unsatisfying report of "dysplasia—unable to grade."

Limits to Colposcopic Grading

An evolving understanding of cervical disease has suggested that colposcopic grading oversimplifies the approach to colposcopic diagnosis of CIN 2,3. Moreover, as borderline cytology leads increasingly often to colposcopy, atypical presentations of CIN 2,3 are becoming more common. Studies of colposcopic grading, especially the RCI, have shown that increasing scores are highly associated with increasing grade of disease. Unfortunately, *the discriminant value of colposcopic grading appears to be suboptimal.*[63] Some lesions with metaplastic or low-grade features contain CIN 2,3. Conversely, some lesions with high-grade features contain CIN 1, condylomatous changes, or atypical metaplasia. In addition, early studies of colposcopic grading used inappropriate statistics. *More recent studies suggest that the correlation between colposcopic impression and biopsy grade is only fair to poor.*[64,65]

Of greatest concern, some women with early CIN 3 may have no visible lesions colposcopically. In the ASC-US/LSIL Triage Study (ALTS), the sensitivity of intake colposcopy to identify CIN 3 that was diagnosed within 2 years of study enrollment (presumed to be present from that time, although sometimes missed) was only 54%.[22] Gage and colleagues analyzed data from the ALTS and found that the sensitivity for identifying CIN 3 improved as the number of biopsies increased.[25] One study suggested that adding random biopsy of colposcopically normal cervix to colposcopically directed biopsies improved sensitivity significantly.[27]

The emerging consensus appears to be that colposcopic grading may be useful to define what portion of a lesion to biopsy and to prioritize sequence as biopsy sites are selected, but that all colposcopic lesions should be biopsied. Management is defined by the highest grade of any lesion. This strategy can increase pathology costs, and some authorities have suggested minimizing this by placing multiple biopsies in a single container. Doing so eliminates the feedback that allows colposcopists to improve their correlation between the colposcopic appearance of a lesion and the ultimate histology. It also risks having the one high-grade lesion missed if one of multiple biopsy specimens in a single specimen container is missed during processing.

Management

Because all CIN 2,3 lesions must be considered to have the potential to evolve into cancer if untreated, therapy is indicated. Cure rates vary according to lesion size, lesion grade, and patient age. The latter is likely a reflection of disease within the endocervical canal. Treatments include cryotherapy, laser ablation, laser conizing, knife conization, and loop electrosurgical excision. Although studies in general have been small and may have difficulty in distinguishing subtle differences among treatments, *various treatments appear to be similarly efficacious in eradicating preinvasive disease,* a proxy measure for preventing cervical cancer.[66–68] *Selection of the appropriate treatment modality depends on operator experience, equipment availability, lesion size, and other factors.* For example, a woman with a large CIN 3 lesion might not be best treated with cryotherapy if the lesion is larger than available cryoprobes. Alternatively, if the lesion extends onto the vagina, laser ablation may be more appropriate, as it can be tailored to encompass the entire lesion with excellent depth control. When microinvasive cancer is suspected, then loop excision and knife conization provide histologic specimens for assessment.

However, *ablative treatments* (e.g., cryotherapy, laser) *can only be employed after rigorously excluding invasive cancer.* When endocervical assessment shows CIN or when colposcopic visualization of the SCJ is unsatisfactory, cancer may be present but unseen. Ablative therapy in these circumstances may result in the later presentation of cancer that was probably missed at initial treatment.[31,32] When cytology or colposcopy suggests cancer, additional histologic material must be collected to better define the diagnosis. Finally, *after prior therapy, skip lesions may be present, and these may contain focal invasive cancer.* In these cases, ablation may result in destruction of cancer that later recurs at an advanced stage, with potentially lethal results. In contrast, excisional treatments (e.g., laser conization, knife conization, loop excision) yield a diagnostic specimen, and occult cancer can be identified, allowing for appropriate radical therapy.

Laser and loop electrosurgical excision offer an advantage over cold-knife conization in that they minimize blood loss by thermal cautery during excision. However, this results in some thermal artifact, at least at the margins.[69,70] In some circumstances, thermal artifact may impair the interpretability of a specimen excised for CIN 2,3. This might alter therapy, as in cases of CIN 2,3 when cytology or colposcopy indicates invasive cancer. Cautery artifact at a focus of possible microinvasion might make interpretation impossible, and concern about undertreatment might lead to radical therapy that would have been unnecessary if the specimen was better preserved. In these cases, either knife conization or wide excision using a large loop may be preferable.

Truly premalignant CIN 2,3 is the histologic expression of high-risk HPV infection. Although occasional low-risk HPV types may cause CIN 2, most CIN 2,3 lesions are associated with high-risk HPV. A positive test does not alter management. Falsely negative HPV tests may occur as a result of sampling or processing errors, so a negative result should not change management. Thus *there is little role for HPV testing in the management of women with untreated CIN 2,3* (Table 13-3, Figure 13-12).

Similarly, *cytology cannot be used to follow untreated CIN 2,3.* The sensitivity of cytology may be as low as 50%.[33] When CIN 3 is present, the next step in oncogenesis is the development of invasive cancer. There is no latitude for error. Repeat cytology may miss a progressive lesion, and cancer may not be identified cytologically until advanced. However as with HSIL, exceptions to this principle exist. The risk of progression to invasive cancer is low before the age of 21 years, and some CIN 2,3 lesions regress, especially in younger women. CIN 2,3 rarely progresses to invasive cancer during the few months of pregnancy. For these reasons, after excluding cancer, *observation of adolescents and young women and of pregnant women appears safe and reasonable approach* (Table 13-4, Figure 13-13).[71]

CIN 2,3 is a premalignant lesion, but it is not cancer. Eradication of the cervical TZ will eliminate cells at risk for progression to malignancy. Removing the uterine fundus can add substantially to the risk of perioperative morbidity, yet it does little to decrease the risk of recurrence, which is usually reflected as later vaginal intraepithelial neoplasia or cancer. One retrospective study of women treated for CIN 3 found recurrences in 3% of women after loop excision and 1% after hysterectomy; this difference was not significant although the study was too small to control for significantly higher-risk lesions in the hysterectomy group.[72] Another study found unsuspected cancers in 8% of women undergoing hysterectomy for CIN 2,3, which suggests that prior conization is mandatory to exclude malignancy.[73] For these reasons, *hysterectomy is never acceptable as the primary therapy for CIN 2,3.*

Management of Positive Excision Margins

Women with CIN 2,3 involving excision margins and those with CIN 2,3 at postprocedure endocervical sampling are at increased risk for persistence compared with those with clear margins.[74–79] In two studies from one center that included 5386 women after conization for CIN 3, recurrence was found in 0.4%

Table 13-3 2006 ASCCP Management Guidelines for Women with CIN 2,3

Initial Management

- Both excision and ablation are acceptable treatment modalities for women with a histological diagnosis of CIN 2,3 and satisfactory colposcopy, except in special circumstances (see below). **(AI)**
- A diagnostic excisional procedure is recommended for women with recurrent CIN 2,3. **(AII)**
- Ablation is unacceptable and a diagnostic excisional procedure is recommended for women with a histological diagnosis of CIN 2,3 and unsatisfactory colposcopy. **(AII)**
- Observation of CIN 2,3 with sequential cytology and colposcopy is unacceptable, except in special circumstances (see below). **(EII)**
- Hysterectomy is unacceptable as primary therapy for CIN 2,3. **(EII)**

Follow-Up after Treatment

- Acceptable post-treatment management options for women with CIN 2,3 include HPV DNA testing at 6 to 12 months. **(BII)**
  - Follow-up using either cytology alone or a combination of cytology and colposcopy at 6-months intervals is also acceptable. **(BII)**
  - Colposcopy with endocervical sampling is recommended for women who are HPV DNA positive or have a repeat cytology result of ASC-US or greater. **(BII)**
  - If the HPV DNA test is negative or if two consecutive repeat cytology tests are "negative for intraepithelial lesion or malignancy," routine screening for at least 20 years commencing at 12 months is recommended. **(AI)**
  - Repeat treatment or hysterectomy based on a positive HPV DNA test is unacceptable. **(EII)**
- If CIN 2,3 is identified at the margins of a diagnostic excisional procedure or in an endocervical sample obtained immediately after the procedure, reassessment using cytology with endocervical sampling at 4-6 months post-treatment is preferred. **(BII)**
  - Performing a repeat diagnostic excisional procedure is acceptable. **(CIII)**
  - Hysterectomy is acceptable if a repeat diagnostic procedure is not feasible.
- A repeat diagnostic excision or hysterectomy is acceptable for women with a histological diagnosis of recurrent or persistent CIN 2,3. **(BII)**

ASCCP, American Society for Colposcopy and Cervical Pathology; *CIN*, cervical intraepithelial neoplasia; *HPV*, human papillomavirus; *DNA*, deoxyribonucleic acid; *ASC-US*, atypical squamous cells of undetermined significance.
From Ref. 71.

Management of Women with a Histological Diagnosis of Cervical Intraepithelial Neoplasia - (CIN 2,3) *

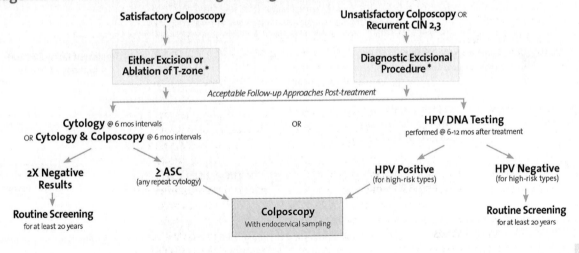

*Management options will vary in special circumstances

Figure 13-12 Reprinted from *The Journal of Lower Genital Tract Disease* Vol. 11 Issue 4, with the permission of ASCCP © American Society for Colposcopy and Cervical Pathology 2007. No copies of the algorithms may be made without the prior consent of ASCCP.

with clear margins and 22% with involved margins, with cancers in 7% of recurrences.[80,81] A positive excision margin is a convenient marker for recurrence, especially when the endocervical margin is involved. However, multiple studies have shown that margin involvement by CIN is not an independent marker for recurrence or persistence.[74-76] *Independent risks for recurrence or persistence of CIN include older age, larger lesions, and higher-grade disease, with risks as high as 50% for older women with large CIN 3 lesions.* Expansion

of the indications for colposcopy to include women with atypical Pap tests has resulted in CIN 2,3 being diagnosed in smaller lesions, and these women may have lower rates of persistence or recurrence than those reported historically. Cold-knife conization can be tailored to encompass large lesions, whereas loop excision may remove lesions in multiple passes, resulting in cut-through margins that do not reflect the true patient margin. These artifactually positive margins are unlikely to have the same significance as true

Table 13-4 2006 ASCCP Management Guidelines for Special Populations of Women with CIN 2,3

Adolescent and Young Women

- For adolescents and young women with a histological diagnosis of CIN 2,3 not otherwise specified, either treatment or observation for as long as 24 months using both colposcopy and cytology at 6-month intervals is acceptable, provided colposcopy is satisfactory. **(BIII)**
  - When a histological diagnosis of CIN 2 is specified, observation is preferred but treatment is acceptable. When a histological diagnosis of CIN 3 is specified, or when colposcopy is unsatisfactory, treatment is recommended. **(BIII)**
- If the colposcopic appearance of the lesion worsens, or if HSIL cytology or a high-grade colposcopic lesion persists for 1 year, repeat biopsy is recommended. **(BIII)**
  - After two consecutive "negative for intraepithelial lesion or malignancy" results, adolescents and young women with normal colposcopy can return to routine cytologic screening. **(BII)**
- Treatment is recommended if CIN 3 is subsequently identified or if CIN 2,3 persists for 24 months. **(BII)**

Pregnant Women

- In the absence of invasive disease or advanced pregnancy, additional colposcopic and cytological examinations are acceptable in pregnant women with a histological diagnosis of CIN 2,3 at intervals no more frequent than every 12 weeks. **(BII)**
  - Repeat biopsy is recommended only if the appearance of the lesion worsens or if cytology suggests invasive cancer. **(BII)**
  - Deferring re-evaluation until at least 6 weeks postpartum is acceptable. **(BII)**
  - A diagnostic excisional procedure is recommended only if invasion is suspected. **(BII)**
  - Unless invasive cancer is identified, treatment is unacceptable. **(EII)**
- Re-evaluation with cytology and colposcopy is recommended no sooner than 6 weeks postpartum. **(CIII)**

ASCCP, American Society for Colposcopy and Cervical Pathology; *CIN*, cervical intraepithelial neoplasia; *HSIL*, high-grade squamous intraepithelial lesion. From Ref. 71.

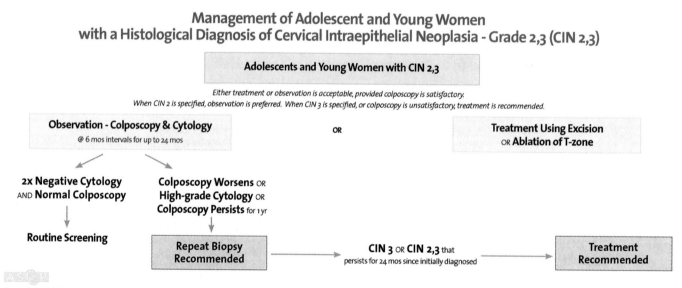

Management of Adolescent and Young Women with a Histological Diagnosis of Cervical Intraepithelial Neoplasia - Grade 2,3 (CIN 2,3)

Figure 13-13 Reprinted from *The Journal of Lower Genital Tract Disease* Vol. 11 Issue 4, with the permission of ASCCP © American Society for Colposcopy and Cervical Pathology 2007. No copies of the algorithms may be made without the prior consent of ASCCP.

positive margins. In addition, postprocedure electrical and chemical cautery can eradicate residual disease at the margin. Women with apparent positive margins at loop excision may not have residual disease, and some women with clear margins may have persistent CIN.[74–76, 82]

Traditional management of involved conization margins has included surveillance, repeat conization, or hysterectomy (see Table 13-3, Figure 13-12).[71] Observation is increasingly preferred, and hysterectomy is almost never required. Strategies for surveillance of women with positive margins include serial cytology, HPV testing, and combination cytology and HPV testing. Combination testing is most sensitive but also most costly. Reassessment with cytology and endocervical sampling

should occur 6 months after the procedure. Many experts include colposcopic assessment as well.[83] The endocervical sampling can be ECC, but including an endocervical brushing with the cytology sample is more sensitive and less painful.[84] This approach is ideal for women who are younger and hope to maintain fertility, as re-excision increases the risk of preterm delivery and pregnancy complications.

Alternatively, when excision margins or postprocedure sampling is positive, conization can be employed to exclude invasive cancer in the canal. Repeat conization provides the greatest reassurance that cancer has been excluded. Such an approach may be most important for women with CIN 3 at the endocervical margin, especially after treatment of large lesions excised after cytology or colposcopy suspicious for invasive cancer. Women may be unwilling to proceed if initial conization failed to provide definitive management, and the residual cervix may be too small to allow safe repeat conization without risk for bladder and vaginal injury.

However, hysterectomy may be considered for women with involved excision margins and other indications for hysterectomy, such as abnormal bleeding or uterine fibroids. Hysterectomy may be most appropriate when the residual cervix is too small for safe excision or because the patient's fear of cancer or other circumstances leads her to decline consent for more conservative management. Vaginal hysterectomy minimizes recovery time and allows the operator to ensure that all involved epithelium is excised, but care is needed to avoid bladder injury after conization. When abnormal bleeding contributes to a decision for hysterectomy, careful assessment must be carried out to exclude endocervical carcinoma as the cause, and if any findings raise suspicions for cancer, re-excision must precede hysterectomy. Women undergoing hysterectomy after conization for CIN 2,3 should be counseled that they may have complications from surgery despite a later finding that no residual disease was present. They also should be advised that pathologic assessment may show occult carcinoma invading deeply into the cervical stroma, with risk for metastasis into parametria and nodal beds. Radiation is required if an occult cancer is present. Survival is not altered provided radiation is initiated promptly and parametrial margins are clear although morbidity may be higher than when primary radiotherapy is administered.[85–87] For that reason, an examination under anesthesia should be done prior to hysterectomy for CIN 2,3 with involved margins, and the planned procedure should be aborted and chemoradiotherapy substituted if parametrial invasion by cancer is found. Radical parametrectomy is also an option for women with occult carcinoma after simple hysterectomy.[88] To minimize the chance that occult carcinoma will be missed when simple hysterectomy is undertaken after conization, the pathologist should be asked to comprehensively section the cervix as for a cone biopsy.

Duration of Follow-Up after Treatment

No therapy for CIN 2,3 (including hysterectomy) achieves cure in all cases. This may be because conservative treatment misses disease extending into the cervical canal above the limit of therapy or laterally beyond the limits of treatment. It may occur because of autoinoculation with persistent carcinogenic HPV in tissues that were not treated. Finally, it may occur because of reinfection with new carcinogenic HPV types. *Persistent untreated CIN 2,3 is likely responsible for most high-grade recurrences within the first or second year after treatment, whereas new viral infections probably account for many low-grade recurrences and some late high-grade recurrences.*

Observation after treatment requires long-term surveillance (see Table 13-3, Figure 13-12).[71] Although most recurrent or persistent CIN is found within the first 1 to 5 years, cancers have been found as long as 20 years after initial therapy.[89,90] A British study of 2244 women followed after treatment for CIN found that the sensitivity of cytology in identifying recurrent or persistent CIN is only 64%. Adding colposcopy improved sensitivity to 91% but reduced specificity from

95% to 88%.[91] A combination of HPV testing and cytology is the most sensitive but the least specific and most costly program for identifying persistent or recurrent CIN.[92] HPV testing alone is highly sensitive, and a single test at 1 year will detect most recurrences, with follow-up HPV testing or cytology identifying most later recurrences. In these circumstances, repeat colposcopy with endocervical sampling using brush cytology or curettage is required if carcinogenic HPV is detected. *Hysterectomy is never indicated for persistent HPV detected after treatment of CIN 2,3 unless recurrent high-grade CIN is found.*

Cytology alone is less sensitive, but it is easily available and generally understood by patients and providers. In addition, few women present with invasive cancers soon after treatment for CIN 2,3, so there is usually time for serial cytologic assessment over many years. With repeated tests comes an improvement in sensitivity. Outcomes are identical whether persistent CIN 2,3 is identified immediately or after a delay, so long as persistent disease is identified and eradicated before invasion occurs. For this reason, *serial cytology testing should be employed 6 and 12 months after treatment, as risk for persistence and recurrence is highest during the first year. Annual cytology should be conducted in subsequent years.* Data are insufficient to determine whether cytology intervals can be extended safely to every 3 years or whether combination HPV testing and cytology is cost-effective after CIN therapy. Colposcopy with endocervical sampling is indicated if cytology results of ASC-US or a more serious lesion is found.

For most patients, retreatment results in long-term cure. *Excision, ablation, and hysterectomy are not indicated for management of carcinogenic HPV in the absence of documented CIN 2,3.* Similarly, although diagnostic excision may be indicated after HSIL or atypical glandular cell (AGC) cytology results, ablation is unacceptable because cancer has not been excluded, and hysterectomy is contraindicated unless diagnostic excision is infeasible. As noted earlier, after prior treatment and subsequent healing, islands of at-risk squamous epithelium may be isolated in the endocervical canal. To avoid undertreatment of these skip lesions, in most cases, *excisional rather than ablational therapy is preferred for recurrent CIN 2,3.* Hysterectomy is also acceptable for women who have completed childbearing.

Management in Adolescent Women

There is a paucity of evidence on the natural history of CIN 2,3 in young women (see Table 13-4, Figure 13-13).[71] High-grade lesions are not uncommon in adolescent women with abnormal colposcopy.[93–96] In these colposcopy studies, rates of CIN 2,3 have ranged from 10% to 35% for ASC-US, 3% to 24% for LSIL, and 52% to 86% for HSIL. The risk of CIN 2,3 does not appear to rise with age among teenagers.[94]

Despite the relatively high risk of high-grade CIN in adolescents with abnormal cytology, outcomes for these women are unclear. The likelihood that young women will develop invasive cervical cancer is very low: there were only 12 cases of cervical cancer annually in 2000 to 2003, and no cervical cancer deaths were reported in women younger than age 20 years in 2000 to 2003.[97] In addition, as noted previously, many cases of CIN 2 will regress, especially in younger women, in whom CIN 2 is often merely an expression of exuberant HPV infection that may be cleared as the immune system is activated. In one nonrandomized, retrospective Norwegian study of women younger than age 30 years with Pap reports showing moderate dysplasia, CIN 2+ was diagnosed in 70% who had immediate colposcopy but in only one third who were followed cytologically for 12 months.[98] This suggests that some 40% of CIN 2+ lesions regressed during the first year. There are no observational studies of frank CIN 3 in young women.

For a clinician managing a women with CIN 2,3 diagnosed before the age of 21 years, the goal of management shifts from eradicating a lesion that may progress to cancer at any time to observing lesions that may regress. Eradication of a lesion destined to regress contributes little to cancer prevention, and it can have substantial morbidity, especially during future pregnancies (Table 13-4).

When young women have unequivocal CIN 3, there is no margin for error. Although cancer is unlikely in the short term, lifetime cancer risk is high, and progression will result in the development of invasive cancer, with potentially devastating consequences. CIN 3 lesions are less likely to regress than lesser lesions. Similarly, when CIN 2,3 is associated with unsatisfactory colposcopy, a frank CIN 3 may be located within the endocervical canal. Although in young women the SCJ is often widely lateral to the cervical os, when it is hidden in the canal (especially in the presence of high-grade disease), treatment is prudent. Even when CIN 2 or CIN 2,3 is found in the presence of satisfactory colposcopy, treatment may be considered. This would be the case, for example, in an older adolescent several years after first intercourse who may have other risk factors for cervical cancer such as smoking and who has been noncompliant with prior appointments for cervical evaluation or follow-up.

However, there is an option for *young women with CIN 2 and CIN 2,3 and satisfactory colposcopy* that avoids the treatment-related risk of cervical insufficiency. *Young women may be observed, but observation requires both cytology and colposcopy at 6-month intervals.* This can continue for as long as 2 years, as most lesions that will regress will do so during that time. As a safety measure, if the lesion being followed develops an increasingly high-grade appearance at any time, or if HSIL cytology persists for 1 year, then repeat biopsy should be undertaken, with treatment if CIN 3 is found. If the lesion persists for 2 years, then treatment is recommended. On the other hand, when regression does occur, as documented by two consecutive normal Pap test results and negative colposcopic examinations, young women can return to annual screening. Apparent partial regression to CIN 1 often represents new HPV infection. This may also be the case when colposcopic lesions resolve but cytology continues to be reported as ASC or LSIL. In these cases, management can follow the new diagnosis.

Management in Pregnancy

The goal of Pap testing during pregnancy is to identify women with invasive cancer that may endanger the life of the mother. When colposcopy during pregnancy identifies CIN 2,3, subsequent diagnosis of a life-threatening cancer is rare. Indeed, *many gynecologic oncologists elect to follow early cancers*

in pregnant women to avoid fetal mortality and the considerable morbidity that results from radical hysterectomy performed when uterine blood flow is increased by pregnancy.[99-101] Preinvasive lesions can be followed until at least 6 weeks postpartum, when eradication can be undertaken with reduced risk.

Clinicians following women with CIN 2,3 during pregnancy (see Table 13-4)[71] may either perform repeat colposcopic and cytologic assessments in an effort to identify occult invasive cancer or defer additional evaluation until the postpartum period. Repeat cytology and colposcopy may be important in identifying the rare occult cancer for women diagnosed early in pregnancy, especially in the older gravida when colposcopy is unsatisfactory, the lesion is large, or CIN 3 is diagnosed. In that case, assessment should be deferred at least 12 weeks to allow the lesion to evolve. At reassessment, biopsy should be repeated only if the lesion's colposcopic appearance is worsening or if cytology suggests invasive cancer. Conversely, when the lesion is identified after the second trimester deferring reassessment until postpartum may be prudent. It also is reasonable when colposcopy is satisfactory, the lesion is modest in size, the colposcopic appearance suggests low or intermediate grade, or when only CIN 2 is diagnosed at biopsy.

A diagnostic excision is rarely indicated during pregnancy. It should be considered only if invasive cancer is suspected on the basis of cytology, colposcopic appearance, or biopsy. Diagnostic excision of the pregnant cervix risks hemorrhage and pregnancy loss. It should be conducted only in an operating room with access to large-bore intravenous lines and blood for transfusion. Pre-excision placement of a cerclage suture may minimize bleeding, and excision can be done with either a scalpel or electrosurgical loop.[102,103] In most cases, the development of a cervical ectropion is one of the changes accompanying pregnancy, and excision may involve only the superficial portion of the cervix rather than deep excision into the endocervical canal—a *coin* biopsy rather than a conventional *cone* biopsy. Because of the substantial risks, treatment of CIN 2,3 is unacceptable during pregnancy.

MANAGEMENT SCENARIOS

Scenario 1

Sentinel Pap: HSIL
Colposcopic findings or histologic cell type if a biopsy was done: CIN 1 or no CIN found
HPV testing for high-risk (oncogenic) HPV types: Not applicable (N/A)
Satisfactory colposcopy: Yes
Fertility desires: Yes

In the 2006 guidelines, three options are considered acceptable for a woman with the above-listed findings. These include either a diagnostic excisional procedure or observation with colposcopy and cytology at 6-month intervals for 1 year or review of the cytology, histology and colposcopy. A review of the rationale supporting these guidelines will help determine the best option for this patient. About 75% of all women with HSIL cytology have CIN 2,3 on biopsy, and 1% to 4% may have invasive cancer, thus it is reasonable to proceed with a diagnostic excision. Women with negative colposcopy after abnormal cytology have substantial rates of subsequent disease, which suggests that lesions were missed. When high-grade CIN is not identified, it may mean that the lesion is small, and diligent biopsy of small lesions improves the sensitivity of colposcopy. However, in ALTS, the sensitivity of initial colposcopy for CIN 3 was only 54%, and the risk of CIN in follow-up after negative colposcopy was 20%. In ALTS, the risk of CIN 3 after two negative Pap tests was only 11%. This argues for colposcopy and biopsy, not immediate treatment. In the 2001 guidelines, when colposcopy was negative after HSIL cytology, review was recommended. This was based on evidence from ALTS that showed that of 433 smears read as >HSIL, 27% were downgraded to LSIL, 23% were downgraded to ASC-US, and 0.3% were read as normal. This suggests a substantial value to reviewing cytology. However, other studies show that most clinical pathologists are less likely to reverse readings on review than research pathologists. Therefore in the 2006 guidelines when colposcopic findings do not reflect HSIL, review of the Pap slide is *acceptable* but not required. The rationale is that some insurers will not pay for review, some labs will not release slides for review, and most pathologists will not reverse an HSIL diagnosis of another pathologist. In the final analysis, with the knowledge that any therapy for CIN may interfere with the ability to carry a pregnancy to term in the future, this woman (who desires future fertility) deserves every opportunity to avoid treatment that is unnecessary. The cytology slides should be reviewed and, if the lesion is downgraded, she should be managed according to the lower-grade reading. She should undergo colposcopy and biopsy, rather than immediate treatment, and because no lesion was found, she should be followed with cytology and colposcopy every 6 months.

Scenario 2

Sentinel Pap: HSIL
Colposcopic findings or histologic cell type if a biopsy was done:
    CIN 1 or no CIN found
HPV testing for high-risk (oncogenic) HPV types: N/A
Satisfactory colposcopy: No
Fertility desires: N/A

This scenario is identical to Scenario 1, except that the colposcopy was not satisfactory (or the ECC was positive for CIN). With an unsatisfactory colposcopy, the SCJ is not visible, and therefore a lesion, if present, may not be apparent. Because 75% of all women with HSIL cytology have CIN 2,3, 1% to 4% may have invasive cancer, and CIN 3 or invasive cancer cannot be excluded without evaluating all the epithelium at risk, this woman must have an excisional conization regardless of her desire for future fertility.

Scenario 3

Sentinel Pap: Any
Colposcopic findings or histologic cell type if a biopsy was done:
    CIN 2,3 on conization; margins positive for CIN 2,3

HPV testing for high-risk (oncogenic) HPV types: N/A
Satisfactory colposcopy: N/A
Fertility desires: Yes

If CIN 2,3 is identified at the margins of a diagnostic excisional procedure or in an endocervical sample obtained immediately after the procedure, reassessment using cytology with endocervical sampling at 4 to 6 months post-treatment is preferred. Recurrences are found in about 25% of women with involved margins, but risk factors include older age and larger lesions. Although repeat conization is also acceptable in this woman, it is likely to affect her future ability to carry a pregnancy and, given this patient's interest in future fertility, conservative follow-up seems most prudent.

COUNSELING SCENARIOS

One of the more difficult counseling scenarios that clinicians experience is the management of a young woman with CIN 2,3 and positive margins on conization. In such cases, both the patient and her physician are concerned about the possibility that she has residual CIN 2,3 and possibly even unrecognized cervical cancer, and there is a natural tendency to want to repeat the conization. Unfortunately, we know that a single conization may double the risk of premature delivery in a future pregnancy, and although no studies on the effect of two or more conizations have been performed, the likelihood is that the risk of prematurity will be even higher. In such cases, several points need to be considered. First, women who were regularly screened before the discovery of CIN 2,3 are very unlikely to have undiscovered invasive cervical cancer. Furthermore, if the patient does have residual CIN 2,3, it is very unlikely to progress to invasive cancer in the following 6 to 12 months of follow-up. In a patient reliable for follow-up, the persistent disease is likely to be discovered and can be treated at that time. The cure rate for treating a persistent lesion immediately is no different than when the same lesion is treated 1 year later. Finally, given the recurrence rate of women with CIN 2,3 and positive margins (about 25%), treating this woman immediately carries a 75% risk of unnecessary treatment, whereas careful follow-up carries little additional risk for the patient.

With this rationale, it would seem easy to convince the patient that watchful waiting is in her best interest. However, in reality, fear of the unknown usually overcomes rational thinking, and both the clinician and the patient often lean toward the decision to do a repeat conization. In the author's experience, this is often due to clinicians' lack of confidence in their own argument not to re-treat. Patients are very astute and can usually read the clinician's body language. If the clinician lacks confidence in his or her recommendation, the patient can usually tell and will then insist on re-treatment. The clinician may rationalize that he or she has given the patient fair and balanced counseling and that the patient has made a choice by which the clinician is bound to abide. However, in the end, it is the clinician's lack of confidence in the recommendation that evolves into a poor clinical decision. The solution to this problem is for the clinician to be convinced and in turn to be convincing in presenting the recommendation. If the patient can be confidently assured that follow-up is in her best interest, she is likely to accept the recommendation.

REFERENCES

1. Davey DD, Neal MH, Wilbur DC, et al. Bethesda 2001 implementation and reporting rates: 2003 practices of participants in the College of American Pathologists Interlaboratory Comparison Program in Cervicovaginal Cytology. Arch Pathol Lab Med 2004;128:1224–1229.

2. Insinga RP, Glass AG, Rush BB. Diagnoses and outcomes in cervical cancer screening: a population-based study. Am J Obstet Gynecol 2004;191:105–113.

3. Jones BA, Novis DA. Cervical biopsy-cytology correlation. A College of American Pathologists Q-Probes study of 22,439 correlations in 348 laboratories. Arch Pathol Lab Med 1996; 120:523–531.

4. Massad LS, Collins YC, Meyer PM. Biopsy correlates of abnormal cervical cytology classified using the Bethesda System. Gynecol Oncol 2001;82:516–522.

5. Solomon D, Davey D, Kurman R, et al, for the Forum Group members and the Bethesda 2001 Workshop. The 2001 Bethesda System: terminology for reporting results of cervical cytology. J Am Med Assoc 2002;287:2114–2119.

6. Kurman RJ, Solomon D. The Bethesda System for Reporting Cervical/Vaginal Cytologic Diagnoses. New York: Springer-Verlag, 1994.

7. Kyrgiou M, Koliopoulos G, Martin-Hirsch P, et al. Obstetric outcomes after conservative treatment for intraepithelial or early invasive cervical lesions: systematic review and meta-analysis. Lancet 2006;367:489–498.

8. Crane JMG. Pregnancy outcome after loop electrosurgical excision procedure: a systematic review. Obstet Gynecol 2003;102:1058–1062.

9. Jakobsson M, Gissler M, Sainio S, et al. Preterm delivery after surgical treatment for cervical intraepithelial neoplasia. Obstet Gynecol 2007;109:309–313.

10. Bruinsma F, Lumley J, Tan J, et al. Precancerous changes in the cervix and risk of subsequent preterm birth. Br J Obstet Gynecol 2007;114:3–4.

11. Kurman RJ, Henson DE, Herbst AL, et al. Interim guidelines for management of abnormal cervical cytology. J Am Med Assoc 1994;271:1866.

12. Sigurdsson K. Quality assurance in cervical cancer screening: the Icelandic experience 1964–1993. Eur J Cancer 1995;31:728–734.

13. Adami HO, Ponten J, Sparen P, et al. Survival trend after invasive cervical cancer diagnosis in Sweden before and after cytologic screening. Cancer 1994;73:140–147.

14. Benedet JL, Anderson GH, Matisic JP. A comprehensive program for cervical cancer detection and management. Am J Obstet Gynecol 1992;166:1254–1259.

15. Nasca PC, Ellish N, Caputo TA, et al. A epidemiologic study of Pap screening histories in women with invasive carcinomas of the uterine cervix. N Y State J Med 1991;91:152–156.

16. Fruchter RG, Boyce J, Hunt M. Missed opportunities for early diagnosis of cancer of the cervix. Am J Public Health 1980;70:418–420.

17. Kinney W, Sung HY, Kearney KA, et al. Missed opportunities for cervical cancer screening of HMO members developing invasive cervical cancer (ICC). Gynecol Oncol 1998;71: 428–430.

18. Irvin WP, Andersen WA, Taylor PT, et al. "See-and-treat" loop electrosurgical excision. Has the time come for a reassessment? J Reprod Med 2002;47:569–574.

19. Numnum TM, Kirby TO, Leath CA, et al. A prospective evaluation of "see and treat" in women with HSIL Pap smear results: is this an appropriate strategy? J Lower Genital Tract Dis 2005;9:2–6.

20. Ferris DG, Hainer BL, Pfenninger JL, et al. "See and treat" electrosurgical loop excision of the cervical transformation zone. J Fam Pract 1996;42:253–257.

21. Shafi MI, Luesley DM, Jordan JA, et al. Randomised trial of immediate versus deferred treatment strategies for the management of minor cervical cytological abnormalities. Br J Obstet Gynaecol 1997;104:590–594.

22. The ASCUS-LSIL Triage Study (ALTS) Group. Results of a randomized trial on the management of cytology interpretations of atypical squamous cells of undetermined significance. Am J Obstet Gynecol 2003;188:1383–1392.

23. Milne DS, Wadehra V, Mennim D, et al. A prospective follow-up study of women with colposcopically unconfirmed positive cervical smears. Br J Obstet Gynaecol 1999;106:38–41.

24. Hellberg D, Nilsson S, Valentin J. Positive cervical smear with subsequent normal colposcopy and histology—frequency of CIN: a long-term follow-up. Gynecol Oncol 1994;53:148–151.

25. Gage JC, Hanson VW, Abbey K, et al, for the ASC-US LSIL Triage Study (ALTS) Group. Number of cervical biopsies and sensitivity of colposcopy. Obstet Gynecol 2006;108: 264–272.

26. Baum ME, Rader JS, Gibb RK, et al. Colposcopic accuracy of obstetrics and gynecology residents. Gynecol Oncol 2006; 103:966–970.

27. Pretorius RG, Zhang WH, Belinson JL, et al. Colposcopically directed biopsy, random cervical biopsy, and endocervical curettage in the diagnosis of cervical intraepithelial neoplasia II or worse. Am J Obstet Gynecol 2004;191:430–434.

28. Wright TC Jr, Massad LS, Dunton CJ, Spitzer M, Wilkinson EJ, Solomon D; for the 2006 ASCCP-Sponsored Consensus Conference. 2006 consensus guidelines for the management of women with abnormal cervical screening tests. J Low Genit Tract Dis. 2007 Oct;11(4):201–222.

29. Stoler MH, Schiffman M, for the ALTS Group. Interobserver reproducibility of cervical cytologic and histologic interpretations: realistic estimates from the ASCUS-LSIL Triage Study. J Am Med Assoc 2001;285:1500–1505.

30. Massad LS, Halperin CJ, Biterman P. Correlation between colposcopically directed biopsy and cervical loop excision. Gynecol Oncol 1996;60:400–403.

31. Townsend DE, Richart RM, Marks E, et al. Invasive cancer following outpatient evaluation and therapy for cervical disease. Obstet Gynecol 1981;57:145–149.

32. Sevin BU, Ford JH, Girtanner RD, et al. Invasive cancer of the cervix after cryosurgery. Pitfalls of conservative management. Obstet Gynecol 1979;53:465–471.

33. Nanda K, McCrory DC, Myers ER, et al. Accuracy of the Papanicolaou test in screening for and follow-up of cervical cytologic abnormalities: a systematic review. Ann Intern Med 2000;132:810–819.

34. Coppleson M, Reid BL. A colposcopic study of the cervix during pregnancy and the puerperium. J Obstet Gynaec Brit Cwlth 1966;73:575–585.

35. Cristoforoni PM, Gerbaldo DL, Philipson J, et al. Management of the abnormal Papanicolaou smear during pregnancy: lessons for quality improvement. J Lower Genital Tract Dis 1999;3:225–230.

36. Benedet JL, Selke PA, Nickerson KG. Colposcopic evaluation of abnormal Papanicolaou smears in pregnancy. Am J Obstet Gynecol 1987;157:932–937.

37. Paraskevaidis E, Koliopoulos G, Kalantaridou S, et al. Management and evolution of cervical intraepithelail neoplasia during pregnancy and postpartum. Eur J Obstet Gynecol Reprod Biol 2002;104:67–69.

38. Woodrow N, Permezel M, Butterfield L, et al. Abnormal cervical cytology in pregnancy: experience of 811 cases. Aust N Z J Obstet Gynaecol 1998;38:161–165.

39. Roberts CH, Dinh TV, Hannigan EV, et al. Management of cervical intraepithelial neoplasia during pregnancy: a simplified and cost-effective approach. J Lower Genital Tract Dis 1998; 2:67–70.

40. Boardman LA, Goldman DL, Cooper AS, et al. CIN in pregnancy: antepartum and postpartum cytology and histology. J Reprod Med 2005;50:13–18.

41. Siddiqui G, Kurzel RB, Lampley EC, et al. Cervical dysplasia in pregnancy: progression versus regression post-partum. Int J Fertil 2001;46:278–280.

42. Kaplan KJ, Dainty LA, Dolinsky B, et al. Prognosis and recurrence risk for patients with cervical squamous intraepithelial lesions diagnosed during pregnancy. Cancer 2004;102:228–232.

43. Richart RM. Natural history of cervical intraepithelial neoplasia. Clin Obstet Gynecol 1967;10:748–784.

44. Richart RM. A modified terminology for cervical intraepithelial neoplasia. Obstet Gynecol 1990;75:131–133.

45. Munoz N, Castellsague X, Berrington de Gonzalez A, et al. Chapter 1: HPV in the etiology of human cancer. Vaccine 2006;24S3:S3/1–S3/10.

46. Maddux HR, Varia MA, Spann CO, et al. Invasive carcioma of the uterine cervix in women age 25 or less. Int J Radiat Oncol Biol Physics 1990;19:701–706.

47. Moscicki AB, Schiffman M, Kjaer S, et al. Chapter 5: updating the natural history of HPV and anogenital cancer. Vaccine 2006;24S3:S42–S52.

48. Ostor AG. Natural history of cervical intraepithelial neoplasia: a critical review. Int J Gynecol Pathol 1993;12:186–192.

49. Brewer CA, Wilczynski SP, Kurosaki T, et al. Colposcopic regression patterns in high-grade cervical intraepithelial neoplasia. Obstet Gynecol 1997;90:617–621.

50. Trimble CL, Piantadosi S, Gravitt P, et al. Spontaneous regression of high-grade cervical dysplasia: effects of human papillomavirus type and HLA phenotype. Clin Cancer Res 2005;11: 4717–4723.

51. McIndoe WA, McLean MR, Jones RW, et al. The invasive potential of carcinoma-in-situ of the cervix. Obstet Gynecol 1984;64:451–458.

52. Tidbury P, Singer A, Jenkins D. CIN 3: the role of lesion size in invasion. Br J Obstet Gynaecol 1992;99:583–586.

53. Eddy DM. Screening for cervical cancer. Ann Intern Med 1990;113:214–226.

54. Richart RM. Natural history of cervical intraepithelial neoplasia. Clin Obstet Gynecol 1967;10:748–784.

55. Kiviat N. Natural history of cervical neoplasia: overview and update. Am J Obstet Gynecol 1996;175:1099–1104.

56. Enomoto T, Haba T, Fujita M, et al. Clonal analysis of high-grade squamous intra-epithelial lesions of the uterine cervix. Int J Cancer 1997;73:339–344.

57. Parker MF, Zahn CM, Vogel KM, et al. Discrepancy in the interpretation of cervical histology by gynecologic pathologists. Obstet Gynecol 2002;100:277–280.

58. Kinney WK, Manos MM, Hurley LB, et al. Where's the high-grade cervical neoplasia? The importance of minimally abnormal Papanicolaou diagnoses. Obstet Gynecol 1998;91: 973–976.

59. Sherman ME, Wang SS, Tarone R, et al. Histopathologic extent of cervical intraepithelial neoplasia 3 lesions in the Atypical Squamous Cells of Undetermined Significance Low-Grade Squamous Intraepithelial Lesion Triage Study: implications for subject safety and lead-time bias. Cancer Epidemiol Biomarkers Prev 2993;12:372–379.

60. Reid R, Scalzi P. Genital warts and cervical cancer. VII. An improved colposcopic index for differentiating benign papillomaviral infections from high-grade cervical intraepithelial neoplasia. Am J Obstet Gynecol 1985;153:611–618.

61. Pogue BW, Kaufman HB, Zelenchuk A, et al. Analysis of acetic acid-induced whitening of high-grade squamous intraepithelial lesions. J Biomed Opt 2001;6:397–403.

62. Walker P, Dexeus S, De Palo G, et al. International terminology of colposcopy: an updated report from the International Federation for Cervical Pathology and Colposcopy. Obstet Gynecol 2003;101:175–178.

63. Jeronimo J, Schiffman M. Colposcopy at a crossroads. Am J Ostet Gynecol 2006;195:349–353.

64. Ferris DG, Litaker MS, for the ALTS Group. Prediction of cervical histologic results using an abbreviated Reid Colposcopic Index during ALTS. Am J Obstet Gynecol 2006;194:704–710.

65. Massad LS, Collins YC. The strength of correlations between colposcopic impression and biopsy histology. Gynecol Oncol 2003;89:424–428.

66. Mitchell MF, Tortolero-Luna G, Cook E, et al. A randomized clinical trial of cryotherapy, laser vaportization, and loop electrosurgical excision for treatment of squamous intraepithelial lesions of the cervix. Obstet Gynecol 1998;92:737–744.

67. Alvarez RD, Helm CW, Edwards RP, et al. Prospective randomized trial of LLETZ versus laser ablation in patients with cervical intraepithelial neoplasia. Gynecol Oncol 1994;52:175–179.

68. Duggan BD, Felix JC, Muderspach LI, et al. Cold-knife conization versus conization by the loop electrosurgical excision procedure: a randomized, prospective study. Am J Obstet Gynecol 1999;180:275–282.

69. Wright TC, Richart RM, Ferenczy A, et al. Comparison of specimens removed by CO2 laser conization and the loop electrosurgical excision procedure. Obstet Gynecol 1992;79:147–153.

70. Messing MJ, Otken L, King LA, et al. Large loop excision of the transformation zone (LLETZ): a pathologic evaluation. Gynecol Oncol 1994;52:207–211.

71. Wright TC Jr, Massad LS, Dunton CJ, Spitzer M, Wilkinson EJ, Solomon D; 2006 American Society for Colposcopy and Cervical Pathology-sponsored Consensus Conference. 2006 consensus guidelines for the management of women with cervical intraepithelial neoplasia or adenocarcinoma in situ. J Low Genit Tract Dis. 2007 Oct;11(4):223–239.

72. Kang SB, Roh JW, Kim JW, et al. A comparison of the therapeutic efficacies of large loop excision of the transformation zone and hysterectomy for the treatment of cervical intraepithelial neoplasia III. Int J Gynecol Cancer 2001;11:387–391.

73. Kesic V, Dokic M, Atanackovic J, et al. Hysterectomy for treatment of CIN. J Low Genit Tract Dis 2003;7:32–35.

74. Lu CH, Liu FS, Kuo CJ, et al. Prediction of persistence or recurrence after conization for cervical intraepithelial neoplasia III. Obstet Gynecol 2006;107:830–835.

75. Moore BC, Higgins RV, Laurent SL, et al. Predictive factors from cold knife conization for residual cervical intraepithelial neoplasia in subsequent hysterectomy. Am J Obstet Gynecol 1995;173:361–368.

76. Kalogirou D, Antoniu G, Karakitsos P, et al. Predictive factors used to justify hysterectomy after loop conization: increasing age and severity of disease. Eur J Gynaec Oncol 1997;18:113–116.

77. Phelps JY, Ward JA, Szigeti J, et al. Cervical cone margins as a predictor for residual dysplasia in post-cone hysterectomy specimens. Obstet Gynecol 1994;84:128–130.

78. Chang DY, Cheng WF, Torng PL, et al. Prediction of residual neoplasia based on histopathology and margin status of conization specimens. Gynecol Oncol 1996;63:53–56.

79. Kobak WH, Roman LD, Felix JC, et al. The role of endocervical curettage at cervical conization for high-grade dysplasia. Obstet Gynecol 1995;85:197–201.

80. Reich O, Pickel H, Lahousen M, et al. Cervical intraepithelial neoplasia III: long-term outcome after cold-knife conization with clear margins. Obstet Gynecol 2001;97:428–430.

81. Reich O, Lahousen M, Pickel H, et al. Cervical intraepithelial neoplasia III: long-term follow-p after cold-knife conization with involved margins. Obstet Gynecol 2002;99:193–196.

82. Murdoch JB, Morgan PR, Lopes A, et al. Histological incomplete excision of CIN after large loop excision of the transformation zone (LLETZ) merits careful follow up, not retreatment. Br J Obstet Gynaecol 1992;99:990–993.

83. Dietrich CS, Yancey MK, Miyazawa K, et al. Risk factors for early cytologic abnormalities after loop electrosurgical excision procedure. Obstet Gynecol 2002;99:188–192.

84. Hoffman MS, Sterghos S, Gordy LW, et al. Evaluation of the cervical canal with the endocervical brush. Obstet Gynecol 1993;82:573–577.

85. Andras EJ, Fletcher GH, Rutledge F. Radiotherapy of carcinoma of the cervix following simple hysterectomy. Am J Obstet Gynecol 1973;115:647–655.

86. Crane CH, Schneider BF. Occult carcinoma discovered after simple hysterectomy treated with postoperative radiotherapy. Int J Radiat Oncol Biol Phys 1999;43:1049–1053.

87. Roman LD, Morris M, Mitchell MF, et al. Prognostic factors for patients undergoing simple hysterectomy in the presence of invasive cancer of the cervix. Gynecol Oncol 1993;50:179–184.

88. Chapman JA, Mannel RS, DiSaia PJ, et al. Surgical treatment of unexpected invasive cervical cancer found at total hysterectomy. Obstet Gynecol 1992;80:931–934.

89. Hellberg D, Nilsson S. 20-year experience of follow-up of the abnormal smear with colposcopy and histology and treatment by conization or cryosurgery. Gynecol Oncol 1990;38: 166–169.

90. Kalliala I, Anttila A, Pukkala E, et al. Risk of cervical and other cancers after treatment of cervical intraepithelial neoplasia: retrospective cohort study. Br Med J 2005;331:1183–1185.

91. Souter WP, Butler JS, Tipples M. The role of colposcopy in the follow up of women treated for cervical intraepithelial neoplasia. Br J Obstet Gynecol 2006;113:511–514.

92. Kreimer AR, Guido RS, Solomon D, et al. Human papillomavirus testing following loop electrosurgical excision procedure identifies women at risk for posttreatment cervical intraepithelial neoplasia grade 2 or 3 disease. Cancer Epidemiol Biomarkers Prev 2006;15:908–914.

93. Economos K, Perez-Veridiano N, Mann M, et al. Abnormal cervical cytology in adolescents: a 15-year experience. J Reprod Med 1994;39:973–976.

94. Wright JD, Davila RM, Pinto KR, et al. Cervical dysplasia in adolescents. Obstet Gynecol 2005;106:115–120.

95. Massad LS, Markwell S, Cejtin HE, et al. Risk of high-grade cervical intraepithelial neoplasia among young women with abnormal screening cytology. J Lower Genital Tract Dis 2005;9:225–229.

96. Case AS, Rocconi RP, Straughn JM, et al. Cervical intraepithelial neoplasia in adolescent women: Incidence and treatment outcomes. 2006;108:1369–1374.

97. SEER Cancer Statistics Review. Available at: *www.seer.cancer.gov/cgi-bin/csr/1975_2003/search.pl#results*. Accessed April 26, 2007.

98. Nygard JF, Nygard M, Skare GB, et al. Pap smear screening in women under 30 in the Norwegian Coordinated Cervical Cancer Screening Program, with a comparison of immediate biopsy vs Pap smear triage of moderate dysplasia. Acta Cytol 2006;50:295–302.

99. Greer BE, Easterling TR, McLennan DA, et al. Fetal and maternal considerations in the management of stage IB cervical cancer during pregnancy. Gynecol Oncol 1989;34:61–65.

100. Duggan B, Muderspach LI, Roman LD, et al. Cervical cancer in pregnancy: reporting on planned delay in therapy. Obstet Gynecol 1993;82:598–602.

101. Sorosky JI, Squatrito R, Ndubisi BU, et al. Stage I squamous cell cervical carcinoma in pregnancy: planned delay in therapy awaiting fetal maturity. Gynecol Oncol 1995;59: 207–210.

102. Hannigan EV, Whitehouse HH, Atkinson WD, et al. Cone biopsy during pregnancy. Obstet Gynecol 1982;60:450–455.

103. Dunn TS, Ginsburg V, Wolf D. Loop-cone cerclage in pregnancy: a 5-year review. Gynecol Oncol 2003;90:577–580.

CASE STUDY 1 QUESTIONS

HISTORY

A 29-year-old gravida II, para II had an LSIL Pap smear 2 years ago but is just now presenting to the colposcopy clinic for evaluation. She is a smoker and has a history of chlamydia.

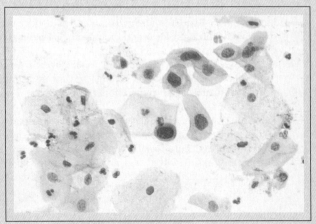

Figure 13-14 This is her Pap smear.

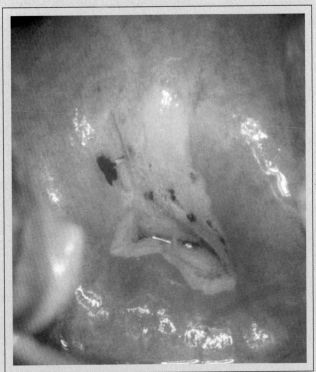

Figure 13-15 This is a colpophotograph of her cervix after the application of 5% acetic acid.

- What do you see?
- Is this an adequate examination?
- Are the findings normal or abnormal?

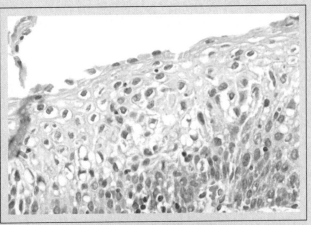

Figure 13-16 This represents a biopsy taken from the 6-o'clock position.

- What is your pathologic diagnosis?
- Based on your diagnosis, what treatment options would be appropriate for this patient?

CASE STUDY 1 ANSWERS

FIGURE 13-14

This slide represents an HSIL Pap smear. The cells in the center of the field are consistent with HSIL with moderate nuclear pleomorphism and nuclear chromatin hyperchromasia.

FIGURE 13-15

An area of acetowhite epithelium near the os extends into the canal. If the SCJ cannot be seen, this would be an unsatisfactory examination. With an endocervical speculum, the SCJ could be seen extending 1 cm into the os.

FIGURE 13-16

The biopsy demonstrates CIN 2 with koilocytosis. In the parabasal area, nuclear crowding is present, and the cells within the epithelium lack some degree of maturation, although maturation is present in the upper half of the epithelium. Some of the cells near the surface show distinct perinucelar halos with binucleation and features of koilocytosis. Appropriate treatment consists of loop excision or a cone biopsy. Laser ablation or cryotherapy is not appropriate because the disease extends more than 5 mm into the os.

CASE STUDY 2 QUESTIONS

HISTORY

This 25-year-old gravida I, para I presents with a Pap test showing HSIL. Last year, she was treated with electrosurgical loop excision for a CIN 3 lesion. The margins of the specimen were positive at that time. She is sexually active and uses condoms for contraception. She smokes one pack of cigarettes a day.

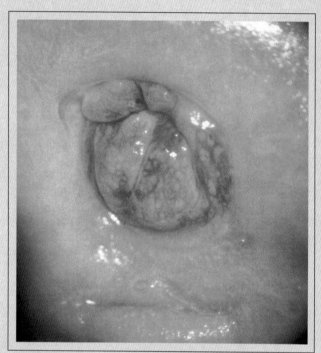

Figure 13-17 This is a colpophotograph of her cervix after the application of 5% acetic acid.

- Is the TZ fully visualized?
- Describe what you see.
- What is the differential diagnosis for this lesion?

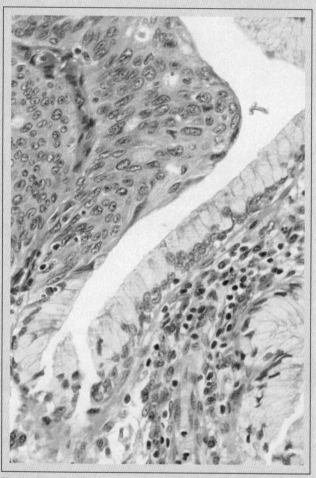

Figure 13-18 This is a biopsy of the most severe colposcopic lesion.

- What is your histologic diagnosis?
- What is the next step in this patient's evaluation?

CASE STUDY 2 ANSWERS

FIGURE 13-17

The TZ is not fully visualized. The ectocervical squamous epithelium ends in an abrupt circular rim characteristic of a previously treated cervix. Acetowhite epithelium with a mosaic pattern is seen medial to this ectocervical rim. The mosaic tiles are irregular in shape and size, and some have a central punctation. This is highly suggestive of a

high-grade lesion, but the possibility must be considered that this is just immature squamous metaplasia.

FIGURE 13-18

An endocervical crypt is seen. At the lower portion of the photomicrograph, normal columnar epithelium is seen with basally placed nuclei and cells in a "picket-fence" arrangement. However, at the upper portion of the crypt, the columnar cells have been replaced by a dysplastic squamous epithelium whose nuclei are disordered and reach to the top of the epithelium. This is a high-grade intraepithelial lesion.

The patient has an unsatisfactory colposcopy and a recurrent high-grade lesion. She needs a cone biopsy for treatment and to exclude the possibility of more advanced disease in the endocervical canal.

CASE STUDY 3 QUESTIONS

HISTORY

This 30-year-old gravida 0, para 0 presents with a Pap smear showing LSIL. She is sexually active and uses condoms for contraception. She has had five previous sexual partners. She smokes two packs of cigarettes a day.

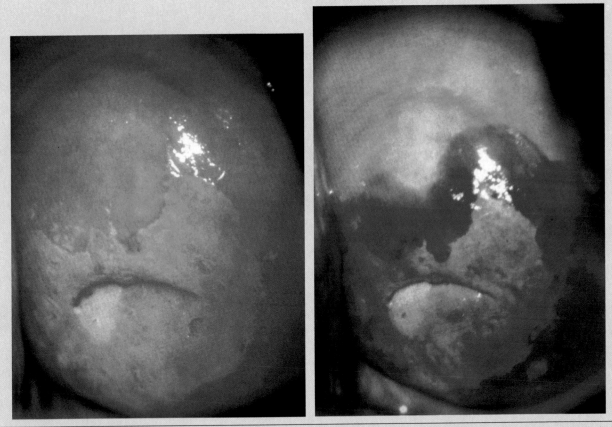

Figure 13-19 and 13-20 Figure 13-19 is a colpophotograph of her cervix after the application of 5% acetic acid. Figure 13-20 is a colpophotograph of her cervix after the application of Lugol's iodine.

- Is the TZ fully visualized?
- Describe what you see.
- What is the most appropriate site for a directed biopsy?

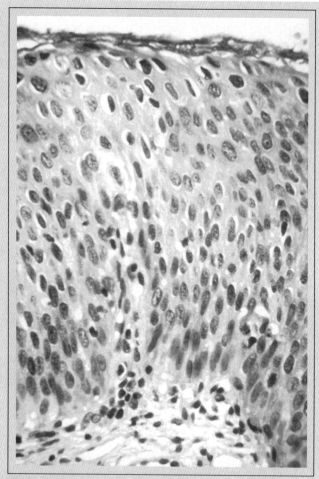

Figure 13-21 This is a biopsy of the most severe colposcopic lesion.

- What is your histologic diagnosis?

CASE STUDY 3 ANSWERS

FIGURES 13-19 AND 13-20

The TZ is not fully visualized. A large area of low-grade acetowhite epithelium with an irregular geographic border replaces most of the TZ. In Figure 13-17, this can be seen as a variegated area of patchy iodine uptake. This is consistent with low-grade CIN. However, at the 7-o'clock position, there is a patch of higher-grade acetowhite epithelium (see Figure 13-17) that is more starkly nonstaining with Lugol's iodine (see Figure 13-18). This appearance of a "lesion within a lesion" is called an *internal margin* and is very highly suggestive of a high-grade lesion. The biopsy should come from this area. Biopsies of the outer lesion may also be obtained.

FIGURE 13-21

The biopsy shows full-thickness change with disordered, hyperchromatic, dysplastic nuclei. This is a CIN 3 lesion.

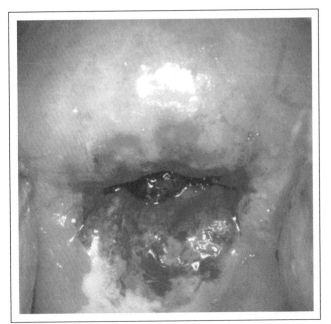

Plate 13-1 Focal area of dense acetowhite epithelium on the posterior lip of the cervix. Biopsy revealed CIN 2.

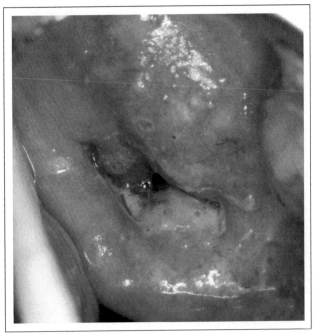

Plate 13-3 Dense acetowhite epithelium at the os consistent with HSIL. The SCJ cannot be seen at 4 o'clock, making this an unsatisfactory examination. Although there is no disease on the anterior lip, the TZ is extensive, as evidenced by the presence of several nabothian cysts.

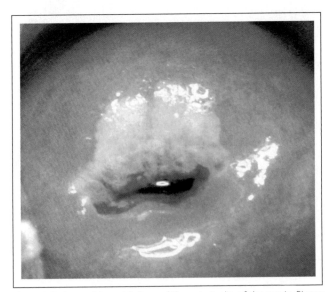

Plate 13-2 Acetowhite epithelium of the anterior lip of the cervix. Biopsy revealed CIN 2.

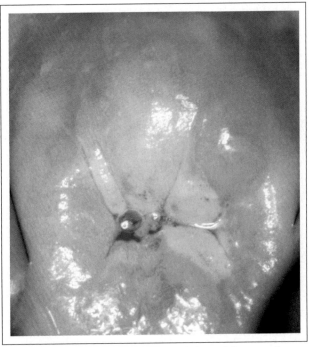

Plate 13-4 HSIL with dense acetowhite epithelium, slight punctation at 12 o'clock, and sharp margins. The SCJ is not seen in this image.

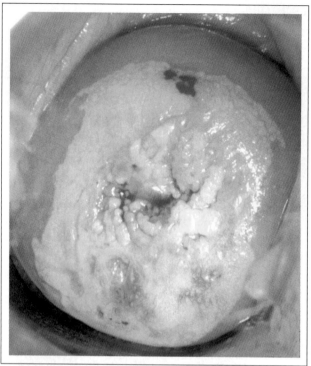

Plate 13-5 This cervix has a large TZ with peripheral immature metaplasia and faint mosaic pattern, along with an area of dense acetowhite epithelium centrally. A biopsy at 9 o'clock revealed metaplasia, whereas a biopsy at 4 o'clock revealed CIN 3.

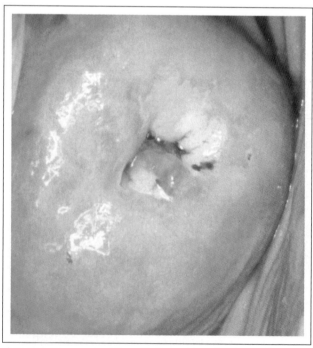

Plate 13-7 Well-defined focal area of acetowhite epithelium at 6 o'clock and, less prominently, at 12 o'clock. Biopsy revealed CIN 2.

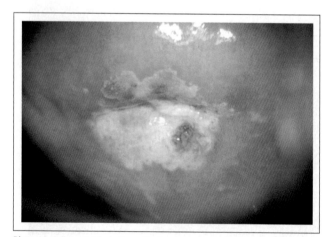

Plate 13-6 Low-grade lesion with fine mosaic on the anterior lip and high-grade lesion with coarse mosaic on the posterior lip. Biopsy at 12 o'clock revealed CIN 1; biopsy at 5 o'clock revealed CIN 3.

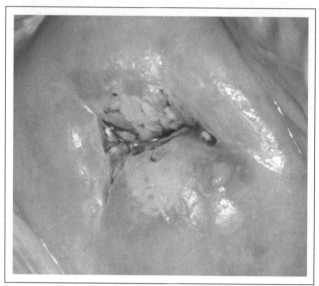

Plate 13-8 Dense acetowhite epithelium surrounding the os. Mucus is also present. The SCJ cannot be seen. Biopsy revealed CIN 3.

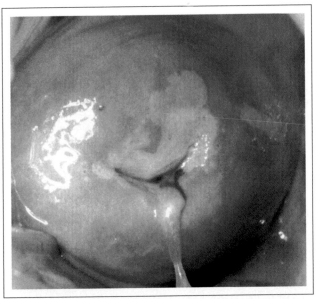

Plate 13-9 Peripheral LSIL with geographic margins and mild, acetowhite epithelium with a central, dense acetowhite lesion. The SCJ is not seen. Peripheral biopsy revealed CIN 1, and central biopsy revealed CIN 2.

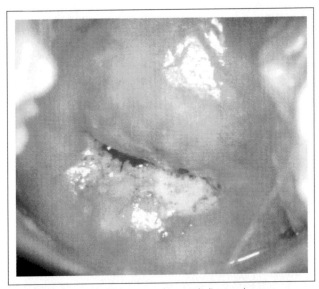

Plate 13-11 HSIL with dense acetowhite epithelium and coarse punctation on the left posterior cervix. The SCJ is not seen.

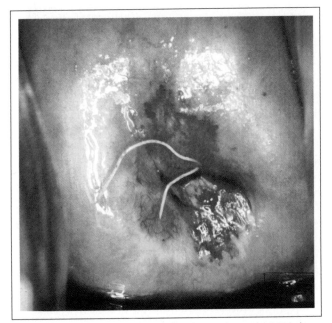

Plate 13-10 Dense acetowhite epithelium is noted near the internal os posteriorly, along with a coarse mosaic pattern. Biopsy revealed CIN 3.

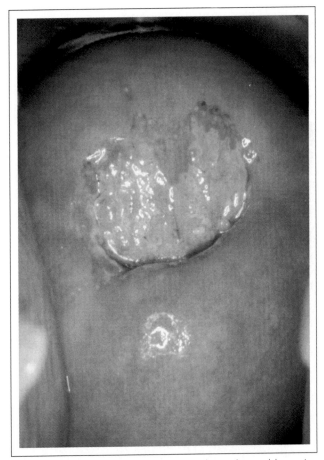

Plate 13-12 Acetowhite epithelium that extends into the canal, becoming a denser acetowhite near the os. Visualization of the upper border of the lesion is important because the most abnormal region of the lesion is usually at the SCJ. The biopsies showed CIN 2.

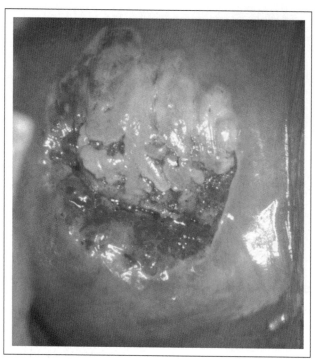

Plate 13-13 CIN 2 lesion of the anterior lip of the cervix.

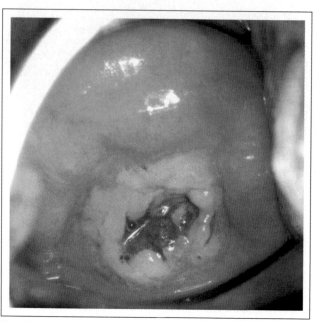

Plate 13-15 Acetowhite epithelium near the os in a patient who had laser treatment 1 year previously. A biopsy at 6 o'clock revealed CIN 2.

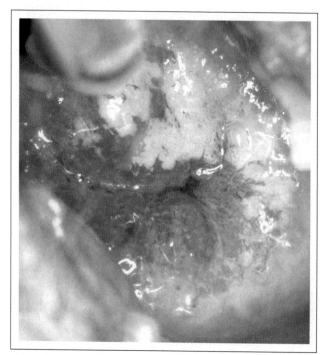

Plate 13-14 HSIL with dense acetowhite epithelium and coarse punctation noted at 2 o'clock.

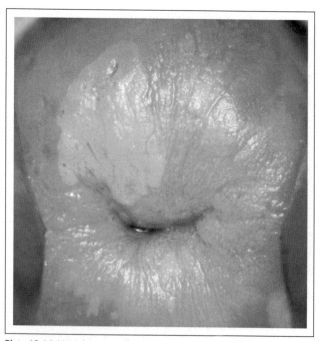

Plate 13-16 Hyperkeratosis after laser surgery gives this cervix its granular appearance. There is a large, well-circumscribed area of acetowhite epithelium at the 9- to 12-o'clock position that represents residual post-treatment CIN.

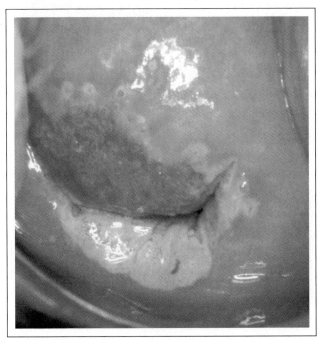

Plate 13-17 Well-demarcated peripheral border of the acetowhite epithelium on the posterior lip of the cervix. CIN 3 was found on biopsy.

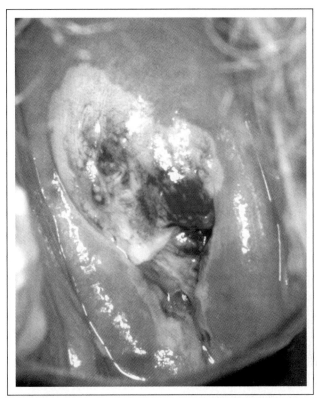

Plate 13-19 High-grade lesion with dense acetowhite epithelium and coarse mosaic that extends into the canal. The upper limits of the lesions could not be seen, and the patient underwent a cone biopsy. The pathology was CIN 3.

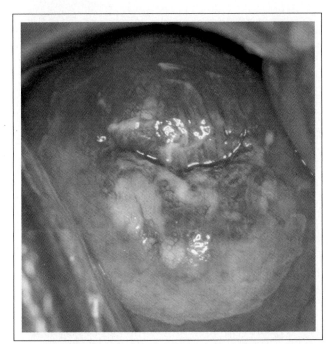

Plate 13-18 Large TZ with mild acetowhite epithelium peripherally and dense acetowhite epithelium with coarse mosaic pattern mainly at 7 and 11 o'clock. Biopsy revealed CIN 3.

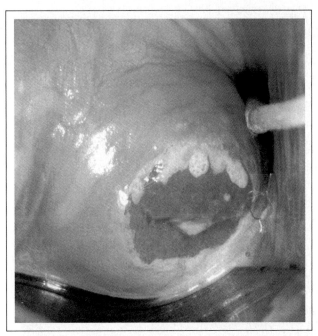

Plate 13-20 Adequate examination with mild acetowhite epithelium anteriorly and a central, 12-o'clock, denser acetowhite area with coarse punctation. A biopsy of the area of punctation revealed CIN 2.

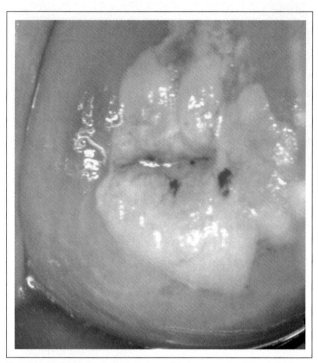

Plate 13-21 Large, high-grade lesion with dense acetowhite epithelium, no vessels, and an inadequate examination.

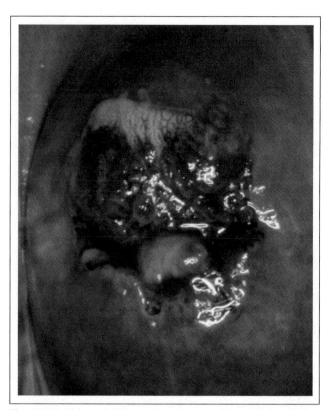

Plate 13-23 High-grade lesion with dense acetowhite epithelium and coarse mosaic on the anterior periphery of the cervix. The SCJ is visible. A plug of mucus is present at the os.

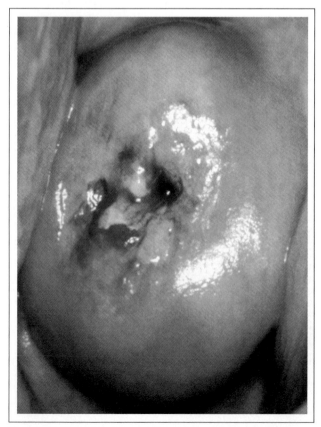

Plate 13-22 High-grade lesion on the posterior lip of the cervix with intermediate acetowhite epithelium, a rolled edge at 6 o'clock, and some bleeding present. The SCJ is not visible.

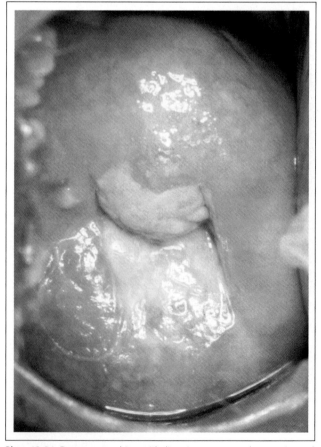

Plate 13-24 Dense acetowhite epithelium is present on the anterior and posterior lips of the cervix. No vessels are seen. The SCJ is not visible.

Squamous Cervical Cancer

R. Kevin Reynolds

INCIDENCE

In much of the world, cervical cancer remains the most common cancer diagnosis in women. The incidence of cervical cancer is substantially lower in nations with universal screening and treatment of preinvasive lesions. Since the early 1960s, cervical cancer incidence in the United States has declined by 87%.[1] Although the reasons for this decline in mortality are complex, the trend has clearly followed the widespread acceptance of Papanicolaou (Pap) smear screening to identify patients with treatable preinvasive disease. *A total of 9710 new diagnoses of cervical cancer and 3700 cervical cancer deaths are estimated to have occurred in the United States in 2006.[2]*

COLPOSCOPIC ASSESSMENT OF INVASIVE AND MICROINVASIVE LESIONS

When a visible lesion is identified on the cervix, or when a squamous intraepithelial lesion is diagnosed on Pap testing, visual and colposcopic inspection of the cervix and vagina with directed biopsy, endocervical assessment with either curettage or brushing for cytology, and bimanual pelvic examination are warranted. Many authors have attempted to distinguish the colposcopic appearance of preinvasive cervical neoplasia from microinvasive or invasive cervical carcinoma.[3,4,5]

The premise on which colposcopy is based is that dysplastic lesions and cancers have visually distinct morphology that can be recognized by the skilled colposcopist. Abnormal colposcopic findings indicative of microinvasive and invasive cervical carcinomas are similar to those described in previous chapters for preinvasive cervical neoplasia. Although microinvasive and invasive cervical carcinomas are often assumed to demonstrate progressively more abnormal findings on a continuum beginning with preinvasive disease, published evidence does not support this assumption. *The most severe lesions do not always demonstrate the most abnormal colposcopic findings. Likewise, a lack of abnormal colposcopic findings does not always indicate an absence of cervical pathology.*

Colposcopic detection of microinvasive and invasive disease can be difficult. Although many authors report that colposcopy is of value in detecting early invasive disease, these same authors report a significant problem with inaccuracy of colposcopic diagnosis.[6,7] In a retrospective review of 180 patients with microinvasive and occult invasive squamous cell carcinoma of the cervix, Benedet defined the accuracy rate of colposcopy as the percentage of patients with a satisfactory colposcopic examination who were correctly diagnosed on the basis of this examination.[7] In this series, patients were correctly identified as having microinvasive carcinoma only 73% of the time. *Patients with occult invasive squamous cell carcinoma of the cervix were accurately detected only 87% of the time.* In a similar population-based study of 61 patients with microinvasive disease, Paraskevaidis and associates reported a colposcopic sensitivity of only 50%.[8] Hopman and coworkers, in a review of the relevant literature, found that *microinvasive disease was missed by colposcopic assessment in nearly 50% of cases.*[9] In one report, all cases of microinvasive carcinoma were underdiagnosed with colposcopic examination.[10] Hopman and colleagues also found interobserver agreement of colposcopic impression about half the time among 23 experienced colposcopists.[11] These studies highlight the limitations of colposcopic assessment in the detection of microinvasive and invasive lesions.

A number of abnormal colposcopic findings are reported to be associated with microinvasive and invasive cervical cancer. These include *atypical vessels, necrosis, ulceration, and exophytic mass* (Figures 14-1 to 14-4). Many abnormal colposcopic findings are also associated with intraepithelial neoplasia, as reported in previous chapters. These include

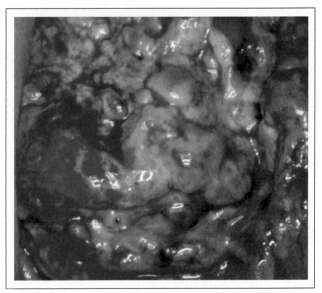

Figure 14-2 Example of necrosis and yellow appearance of the cervical epithelium.

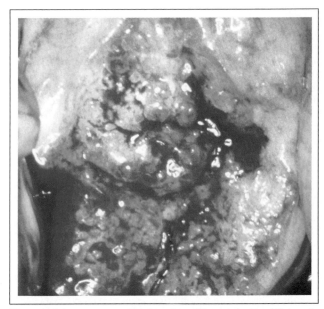

Figure 14-3 Large cancer with ulceration of the anterior lip of the cervix; overall yellow, necrotic appearance, and friability.

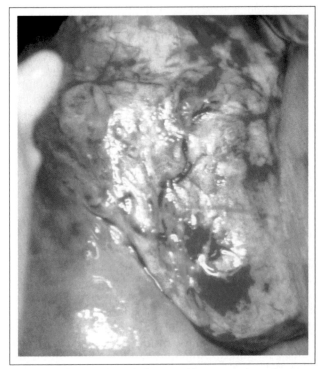

Figure 14-1 Cancer with cervical mass and large atypical vessels present.

acetowhite epithelium, punctation, mosaic, atypical vessels, and keratosis. Some colposcopic findings, such as unusual friability, necrosis, ulceration, and exophytic mass, may also be associated with benign conditions such as infections and trauma. Atypical vessels are surface capillaries that have unusual patterns such as hairpin loops, abnormal branching, commas, star bursts, and corkscrews. Nabothian cysts may have surface vascularity, but these can be distinguished from atypical vascular patterns because of the normal pattern of vessel arborization and the characteristic hemispheric contour of the cyst (Figures 14-5 and 14-6). *Necrosis of neoplastic tissue may be noted by a color change*

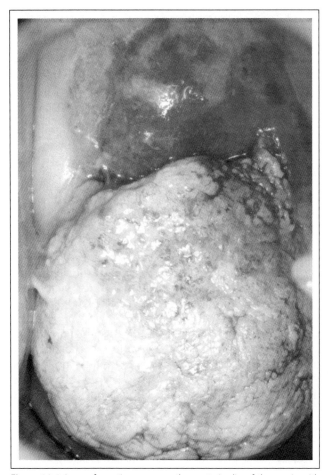

Figure 14-4 Large, fungating mass on the posterior lip of the cervix with dense acetowhite epithelium and atypical vessels. (Image provided by Dr. Vesna Kesic.)

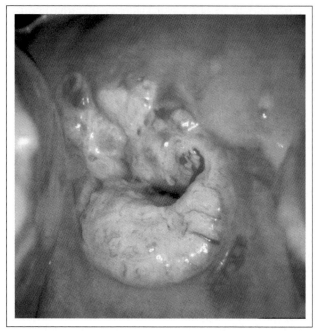

Figure 14-6 Nonbranching atypical vessels on the surface of a raised acetowhite mass on the posterior lip of the cervix. Two nabothian cysts are also present at 2 o'clock.

resulting in a yellow-to-tan appearance, often associated with friability (Figure 14-7). Invasive lesions may demonstrate endophytic growth, leading to ulceration, or exophytic growth, resulting in an irregularly shaped mass protruding from the cervical surface.

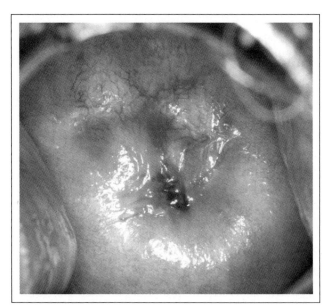

Figure 14-5 Normal, arborizing vessels and nabothian cysts.

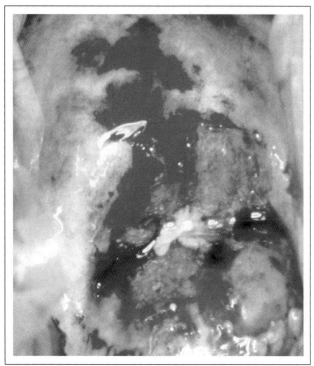

Figure 14-7 Cancer with necrosis, friability, and a diffuse yellow appearance.

263

Many authors report a constellation of these findings that may be more indicative of microinvasive or invasive disease. In a review of 46 patients with microinvasive and invasive carcinoma, Sugimori and coworkers reported thick, white, elevated lesions with sharply demarcated margins in 85% of patients with microinvasive disease, whereas this condition was noted in only 41% of patients with carcinoma *in situ*.[6] They demonstrated that when mosaic, punctation, and acetowhite epithelium were noted, microinvasive carcinoma was more likely when the lesion encompassed the circumference of the external os and when the lesion was sharply demarcated. Other studies have not confirmed these observations.[12,13] Liu and coworkers reported that 40% of patients with microinvasive cancer demonstrated mosaic, punctation, and acetowhite epithelium; 37% were found to have only two of these abnormalities; 18% had only one; and 5% had no abnormal colposcopic findings at all.[5] In a retrospective review of 228 patients, Noda evaluated the ability of colposcopy to discriminate among dysplasia, carcinoma *in situ*, and microinvasive carcinoma.[4] Twenty-five percent of patients with microinvasive disease had lesions that demonstrated a mosaic pattern, 14% harbored punctation, 25% had acetowhite epithelium, and 50% showed keratosis. *The triad of mosaic, punctation, and acetowhite epithelium appeared in approximately 20% of patients with microinvasive carcinoma.* Paraskevaidis and colleagues reported that *34% of patients with microinvasive disease had no abnormal colposcopic findings.*[8]

It has long been believed that the pathognomonic colposcopic finding indicative of microinvasive or invasive disease is the presence of atypical vessels.[9] Koller first described atypical vessels as vessels that are 2 to 10 times wider than normal capillaries and are irregular in width, shape, and course.[14] Authors have reported wide ranges in the presence of atypical vessels in microinvasive cancer, from 0% to approximately 80% of patients. Several reported that the frequency of atypical vessels increased with increasing depth of invasion.[4,5,9] Liu and associates reported that 32% of patients with invasion of less than 3 mm in depth had atypical vessels, whereas 100% of patients with invasion of 3 to 5 mm had atypical vessels.[5] Van Meir and colleagues reported that atypical vessels were not found in any patients with less than 3 mm of invasion but were found in all patients with 3 to 5 mm of invasion.[13] *One proposed explanation for the lack of atypical vessels with microinvasive disease is that neovascularization may not be necessary for the development of small lesions.*[5] Folkman indicated that tumors as large as 2 to 3 mm in diameter can survive by diffusion alone without requiring angiogenesis.[15]

ADDITIONAL DIAGNOSTIC BIOPSY PROCEDURES

Following colposcopic assessment with directed biopsies, additional biopsy material may be required to accurately stage the cervical lesion. *If the colposcopically directed biopsy reveals a lesion invading more than 5 mm below the basement membrane, no further histologic data are required to stage the lesion. If invasion less than or equal to 5 mm below the basement membrane is detected, complete assessment of the cervical portio is required to rule out the presence of deeper invasion.* Treatment by conization should be reserved for special cases that are discussed in detail later in this chapter. *Ablative therapy, such as cryocautery or CO_2 laser ablation, is always contraindicated once invasion is documented.*[16]

HISTOPATHOLOGY

The American Joint Commission on Cancer (AJCC), in cooperation with the American College of Surgeons and the American Cancer Society, has proposed universal adoption of the World Health Organization (WHO) system, the International Histological Classification of Tumors.[17] The AJCC classification of cervical cancer types is divided into three major categories: *squamous carcinoma, adenocarcinoma, and other types* (Table 14-1). The squamous types are divided into preinvasive and invasive groups, and the invasive category can be further subdivided into keratinizing, nonkeratinizing, and verrucous types. Squamous cancer accounts for at least 75% of cervical cancers; it is discussed later in this chapter.[1] Adenocarcinoma will be addressed in Chapter 15.

Table 14-1 American Joint Committee on Cancer Classification of Cervical Cancer Histopathology

Cervical intraepithelial neoplasia, grade 3
Squamous cell carcinoma *in situ*
Squamous cell carcinoma
Invasive
Keratinizing
Nonkeratinizing
Verrucous
Adenocarcinoma *in situ*
Adenocarcinoma
Invasive carcinoma
Endocervical carcinoma
Endometrioid carcinoma
Clear cell carcinoma
Adenosquamous carcinoma
Adenoid cystic carcinoma
Small-cell carcinoma (neuroendocrine)
Undifferentiated carcinoma

Data from Fleming ID, Cooper JS, Henson DE, et al (eds). AJCC Cancer Staging Handbook. Philadelphia: Lippincott-Raven, 1998.

Invasive squamous cervical cancer is usually composed of compact nests of neoplastic squamous cells invading the subepithelial stroma. The size, shape, and degree of keratinization vary widely. At least two systems for grading of squamous carcinoma are currently used. *The AJCC system defines the grades as well differentiated (G1), moderately differentiated (G2), poorly differentiated (G3), or undifferentiated (G4).*[17] For practical reasons, the older morphologic grading system proposed by Reagan and Ng is more widely used. Using the Reagan and Ng nomenclature, well-differentiated carcinoma is called *large-cell keratinizing type*, moderately differentiated carcinoma is defined as *large-cell nonkeratinizing type*, and poorly differentiated tumors are termed *small-cell nonkeratinizing type.*[18] Small-cell nonkeratinizing tumors are of squamous origin and are distinct from small-cell neuroendocrine tumors. When small cells predominate in a tumor, immunohistochemical analysis aids in determining the correct cell type.

In well-differentiated squamous carcinoma of the cervix, the most prominent feature is the presence of keratin, often deposited in keratin pearls. Keratin pearls are eosinophilic, concentric whorls surrounded by epithelial nests (Figure 14-8). Well-differentiated squamous carcinoma cells are usually oval or polygonal in shape and have distinct intercellular bridges. Nuclei are usually large, hyperchromatic, and irregularly shaped.[1,19]

The cells and nuclei of moderately differentiated tumors are more pleomorphic, and mitotic figures are more frequent. Cellular borders and intercellular bridges are less distinct. Dyskeratosis and abnormal intracellular keratin formation are often present, but keratin pearl formation is rare (Figure 14-9).

Poorly differentiated carcinomas are characterized by large, irregular nuclei; frequent mitotic figures; minimal cytoplasm; and areas of necrosis. Cells may be oval or fusiform in shape. Keratin formation is rare or absent. The differential diagnosis for cells with these characteristics includes small-cell neuroendocrine and sarcoma tumor types. Immunohistochemical analysis may be required to reach the correct diagnosis.[1,19]

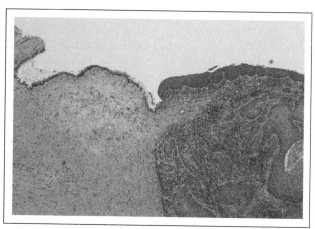

Figure 14-9 Large-cell, nonkeratinizing carcinoma.

The presence of lymph-vascular space invasion (LVSI) has significant impact on treatment planning and prognosis, which are discussed later in this chapter. *LVSI is diagnosed when malignant cells are detected in a lumen that is lined with endothelial cells* (Figure 14-10). The differential diagnosis includes tissue-processing artifact, in which retraction of tissue during fixation causes an apparent lumen.[1] Unlike true LVSI, a lining of endothelial cells will not be seen at the border of the lumen.

Discriminating between dysplastic and microinvasive lesions can be difficult, particularly if the biopsy specimen has been cut tangentially. When squamous carcinoma first breeches the basement membrane, the invading squamous cells appear better differentiated than adjacent dysplastic epithelial cells. The cells are larger and contain more abundant eosinophilic cytoplasm and occasional keratin pearl formation. The leading edge of the invasive focus appears ragged, with neoplastic cells appearing to drop off the epithelium and into the stroma.[1,20] *A marked, local, acute inflammatory response is often noted surrounding the site of invasion. By convention, the depth of stromal invasion is measured perpendicularly*

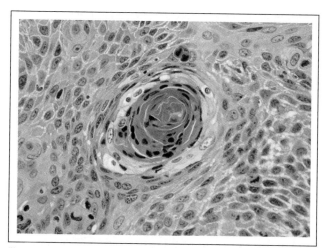

Figure 14-8 Keratin pearls demonstrating eosinophilic, concentric whorls surrounded by epithelial nests.

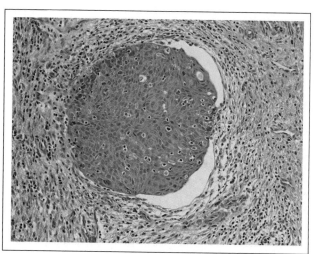

Figure 14-10 Histology demonstrating lymphovascular space invasion.

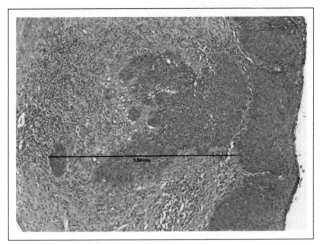

Figure 14-11 Microinvasion.

from the nearest basement membrane to the base of the lesion (Figure 14-11). If the origination site of the tumor is not obvious, depth is measured from the basement membrane of the nearest surface epithelium. If the invasive focus arises from the base of a gland, depth is measured from the site of origin of the invasive focus to the deepest portion of the invasive lesion.

An unusual variant of squamous cervical carcinoma is *verrucous carcinoma. This tumor is usually associated with human papillomavirus (HPV) type 6, and its papillary appearance is often mistaken clinically for a giant condyloma.*[21,22] The tumor is exophytic in nature. Microscopic features include bland-appearing cells with a low mitotic index and an undulating surface (Figure 14-12). Fibrovascular cores are absent in the papillary structure of the tumor, which offers a useful distinction in comparison with the prominent fibrovascular cores noted in condyloma. The stromal-epithelial interface is often described as having a pushing border with a broad, smooth appearance. These tumors tend to recur locally, and distant metastasis is uncommon.[21–23]

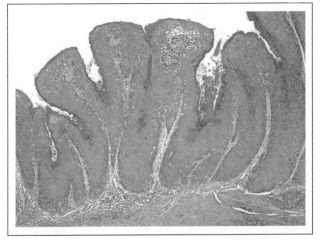

Figure 14-12 Verrucous carcinoma.

STAGING OF CERVICAL CANCER

Patients must be staged to determine appropriate treatment and to offer accurate counsel regarding prognosis. Figure 14-13 demonstrates a pictorial description of clinical staging for cervical cancer. Two staging systems are in widespread use today. The more commonly used international standard for staging is defined by the International Federation of Gynecology and Obstetrics (FIGO) in conjunction with the WHO.[17] The FIGO cervical cancer staging criteria were revised in 1995 (Table 14-2). By convention, when there is disagreement regarding staging, the less advanced stage is chosen for statistical consistency. *Stage is based primarily on clinical examination that includes bimanual pelvic and rectovaginal examination. When determining stage with the FIGO system, tests that may be used include biopsy, colposcopy, intravenous pyelogram (IVP), chest x-ray, cystoscopy, and sigmoidoscopy.* Tests that may not be considered when assigning the stage include computed tomography (CT), magnetic resonance imaging (MRI), lymphangiogram, and surgical findings from laparoscopy and laparotomy. *By convention, once a patient has been staged, the stage is not changed even if subsequent testing or surgery indicates that the tumor is more or less advanced than was originally believed.* Tests should be used selectively based on the physical examination. For example, cystoscopy or sigmoidoscopy is recommended when the clinical examination suggests a stage III or stage IV lesion, but it is not cost-effective for stage I and stage II lesions because of low yield.[24] Although not considered for staging purposes, CT scans may occasionally be useful for treatment planning. CT scanning of the abdomen and pelvis is unlikely to detect lymphadenopathy for stage 1B1 lesions owing to the low expected incidence of lymphatic metastases, but it would be much more likely to identify lymph node metastases in larger stage IB2, stage II, and stage III lesions where para-aortic node metastases occur in 18% to 33% of patients.[25] Lymphangiography and MRI scans are considered optional and are not routinely ordered. Positron emission tomography (PET) scans provide an image associated with biological function and are becoming more widely used for initial treatment planning of patients who will receive radiation therapy for disease beyond the cervix.[26] Although PET scan is now accepted and approved for treatment planning, the test result does not alter the FIGO stage. The role of PET scan for surveillance of patients after treatment is currently being investigated.

The AJCC, using the tumor, nodes, and metastasis (TNM) staging system, has defined a parallel staging system.[17] The American College of Surgeons requires use of the AJCC system for accreditation of tumor registries. The AJCC definition of the tumor categories corresponds to the FIGO staging system. When surgery is the primary treatment, the histologic findings permit the case to be assigned a pathologic stage that is designated postsurgical TNM (pTNM). A comparison of the FIGO and AJCC staging systems is presented in Tables 14-2 and 14-3.

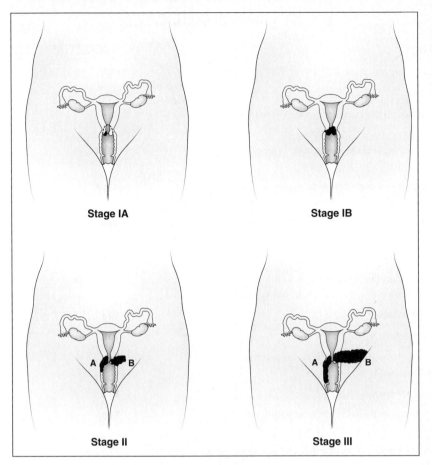

Stage IA

Stage IB

Stage II

Stage III

Figure 14-13 Pictorial description of clinical staging for cervical cancer. This figure illustrates findings that the examiner may appreciate on bimanual and rectovaginal examination. The dotted line in the stage IA diagram illustrates the line of resection for a cold-knife cone biopsy. The A and B substages for stages II and III disease are represented on the patient's right and left sides, respectively.

Both the FIGO and AJCC staging systems are applicable to all histologic types, including glandular neoplasms. However, the microinvasive cancer entity has not been defined for adenocarcinoma, primarily because of controversy regarding the lack of a reproducible reference point for measurement of lesion depth. This contrasts with squamous lesions, for which depth is measured perpendicular to the nearest basement membrane to determine depth of invasion.

Surgical staging to obtain pelvic and para-aortic nodes before treatment has been evaluated in several clinical trials. An extrafascial surgical approach has been shown to cause less radiation-associated morbidity.[27] *Surgical staging has not been shown to improve survival.*[28] With the exception of clinical trials, surgical staging is not routinely performed.

TREATMENT OF CERVICAL CANCER

Disease confined to the cervix is defined as stage I. The substage (i.e., IA1, IA2, IB1, IB2) is based on depth and diameter of invasion within the cervix. This correlates well with likelihood of metastases as well as survival.

Microinvasive Carcinoma, Stages IA1 and IA2

Stage IA lesions are referred to as *microinvasive. Cancer is deemed microinvasive when lymph node metastases and recurrences are rare.* Because many women who develop cervical cancer are in their reproductive years, it is helpful to define a group of patients with little risk of recurrence so that fertility-sparing treatment may be considered. The definition of microinvasive cervical carcinoma has been a point of controversy and confusion for many years. Three widely accepted definitions of microinvasive disease that have been used are those of FIGO, the Society of Gynecologic Oncologists (SGO), and a Japanese definition.[29] The FIGO definition specifies tumor depth and width, whereas the SGO definition specifies tumor depth but excludes multifocal lesions and LVSI. The Japanese definition specifies tumor depth, confluence, and cell type and excludes LVSI. The one variable that is specified in each of the three definitions is depth of invasion, although the actual depth varies for each definition. Many studies have analyzed the risk of metastasis to lymph nodes based on depth of invasion within the cervical lesion. Collectively, the data indicate that *invasion of less than or equal to 3 mm beyond the basement membrane carries a 0.5% risk of nodal metastasis, whereas the risk of nodal spread when the depth of invasion is greater than*

Table 14-2 Cervical Cancer Staging: International Federation on Gynecology and Obstetrics and American Joint Committee on Cancer Systems

FIGO Stage	Primary Tumor	AJCC TNM
—	Primary tumor cannot be assessed	TX
0	Carcinoma *in situ*	Tis
I	Carcinoma confined to the cervix (disregard extension to corpus)	T1
IA1	Measurable invasion ≤3 mm in depth and 7 mm in diameter	T1a1
IA2	Measurable invasion >3 and ≤5 mm in depth as well as ≤7 mm in diameter	T1a2
IB1	Lesion of ≤5 mm in depth and/or >7 mm in diameter, but ≤ 4 cm in diameter	T1b1
IB2	Lesion of >4 cm in diameter	T1b2
II	Tumor extends beyond the cervix but not to the pelvic wall; tumor may involve vagina, but not the lower third	T2
IIA	No parametrial involvement	T2a
IIB	Parametrial involvement	T2b
III	Tumor extends to the pelvic wall or may involve the lower third of the vagina	T3
IIIA	No extension to pelvic wall	T3a
IIIB	Extension to pelvic wall; includes all cases with hydronephrosis or nonfunctioning kidney	T3b
IV	Spread beyond true pelvis or involvement of bladder or rectal mucosa	T4
IVA	Tumor invades bladder or rectal mucosa and/or extends beyond true pelvis; bullous edema is not sufficient to classify invasion	T4a
IVB	Distant metastases	T4b
FIGO Stage	**Regional Lymph Nodes**	**AJCC TNM**
—	Regional lymph nodes cannot be assessed	NX
—	No regional lymph node metastasis	N0
—	Regional lymph node metastasis	N1
FIGO Stage	**Distant Metastasis**	**AJCC TNM**
—	Distant metastasis cannot be assessed	MX
—	No distant metastasis	M0
—	Distant metastasis, including para-aortic node metastases	M1

AJCC, American Joint Committee on Cancer; FIGO, International Federation of Gynecology and Obstetrics; TNM, tumor, nodes, and metastasis.
Data from Fleming ID, Cooper JS, Henson DE, et al (eds). AJCC Cancer Staging Handbook. Philadelphia: Lippincott-Raven, 1998.

3 mm is 8.2%.[30] Only 1 of 397 patients with cervical stromal invasion less than or equal to 3 mm was found to have lymph node metastasis.[31] *These data support the practice of offering conservative surgery, including fertility-sparing cervical conization, to patients with invasion measuring less than or equal*

to 3 mm. Simple hysterectomy would be recommended for patients not wishing to preserve their fertility.

Another predictor of metastatic disease and recurrence in patients with microinvasive cervical carcinoma is the presence of LVSI. In 1994, the Gynecologic Oncology Group

Table 14-3 Cervical Cancer Stage Grouping, American Joint Committee on Cancer System

Stage	T	N	M
Stage 0	Tis	N0	M0
Stage IA1	T1a1	N0	M0
Stage IA2	T1a2	N0	M0
Stage IB1	T1b1	N0	M0
Stage IB2	T1b2	N0	M0
Stage IIA	T2a	N0	M0
Stage IIB	T2b	N0	M0
Stage IIIA	T3a	N0	M0
Stage IIIB	T1	N1	M0
	T2	N1	M0
	T3a	N1	M0
	T3b	Any N	M0
Stage IVA	T4	Any N	M0
Stage IVB	Any T	Any N	M1

Data from Fleming ID, Cooper JS, Henson DE, et al (eds). AJCC Cancer Staging Handbook. Philadelphia: Lippincott-Raven, 1998.

analyzed the risk of nodal metastases in the presence of LVSI.[32] In patients with 3 to 5 mm of invasion and LVSI, 15.6% had pelvic node metastasis, whereas only 0.9% of patients had evidence of pelvic node metastases in the absence of LVSI. Van Nagell and coworkers reported no nodal metastases and no recurrences in 17 patients with invasion of less than 3 mm and LVSI. However, 25% of patients with stromal invasion from 3.1 to 5 mm and LVSI developed recurrent disease.[31] Creasman and colleagues reviewed 114 patients with microinvasive cervical carcinoma and reported that 2 of 25 patients with less than 1 mm of invasion had lymph-vascular involvement and that neither patient developed recurrent disease.[32] Although each of these studies has a small number of patients, the data suggest that *the presence of LVSI and stromal invasion greater than 3 mm carries a significant risk of recurrence. The risk of recurrence appears to be low with invasion of less than 3 mm, despite the presence of LVSI.*

Stage IA1

Accepted surgical treatments for microinvasive disease include simple hysterectomy, using either the abdominal or the vaginal approach, or cervical cone biopsy, using cold-knife conization or the loop electrocautery excision procedure (LEEP). Tseng and associates reported on 12 patients with microinvasive cervical carcinoma of less than 3 mm of invasion who were managed with cold-knife conization alone and developed no recurrences after a mean follow-up of 6.7 years.[33] In a

prospective study of the management of 29 patients with microinvasive cervical carcinoma managed by LEEP, all patients had a depth of invasion of less than 3 mm, and no patient was noted to have LVSI. After 25 months of follow-up, none of these patients developed recurrence.[34] However, a case of widespread lymph node metastasis in a patient with microinvasive cervical carcinoma measuring 0.8 mm has been reported.[35] In another report, a patient with 0.2 mm of invasion and positive LVSI demonstrated bulky pelvic lymph node metastases at the time of laparotomy.[31] *Patients must be informed of the slight but ever-present risk of recurrent disease despite appropriate conservative management.*

Stage IA2

Stage IA2 is defined as invasion of greater than 3 mm but less than 5 mm in depth and tumor diameter no greater than 7 mm in width. Appropriate treatment for this stage includes radical hysterectomy with pelvic lymphadenectomy, modified radical hysterectomy with pelvic lymphadenectomy, or radiation therapy. In carefully selected individuals who wish to retain their fertility, a radical vaginal trachelectomy may be offered. Details are presented in the Fertility Preservation section later in this chapter. *Although radical hysterectomy* (Table 14-4) *results in excellent long-term survival for patients with stage IA2 disease, a modified radical hysterectomy may also prove to be curative, with fewer potential complications and less morbidity,*[36] especially with regard to urinary tract dysfunction.[37] Several studies suggest that tumor volume less than or equal to 1 cm can be successfully treated with a modified radical approach with survival rates comparable to a full radical hysterectomy. In a retrospective review, Magrina and coworkers reported that 47 patients with tumor volume less than or equal to 2 cm treated with a modified radical hysterectomy had a 5-year survival of 100% with no recurrences.[38] *These studies suggest that a modified radical hysterectomy provides adequate disease resection. However, because no consensus definition of appropriate tumor size or volume has been accepted to define the patient population best suited for this approach, modified radical hysterectomy is not used by many oncologists.*

Other suggested indications for modified radical hysterectomy include microinvasion with lymph-vascular invasion, adjuvant hysterectomy following radiation therapy with small-volume residual carcinoma, or medial parametrial thickening or a positive endocervical curettage.[29] Although this approach has been reported to be a reasonable option, it must be understood that no advantage in performing a modified radical hysterectomy has been shown for patients with these indications.

Stage IA2 lesions may also be treated with intracavitary radiation therapy alone.[19,39,40] Although some authors report that external pelvic radiotherapy is not required for these tumors, patients with 3 to 5 mm of invasion and LVSI will have an 8.2% risk of pelvic nodal metastasis. Consideration should be given to treating these patients with both external radiation therapy and intracavitary implants.

Table 14-4 Comparison of Hysterectomy Types

Anatomic Structure	Extrafascial	Modified Radical	Radical
Uterus	Removed	Removed	Removed
Ovaries	Optional removal	Optional removal	Optional removal
Cervix	Removed	Removed	Removed
Vaginal margin	None	1–2 cm margin	>2–3 cm margin
Ureters	Not mobilized	Dissected through broad ligament	Dissected through broad ligament
Cardinal ligaments	Divided at uterine border	Divided where ureter transits the broad ligament	Divided at pelvic sidewall
Uterosacral ligaments	Divided at cervical border	Partially resected	Divided near sacral origin
Bladder	Mobilized to base of cervix	Mobilized to upper vagina	Mobilized to middle vagina
Rectum	Not mobilized	Mobilized below cervix	Mobilized below middle vagina

Stages IB and IIA

Stage IB or IIA cervical cancer is effectively treated with either radical pelvic surgery or radiation therapy, with nearly equal survival rates.[41–43] The surgical approach is preferred in younger patients because of the ability to preserve ovarian function and vaginal pliability for sexual function.[44–46] The choice between surgical or radiation therapy depends on tumor characteristics, the medical condition of the patient, and the preferences of the patient and her treating physicians. *Preferences are often based on the difference in treatment-related complications rather than on differences in the likelihood of long-term survival.*[19] Acute surgery-related complications include intraoperative bleeding and postoperative infection. Delayed postsurgical complications include vesicovaginal and ureterovaginal fistulae that occur in fewer than 2% of cases.[47–49] Loss of ovarian function occurs in as many as 40% of surgically treated cervical cancer patients despite ovarian preservation.[50,51] In comparison, radiation-associated complications include diarrhea in both the acute and the chronic setting, as well as stricture or fistula formation that is prone to occur 2 or more years after treatment. The incidence of chronic diarrhea may range between 3% and 40% depending on the volume of small bowel radiated and the total radiation dose. The likelihood of stricture or fistula formation varies with the radiation dose administered and the medical condition of the patient. Strictures, perforation, and formation of fistulae occur in about 5% of patients who undergo pelvic radiation.[52] *With the exception of carefully selected individuals with stage IB1 lesions smaller than 2 cm in whom fertility preservation is desired, the surgical procedure*

of choice for the treatment of stage IB or stage IIA cervical cancer is radical hysterectomy with pelvic lymphadenectomy. A radical hysterectomy differs from a simple, or extrafascial, hysterectomy by including resection of the cardinal and uterosacral ligaments and removal of the upper portion of the vagina.[29,53,54] Several hysterectomy techniques are compared in Table 14-4. Simple extrafascial hysterectomy has no place in the treatment of invasive cervical cancer, with the exception of combined radiation and surgery protocols for unusual tumor distributions such as the so-called barrel-shaped cervix.[55–57]

Radiation therapy for stage IB and stage IIA cervical cancer treatment usually includes external beam treatment and intracavitary implants. External beam radiotherapy (teletherapy) is administered in daily fractions for approximately 5 weeks. In addition, intracavitary implants are recommended, using either the low-dose-rate afterloading technique or the more recently developed high-dose-rate afterloading technique.[19] Specific doses and treatment schedules vary although clinical outcomes for the various regimens are generally similar.

Stages IIB and III

In the past, patients with stage IIB and stage III tumors were treated with radiation therapy alone. Standard radiation therapy treatment includes external radiation therapy to the pelvis using a daily four-field box technique, typically administering 4500 to 5000 cGy. An additional boost to areas with bulky tumor is often necessary. *In addition to external radiation therapy, an intracavitary implant is required to attain a tumoricidal dose of radiation.* Intracavitary therapy using a tandem and ovoid application for small tumors or an interstitial template for large tumors allows optimization of the final radiation dose to the tumor while minimizing the dose to the bladder and rectum.

In 1999, the National Cancer Institute issued a clinical announcement citing five clinical trials, all of which demonstrated significant improvement of survival rates for patients treated with radiation and concurrent chemotherapy. The five trials did not use the same chemotherapy drugs, schedules, or dosages, although cisplatin was included in all five protocols.[58-60] *A combination of radiation and chemotherapy has become the standard approach for treatment of patients with locally advanced cervical cancer.* However, optimization of the chemotherapy drug regimens, dosages, and schedules requires further study.

Patients with pelvic lymph node metastasis or with bulky cervical primary lesions have a significant risk of metastasis to the para-aortic nodes. Patients with stage IIB lesions have involved para-aortic nodes in 12.8% of cases.[19] Para-aortic nodes are not included in the standard pelvic port for radiation therapy, potentially resulting in undertreatment of these patients. The Radiation Therapy Oncology Group reported on a clinical trial in which patients were randomized to receive either standard pelvic radiotherapy or para-aortic node radiation in addition to standard pelvic radiotherapy. The 5-year survival for those who received para-aortic node radiation was 67% versus 55% in the control group.[61] Severe or life-threatening toxicities were four times more likely in the group receiving para-aortic radiation. A similar randomized trial reported by the European Organization for Research on Treatment of Cancer did not show survival benefit for patients receiving para-aortic radiation.[62] Until further studies can resolve this conflict, *there seems to be little justification for empirically treating the para-aortic nodes in patients with stage IIB or stage III lesions unless metastasis has been clearly documented.*

Stage IV and Recurrent Cervical Cancer

Treatment of stage IVA disease involving the bladder or the rectal mucosa may include either combined chemotherapy and radiation or pelvic exenteration, an ultraradical surgical procedure that removes the uterus, tubes, ovaries, vagina, bladder, and rectum.[63,64] Exenteration is usually reserved for patients with vesicovaginal or rectovaginal fistula before treatment. Treatment of widely metastatic disease (stage IVB) is individualized and includes combinations of radiation and chemotherapy, depending on location and extent of metastases. *The most active chemotherapeutic drugs include cisplatin, fluorouracil, ifosfamide, and bleomycin.*[19] *The most active combination therapy is cisplatin and topotecan.*[65] Long-term survival is unlikely. In patients with distant metastases, surgery is indicated only for palliation. Treatment of recurrent cervical cancer that is confined to the pelvis is based on the type of treatment originally administered. Patients who were initially treated with surgery may be treated with radiation therapy to the pelvis or to other sites of metastasis.

Central pelvic recurrence in patients previously treated with radiation may be amenable to pelvic exenteration.[64] Reconstructive surgical techniques allow restoration of bladder, rectal, and vaginal function via continent urinary conduit formation, low rectal reanastomosis, and vaginoplasty, respectively. Figure 14-14 presents a summary diagram for the management of cervical cancer.

FERTILITY PRESERVATION OPTIONS FOR CERVICAL CANCER PATIENTS

As many as 43% of cervical cancer cases in the United States are diagnosed during the reproductive years, and many of the young women afflicted with this diagnosis would like to retain their fertility.[66] In 1994, Dargent was the first to describe the *radical vaginal trachelectomy procedure that removed the cervix along with the attached ligaments and a wide vaginal margin. In addition, pelvic lymph nodes are removed laparoscopically. This procedure preserves the uterine corpus and its blood supply.* A permanent cervical cerclage is placed at completion of the procedure to reduce the risk of subsequent cervical incompetence during pregnancy.[67]

Candidates for this operation are individuals with small cervical lesions and low risk of metastases. Key criteria include strong desire for fertility, age younger than 40 years, and limited extent of tumor.[66] The lesions should either be patients with stage IA1 disease who are not candidates for more conservative therapy because they have lymph-vascular space invasion, or those with stage IB1 lesions less than 2 cm in diameter. The data reported to date are predominantly on the treatment of squamous cancer, but locally confined adenocarcinoma has also been treated in addition to a small number of patients with tumors larger than 2 cm.

Darsun reviewed outcome data from seven institutions: a combined recurrence rate of 4.2% with median follow-up of 48 months was reported, which is comparable with historical data for survival after radical hysterectomy.[66] Six institutions have reported pregnancy outcome data following radical trachelectomy. *Of the 310 pregnancies reported, 16% ended with spontaneous abortion, 1.3% were ectopic pregnancies, 10% resulted in second-trimester loss, and 72% resulted in delivery after 37 weeks of gestation.*[68] The incidence of spontaneous abortion and secondary infertility do not appear to be increased in these patients. Optimal prenatal management to prevent or minimize second- and early third-trimester losses requires further study.

SURVIVAL

The 5-year survival of patients with microinvasive squamous carcinoma of the cervix (stage IA1) is 99%, even when conservative surgical therapy is used to preserve fertility.[19] *Patients with larger*

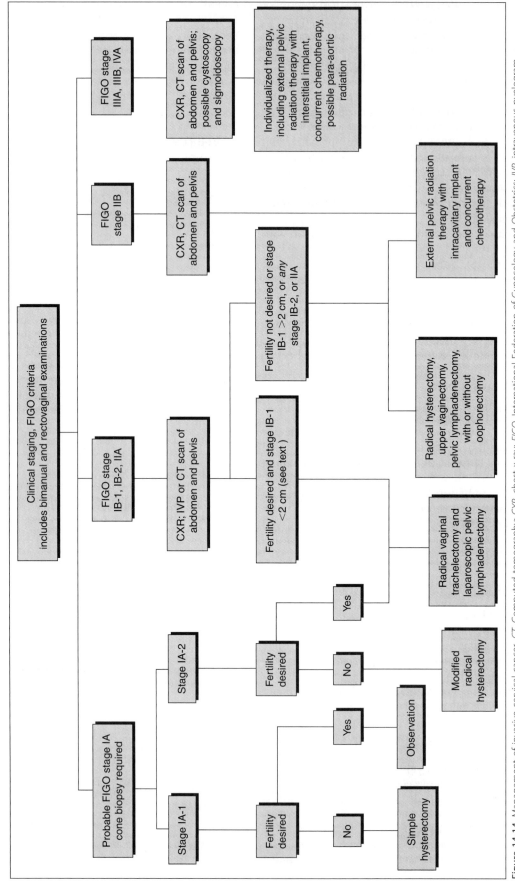

Figure 14-14 Management of invasive cervical cancer. *CT,* Computed tomography; *CXR,* chest x-ray; *FIGO,* International Federation of Gynecology and Obstetrics; *IVP,* intravenous pyelogram.

lesions still confined to the cervix (stages IA2, IB1, and IB2) have an approximately 90% likelihood of 5-year survival following treatment with either surgery or radiation.[41,42] In the subset of patients who are treated surgically and who have no evidence of lymph node metastases, 96% survive 5 years. *However, when disease extends beyond the cervix, 5-year survival falls to 65% for patients with stage II lesions, to 45% for patients with stage III lesions, and to less than 10% for patients with stage IV lesions. Recurrent disease in the pelvis that is treated with radiation results in long-term survival of as many as 45% of patients.* Pelvic exenteration for women whose recurrence is limited to the central pelvis can potentially salvage as much as 60% of patients.[64] Approximately 10% to 15% of patients with metastatic recurrent cervical cancer treated with chemotherapy have objective responses. Progression-free intervals are typically no longer than 1 year.[19]

REFERENCES

1. Ferenczy A, Winkler B. Carcinoma and metastatic tumors of the cervix. In: Kurman RJ (ed). Blaustein's Pathology of the Female Genital Tract, ed 3. New York: Springer Verlag, 1987.

2. Jemal A, Siegel R, Ward E, et al. Cancer statistics: 2006. CA Cancer J Clin 2006;56:106–130.

3. Hinselmann H. Verbesserung der inspektionsmoglichkeiten von vulva, vagina und portio. Munch Med Wschr 1925;1733.

4. Noda S. Colposcopic differential diagnosis of dysplasia, carcinoma in situ and microinvasive carcinoma of the cervix. Aust N Z J Obstet Gynaecol 1981;21:37–42.

5. Liu WM, Chao KC, Wang KI, et al. Colposcopic assessment in microinvasive carcinoma of the cervix. Zhonghua Yi Xue Za Zhi (Taipei) 1989;43:171–176.

6. Sugimori H, Matsuyama T, Kashimura M, et al. Colposcopic findings in microinvasive carcinoma of the uterine cervix. Obstet Gynecol Survey 1979;34:804–807.

7. Benedet JL, Anderson GH, Boyes DA. Colposcopic accuracy in the diagnosis of microinvasive and occult invasive carcinoma of the cervix. Obstet Gynecol 1985;65:557–562.

8. Paraskevaidis E, Kitchener HC, Miller ID, et al. A population-based study of microinvasive disease of the cervix-a colposcopic and cytologic analysis. Gynecol Oncol 1992;45:9–12.

9. Hopman EH, Kenemans P, Helmerhorst TJM. Positive predictive rate of colposcopic examination of the cervix uteri: an overview of literature. Obstet Gynecol Survey 1998;53:97–106.

10. Edebiri AA. The relative significance of colposcopic descriptive appearances in the diagnosis of cervical intraepithelial neoplasia. Int J Gynecol Obstet 1990;33:23–29.

11. Hopman EH, Voorhorst FJ, Kenemans P, et al. Observer agreement on interpreting colposcopic images of CIN. Gynecol Oncol 1995;58:206–209.

12. Choo YC, Chan OLY, Hsu C, et al. Colposcopy in microinvasive carcinoma of the cervix: an enigma of diagnosis. Br J Obstet Gynaecol 1994;91:1156–1160.

13. Van Meir JM, Wielenga G, Drogendijk A. Colposcopic analysis of 20 patients with microinvasive carcinoma of the uterine cervix. Obstet Gynecol Surv 1979;34:872–873.

14. Koller O. The Vascular Patterns of the Uterine Cervix. Philadelphia: FA Davis, 1963.

15. Folkman J. Tumor angiogenesis: therapeutic implications. New Engl J Med 1971;285:1182.

16. Follen M. Preinvasive squamous lesions of the female lower genital tract. In: Gershenson DM, DeCherney AH, Curry SJ, Brubaker L (eds). Operative Gynecology, 2nd Edition. Philadelphia: Saunders, 2001.

17. Cervix uteri. In: Fleming ID, Cooper JS, Henson DE, et al (eds). AJCC Cancer Staging Handbook. Philadelphia: Lippincott-Raven, 1998.

18. Reagan JW, Ng ABP. The cellular manifestations of uterine carcinogenesis. In: Norris NJ, Hertig AT, Abell MR (eds). The Uterus. Baltimore: Williams & Wilkins, 1973.

19. Stehman FB, Perez CA, Kurman RJ, et al. Uterine cervix. In: Hoskins WJ, Perez CA, Young RC (eds). Principles and Practice of Gynecologic Oncology. Philadelphia: Lippincott-Raven, 1997.

20. Cherry CP, Glucksmann A. Lymphatic embolism and lymph node metastasis in cancers of the vulva and uterine cervix. Cancer 1955;8:564–575.

21. Okagaki T, Clark BA, Zachow KR. Presence of human papillomavirus in verrucous carcinoma of the vagina: immunohistochemical, ultrastructural, and DNA hybridization studies. Arch Pathol Lab Med 1984;108:567–570.

22. Rando RF, Sedlacek TV, Hunt J, et al. Verrucous carcinoma of the vulva associated with an unusual type 6 human papillomavirus. Obstet Gynecol 1986;67(3 suppl):70S–75S.

23. Kashimura M, Tsukamoto N, Matsuyama K, et al. Verrucous carcinoma of the uterine cervix: report of a case with follow-up of 6½ years. Gynecol Oncol 1984;19:204–215.

24. Shingleton HM, Fowler WCJr, Koch GG. Pretreatment evaluation in cervical cancer. Am J Obstet Gynecol 1971;110: 385–389.

25. Lagasse LD, Creasman WT, Shingleton HM, et al. Results and complications of operative staging in cervical cancer: experience of the Gynecologic Oncology Group. Gynecol Oncol 1980;9:90–98.

26. Rajendran JG, Greer BE. Expanding role of positron emission tomography in cancer of the uterine cervix. J Natl Compr Canc Netw 2006;4:463–469.

27. Berman ML, Lagasse LD, Watring WG, et al. The operative evaluation of patients with cervical carcinoma by an extraperitoneal approach. Obstet Gynecol 1977;50:658–664.

28. Nelson JH, Macasaet MA, Lu T, et al. The incidence and significance of para-aortic lymph node metastases in invasive carcinoma of the cervix. Am J Obstet Gynecol 1974;118: 749–756.

29. Morrow CP, Curtin JP. Surgery for cervical neoplasia. In: Gynecologic Cancer Surgery. New York: Churchill Livingstone, 1996, p 472.

30. Cavanagh D, Ruffalo EH, Marsden DE. Gynecologic Cancer: A Clinico-Pathologic Approach. East Norwalk, CT: Appleton-Lange, 1985, p 79.

31. Van Nagell JR, Greenwell N, Powell DF, et al. Microinvasive carcinoma of the cervix. Am J Obstet Gynecol 1983;145: 981–991.

32. Creasman WT, Fetter BF, Clarke-Pearson DL, et al. Management of stage IA carcinoma of the cervix. Am J Obstet Gynecol 1985;153:164–172.

33. Tseng CJ, Horng SG, Soong YK, et al. Conservative conization for microinvasive carcinoma of the cervix. Am J Obstet Gynecol 1997;176:1009–1010.

34. Paraskevaidis E, Kalantaridou SN, Kaponis A, et al. Surgical management of early stage cervical cancer: ten years experience from one Greek health region. Eur J Gynaecol Oncol. 2002; 23(4):341–344.

35. Collins HS, Burke TW, Woodward JE, et al. Widespread lymph node metastases in a patient with microinvasive cervical carcinoma. Gynecol Oncol 1989;34:219.

36. Photopulos GJ, Vander Zwagg R. Class II radical hysterectomy shows less morbidity and good treatment efficacy compared to class III. Gynecol Oncol 1991;40:21.

37. Magrina JF, Goodrich MA, Weaver AL, et al. Modified radical hysterectomy: morbidity and mortality. Gynecol Oncol 1995; 59:277.

38. Magrina JF, Goodrich MA, Lidner TK, et al. Modified radical hysterectomy in the treatment of early squamous cervical cancer. Gynecol Oncol 1999;72:183–186.

39. Nelson JH Jr, Averette HE, Richart RM. Detection, diagnostic evaluation and treatment of dysplasia and early carcinoma of the cervix. CA Cancer J Clin 1975 May-Jun; 25(3):134–151.

40. Seski JC, Abell MR, Morley GW. Microinvasive squamous carcinoma of the cervix: definition, histologic analysis, late results of treatment. Obstet Gynecol 1977;50:410–414.

41. Newton M. Radical hysterectomy or radiotherapy for stage I cervical cancer. Am J Obstet Gynecol 1975;123:535–542.

42. Morley GW, Seski JC. Radical pelvic surgery versus radiation therapy for stage I carcinoma of the cervix (exclusive of microinvasion). Am J Obstet Gynecol 1976;126:785–798.

43. Roddick JW Jr, Greenelaw RH. Treatment of cervical cancer. A randomized study of operation and radiation. Am J Obstet Gynecol 1971;119:754–764.

44. Webb GA. The role of ovarian conservation in the treatment of carcinoma of the cervix with radical surgery. Am J Obstet Gynecol 1975;122:476–484.

45. Abitbol NM, Davenport JH. Sexual dysfunction after therapy for cervical carcinoma. Am J Obstet Gynecol 1974;119: 181–189.

46. Seibel M, Freeman MG, Graves WL. Carcinoma of the cervix and sexual function. Obstet Gynecol 1979;55:484–487.

47. Allen HH, Collins JA. Surgical management of carcinoma of the cervix. Am J Obstet Gynecol 1977;127:741–744.

48. Artman LE, Hoskins WJ, Bibro MC, et al. Radical hysterectomy and pelvic lymphadenectomy for stage IB carcinoma of the cervix: 21 years experience. Gynecol Oncol 1987;28:8–13.

49. Hoskins WJ, Ford JH Jr, Lutz MH, et al. Radical hysterectomy and pelvic lymphadenectomy for the management of early invasive cancer of the cervix. Gynecol Oncol 1976;4:278–290.

50. Anderson B, LaPolla J, Turner D, et al. Ovarian transposition in cervical cancer. Gynecol Oncol 1993;4:206–214.

51. Feeney DD, Moore DH, Look KY, et al. The fate of the ovaries after radical hysterectomy and ovarian transposition. Gynecol Oncol 1995;56:3–7.

52. Letschert JG. The prevention of radiation induced small bowel complications. Eur J Cancer 1995;31A:1361–1365.

53. Extraperitoneal pelvic lymph node dissection with modified radical hysterectomy. In: Gallup DG, Talledo OE (eds). Surgical Atlas of Gynecologic Oncology. Philadelphia: Saunders, 1994.

54. Radical hysterectomy with pelvic lymph node dissection. In: Gallup DG, Talledo OE (eds). Surgical Atlas of Gynecologic Oncology. Philadelphia: Saunders, 1994.

55. Hopkins MP, Peters WA 3rd , Anderson W, et al. Invasive cervical cancer treated initially by standard hysterectomy. Gynecol Oncol 1990;36:7–12.

56. Nelson AJ 3rd, Fletcher GH, Wharton JT. Indications for adjunctive conservative extrafascial hysterectomy in selected cases of carcinoma of the uterine cervix. AJR Am J Roentgenol 1975;123:91–99.

57. Gallion HH, Van Nagell JR Jr, Donaldson ES, et al. Combined radiation therapy and extrafascial hysterectomy in the treatment of stage IB barrel-shaped cervical cancer. Cancer 1985;56:262–265.

58. Whitney CW, Sause W, Bundy BN, et al. Randomized comparison of fluorouracil plus cisplatin versus hydroxyurea as an adjunct to radiation therapy in stages IIB-IVA carcinoma of the cervix with negative para-aortic nodes. A Gynecologic Oncology Group and Southwest Oncology Group study. J Clin Oncol 1999;17:1339–1348.

59. Morris M, Eifel PJ, Lu J, et al. Pelvic radiation with concurrent chemotherapy versus pelvic and para-aortic radiation for high-risk cervical cancer: a randomized Radiation Therapy Oncology Group clinical trial. New Engl J Med 1999;340:1137–1343.

60. Rose PG, Bundy BN, Watkins EB, et al. Concurrent cisplatin-based chemoradiation improves progression-free and overall survival in advanced cervical cancer: results of a randomized Gynecologic Oncology Group study. New Engl J Med 1999;340:1144–1153. Erratum in: N Engl J Med 1999;341(9):708.

61. Rotman M, Choi K, Guse C, et al. Prophylactic irradiation of the para-aortic node chain in stage IIB and bulky stage IB carcinoma of the cervix: Initial results of RTOG 7920. Int J Radiat Oncol Biol Phys 1990;19:513–521. Erratum in: Int J Radiat Oncol Biol Phys 1991;20(1):193.

62. Haie C, Pejovic MH, Gerbaulet A, et al. Is prophylactic para-aortic irradiation worthwhile in the treatment of advanced cervical carcinoma? Results of controlled clinical trial of the EORTC radiotherapy group. Radiother Oncol 1988;11: 101–112.

63. Million RR, Rutledge F, Fletcher GH. Stage IV carcinoma of the cervix with bladder invasion. Am J Obstet Gynecol 1972;113:239–246.

64. Morley GW, Hopkins MP, Lindenauer SM, et al. Pelvic exenteration, University of Michigan: 100 patients at 5 years. Obstet Gynecol 1989;74:934–943.

65. duPont NC, Monk BJ. Chemotherapy in the management of cervical carcinoma. Clin Adv Hematol Oncol 2006;4: 279–286.

66. Dursun P, LeBlanc E, Nogueira MC. Radical vaginal trachelectomy (Dargent's operation): a critical review of the literature. Eur J Surg Oncol 2007 Oct; 33(8):933–941

67. Dargent D. Radical vaginal hysterectomy. In: Smith JR, Del Priore G, Curtin J, et al (eds). An Atlas of Gynecologic Oncology. London: Martin Dunitz, 2001.

68. Plante M, Renaud M-C, Hoskins IA, et al. Vaginal radical trachelectomy: a valuable fertility-preserving option in the management of early-stage cervical cancer. A series of 50 pregnancies and review of the literature. Gynecol Oncol 2005;98:3–10.

CASE STUDY 1 QUESTIONS

HISTORY

A 63-year-old gravida 2, para 2 is referred to you. Her last Pap smear and gynecologic examination were 30 years ago during her last pregnancy.

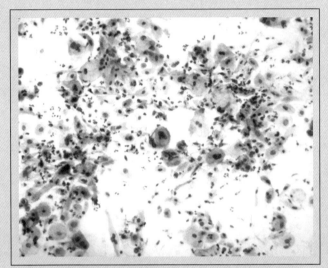

Figure 14-15 This is her Pap smear.

• Describe what you see.

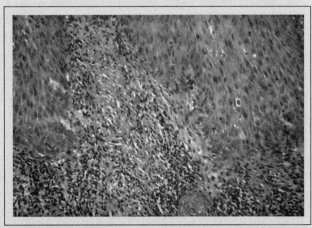

Figure 14-17 This is a biopsy of the cervix at the 6-o'clock position.

• What is your diagnosis?
• What is the appropriate next step in this patient's management?

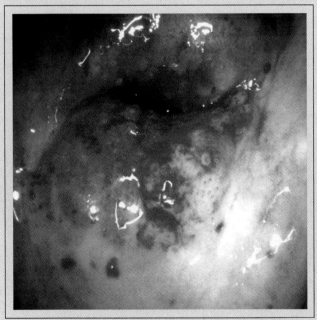

Figure 14-16 This is a photograph of her colposcopic findings.

• What do you see?

CASE STUDY 1 ANSWERS

FIGURE 14-15

There are several keratinized cells with larger hyperchromatic nuclei and pink cytoplasm. The shape of the cells is elongated and bizarre, suggestive of malignancy.

FIGURE 14-16

The cervix is atrophic, which makes the colposcopic findings less prominent. Acetowhite epithelium is seen with coarse punctation. Some of the punctation tends to be slightly linear or comma shaped. The borders of the lesions are not well seen. This is a high-grade lesion.

FIGURE 14-17

Although the surface of the lesion is not seen in this view, there are spindle-shaped, crowded, hyperchromatic nuclei extending toward the surface of the epithelium, suggestive of a high-grade lesion. However, at the bottom, a small tongue of neoplastic epithelium can be seen below the basement membrane. This is a microinvasive lesion.

The next step in the patient's management is a cone biopsy. When microinvasive cancer is seen on a punch biopsy, one can never be certain that frankly invasive cancer is not present elsewhere in the cervix. In the postmenopausal patient, treatment with an extrafascial hysterectomy following the cone biopsy is appropriate. Bypassing the cone biopsy and treating the patient with an extrafascial hysterectomy could potentially compromise treatment if she turns out to have an occult or frankly invasive cancer because it would eliminate the ability to treat her with a radical hysterectomy.

CASE STUDY 2 QUESTIONS

HISTORY

A 30-year-old gravida 0, para 0 is referred to you for evaluation of a Pap smear showing atypical squamous cells of undetermined significance.

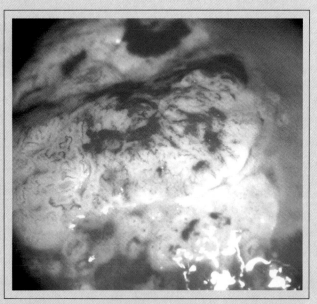

Figure 14-18 This is a close-up photograph of her colposcopic findings.

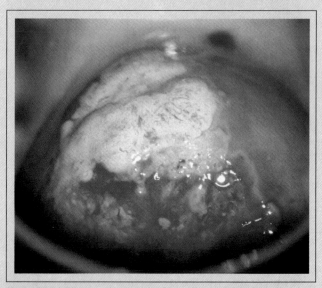

Figure 14-19 This is a photograph of her colposcopic findings.

• Describe what you see.

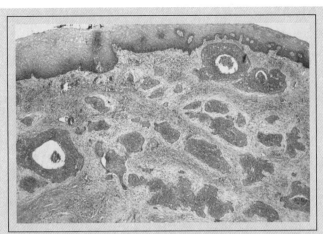

Figure 14-20 This is a biopsy of the cervix from the friable area with atypical vessels.

- What is the diagnosis?
- What is the proper management of this case?

CASE STUDY 2 ANSWERS

FIGURES 14-18 AND 14-19

On the anterior lip of the cervix, there is a dense, raised, acetowhite lesion with atypical vessels, including comma shapes and curlicues. This is consistent with an invasive cancer.

FIGURE 14-20

This is a frankly invasive cancer, with infiltrating cancer seen throughout under the basement membrane.

This woman needs to be treated with a radical hysterectomy. For a FIGO stage I lesion, pelvic radiation is inappropriate because it will irradiate her ovaries and cause premature menopause. If she still desires to retain her fertility, a woman with a lesion of 2 cm may be offered a radical vaginal trachelectomy procedure. Less aggressive therapy (cone biopsy or simple hysterectomy) would not be curative.

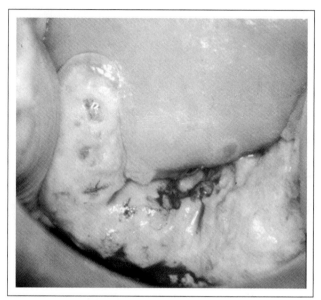

Plate 14-1 Large, raised cancer, yellow in appearance, on the posterior lip of the cervix. There is an ulcer at 6 o'clock and atypical vessels throughout the mass.

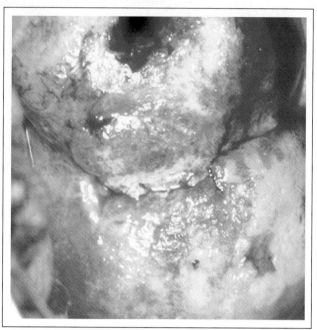

Plate 14-3 Mass on the anterior lip of cervix with atypical vessels and yellow appearance. There is also leukoplakia of the posterior lip of the cervix.

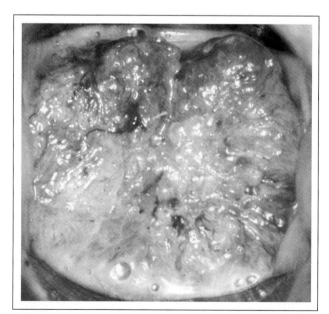

Plate 14-2 Fungating cancer with obliteration of the os and multiple atypical vessels.

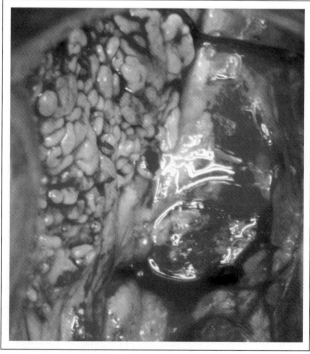

Plate 14-4 Papillary tumor of the cervix.

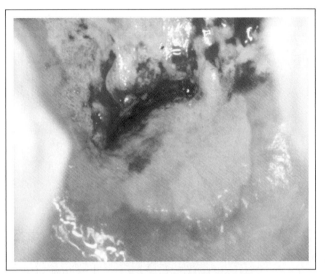

Plate 14-5 Example of microinvasive cancer. There is dense acetowhite epithelium and coarse punctation with a rolled edge at 10 o'clock. Contact bleeding is present on the upper right cervix.

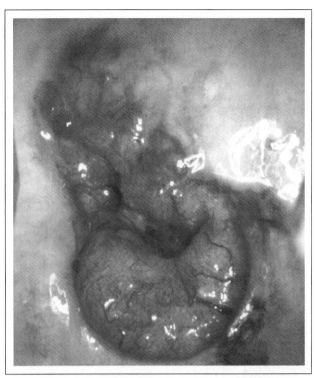

Plate 14-7 Raised fleshy mass almost circumferentially involving the central cervix. Note the multiple atypical vessels. This is Figure 14.6 before the application of 5% acetic acid.

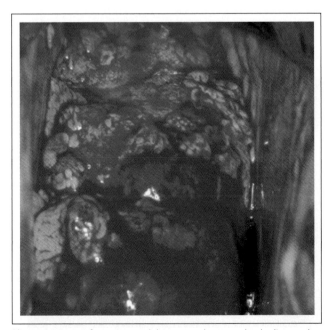

Plate 14-6 Large, fungating, nodular cancer that completely distorts the normal cervical anatomy, accompanied by bleeding.

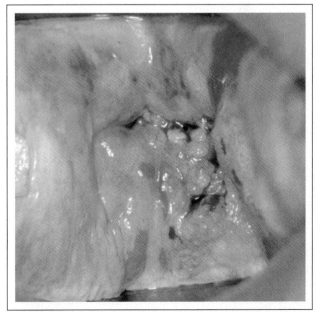

Plate 14-8 Irregular surface contour of a cancer involving primarily the central, posterior portion of the cervix. (Image provided by Dr. Vesna Kesic.)

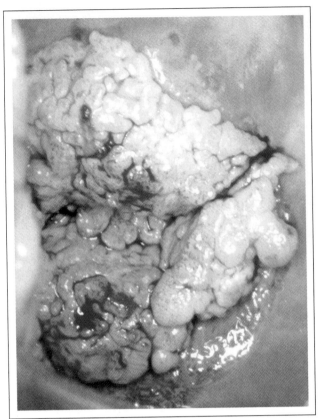

Plate 14-9 Cervical cancer with an encephaloid appearance and scattered atypical vessels. This could be confused with a condyloma.

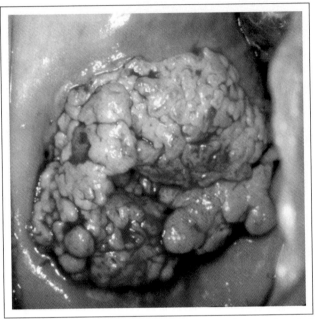

Plate 14-11 Cancer with encephaloid appearance and scattered atypical vessels.

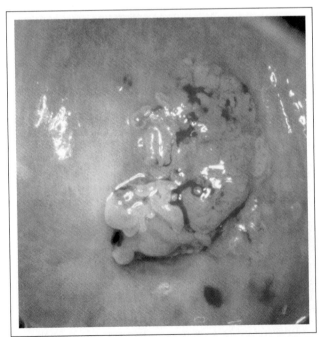

Plate 14-10 Papillary cancer with atypical vessels. (Image provided by Dr. Vesna Kesic.)

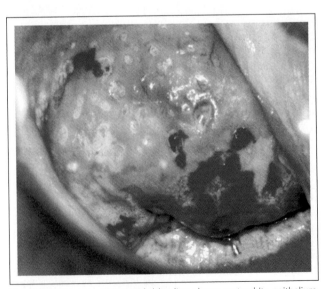

Plate 14-12 Invasive cancer with bleeding, dense acetowhite epithelium, and superficial spread on the anterior aspect of the cervix.

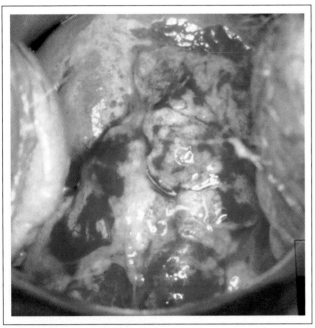

Plate 14-13 Cancer with an irregular, papillary surface; dense acetowhite epithelium; and atypical vessels.

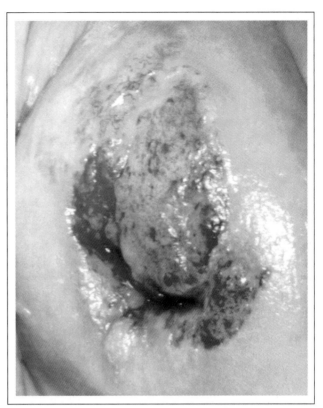

Plate 14-15 Bizarre vessels over the entire cervix and a nodule at 7 o'clock.

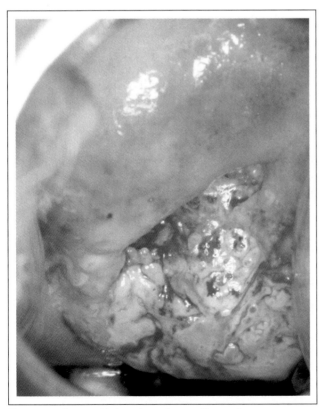

Plate 14-14 Cancer with irregular, yellow papillary surface.

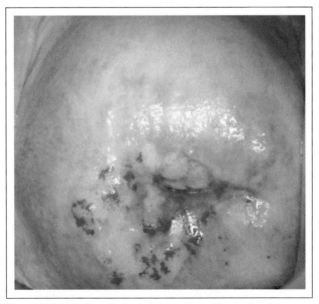

Plate 14-16 Multiple atypical vessels in a patient with microinvasive carcinoma.

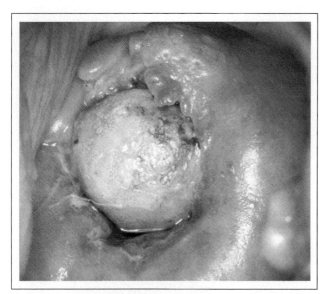

Plate 14-17 Large endocervical mass with acetowhite epithelium, mosaic, and papillary necrosis. Biopsy showed invasive cancer.

CHAPTER 15

Cervical Glandular Disease: Adenocarcinoma *In Situ* and Adenocarcinoma

V. Cecil Wright

KEY POINTS

- The incidence of glandular disease is increasing in young women, particularly those younger than 35 years old.
- Approximately 46% to 72% of glandular cases contain a coexisting squamous lesion.
- Atypical glandular cells are reported in 41% to 71% of cases of cervical adenocarcinoma and adenocarcinoma *in situ* (AIS).
- Oncogenic HPV deoxyribonucleic acid (DNA) viral types are found in 64% to 89% of cases adenocarcinoma and AIS; viral type 16 is most common in AIS and viral type 18 in adenocarcinoma.
- The most common presentation is a papillary expression resembling an immature transformation zone (TZ). The criteria for evaluating the squamous lesion are not applicable for glandular lesions. Punctation, mosaicism, and corkscrew-like blood vessels as seen in squamous disease are not seen in glandular lesions.
- All patients with atypical glandular cytology are referred for colposcopy.
- Colposcopy cannot differentiate between AIS and an adenocarcinoma.
- Most glandular lesions lie within or close to the TZ.
- The diagnosis of AIS is made on an excisional biopsy. In order to be certain that no coexisting adenocarcinoma exists, the specimen must have negative margins.
- Conservative management is an acceptable option in a woman with AIS with negative histologically proved margins.

Adenocarcinoma *in situ* (AIS) of the uterine cervix was first described in 1953 by Fridel and McKay.[1] The incidence ratio of AIS to cervical intraepithelial neoplasia, grade 3 (CIN 3) (severe dysplasia/carcinoma *in situ*) has been reported as 1:26 to 1:237.[2,3] *Approximately 46% to 72% of glandular lesions (adenocarcinoma or AIS) contain a coexisting squamous lesion and are termed* mixed disease.[2,4] The difference between the proportion of AIS (2% of *in situ* lesions) and the proportion of adenocarcinoma cases (23–25% of all cervical cancers) is striking.[3,5] The squamous components (of

both *in situ* and invasive disease) appear to remain separate and distinct from the glandular lesions.[6] AIS is found in women between 18 and 75 years with an mean age range of 35 to 38.8 years.[3,7] Women with mixed disease are 5 to 6 years younger than those with pure AIS.[8] This is because cytology is better at identifying squamous than glandular disease, hence the unexpected cases of glandular histology when investigating abnormal squamous cytology.[8] *The early diagnosis of AIS continues to represent a challenge for clinicians because of the lack of clinical findings, the absence of cytologic evidence of glandular disease, and the fact that clinicians may be unfamiliar with the colposcopic signs of glandular disease.*[6]

RISK FACTORS AND EPIDEMIOLOGY

The stimulus to disease development relates to many factors including reserve cell hyperplasia, human papillomavirus (HPV) infection, hormones, and obesity.

Reserve Cell Hyperplasia

The subcolumnar reserve cells in cervical epithelium are analogous to stem cells in the hemopoietic system and represent undifferentiated bipotential cells (Figure 15-1). A proliferation of reserve cells without maturation is called *reserve cell hyperplasia.* Reserve cell hyperplasia is observed in the metaplastic process, during which stratified squamous epithelium replaces columnar epithelium on the surface epithelium and in the glandular crypts. Atypical reserve cells have been observed in both squamous and glandular disease. This supports the theory that the reserve cell has a potential to differentiate into a squamous cancer cell or an adenocarcinoma cell.[9,10] This would explain the association of glandular lesions with normal metaplasia or glandular lesions coexisting with squamous disease. One explanation for the disparity in incidence of squamous disease and

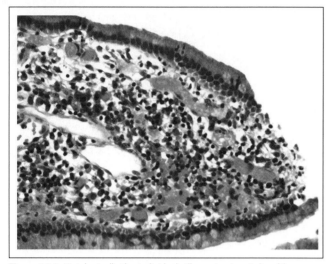

Figure 15-1 Histologically the individual villous structure is lined by a single layer of tall columnar cells with basally situated nuclei. It contains a central vascular network. Reserve cells lie beneath the columnar cells (hematoxylin-eosin stain, high magnification).

glandular disease may be the tendency for reserve cells to show a preference to develop into squamous cells. Reserve cells proliferate as a result of external stimulation as injury of columnar epithelium, changes toward an acidic vaginal pH (normal 3.8–4.2), hormonal stimuli, and pregnancy.[11]

Hormone Stimulation

The increased incidence of adenocarcinoma of the cervix, particularly in young women, may be related to the long-term use of the oral contraceptive pill (OCP).[12,13] Other authors have found no relationship between the use of OCPs and cervical adenocarcinoma or squamous cell cancer.[14,15] Obesity appears to be a risk factor for adenocarcinoma but not squamous disease. This, in combination with the association of OCP use with glandular disease in some studies, suggests there may be a hormonally associated process for the development of glandular disease.[16] Further study is needed.

Association of High-Risk Human Papillomavirus Deoxyribonucleic Acid Viral Types

Using polymerase chain reaction (PCR)-based tests, oncogenic (high-risk) HPV deoxyribonucleic acid (DNA) is found in 99.7% of squamous cell cervical cancers.[17,18] In cervical glandular disease (AIS and adenocarcinoma) the correlation is less pronounced, with high-risk HPV DNA types found in 64% to 89% of cases.[19] *Viral types 16 and 18 predominate in AIS and adenocarcinoma, with type 18 being more common in adenocarcinoma and type 16 in AIS lesions.*[20,21] *The frequency of HPV DNA-negative adenocarcinomas increases with age.* HPV was identified in 89% of women

younger than age 40 but only in 43% of women older than 60 years.[20] The most common HPV types detected in mucinous adenocarcinomas were HPV 16 (50%), HPV 18 (40%), HPV 45 (10%), HPV 52 (2%), and HPV 35 (1%). Multiple HPV types were detected in 9.7% of the cases.[22] HPV was not detected in any nonmucinous adenocarcinomas including clear cell, serous, and mesonephric carcinomas.[22]

NATURAL HISTORY

Adenocarcinoma *In Situ*: The Precancerous Lesion

Many studies confirm that AIS is a preinvasive lesion that progresses to cervical adenocarcinoma if left untreated.[3,4,7,23] *Women diagnosed with AIS are 10 to 20 years younger than those with invasive disease.*[3,7,24] The AIS component is frequently found within the same specimen as the adenocarcinoma with similar recognizable histologic features.[4,23] Foci of microscopic invasive disease are seen arising from AIS areas.[4] The rate of progression of AIS to a glandular cancer is not altered by the presence of a squamous component. Finally, similar high-risk HPV DNA viral types are found in both AIS and adenocarcinoma.[20–22]

SCREENING

Cytology

The identification of abnormal glandular cells on cervical cytology is a significant finding. *Cytologic screening is less effective in preventing adenocarcinoma than squamous cell carcinoma of the cervix.*[25–27] This relates to the sensitivity of detection (the percentage of smears demonstrating a high-grade abnormality, either squamous or glandular) and to sampling and screening/diagnostic errors (smears on review demonstrating positive cytology that were originally missed).[28] Unfortunately, an alternative screening test for AIS with better performance characteristics is not available. Atypical glandular cells (AGCs) are reported cytologically in only 41% to 71% of AIS cases.[8,27–29] *The remaining cases of glandular disease are recognized in the course of the evaluation of women with abnormal squamous cytology, particularly in women with mixed disease. AIS can be found buried under normal metaplastic and dysplastic squamous epithelium in 60% of cases, making the glandular component inaccessible to cytologic sampling* (Figure 15-2).[4] Devices such as the extended spatula, endocervical brush, and broom enable sampling of the ectocervix, transformation zone (TZ), and endocervix and appear to have the lowest false-negative rates.[30–32] However, both the benign and neoplastic cytologic patterns produced by these sampling devices are different that those typical of conventional cytology and may require the cytopathologist to retrain.[33,34] Other causes of

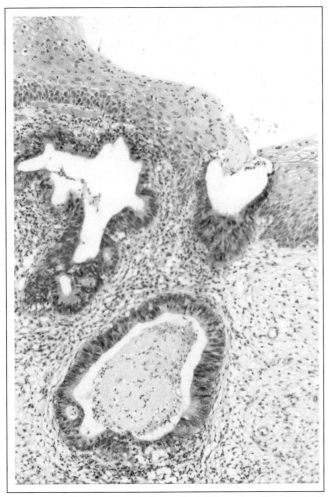

Figure 15-2 AIS disease in cervical crypts buried beneath surface dysplastic epithelium (hematoxylin-eosin stain, intermediate magnification).

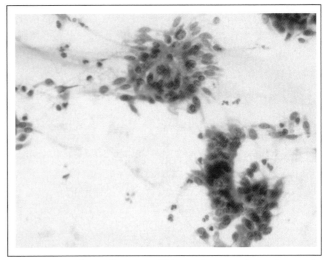

Figure 15-3 Cytology reflecting an AIS lesion demonstrating nuclear atypia, overlapping of cells (pseudostratification), sheets, strips or rosette formations, peripheral featuring, and chromatin clumping.

The cytologic features of AIS/adenocarcinoma are well described. These include nuclear atypia, overlapping of cells (pseudostratification), sheets, strips or rosette formations, peripheral featuring, and chromatin clumping in a clear background (Figure 15-3).[29,38,39] When a cytologic smear is reported as endocervical AIS, a glandular lesion (AIS or adenocarcinoma) will be found in 96% of cases, with the majority (more than 80%) being AIS cases.[28,39]

Adjunct Diagnostic/Screening Tools

Evidence suggests that adjunct diagnostic tools such as HPV testing and immunohistochemistry for molecular markers such as p16 (INK4A) are of value to further evaluate abnormal cytology.[40–43] Overexpression of p16 is induced by HPV oncoprotein E7 and distinguishes intraepithelial lesions from benign lesions.[40] Investigation using p16 (INK4A) has been evaluated in AGC. HPV DNA was detected in 93% of women with HSIL associated with AGC and in 71% of women with AIS cytology.[41] Other studies demonstrate p16 immunocytochemical stain to identify cytology related to HPV.[42] However, not all glandular cases test positive for the molecular marker.[41,43]

Detection of high-risk HPV DNA has been used in investigating women with AGC. Studies indicate that HPV DNA testing might be an effective screening test in the initial management of cytologic atypical glandular cells (AGC-NOS).[43–45]

COLPOSCOPIC FINDINGS

Normal Columnar Epithelium

Columnar epithelium lines the surface of the cervix and its associated endocervical crypts between the squamocolumnar junction and the histologic internal os (Figure 15-4).

atypical glandular cells include columnar and squamous epithelium undergoing reactive and regenerative changes; Arias-Stella changes in the cervix (a rare pregnancy change of endocervical crypts characterized by enlarged hyperchromatic nuclei of irregular shape with abundant cytoplasm, with or without increased secretory activity, without mitotic changes); cervical polyps; mesonephric duct hyperplasia; tubal or serous metaplasia; cervical endometriosis; microglandular hyperplasia; and endocervical changes associated with an intrauterine device.[35]

The Bethesda System 2001 assigned categories for abnormal glandular cytology.[36] This subclassification includes AGC (specify endocervical, endometrial, or not otherwise specified [AGC-NOS]); AGC-favor neoplastic (specify endocervical or not otherwise specified); endocervical AIS; and adenocarcinoma. These represent significant categories in that *AGC-NOS reporting demonstrates histologic-proven invasive cancer, AIS, or CIN 2,3 in 9% to 41% of cases, and in AGC-favor neoplasia reported cytology as many as 96% will have a significant histologic lesion comprising invasive cancer, AIS, or CIN 2,3.*[37]

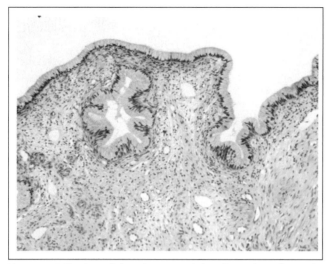

Figure 15-4 Histology of the columnar epithelium lining the surface and underlying endocervical crypts is similar (hematoxylin-eosin stain, low magnification).

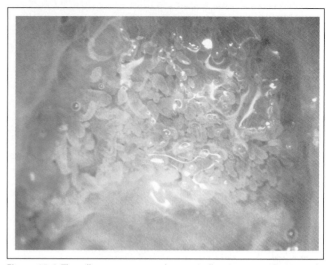

Figure 15-6 The villous structures colposcopically appear translucent and remain so after the application of 3% to 5% acetic acid in the absence of metaplasia. (From Wright VC. Principles of Cervical Colposcopy. Figure 5.3. Houston: Biomedical Communications, 2004, p 5–5.)

The endocervical crypts lie below, at, or above the anatomical internal os. The columnar epithelium becomes continuous with the endometrial epithelium at the internal os. The location of columnar epithelium on the ectocervix is embryologically determined and is termed an *ectopy*. Ectopy contains villous structures (Figure 15-5) with a central vascular core that is responsible for the angioarchitecture seen in glandular disease.[6] Surface epithelium that extends into the cervical stroma forming crypts is lined by the same surface columnar epithelium (see Figure 15-4) and is susceptible to the same benign (metaplasia) or disease process (squamous or glandular) that affects the surface epithelium.

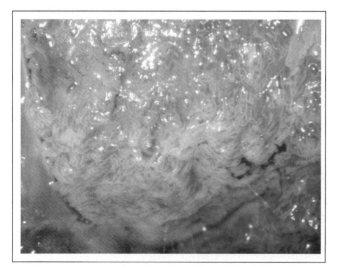

Figure 15-5 A colpophotograph of the villous structures of an ectopy. Frequently no angioarchitecture is seen colposcopically. (From Wright VC. Color Atlas of Colposcopy. Figure 6.1. Houston: Biomedical Communications, 2003, p 6–32.)

Colposcopically the villous structures demonstrate translucence that is retained after the application of 3% to 5% acetic acid in the absence of metaplasia and glandular disease (Figure 15-6). The histologic structure of the cervical columnar epithelium and associated crypts consist of a single layer of tall secretory cylindrical cells with basally situated nuclei (see Figure 15-4). Ciliary cells account for 4% to 6% of the total population. The primitive stem cells (reserve cells) lie below the basal layer (see Figure 15-1).[46–48]

Presentations of Adenocarcinoma *In Situ* and Adenocarcinoma

There is no single colposcopic appearance that characterizes glandular lesions. In many cases the colposcopic appearances mimic other lesions.[6] Colposcopy cannot differentiate between AIS and cervical adenocarcinoma. *The diagnosis of AIS requires an excised conization specimen with negative margins that demonstrates AIS in the absence of adenocarcinoma. Most AIS lesions are located within the TZ or its immediate proximity.* Features of glandular disease have been described to alert the colposcopist to suspect a glandular lesion.[6] *The standard colposcopic criteria commonly used to identify and grade squamous lesion, including vascular patterns (mosaic, punctuation, corkscrew vessels), surface contour, color tone, and the margin of the lesion, are not applicable to glandular lesions.*[6,49,50]

When glandular disease can be colposcopically identified, its appearance is most commonly manifest in one of three ways.[6,51] *The most common manifestation (85%) appears after the application of 3% to 5% acetic acid and resembles immature metaplasia.* The diseased villous structures assume a white color resembling the fused-appearing villous structures of immature metaplasia (Figure 15-7). *The second most common manifestation is variegated (patchy) red and white*

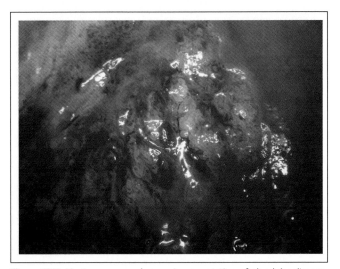

Figure 15-7 Most common colposcopic presentation of glandular disease (in this case, AIS). After the application of 3% to 5% acetic acid, the involved diseased villi assume a white color resembling metaplasia found in an immature TZ. (From Wright VC. Principles of Cervical Colposcopy. Figure 10.11. Houston: Biomedical Communications, 2004, p 10–9.)

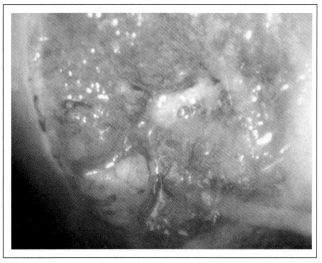

Figure 15-9 The least common colposcopic presentation of glandular disease (in this case, AIS) is a single, isolated, densely acetowhite and elevated lesion that may or may not be in contact with the squamocolumnar junction. (From Wright VC. Principles of Cervical Colposcopy. Figure 10.28. Houston: Biomedical Communications, 2004, p 10–13.)

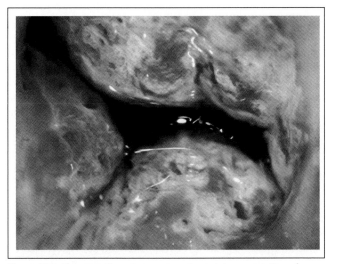

Figure 15-8 The second most common colposcopic presentation of glandular disease (in this case, AIS) is variegated (patchy) red and white areas resembling an immature transformation zone. (From Wright VC. Principles of Cervical Colposcopy. Figure 10.22. Houston: Biomedical Communications, 2004, p 10–11.)

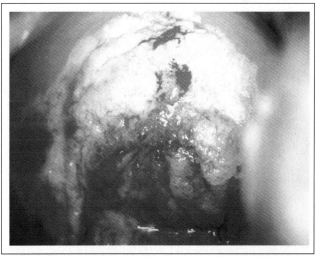

Figure 15-10 A colpophotograph of the surface topography of AIS demonstrating acetowhite papillary formations overlying columnar epithelium. (From Wright VC. Color Atlas of Colposcopy. Figure 11.20. Houston: Biomedical Communications, 2003, p 11–72.)

areas resembling an immature TZ (Figure 15-8). *Finally, a glandular lesion may be manifested as a single, isolated, densely acetowhite and elevated lesion that may or may not be in contact with the squamocolumnar junction* (Figure 15-9).

Surface Topography Compared with Colposcopic Mimics

Papillary growths must be differentiated from the normal papillary glandular mucosa (see Figures 15-5 and 15-6), AIS (see Figures 15-7 and 15-10), adenocarcinoma (Figure 15-11),

metaplasia (Figure 15-12), condylomata (Figure 15-13), squamous cell carcinoma (Figure 15-14), and microglandular hyperplasia (Figure 15-15). AIS may exhibit papillary excrescences that may appear as single structures or clumped masses after the application of acetic acid (Figures 15-16 and 15-17). Papillary adenocarcinomas may demonstrate individual villous structures that appear elongated and taper to a narrow tip that projects in multiple directions. When viewed sagittally, loop blood vessels may be visible in the individual excrescences. When viewed end on, they can be seen as single dots on the villous

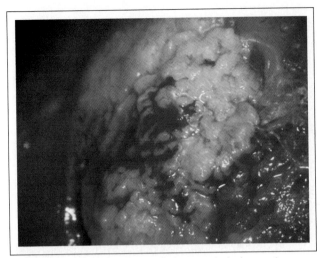

Figure 15-11 A colpophotograph of a large cervical adenocarcinoma, which is very dense acetowhite with fused-appearing papillary excrescences. (From Wright VC. Color Atlas of Colposcopy. Figure 11.31. Houston: Biomedical Communications, 2003, p 11–74.)

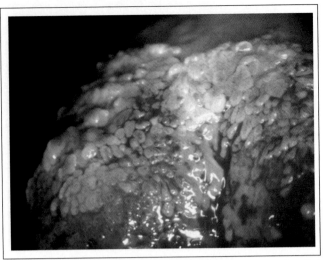

Figure 15-13 A colpophotograph of fused papillary excrescences of cervical condylomata that mimic a glandular lesion. Note the dot-like angioarchitecture in the tips of some of the excrescences. This is also seen in glandular lesions. (From Wright VC. Color Atlas of Colposcopy. Figure 15.4. Houston: Biomedical Communications, 2003, p 15–111.)

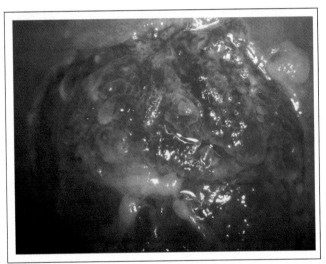

Figure 15-12 A colpophotograph of a fused acetowhite papillary excrescences of immature metaplasia that mimics a glandular lesion. (From Wright VC. Principles of Cervical Colposcopy. Figure 6.1. Houston: Biomedical Communications, 2004, p 6–6.)

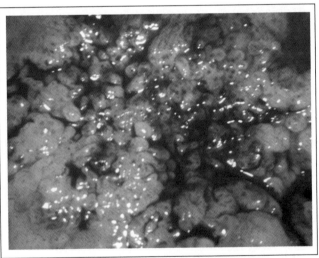

Figure 15-14 A colpophotograph of the fused-appearing papillary excrescences of a squamous cell carcinoma with dot-like angioarchitecture in the tips of the excrescences, which resembles a glandular lesion. (From Wright VC. Principles of Cervical Colposcopy. Figure 7.74. Houston: Biomedical Communications, 2004, p 7–28.)

tips (Figure 15-18). In other papillary adenocarcinomas, the projections are observed to clump into large, dense acetowhite masses with loss of transparency (Figure 15-19).

Epithelial budding formations are seen in AIS (Figure 15-20), metaplasia (Figure 15-21), and condylomata (Figure 15-22). In AIS the enlarging villi become swollen, rounded, or scalloped or have serrated edges (see Figure 15-20).

Some lesions appear to overlie columnar epithelium and demonstrate a band of normal columnar epithelium between the squamous border and the lesion. In this case, the differential diagnosis includes AIS (see Figure 15-9), adenocarcinoma (Figure 15-23), metaplasia (Figure 15-24), condylomata (Figure 15-25), and microglandular hyperplasia (Figure 15-26). AIS can manifest itself as a single, elevated, well-demarcated lesion with an irregular surface overlying columnar epithelium (see Figure 15-9). Alternately, it may exhibit clumped villi in discrete masses that resemble an immature TZ overlying columnar epithelium after dilute acetic acid application (see Figure 15-16).

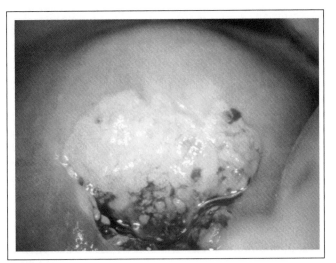

Figure 15-15 A colpophotograph of the acetowhite fused papillary excrescences of microglandular hyperplasia (MGH) mimicking a glandular lesion. MGH lesions are usually devoid of an angioarchitectural pattern colposcopically. (From Wright VC. Principles of Cervical Colposcopy. Figure 14.2. Houston: Biomedical Communications, 2004, p 14–2.)

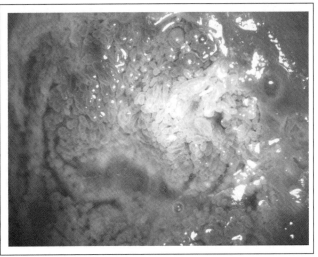

Figure 15-17 This colpophotograph illustrates individual acetowhite villous structures of an AIS lesion in the patient's upper left cervical quadrant. (From Wright VC. Principles of Cervical Colposcopy. Figure 10.6. Houston: Biomedical Communications, 2004, p 10–7.)

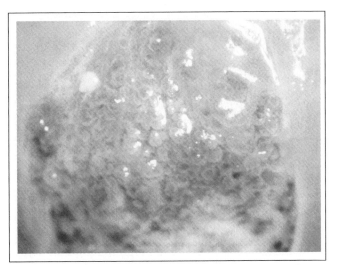

Figure 15-16 A colpophotograph of groups of acetowhite single villous structures of an AIS lesion on the anterior cervical lip. (From Wright VC. Principles of Cervical Colposcopy. Figure 10.6. Houston: Biomedical Communications, 2004, p 10–7.)

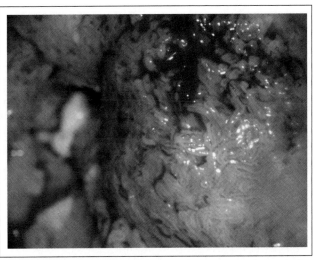

Figure 15-18 A papillary cervical adenocarcinoma is seen colposcopically. Numerous villous-like individual excrescences are seen, which appear similar to the villous structure of an ectopy. Dot-like and looped angioarchitecture is visible colposcopically. (From Wright VC. Principles of Cervical Colposcopy. Figure 10.64. Houston: Biomedical Communications, 2004, p 10–25.)

In contrast, *except in previously treated patients, squamous lesions (intraepithelial and cancer) are always in contact with the squamous border* (Figure 15-27). Adenocarcinoma is also observed overlying columnar epithelium and not in contact with the squamous border, regardless of whether it is expressed as papillary formations or dense acetowhite masses (see Figure 15-23).

When a variegated (patchy) red and white surface is seen, the colposcopist must differentiate between AIS (see Figures 15-8 and 15-28), adenocarcinoma (Figure 15-29), and metaplasia (Figure 15-30).

Blood Vessel Patterns Compared with Colposcopic Mimics

In AIS and adenocarcinoma, a variety of blood vessel patterns can be encountered. *The most common varieties are waste thread–like, tendril-like, root-like, character writing–like, and multiple dot-like vessels.* Waste thread vessels (Figure 15-31) are those that assume peculiar configurations similar to dropping a piece of thread on the floor. These curious formations are seen in AIS (Figure 15-32), adenocarcinoma (Figure 15-33), condylomata (Figure 15-34),

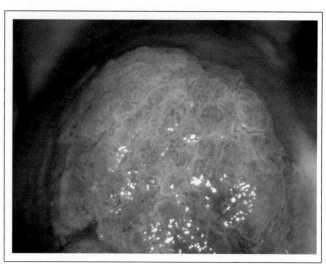

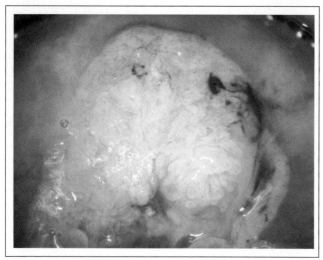

Figure 15-19 Colposcopy demonstrates a papillary adenocarcinoma with dense acetowhite fused papillary excrescences and loss of transparency. (From Wright VC. Principles of Cervical Colposcopy. Figure 10.51. Houston: Biomedical Communications, 2004, p 10–21.)

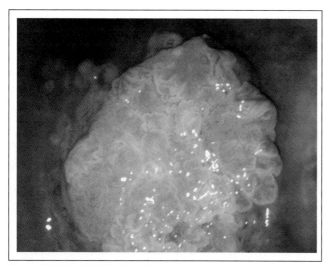

Figure 15-20 Epithelial budding formations are seen colposcopically in this AIS lesion. The enlarged villi appear swollen, rounded, scalloped, or serrated. (From Wright VC. Principles of Cervical Colposcopy. Figure 10.16. Houston: Biomedical Communications, 2004, p 10–10.)

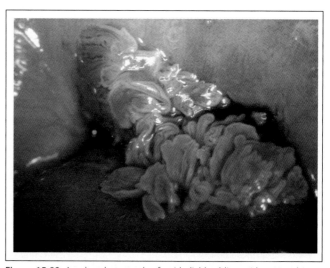

Figure 15-21 A colpophotograph of immature metaplasia with epithelial budding formations similar to those seen in AIS. (From Wright VC. Color Atlas of Colposcopy. Figure 7.4. Houston: Biomedical Communications, 2003, p 7–37.)

Figure 15-22 A colpophotograph of epithelial budding with serrated formations of cervical condylomata. (From Wright VC. Principles of Cervical Colpopscopy. Figure 11.16. Houston: Biomedical Communications, 2004, p 11–8.)

and squamous cell cancer (Figure 15-35). Tendril-like vessels resemble the filiform shoots of climbing plants that reach for and then spiral around nearby structures to support the plant (Figure 15-36). Such vessels are seen in glandular disease (see Figures 15-32 and 15-33), condylomata (Figure 15-37), and squamous cell cancer (see Figure 15-35). Root-like vessels, some tapering like the tap root of a plant (Figure 15-38) and others like a tuberous root (similar to ginger root), are swollen and bulging (Figure 15-39). Such vessels are seen in a matured TZ and adenocarcinoma (Figures 15-40 and 15-41). Character

writing–like vessel configurations occur in AIS (Figure 15-42), adenocarcinoma (Figure 15-43), condylomata (Figures 15-44 and 15-45), and immature metaplastic squamous epithelium (Figure 15-46). Single and multiple dot-like vessels do not represent punctuation in which the blood vessels become entrapped within the dysplastic epithelium. In glandular disease, dots are formed within the tips of the papillary projections by vessels that course through the villous projections and bend sharply in their tips. When they proliferate at the tip, single or multiple dots are seen. Such formations are seen

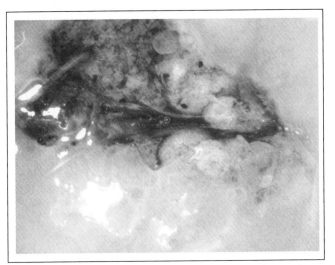

Figure 15-23 A colpophotograph of a papillary appearing adenocarcinoma overlying columnar epithelium. In some areas, it is not in contact with the squamous border. (From Wright VC. Principles of Cervical Colposcopy. Figure 10.66. Houston: Biomedical Communications, 2004, p 10–26.)

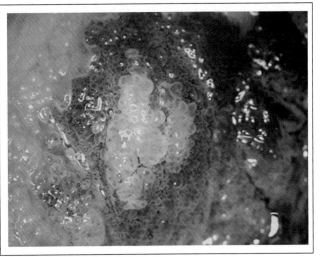

Figure 15-25 Papillary acetowhite formations of a cervical condylomata are seen in this colpophotograph overlying columnar epithelium and not in contact with the squamous border. (Courtesy V.C. Wright.)

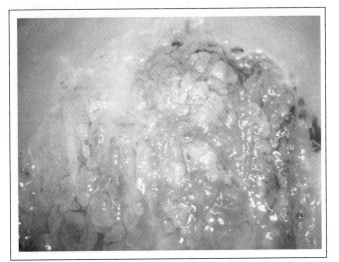

Figure 15-24 Clumps of acetowhite immature metaplastic epithelium are seen overlying columnar epithelium in this colpophotograph. It mimics a glandular lesion. (Courtesy V.C. Wright.)

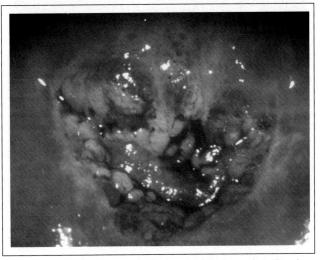

Figure 15-26 A colpophotograph of microglandular hyperplasia. Fused masses of papillary appearing structures are seen overlying columnar epithelium. It mimics a glandular lesion (AIS, adenocarcinoma). (From Wright VC. Principles of Cervical Colposcopy. Figure 14.5. Houston: Biomedical Communications, 2004, p 14–3.)

in glandular disease (Figures 15-47 and 15-48), squamous cell carcinoma (see Figure 15-14), metaplasia (see Figure 15-12), and condylomata (see Figures 15-25 and 15-49).

Mixed Squamous and Glandular Disease

More than 80% of the squamous lesions found in mixed disease will be CIN 3. Furthermore, the AIS component can be destroyed during ablative treatment (e.g., cryotherapy, laser) along with the more distal squamous lesion without the glandular lesion ever being recognized. Despite this possibility, studies of consecutive women who had routine electrosurgical excision found that the proportion of AIS cases did not exceed 2%.[52] In mixed disease the squamous component is usually colposcopically visible. The glandular lesion can abut the squamous lesion (Figures 15-50 to 15-52), be sandwiched between two squamous lesions (Figures 15-53 to 15-55), or lie above the squamous lesion (on the canal side) (Figures 15-56 to 15-60).

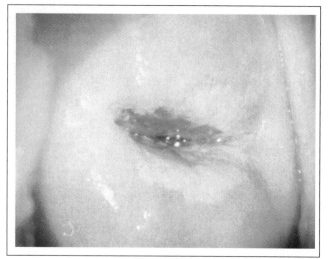

Figure 15-27 A colpophotograph of a CIN 3 lesion demonstrating acetowhiteness from border to border. (From Wright VC. Principles of Cervical Colposcopy. Figure 7.43. Houston: Biomedical Communications, 2004, p 7–21.)

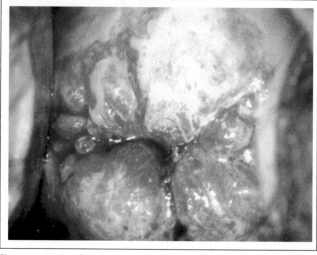

Figure 15-29 A colposcopic image of a cervix at 37 weeks of pregnancy demonstrating patchy (variegated) red and white areas that are scattered over the columnar epithelium. It mimics a TZ. Biopsy confirmed a cervical adenocarcinoma. (From Wright VC. Color Atlas of Colposcopy. Figure 11.29. Houston: Biomedical Communications, 2003, p 11–74.)

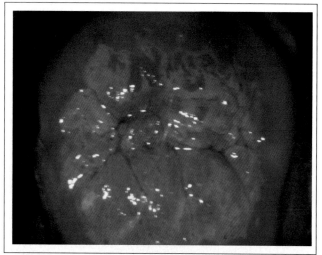

Figure 15-28 Colposcopic image of a variegated (patchy) red and white AIS lesion involving four quadrants of the ectocervix. It mimics an immature TZ. (From Wright VC. Principles of Cervical Colposcopy. Figure 10.19. Houston: Biomedical Communications, 2004, p 10–11.)

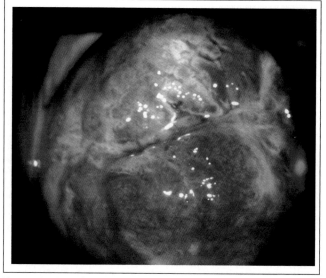

Figure 15-30 A colpophotograph of immature metaplasia demonstrating a patchy (variegated) red and white surface similar to that seen in glandular disease. (From Wright VC. Color Atlas of Colposcopy. Figure 6.14. Houston: Biomedical Communications, 2003, p 6–10.)

Mimics of lesions lying central to a squamous lesion include immature metaplastic epithelium, with the squamous intraepithelial lesion being located peripherally (Figures 15-61 and 15-62). *Colposcopy cannot always differentiate between AIS and immature metaplasia, hence the colposcopist is well advised to biopsy the "metaplastic/AIS"–appearing component.*

HISTOLOGY OF ADENOCARCINOMA *IN SITU*

Ayer et al.[53] subclassified AIS into three subtypes: endocervical, endometroid, and intestinal (mucinous). The endocervical type is found as a pure type, not admixed with the others in 57%. The endometrioid type occurs as a pure type in 4% of cases. The intestinal type appears not to be found alone in its pure form. The endocervical type is associated with other types in 39% of cases (intestinal type, 26%; endometrioid type, 10%; and both intestinal and endometrioid types, 3%).[54] Colposcopy cannot differentiate among the different histologic types.[6]

The endocervical type demonstrates enlarged nuclei, nuclear crowding, hyperchromasia, coarse chromatin, nuclear pseudostratification, and apoptosis (Figures 15-63 and 15-64). There is decreased mucin production confined

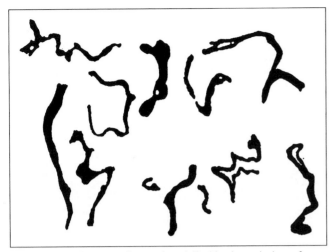

Figure 15-31 Schematics of waste thread–like blood vessels drawn from actual colpophotographs. (From Wright VC, Shier RM [eds]. Basic and Advanced Colposcopy: A Practical Handbook for Diagnosis, ed 2. Figure 12-9. Houston: Biomedical Communications, 1995, p 12–7.)

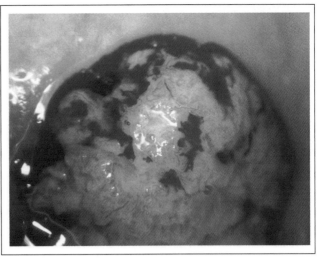

Figure 15-33 Colposcopy demonstrates a friable, papillary cervical adenocarcinoma containing waste thread–like and tendril-like vessels. It is patchy red and acetowhite. (From Wright VC. Principles of Cervical Colposcopy. Figure 10.50. Houston: Biomedical Communications, 2004, p 10–21.)

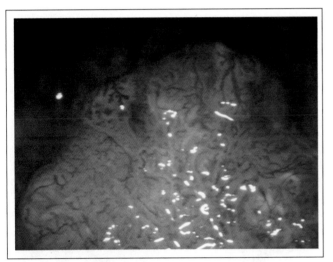

Figure 15-32 A colpophotograph of an AIS lesion demonstrating a variety of blood vessel patterns including character writing–like, tap root–like, waste thread–like, and tendril-like patterns. (From Wright VC. Principles of Cervical Colposcopy. Figure 10.35. Houston: Biomedical Communications, 2004, p 10–16.)

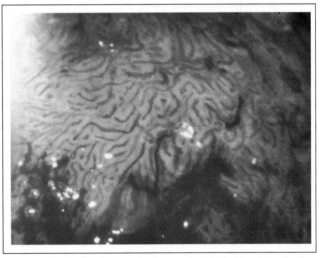

Figure 15-34 A colpophotograph of waste thread–like blood vessels of a cervical condylomata that mimics glandular disease. (From Wright VC. Principles of Cervical Colposcopy. Figure 11.18. Houston: Biomedical Communications, 2004, p 11–8.)

only to luminal accumulations, as demonstrated by Alcian blue negative staining (Figures 15-65 and 15-66). The intestinal (mucinous) subtype demonstrates large vacuoles in an irregular honeycomb pattern producing excessive mucus (Figures 15-67 to 15-69). Such areas are easily identified by Alcian blue staining (Figures 15-70 and 15-71). The endometroid type histologically resembles endometrial carcinoma, and intracellular mucin is absent (Figure 15-72). The most common surface expressions seen histologically (comprising 85% of cases) are papillary formations (Figures 15-73 to 15-75). Other patterns include cribiform

formations (Figure 15-76) and exophytic budding (see Figures 15-20 and 15-63).[54]

Crypt Involvement, Linear Length, Skip Lesions, and Disease Location

Glandular lesions can extend into the superficial and deep cervical crypts (Figure 15-77). Crypt extension averages 2.5 mm and is usually no more than 4 mm with a maximum of 6 mm.[4,55,56] Women younger than age 36 have a lesser depth of crypt extension.[56] In mixed disease, both

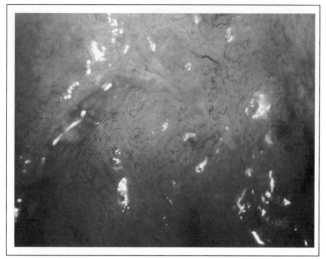

Figure 15-35 A colpophotograph of waste thread–like and corkscrew-like angioarchitecture in a cervical squamous carcinoma. (From Wright VC. Principles of Cervical Colposcopy. Figure 7.20. Houston: Biomedical Communications, 2004, p 7–14.)

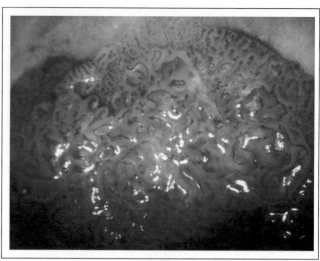

Figure 15-37 A colpophotograph of a cervical condylomata demonstrating tendril-like, waste thread–like, and dot-like angioarchitecture. (From Wright VC. Principles of Cervical Colposcopy. Figure 11.1. Houston: Biomedical Communications, 2004, p 11–6.)

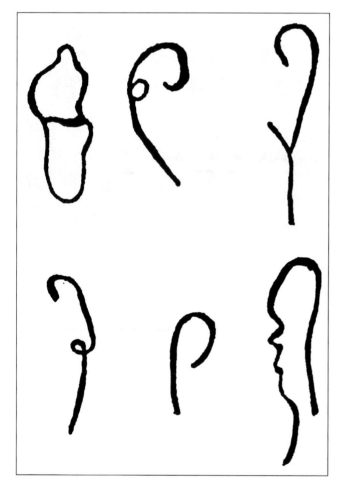

Figure 15-36 Schematics of tendril-like blood vessels. (From Wright VC, Lickrish GM, Shier RM [eds]. Basic and Advanced Colposcopy: A Practical Handbook for Diagnosis, ed 2. Figure 12.5. Houston: Biomedical Communications, 1995, p 12–7.)

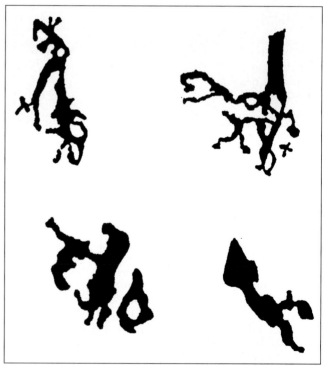

Figure 15-38 Schematics of root-like vessels. (From Wright VC, Lickrish GM, Shier RM [eds]: Basic and Advanced Colposcopy: A Practical Handbook for Diagnosis, ed 2. Figure 12.11. Houston: Biomedical Communications, 1995, p 12–7.)

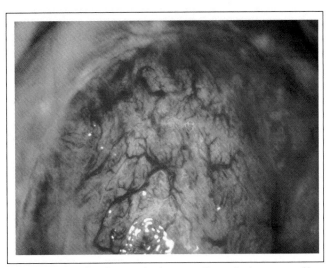

Figure 15-39 A colpophotograph of tap root–like and tuberous root–like blood vessels in a mature TZ. (From Wright VC. Color Atlas of Colposcopy. Figure 7.28. Houston: Biomedical Communications, 2003, p 7–44.)

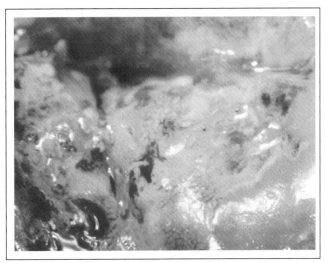

Figure 15-41 Irregular, dilated, tuberous root–like angioarchitecture in a cervical adenocarcinoma seen colposcopically. Character writing–like vascular forms are interspersed. (From Wright VC, Lickrish GM, Shier RM [eds]. Basic and Advanced Colposcopy: A Practical Handbook for Diagnosis, ed 2. Figure 12-23. Houston: Biomedical Communications, 1995, p 13–11.)

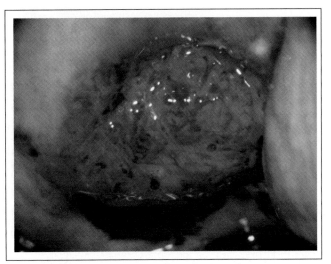

Figure 15-40 Enlarged, tuberous root–like blood vessels seen colposcopically in a cervical adenocarcinoma. (From Wright VC. Color Atlas of Colposcopy. Figure 11.25. Houston: Biomedical Communications, 2003, p 11–73.)

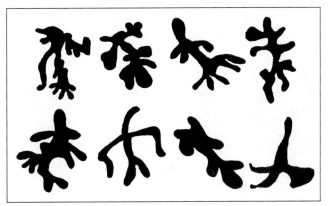

Figure 15-42 Schematics of character writing–like blood vessels. (From Wright VC. Understanding Cervical Glandular Disease CD-ROM. Image 143. Houston: Biomedical Communications, 2004.)

the glandular and squamous component can occupy the same crypt (Figure 15-78). Glandular disease in the crypts can be covered by normal metaplastic or dysplastic epithelium (see Figures 15-2 and 15-79). Buried disease occurs in 60% of cases.[55,56] Skip lesions (multifocal) are foci involving different portions of endocervical mucosa. By definition this represents a complete normal radial histologic section separating two areas of disease. The finding of both normal and involved crypts within the same slide does not meet the definition of multifocal.[55,56] Skip lesions are uncommon (6.5–15%), but when they do exist, they rarely interfere with colposcopic assessment, nor do they increase the chance of residual disease.[6,7]

Most glandular lesions are located within the transformation zone.[7,55,57] *Many of the lesions are small (see Figure 15-17) and easily overlooked.*[6–8] The linear length of AIS lesions (the distance over the tissue surface between caudal and cephalic edges) usually does not exceed 15 mm see (Figures 15-8, 15-68, 15-73, and 15-74).[8,56,57] Women aged 36 years or older have a greater linear length and volume of disease than women younger than 36 years.[56]

AIS can involve a single cervical quadrant (see Figures 15-9 and 15-17) or multiple cervical quadrants (see Figure 15-28). In 48% of lesions, one quadrant is involved, compared with 10% involving all four quadrants. Ectocervical expression of AIS disease occurs in 53% of cases, the endocervical canal alone is involved in 5% of cases, and contiguous involvement occurs in 38% of cases. Consequently, *95% of AIS cases are available for partial or complete colposcopic scrutiny.*[58,59]

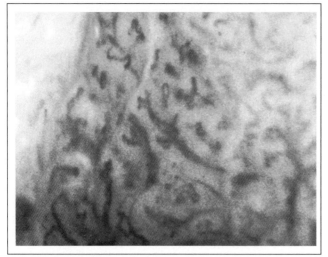

Figure 15-43 A colpophotograph of character writing–like blood vessels in a cervical adenocarcinoma. (From Wright VC. Principles of Cervical Colposcopy. Figure 10.59. Houston: Biomedical Communications, 2004, p 10–23.)

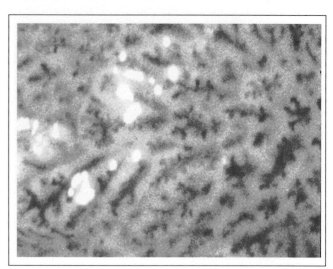

Figure 15-45 High colposcopic magnification of character writing–like blood vessels seen in cervical condylomata. (From Wright VC. Principles of Cervical Colposcopy. Figure 11.9. Houston: Biomedical Communications, 2004, p 11–6.)

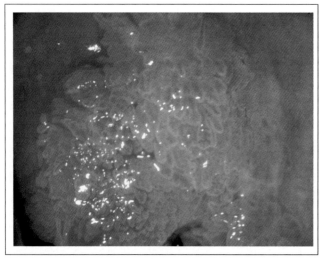

Figure 15-44 Character writing–like blood vessels seen colposcopically within the papillary excrescences of a cervical condylomata mimicking glandular disease. (From Wright VC. Principles of Cervical Colposcopy. Figure 11.8. Houston: Biomedical Communications, 2004, p 11–5.)

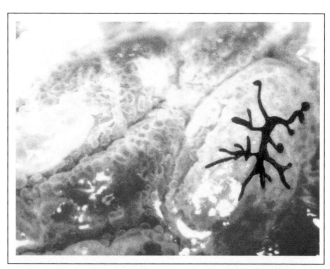

Figure 15-46 Inked-in colposcopic image of character writing–like blood vessels in immature metaplasia. (From Wright VC. Principles of Cervical Colposcopy. Figure 6.32. Houston: Biomedical Communications, 2004, p 6–17.)

MANAGEMENT

Rationale

AGC on Papanicolaou (Pap) smear must be vigorously investigated to identify significant pathology. When a diagnosis of AIS is made on punch biopsy, *an excisional conization is necessary to exclude adenocarcinoma. Adenocarcinoma cannot be excluded unless the excised specimen has negative margins.* AIS must be treated because it is a precursor of cervical adenocarcinoma. In planning therapy for women with histologically diagnosed AIS, consideration must be given to the following variables: (1) patient's age; (2) lesion location; (3) three-dimensional geometry (linear length and crypt involvement);

(4) potential for buried disease; (5) mixed disease (presence of a squamous component); (6) status of the margins after excision; (7) patient's desire for fertility; and (8) patient's compliance.[59] When the diagnosis of adenocarcinoma is made, the patient should be referred to a gynecologic oncologist for staging and appropriate management.

Algorithms

According to the Bethesda 2001 classification system, glandular cytologic abnormalities are subclassified into the following categories[36,60]:

- Atypical glandular cells (AGC) (specify endocervical, endometrial, or not otherwise specified [AGC-NOS])

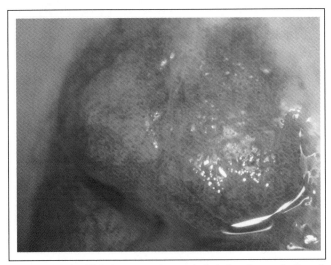

Figure 15-47 An AIS lesion seen colposcopically before the application of 3% to 5% acetic acid displaying dot-like angioarchitecture. (From Wright VC. Principles of Cervical Colposcopy. Figure 10.30. Houston: Biomedical Communications, 2004, p 10–14.)

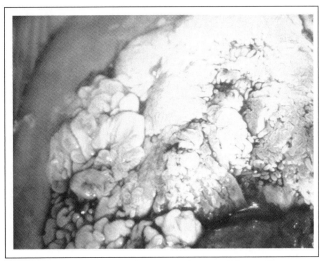

Figure 15-49 Dot-like angioarchitecture in the tips of the papillary excrescences from a cervical condylomata seen colposcopically. (From Wright VC. Principles of Cervical Colposcopy. Figure 11.26. Houston: Biomedical Communications, 2004, p 11–10.)

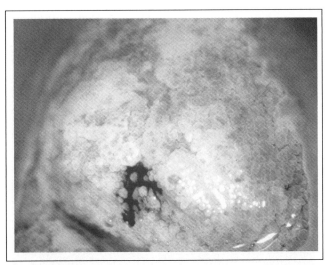

Figure 15-48 A colpophotograph of Figure 13-47 after the application of 3% to 5% acetic acid. Numerous single and multiple dot-like blood vessel formations are seen. (From Wright VC. Principles of Cervical Colposcopy. Figure 10.34. Houston: Biomedical Communications, 2004, p 10–15.)

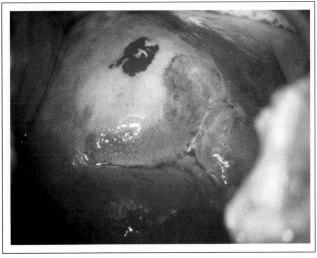

Figure 15-50 The colpophotograph demonstrates a variegated red and white AIS lesion located beside an acetowhite squamous intraepithelial lesion. (From Wright VC. Principles of Cervical Colposcopy. Figure 10.46. Houston: Biomedical Communications, 2004, p 10–19.)

- AGC favor (specify endocervical or not otherwise specified)
- Endocervical adenocarcinoma *in situ* (AIS)
- Adenocarcinoma

2006 American Society for Colposcopy and Cervical Pathology (ASCCP) Guidelines for the Management of Cytologic Glandular Abnormalities

The ASCCP guidelines for management of cytologic glandular abnormalities are as follows (Figure 15-80)[61]:

- Colposcopy with endocervical sampling is *recommended* for women with all subcategories of AGC and endocervical AIS. (AII)

- Endometrial sampling is *recommended* in conjunction with colposcopy and endocervical sampling in women 35 years and older with all subcategories of AGC and AIS. (BII)
- Endometrial sampling is also *recommended* for women younger than 35 years with clinical indications suggesting they may be at risk for neoplastic endometrial lesions. These include unexplained vaginal bleeding or conditions suggesting chronic anovulation.
- It is *recommended* that women with atypical endometrial cells be initially evaluated with endometrial and endocervical sampling. Colposcopy can be either

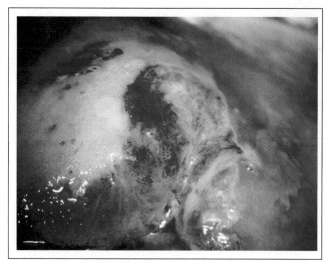

Figure 15-51 A higher magnification of Figure 15-50. (From Wright VC. Principles of Cervical Colposcopy. Figure 10.46. Houston: Biomedical Communications, 2004, p 10–19.)

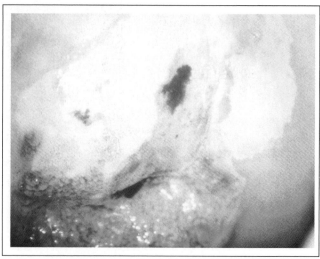

Figure 15-53 Colposcopically a variegated red and white AIS lesion separates two acetowhite squamous intraepithelial lesions. (From Wright VC. Color Atlas of Colposcopy. Figure 11.4. Houston: Biomedical Communications, 2003, p 11–67.)

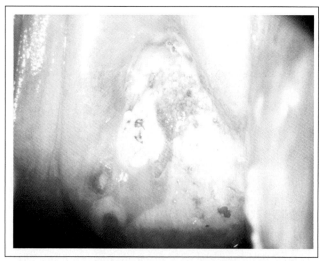

Figure 15-52 A colpophotograph of a mixed lesion seen colposcopically. Centrally and to the left is an elevated, densely acetowhite AIS lesion (proven on excision). It is separated by normal-appearing columnar epithelium from a much larger, densely acetowhite microinvasive squamous cell cancer (seen on the right). (From Wright VC. Principles of Cervical Colposcopy. Figure 10.37. Houston: Biomedical Communications, 2004, p 10–16.)

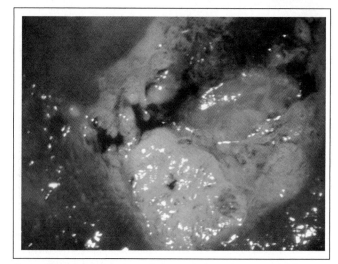

Figure 15-54 A colpophotograph demonstrates a dense, acetowhite lesion with atypical blood vessels located centrally (between 5 and 9 o'clock). From 2 to 5 o'clock and 9 to 12 o'clock are high-grade squamous lesions separated by the AIS component. Histologic diagnosis was confirmed on an excisional specimen. (From Wright VC. Color Atlas of Colposcopy. Figure 11.5. Houston: Biomedical Communications, 2003, p 11–68.)

performed at the initial evaluation or deferred until the results are known. If no endometrial pathology is identified, colposcopy is *recommended*. (AII)

- If not already obtained, HPV DNA testing *at the time of colposcopy* is *preferred* in women with atypical endocervical, endometrial, or glandular cells not otherwise specified (NOS). (CIII)
- The use of HPV DNA testing alone or a program of repeat cervical cytology is *unacceptable* for the *initial triage* of all subcategories of AGC and AIS. (EII)
- In pregnant women, the initial evaluation of AGC should be identical to that of non-pregnant women, except that

endocervical curettage and endometrial biopsy are *unacceptable*. (BII)

- For asymptomatic *premenopausal women* with *benign endometrial cells, endometrial stromal cells, or histiocytes*, no further evaluation is recommended. (BII)
- For *postmenopausal women* with *benign endometrial cells*, endometrial assessment is recommended regardless of symptoms. (BII)
- For *post-hysterectomy patients* with a cytologic report of *benign glandular cells*, no further evaluation is recommended. (BII)

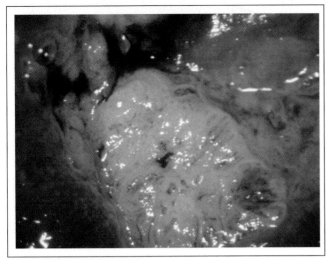

Figure 15-55 A colposcopic higher magnification of Figure 15-54 demonstrating small root-like and waste thread–like blood vessels in the AIS component. (From Wright VC. Color Atlas of Colposcopy. Figure 11.6. Houston: Biomedical Communications, 2003, p 11–68.)

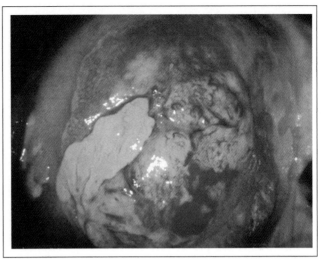

Figure 15-57 The colpophotograph demonstrates a well-defined, high-grade squamous lesion from 6 to 10 o'clock. A variegated red (dark blood vessels) and white AIS lesion occupies the endocervical canal. Histologically the lesions were confirmed on excisional biopsy. (From Wright VC. Principles of Cervical Colposcopy. Figure 11.7. Houston: Biomedical Communications, 2004, p 11–69.)

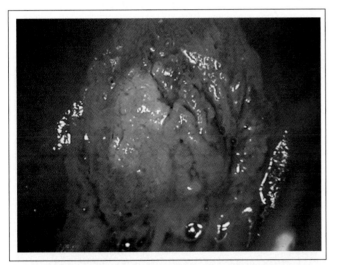

Figure 15-56 The colpophotograph demonstrates a fusing papillary, densely acetowhite AIS lesions centrally on the anterior cervix. Peripherally encircling it from 9 to 3 o'clock is an associated low-grade squamous intraepithelial lesion. (From Wright VC. Principles of Cervical Colposcopy. Figure 10.42. Houston: Biomedical Communications, 2004, p 10–18.)

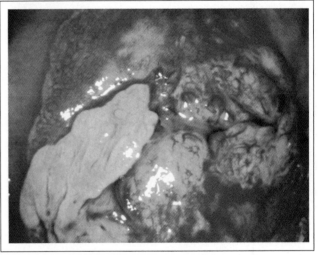

Figure 15-58 A higher colposcopic photograph of Figure 15-57. Numerous root-like and character writing–like blood vessels can be seen in the AIS component. (From Wright VC. Understanding Cervical Glandular Disease CD-ROM. Image 114. Houston: Biomedical Communications, 2004.)

Subsequent Management

The ASCCP guidelines for subsequent management are as follows (Figure 15-81)[61]:

- The recommended post-colposcopy management of women of known HPV DNA status with either atypical endocervical, endometrial, or glandular cells NOS who do not have histologically diagnosed CIN or glandular neoplasia is to repeat cytological testing combined with HPV DNA testing at 6 months if they are HPV DNA positive and at 12 months if they are HPV DNA negative. (CII)
- Referral to colposcopy is recommended for women who subsequently test positive for high-risk (oncogenic) HPV DNA or who are found to have ASC-US or greater on their repeat cytological tests. If both tests are negative, women can return to routine cytologic testing. (BII)
- The recommended postcolposcopy management of women of unknown HPV status with atypical endocervical, endometrial or glandular cells NOS who do not have CIN 2,3 or grandular neoplasia identified histologically is to repeat cytological testing at 6-month intervals. After 4 consecutive "negative for intraepithelial lesion or malignancy" results are obtained, women can return to routine cytological testing. (CIII)
- If CIN, but no glandular neoplasia, is identified histologically during the initial workup of a woman with

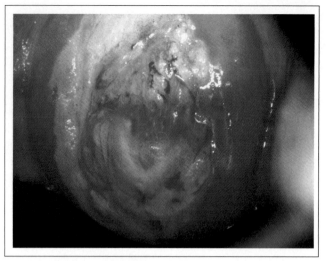

Figure 15-59 Colposcopy demonstrates an AIS lesion (variegated red and white resembling an immature metaplastic TZ) centrally surrounded by a high-grade squamous lesion peripherally from 6 to 12 o'clock. (From Wright VC. Principles of Cervical Colposcopy. Figure 10.9. Houston: Biomedical Communications, 2004, p 10–8.)

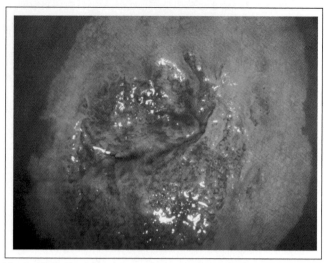

Figure 15-61 The colpophotograph demonstrates a high-grade (CIN 2) acetowhite lesion peripherally. Centrally located is immature metaplasia (variegated red and white). The total image is an excellent mimic of mixed disease. Such lesions should always be biopsied, because colposcopy cannot differentiate between a glandular lesion and metaplasia. (From Wright VC. Principles of Cervical Colposcopy. Figure 7.32. Houston: Biomedical Communications, 2004, p 7–18.)

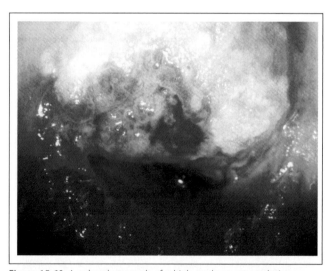

Figure 15-60 A colpophotograph of a high-grade squamous lesion peripherally on the anterior cervix. Below and extending into the endocervical canal is a variegated adenocarcinoma component. (From Wright VC. Color Atlas of Colposcopy. Figure 11.30. Houston: Biomedical Communications, 2003, p 11–74.)

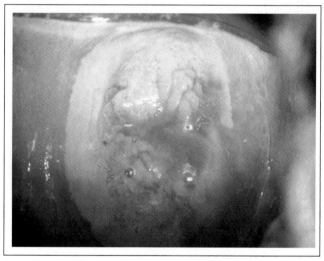

Figure 15-62 A colpophotograph mimicking mixed disease. The high-grade acetowhite squamous lesion is located peripherally, and the variegated red and white area centrally on biopsy was immature metaplasia. (Courtesy V.C. Wright.)

atypical endocervical, endometrial, or glandular cells NOS, management should be according to the 2006 Consensus Guidelines for the Management of Women with Cervical Intraepithelial Neoplasia. If invasive disease is not identified during the initial colposcopic workup, it is recommended that women with atypical endocervical or glandular cells "favor neoplasia" or endocervical AIS undergo a diagnostic excisional procedure. (AII)

- It is *recommended* that the type of diagnostic excisional procedure used in this setting provide an intact specimen with interpretable margins. (BII) Concomitant endocervical sampling is *preferred*. (BII)

TREATMENT DECISIONS

Specimen Guidelines

When AIS is found on cytology or on biopsy, it is necessary to have an excisional procedure that produces a specimen with negative margins to be certain that no unrecognized adenocarcinoma is present. To account for the distribution of disease (crypt involvement, disease location, linear length of disease), *the specimen should be cylindric in shape,* similar to the recommendations for squamous intraepithelial lesions.[35,62,63] It is

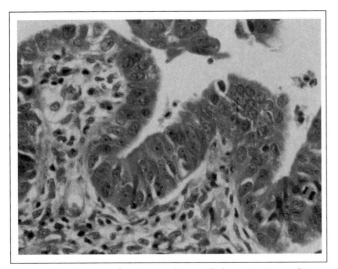

Figure 15-63 Histology of endocervical-type AIS demonstrating nuclear enlargement, pseudostratification, coarse chromatin, reduced nuclear: cytoplasmic ratio, and mitotic activity (hematoxylin-eosin stain, high-power magnification). (From Wright VC. *Understanding Cervical Glandular Disease* CD-ROM. Image 58. Houston: Biomedical Communications, 2004.)

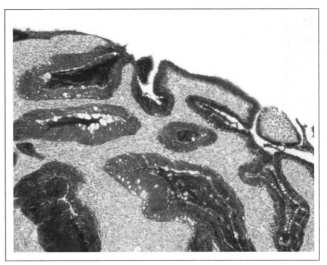

Figure 15-65 Histology of the distribution of mucin stained in normal endocervical columnar epithelium (periodic acid–Schiff [PAS] stain after diatase and Alcian blue, low-power magnification). (From Wright VC. *Understanding Cervical Glandular Disease* CD-ROM. Image 7. Houston: Biomedical Communications, 2004.)

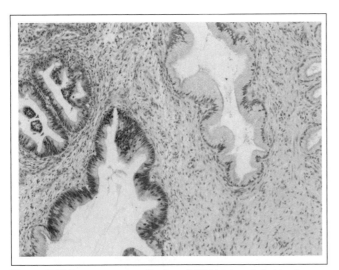

Figure 15-64 Low-power magnification of AIS histology (left side of microphotograph). It is separated abruptly from normal columnar epithelium. In comparison, on the right are normal crypts lined by tall columnar epithelium with basally situated nuclei (hematoxylin-eosin stain). (Courtesy V.C. Wright.)

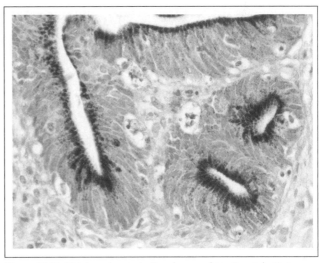

Figure 15-66 Histology demonstrating decreased mucin production confined to luminal acuminations in endocervical type of AIS (PAS stain after diatase and Alcian blue, low-power magnification). (Courtesy V.C. Wright.)

recommended that the procedure be done under colposcopic guidance, noting the lower lesion border and estimating the upper margin (the entire potential linear length).[35,55,63] These observed parameters serve as a guide for determining the dimensions of the cylindric specimen. *The scalpel (cold knife) is preferred over the electrosurgical loop due to cautery artifact that may interfere with histologic interpretation of the specimen.* However, loop excision is acceptable.[52] An alternative to a cold-knife excision involves the use of a high-energy pulsed carbon dioxide laser or electrosurgical needle for the lateral excision followed by a scalpel to sever the apex of the specimen transversely. This approach is associated with fewer postoperative complications than a procedure performed with a scalpel alone.[59,63]

2006 ASCCP Guidelines for the Management of Histologic Glandular Abnormalities

The ASCCP guidelines for management of histologic glandular abnormalities are as follows (Figure 15-82)[64]:

* Hysterectomy is preferred for women who have completed childbearing and have a histological diagnosis of AIS on a specimen from a diagnostic excisional procedure. (CII)

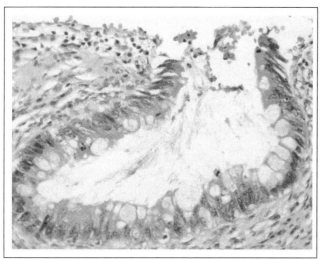

Figure 15-67 Histology of intestinal type of AIS demonstrating the presence of abundant intracytoplasmic mucin vacuoles with variable-sized, clear nuclei with enlarged nucleoli (hematoxylin-eosin stain, high magnification). (Courtesy V.C. Wright.)

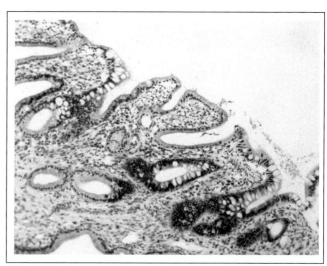

Figure 15-69 Histology of the surface AIS intestinal-type lesion depicted in Figure 15-68 (hematoxylin-eosin stain, low magnification). (From Wright VC. Principles of Cervical Colposcopy. Figure 10.8. Houston: Biomedical Communications, 2004, p 10–8.)

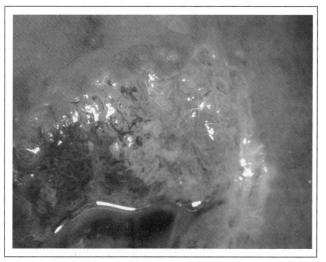

Figure 15-68 A colpophotograph of an AIS lesion after 3–5% acetic acid of the intestinal type histology. It appears acetowhite and papillary, resembling an immature TZ. (From Wright VC. Principles of Cervical Colposcopy. Figure 10.7. Houston: Biomedical Communications, 2004, p 10–8.)

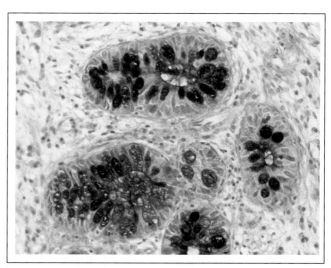

Figure 15-70 Histology of intestinal-type AIS with PAS stain after diatase and Alcian blue. The Alcian blue–positive goblet cells stain abundantly for mucin in this histologic type (intermediate magnification). (Courtesy V.C. Wright.)

- Conservative management is *acceptable* if future fertility is desired. (AII)
- If conservative management is planned and the margins of the specimen are involved or endocervical sampling obtained at the time of excision contains CIN or AIS, re-excision to increase the likehood of complete excision is preferred. Reevaluation at 6 months using a combination of cervical cytology, HPV DNA testing, and colposcopy with endocervical sampling is acceptable in this circumstance. Long-term follow up is recommended for women who do not undergo hysterectomy (CIII).

Negative Specimen Margins

Most studies indicate that if the excised specimen's margins are negative, then conservative management is possible in women who desire future childbearing.[8,58,65–67] However, negative margins are associated with persistent AIS in 8.3% to 50% of cases.[58,66–72] These findings suggest conization should not necessarily be considered a definitive treatment for AIS despite the presence of negative margins. However, studies have rarely identified adenocarcinoma when specimen margins are reported as negative.[68,73,74]

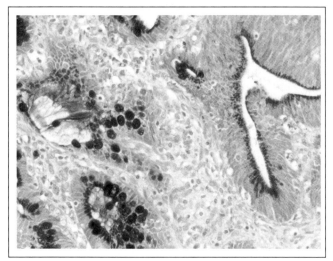

Figure 15-71 Histology of AIS with PAS stain after diatase and Alcian blue. Intestinal type is demonstrated on the left (staining of mucin producing goblet cells) and endocervical type on the right (luminal acuminations of mucin containing cytoplasm). Both histologic types were found in the same specimen (intermediate magnification). (Courtesy V.C. Wright.)

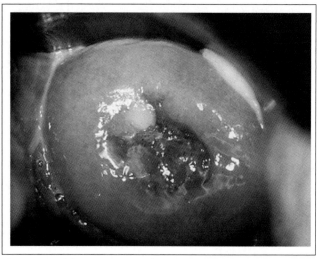

Figure 15-73 Colposcopic image of a mixed lesion. The high-grade squamous lesion is densely acetowhite. Below and involving the endocervical canal, the columnar epithelium is variegated and papillary. This AIS lesion resembles the villous structures of an ectopy. (Courtesy V.C. Wright.)

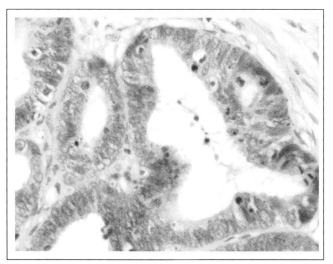

Figure 15-72 Histology of endometroid type resembling endometroid carcinoma (hematoxylin-eosin stain, intermediate magnification). (Courtesy V.C. Wright.)

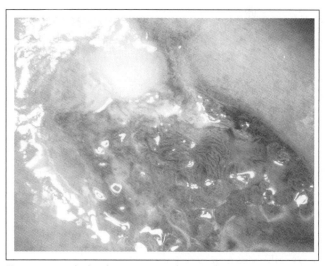

Figure 15-74 A high colposcopic magnification of Figure 15-74. The papillary AIS component is well visualized, as well as the afferent and efferent angioarchitecture within the villous components. When viewed head-on, they will appear as dot-like vessels. (From Wright VC. Principles of Cervical Colposcopy. Figure 10.43. Houston: Biomedical Communications, 2004, p 10–19.)

For the conservatively managed woman, follow-up should consist of cytology, colposcopy, and endocervical curettage every 6 months.[63,68,74] Women who choose to be followed conservatively must be counseled about the importance of compliance and the potential risks of undetected disease, despite negative follow-up findings.[69,73] Once the desire for future childbearing is resolved, extrafascial hysterectomy has been advocated. The question remains whether this is necessary in the compliant patient with no evidence of persistent disease. More long-term studies are necessary to address this issue.[63]

Positive Specimen Margins

Persistent AIS is present in 12.5% to 80% of women with positive conization margins.[56,58,66,71–77] *Some studies found adenocarcinoma in 12.5% to 50% of cases with positive margins*[58,66,68]; however, other studies did not identify adenocarcinoma in such cases.* When positive margins are identified, repeat excision is recommended to exclude the diagnosis of

---

*References 8, 56, 58, 65, 69, 71, 76.

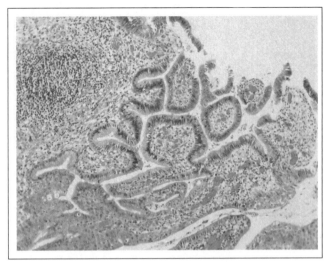

Figure 15-75 Histology of the papillary structures of endocervical type AIS shown in Figure 15-74. Note the centrally placed blood vessels within the individual villi. Colposcopically they appear as dot-like angioarchitecture. (Courtesy V.C. Wright.)

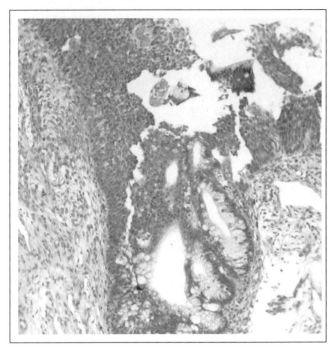

Figure 15-77 Histology of an AIS lesion (mostly intestinal type) within an endocervical crypt. It is covered by dysplastic epithelium, making the lesion colposcopically inaccessible (hematoxylin-eosin stain, intermediate magnification). (Courtesy V.C. Wright.)

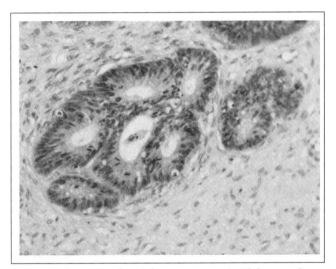

Figure 15-76 Histology of a cribiform pattern seen in AIS (hematoxylin-eosin stain, high magnification). (Courtesy V.C. Wright.)

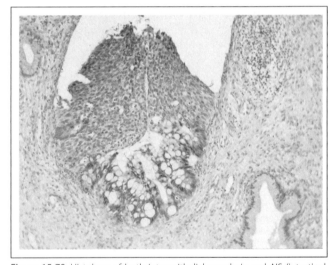

Figure 15-78 Histology of both intraepithelial neoplasia and AIS (intestinal type) within the same crypt (hematoxylin-eosin stain, low magnification). (Courtesy V.C. Wright.)

adenocarcinoma regardless of the woman's desire for future childbearing. If future fertility is desired, repeat excision should precede conservative follow-up. *If fertility is not an issue, repeat excision producing negative margins is recommended before an extrafascial hysterectomy as definitive treatment.* Failure to do so may result in inappropriate surgery (extrafascial hysterectomy instead of radical hysterectomy), should adenocarcinoma be found in the extirpated uterine cervix.[63]

MANAGEMENT SCENARIOS

Scenario 1

Sentinel Pap: High-grade squamous intraepithelial lesion (HSIL)

Colposcopic findings or biopsy result (if a biopsy was done): CIN 3 on colposcopy and on biopsy. Endocervical curettage (ECC) was positive for high-grade CIN

HPV testing for high-risk (oncogenic) types: Not applicable (N/A) for HSIL cytology

Satisfactory colposcopy: No

Fertility desires: Yes

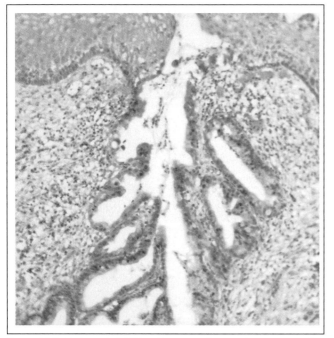

Figure 15-79 Endocervical AIS involving an endocervical crypt covered by normal metaplastic epithelium, making the AIS lesion not accessible for colposcopy (hematoxylin-eosin stain, intermediate magnification). (From Wright VC. Understanding Cervical Glandular Disease CD-ROM. Image 11. Houston: Biomedical Communications, 2004.)

This case indicates that this woman needs an excisional procedure to exclude malignancy because of unsatisfactory colposcopy and a positive ECC. The scalpel was chosen for the excisional procedure. The final pathology of the excised specimen was reported as mixed disease (AIS + HSIL/CIN 3) with negative specimen margins.

One reason that mixed lesions occur unexpectedly is because the colposcopist is unfamiliar with colposcopic patterns of glandular disease. Glandular disease may also be hidden under metaplastic or dysplastic epithelium, or the glandular lesion may be entirely within the endocervical canal. Fortunately, this specimen had negative margins. Because this woman desires future fertility, conservative management is recommended. Although AIS has been described in hysterectomy specimens with negative margins, the finding of a cancer in the hysterectomy specimen is rare in a thoroughly analyzed excisional specimen. In women not desirous of future fertility, extrafascial hysterectomy is recommended.[78] Because most mixed lesions are associated with HSIL cytology or CIN 3 histology, the possibility of a glandular lesion should always be considered in this situation.

Scenario 2

Sentinel Pap: AGC-NOS
Colposcopic findings or biopsy result (if a biopsy was done): No squamous or glandular disease is identified
HPV testing for high-risk (oncogenic) HPV types: Not applicable for initial triage; however, such testing is preferred at the time of colposcopy for future uses, as described for follow-up
Satisfactory colposcopy: Yes
Fertility desires: No

The initial investigation of abnormal glandular cytology in this category is the same for the other glandular case scenarios, except that HPV DNA testing is preferred at the time of colposcopy in the AGC-NOS category. Because no squamous or

Initial Workup of Women with Atypical Glandular Cells (AGC)

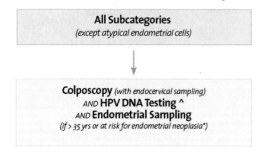

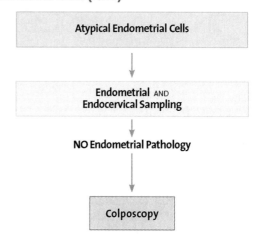

^ *If not already obtained. Test only for high-risk (oncogenic) types.*
* *Includes unexplained vaginal bleeding or conditions suggesting chronic anovulation.*

Figure 15-80 Reprinted from *The Journal of Lower Genital Tract Disease* Vol. 11 Issue 4, with the permission of ASCCP © American Society for Colposcopy and Cervical Pathology 2007. No copies of the algorithms may be made without the prior consent of ASCCP.

Subsequent Management of Women with Atypical Glandular Cells (AGC)

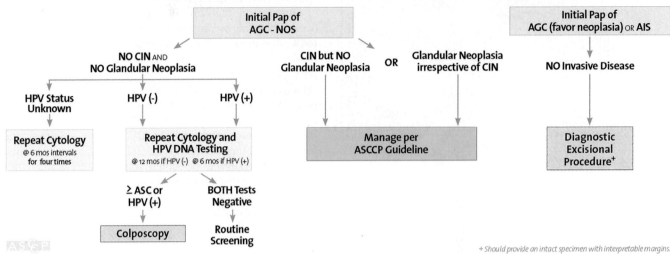

+ Should provide an intact specimen with interpretable margins. Concomitant endocervical sampling is preferred.

Figure 15-81 Reprinted from *The Journal of Lower Genital Tract Disease* Vol. 11 Issue 4, with the permission of ASCCP © American Society for Colposcopy and Cervical Pathology 2007. No copies of the algorithms may be made without the prior consent of ASCCP.

Management of Women with Adenocarcinoma *in-situ* (AIS) Diagnosed from a Diagnostic Excisional Procedure

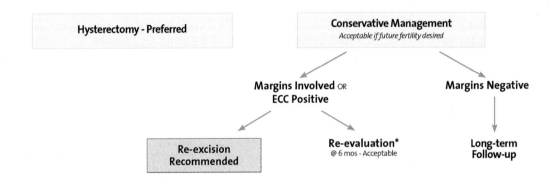

* Using a combination of cytology, HPV testing, and colposcopy with endocervical sampling

Figure 15-82 Reprinted from *The Journal of Lower Genital Tract Disease* Vol. 11 Issue 4, with the permission of ASCCP © American Society for Colposcopy and Cervical Pathology 2007. No copies of the algorithms may be made without the prior consent of ASCCP.

glandular disease was identified during the workup, cytology combined with HPV DNA testing can be repeated at 6-month intervals if the HPV DNA test is positive and at 12 months if the HPV DNA test is negative; if both tests are negative, the patient can resume routine screening. If cytology is reported as ASC or AGC or greater or if the HPV DNA test is positive, the patient should be referred to an expert colposcopist. Women whose repeat cytology shows AGC or HSIL should undergo a diagnostic excision, preferably by an expert.[60]

Scenario 3

Sentinel Pap: Any glandular abnormality
Colposcopic findings or biopsy result (if a biopsy was done): Cervical AIS or adenocarcinoma
HPV testing for high-risk (oncogenic) HPV types: Not applicable in the category as an initial triage
Satisfactory colposcopy: No
Fertility desires: N/A

All cases with glandular cytologic abnormality are referred for colposcopy. The initial investigation is similar, except for cytology indicating atypical endometrial cells. If the initial biopsy was a cervical adenocarcinoma, the woman is referred to a gynecologic oncologist for cancer staging and treatment. If the initial biopsy was AIS, an excisional procedure is required, preferably by scalpel, although an electrosurgical excision procedure is acceptable.[52,79]

Scenario 4

Sentinel Pap: AGC-favor neoplasia or AIS
Colposcopic findings or biopsy result (if a biopsy was done): Any, except adenocarcinoma
HPV testing for high-risk (oncogenic) HPV types: N/A in this category as initial triage
Satisfactory colposcopy: N/A
Fertility desires: No

All women with AGC-favor neoplasia or AIS cytology must be evaluated with colposcopy, biopsy, and ECC. Endometrial sampling is recommended in women older than 35 years and in younger women with unexplained vaginal bleeding. Because colposcopy cannot differentiate between AIS and adenocarcinoma,[6,76] an excisional procedure is required, preferably performed with a scalpel (although other techniques are acceptable).[52,79] If the excised specimen contains adenocarcinoma, clinical staging and treatment by a gynecologic oncologist is recommended. If the excised specimen contains AIS with negative margins, an extrafascial hysterectomy is indicated. If the excised specimen contains positive margins, a repeat conization is recommended to exclude the possibility of a coexisting adenocarcinoma. Regardless of how the patient is treated for her AIS, long-term surveillance for at least 10 years is recommended.[60,79,80]

Scenario 5

Sentinel Pap: AGC-favor neoplasia or AIS
Colposcopic findings or biopsy result (if a biopsy was done): Any except adenocarcinoma
HPV testing for high-risk (oncogenic) HPV types: N/A in this category as initial triage
Satisfactory colposcopy: N/A
Fertility desires: Yes

The initial management of this case is identical to Scenario 4, with the exception of this woman's desires to retain her potential for future fertility. Nevertheless, the risk of AIS and invasive cancer are high enough that a large and deep conization is required despite the potential effect that a conization might have on her future reproductive potential. When considering a conservative approach, the status of the conization margins is critical. Women with a positive endocervical margin should have a repeat conization because of their very high risk of residual disease. Only those with a negative endocervical margin should be offered conservative management. If adenocarcinoma is diagnosed, the woman would be staged and treated appropriately.

Following the conization, women with negative margins on the cone may be offered conservative management. Those with positive margins must undergo a repeat conization to definitively exclude cancer before any consideration is given to conservative management.

COUNSELING SCENARIOS

Many elements of counseling a woman who has a glandular abnormality are similar to those of squamous disease. However, the type of therapy that is preferred (knife conization), the recommended depth of conization, and its potential effect on fertility are unique considerations of glandular disease. The possibility that hysterectomy may be recommended and the fact that there is a greater risk of a final diagnosis of invasive cancer may be particularly concerning to the patient. Other concerns include loss of childbearing and interference with sexual activity. Conservative management is possible in a woman diagnosed with an AIS lesion who desires future fertility. Women diagnosed with cervical adenocarcinoma will require a referral to a gynecologic oncologist for treatment and counseling. Educational materials explaining the investigative procedures, diagnosis, and follow-up management strategies may serve to reduce apprehension.

REFERENCES

1. Friedell GH, McKay DG. Adenocarcinoma in situ of the endocervix. Cancer 1953;6:887–897.
2. Jaworski RC. Endocervical glandular dysplasia, adenocarcinoma in situ and early invasive (microcarcinoma) of the uterine cervix. Semin Diag Path 1990;7:190–204.
3. Plaxe SC, Saltzstein SL. Estimation of the time of the preclinical phase of cervical adenocarcinoma suggests there is ample opportunity for screening. Gynecol Oncol 1999;75:55–61.
4. Colgan TJ, Lickrish GM. The topography and invasive potential of cervical adenocarcinoma in situ, with or without associated squamous dysplasia. Gynecol Oncol 1990:36:246–249.
5. Liu S, Semenciw R, Moa Y. Cervical cancer: The increasing incidence of adenocarcinoma and adenosquamous carcinoma in young women. CMAJ 2001;164:1151–1154.
6. Wright VC. Colposcopy of adenocarcinoma in situ and adenocarcinoma of the uterine cervix. Differentiation from other cervical lesions. J Lower Genital Tract Dis 1999;3:83–87.
7. Östör AG, Duncan A, Quinn M, et al. Adenocarcinoma in situ of the uterine cerviz. An experience with 100 cases. Gynecol Oncol 2000;79:207–210.
8. Cullimore JE, Luesley DM, Rollason TP, et al. A prospective study of conization of the cervix in the management of cervical glandular neoplasia (CIGN). A preliminary report. Br J Obstet Gynecol 1992;99:314–318.
9. Beyer-Boon ME, Verdonk GW. The identification of atypical reserve cells in smears of patients with malignant and premalignant changes in the squamous and glandular epithelium of the uterine cervix. Acta Cytol 1978;22:305–311.
10. Kudo R, Sagae S, Hayakawa O, et al. Morphology of adenocarcinoma in situ and microinvasive carcinoma of the uterine cerviz. A cytologic and ultrastructural study. Acta 1991;35:109–116.

11. von Haam E, Old JW. Reserve cell hyperplasia, squamous metaplasia and epidermidization. In: Gray LA (ed). Dysplasia, Carcinoma In Situ and Microinvasive Carcinoma of the Cervix Uteri. Springfield, IL: Charles C Thomas, 1964, pp 41–82.

12. Jones MW, Silverberg SG. Cervical adenocarcinoma in young women: possible relationship to microglandular hyperplasia and use of oral contraceptives. Obstet Gynecol 1989;73:f984–988.

13. Brinton LA, Reeves WC, Herrero R, et al. Oral contraceptive use and risk of invasive cervical cancer. Int J Epidemiol 1990;19:4–11.

14. Silcox PBS, Thorton-Jones H, Murphy M. Squamous and adenocarcinoma of the uterine cervix: a comparison using routine data. Br J Cancer 1987;55:321–325.

15. Horowitz IR, Jacobson LP, Zucker PK, et al. Epidemiology of adenocarcinoma of the cervix. Gynecol Oncol 1988;31:25–31.

16. Parazzini F, La Vecchia C. Epidemiology of adenocarcinoma of the cervix. Gynecol Oncol 1990;39:40–46.

17. Bosch FX, Manos MM, Munoz N, et al. Prevalence of human papillomavirus in cervical cancer: a worldwide perspective. JNCI 1995;87:792–802.

18. Walboomers JMM, Jacobs MV, Manos MM, et al. Human papillomavirus is a necessary cause of invasive cervical cancer worldwide. J Pathol 1999;189:12–19.

19. Kado S, Kawamata Y, Shono Y, et al. Detection of human papillomaviruses in cervical neoplasia using multiple sets of generic polymerase chaon reaction primers. Gynecol Oncol 2001;81:47–52.

20. Andersson S, Rylander E, Larrsson R, et al. The role of human papillomavirus in cervical adenocarcinoma carcinogenesis. Eur J Cancer 2001;37:246–250.

21. Riethdorf S, Riethdorf L, Milde-Langosch K, et al. Differences in HPV 16 and HPV 18 E6/E7 oncogenic expression between in situ and invasive adenocarcinoma of cervix uteri. Virchows Arch 2000;437:491–500.

22. Pirog EC, Kleter B, Olgac S, et al. Prevalence of human papillomavirus in different histological subtypes of cervical adenocarcinoma. Am J Pathol 2000;157:1055–1060.

23. Anderson MC. Glandular lesions of the cervix: Diagnostic and therapeutic dilemmas. Baillières Clin Obstet Gynecol 1995;9:105–119.

24. Gloor E, Ruzicka J. Morphology of adenocarcinoma in situ of the uterine cervix; a study of 14 cases. Cancer 1982;49:294–298.

25. Shin CH, Schorge JO, Lee KR, et al. Cytologic and biopsy findings leading to conization in adenocarcinoma in situ of the cervix. Obstet Gynecol 2002;100:271–276.

26. Renshaw AA, Mody DR, Lozano RL, et al. Detection of adenocarcinoma in situ of the cervix in Papanicolaou tests: comparison of diagnostic accuracy with high-grade lesions. Arch Pathol Lab Med 2004;128:153–157.

27. Laverty CR, Farnsworth A, Thurloe T, et al. The reliability of a cytological prediction of cervical adenocarcinoma in situ. Aust NZ J Obstet Gynecol 1998;28:307–312.

28. Schooland M, Segal A, Allpress S, et al. Adenocarcinoma in Situ of the Cervix. Cancer 2002;96:319–23.

29. Ayer B, Pacey F, Greenberg et al. The cytologic diagnosis of adenocarcinoma in situ of the cervix and related lesions. I. Adenocarcinoma in situ. Acto Cytol 1987;31:394–411.

30. Alons-van Kordelaar JJM, Boon ME. Diagnostic accuracy of cervical lesions studied in spatula-cytobrush smears. Acta Cytol 1988;32:801–806.

31. Buntinx F, Brouwers M. Relation between sampling devices and detection abnormally in cervical smears: a metaanalysis of randomized and quasi-randomised studies. Br Med J 1996;313:1285–1290.

32. Boon ME, de Graaf Guilloud JC, Rietveld WJ. An analysis of five sampling methods for preparation of cervical smears. Acta Cytol 1989;33:843–848.

33. Novotny DB, Maygarden SJ, Johnson DE, et al. Tubal metaplasia. A frequent potencial pitfall in the cytodiagnosis of endocervical glandular dysplasia on cervical smears. Acta Cytol 1992;36:1–10.

34. Wilbur DC. Endocervical glandular atypia: a new problem for the cytopathologist. Diagn Cytopathol 1995;13:463–469.

35. Lickrish GM, Colgan T. Management of adenocarcinoma in situ of the uterine cervix. In: Wright VC, Lickrish GM, Shier RM (eds). Basic and Advanced Colposcopy—a Practical Handbook for Treatment, ed 2. Houston: Biomedical Communications, 1995, pp 30–33.

36. Solomon D, Davey D, Kurman R, et al. The 2001 Bethesda System: terminology for reporting of cervical cytology. J Am Med Assoc 2002;287:2114–2119.

37. Levine L, Lucci JA 3rd, Dinh TV. Atypical glandular cells: new Bethesda terminology and management guidelines. Obstet Gynecol Survey 2003;58:399–403.

38. Keyhani-Rofafga S, Brewer J, Prokorym P. Comparative cytological findings of in situ and invasive adenocarcinoma of the uterine cervix. Diagn Cytol Pathol 1995;12:120–125.

39. Roberts JM, Thurloe JK, Bowditch RC, et al. Subdividing atypical glandular cells of undetermined significance according to the Australian Modified Bethesda System. Cancer 2000;90:87–96.

40. Vinokurova S, Wentzensen N, von Knebel Doeberitz M. Analysis of p16 INK4a and integrated genomes as progression markers. Methods Mol Med 2005;119:73–83.

41. Derchain SF, Rabelo-Santos SH, Sarian Lo, et al. Human papillomavirus DNA detection and histological findings in women referred for atypical glandular cells or adenocarcinoma in situ in their Pap smears. Gynecol Oncol 2004;95:618–623.

42. Nieh S, Chen SF, Chu TY, et al. Expression of p16 INK4A in Pap smears containing atypical glandular cells from the uterine cervix. Acta Cytol 2004;48:173–180.

43. Schorge JO, Lea JS, Elias KJ, et al. P16 as a molecular marker of cervical adenocarcinoma. Am J Obstet Gynecol 2004;190:668–673.

44. Irvin W, Evans SR, Andersen W, et al. The utility of HPV DNA triage in the management of cytological AGC. Am J Obstet Gynecol 2005;193:559–565.

45. Oliveira ER, Dercgain SF, Rabelo-Santos SH, et al. Detection of high-risk human papillomavirus (HPV) DNA by Hybrid Capture II in women referred due to atypical glandular cells in primary screening. Diagn Cytopathol 2004;31:19–22.

46. Hafez ESE. Structural and ultrastructural parameters of the uterine cervix. Obstet Gynecol Survey 1982;507–516.

47. Phillip E. Normal endocervical epithelium. J Reprod Med 1975;14:188–191.

48. Fluhman CF, Dickman Z. The basic pattern of glandular structures of the cervix uteri. Obstet Gynecol 1958;11:543–545.

49. Kolstad P, Stafl A. Terminology and definitions. In: Kolstad P, Stafl A, Atlas of Colposcopy. Oslo, Universitetsforlaget, 1972, pp 21–25.

50. Reid R, Scalzi P. Genital warts and cervical cancer—VII. An improved colposcopic index for differentiating benign papillomaviral infections from high-grade cervical intraepithelial neoplasia. Am J Obstet Gynecol 1985;153:61–68.

51. Wright VC, Shier RM. Why adenocarcinoma in situ is often missed by colposcopists. In: Wright VC, Shier RM (eds).

Colposcopy of Adenocarcinoma In Situ and Adenocarcinoma of the Cervix. Houston: Biomedical Communications, 2000, pp 1–4.

52. Murdoch JB, Grimshaw RN, Monaghan JM. Loop diathermy excision of the abnormal transformation zone. Int J Gynecol Cancer 1991;1:105–109.

53. Ayer B, Pacey F, Greenberg M. The cytologic diagnosis of adenocarcinoma in situ of the cervix uteri and related lesions. II. Microinvasive adenocarcinoma Acta Cytol 1988;32:318–324.

54. Jaworski RC, Pacey NF, Greenberg M, et al. The histological diagnosis of adenocarcinoma in situ and related lesions of the cervix uteri. Cancer 1988;61:1171–1181.

55. Bertrand M, Lickrish GM, Colgan TJ. The anatomical distribution of cervical adenocarcinoma in situ. Am J Obstet Gynecol 1987;1:21–26.

56. Nicklin JL, Wright RG, Bell JR, et al. A clinicopathological study of adenocarcinoma of the cervix. The influence of HPV infection and other factors, and the role of conservative surgery. Obstet Gynecol 1991;2:179–183.

57. Andersen ES, Arffman E. Adenocarcinoma in situ of the uterine cervix. A clinical-pathologic study of 36 cases. Gynecol Oncol 1989;35:1–7.

58. Muntz HG, Bell DA, Lage JM, et al. Adenocarcinoma in situ of the uterine cervix. Obstet Gynecol 1992;80:935–939.

59. Wright VC. Squamous and glandular intraepithelial neoplasia: identification and current management approaches. Salúd Publica Mex 2003;45:S417–S429.

60. Apgar B, Zoschnick, Wright T. The 2001 Bethesda System Terminology. AM Fam Physician 2003;68:1992–8.

61. Wright TC Jr, Massad LS, Dunton CJ, Spitzer M, Wilkinson EJ, Solomon D; for the 2006 ASCCP-Sponsored Consensus Conference. 2006 consensus guidelines for the management of women with abnormal cervical screening tests. J Low Genit Tract Dis 2007 Oct; 11(14):201–222.

62. Wright VC, Davies E, Riopelle MA. Laser cylindrical excision to replace conization. Am J Obstet Gynecol 1984;150: 704–709.

63. Wright VC, Dubuc-Lissoir J, Ehlen T, et al. Guidelines on adenocarcinoma in situ of the cervix. Clinical features and review of management. J Soc Gynaecol Can 1999;77:699–706.

64. Wright TC Jr, Massad LS, Dunton CJ, Spitzer M, Wilkinson EJ, Solomon D; 2006 American Society for Colposcopy and Cervical Pathology-sponsored Consensus Conference. 2006 consensus guidelines for the management of women with cervical intraepithelial neoplasia or adenocarcinoma in situ. J Low Genit Tract Dis 2007 Oct; 11(4):223–39.

65. McHale MT, Le TD, Burger RA, et al. Fertility sparing treatment for in situ and early invasive adenocarcinoma of the cerviz. Obstet Gynecol 2001;98:726–731.

66. Denehy TR, Gregori CA, Breen JL. Endocervical curettage, cone margins and residual adenocarcinoma in situ of the cervix. Obstet Gynecol 1997;90:1–6.

67. Weisbrot IM, Stabinsky C, Davis AM. Adenocarcinoma in situ of the uterine cervix. Cancer 1972;29:1179–1187.

68. Wildrich T, Kennedy AW, Myers TM, et al. Adenocarcinoma in situ of the cervix. Management and outcome. Gynecol Oncol 1996;11:304–308.

69. Wolf JK, Levenback C, Malpica A, et al. Adenocarcinoma in situ of the cervix. Significance of cone biopsy margins. Obstet Gynecol 1996;88:82–86.

70. Im DO, Duska LR, Rosenshein NB. Adequacy of conization margins in adenocarcinoma in situ as a predictor of residual disease. Gynecol Oncol 1995;59:179–182.

71. Luesley DM, Jordan JA, Woodman CBJ, et al. A retrospective review of adenocarcinoma in situ and glandular atypia of the uterine cervix. Br J Obstet Gynecol 1987;94:699–703.

72. Hopkins MP, Roberts JA, Schmidt RW. Cervical adenocarcinoma in situ. Obstet Gynecol 1988;71:842–844.

73. Poynor EA, Barakat RR, Hoskins WJ. Management follow-up of patients with adenocarcinoma in situ of the uterine cervix. Gynecol 1995;57:158–164.

74. Kennedy AW, Tabbakh GH, Biscotti CW, et al. Invasive adenocarcinoma of the cervix following LLETZ (large loop excision of the transformation zone). Gynecol Oncol 1995;58:274–277.

75. Christopherson WM, Nealson N, Gray LA. Noninvasive precursor lesions of adenocarcinoma and mixed adenosquamous carcinoma of the cervix uteri. Cancer 1981;48:768–773.

76. Kennedy AW, Biscotti CV. Further study of the management of cervical adenocarcinoma in situ. Gynecol Oncol 2002;86: 361–364.

77. Östör AG. Natural history of cervical intraepithelial neoplasia. A critical review. Int J Gynecol Oncol 1993;12:186–192.

78. Piver MS, Rutledge FN, Smith PJ. Five classes of extended hysterectomy of women with cervical cancer. Obstet Gynecol 1974;44:265–269.

79. Bryson P, Stulberg R, Shepherd L, et al. Is electrosurgical loop excision with negative margins sufficient treatment for cervical ACIS? Gynecol Oncol 2003;93:465–468.

80. Hwang DM, Lickrish GM, Chapman W, et al. Long-term surveillance is required for all women treated for cervical adenocarcinoma in situ. J Lower Genit Tract Dis 2004;8:125–131.

CASE STUDY

A 35-year-old woman was referred for colposcopy because cervical cytology was reported as HSIL. She desired more children. Figure 15-83 illustrates the colposcopic image. Describe what you see. A representative biopsy of the lesion is seen in Figure 15-84. Describe what you see. What would you do next?

The colpophotograph demonstrates a mixed lesion (containing glandular and squamous components). The glandular lesion appears like columnar epithelium that has turned mildly acetowhite. It is separating two CIN 3 lesions at the 5- to 7-o'clock position. The histology as depicted in Figure 15-84 demonstrates the AIS component as appearing papillary with centrally placed angioarchitecture and histologically features as previously described (see Figure 15-63). The CIN 3 component demonstrates full-thickness loss of maturation, increased cellularity, dense cytoplasm, and an intact basement membrane.

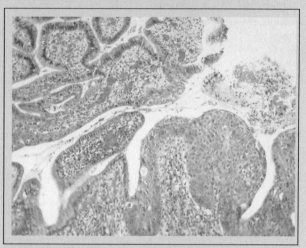

Figure 15-84 Histology of image of Figure 15-83. The AIS component appears papillary with centrally placed angioarchitecture and features of AIS as previously described in Figures 15-63 and 15-64. The HSIL/CIN 3 component demonstrates full-thickness loss of maturation with malignant cells, increased cellularity, dense cytoplasm, and an intact basement membrane.

What should be done next? Colposcopy cannot differentiate between AIS and cervical adenocarcinoma. Therefore an excisional procedure is required. Because the final histology was AIS/CIN 3 with negative specimen margins and the patient has a desire for fertility, a program of conservative follow-up was discussed with her.

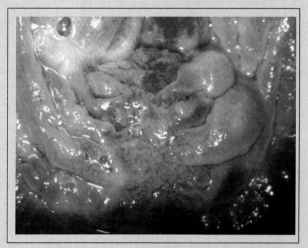

Figure 15-83 A mixed lesion (glandular and squamous) seen colposcopically. The glandular lesion (AIS) on histology, which appears as faint acetowhite columnar epithelium, is separating two acetowhite (HSIL) lesions. (From Wright VC. Principles of Cervical Colposcopy. Figure 10.45. Houston: Biomedical Communications, 2004, p 10–19.)

CHAPTER 16

Vagina: Normal, Premalignant, and Malignant

Barbara S. Apgar • Gregory L. Brotzman*

KEY POINTS

- Vaginal carcinoma constitutes 0.3% of incident cancers and 0.3% of cancer deaths among U.S. women.
- Vaginal intraepithelial neoplasia (VaIN) is identified more frequently in younger women and is usually associated with human papillomavirus (HPV) infection.
- VaIN 1 and VaIN 2 are representative of more benign viral proliferation, whereas VaIN 3 may be a true cancer precursor.
- Approximately 36% to 48% of women with VaIN have concurrent cervical intraepithelial neoplasia (CIN).
- VaIN presents most commonly in women who have undergone hysterectomy for CIN 3. Presenting lesions are usually located on the anterior or posterior vaginal walls and may be hidden by the vaginal speculum.
- Women who have had hysterectomies for benign disease do not need continued Pap screening.
- Vaginal colposcopy is more technically difficult than cervical colposcopy. The application of half-strength Lugol's solution to the vaginal mucosa after examination with 5% acetic acid may be helpful in identifying multifocal areas of epithelial change or areas that are difficult to detect by gross visual inspection.
- Vascular patterns tend to be absent in VaIN 1 but present in VaIN 3. Lesions that are raised, exophytic, or nodular or exhibit abnormal or atypical vessels should raise suspicion for invasion.
- Treatment for VaIN should be individualized. VaIN therapies may include observation of VaIN 1, surgical excision, ablation, radiation, and topical chemotherapy. The treatments are modified and influenced by the size, location, and number of the lesions; the age and health status of the patient; the need to preserve vaginal function; and the patient's compliance with follow-up appointments.
- If there is any suspicion of invasion, or if the patient is older than 40 to 50 years, the treatment of choice for VaIN 3 is partial vaginectomy, with cure rates approaching 90%.
- About 5% of women treated with intravaginal fluorouracil develop chronic vaginal ulcers lasting longer than 6 months.

---

*A very special thank you to Burton Krumholz, M.D. for allowing us to use his images and portions of his text from the first edition of this work in this current chapter on VaIN.

The vagina connects the uterine cervix with the vestibule of the vulva. In the resting position, the vagina forms a fibromuscular tube that is flattened from anterior to posterior,[1] with the exception of the cranial end, where the vagina surrounds the cervix. The deeply recessed vagina areas surrounding the cervix are called the *fornices*. The entire length of the vagina is located between the rectum posteriorly and the urinary bladder and urethra anteriorly. The posterior wall measures about 11 cm in length, whereas the anterior wall measures only 8 cm. The posterior vaginal fornix is adjacent to the pouch of Douglas, which is lined by peritoneum and allows for communication to the lowest point of the peritoneal cavity. The vagina is very elastic and reaches its maximum elasticity during childbirth.

The boundary between the vulva and vagina is called Hart's line.[2] *It can be clearly demarcated by the application of dilute Lugol's solution.* This boundary demonstrates clear histologic differences between the vaginal and the vulvar epithelia. Histologically, the vaginal wall consists of three layers: the epithelial layer, the muscular coat, and the vaginal fascia. The epithelial layer consists of a stratified squamous epithelium and a lamina propria that is subject to age and hormonal influences. The lamina propria contains a dense network of elastic fibers that continue to proliferate until about the age of 40 years. In older women, the fibers often exist only in fragments. The vaginal epithelium forms transverse folds called *rugae*. Historically, it was understood that the vaginal epithelium had few, if any, glands. *More recent descriptions of the vaginal epithelium reveal the presence of glandular elements or their metaplastic counterpart in 3% to 4% of women. These areas have been described as* adenosis, *although they represent normal vaginal variants or remnants from embryologic development* (Figure 16-1). These areas may also be described as a *vaginal transformation zone*.[3] Although the cyclic hormonal changes in the vaginal epithelium are less pronounced than those in the endometrium, they are apparent on cytologic examination. Glycogen content is highest during ovulation and is significantly decreased in estrogen deficiency states.

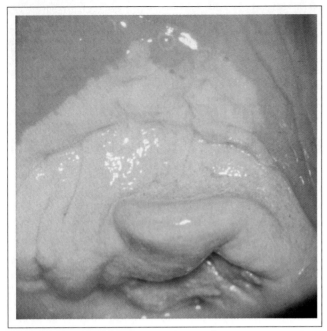

Figure 16-1 Cervical deformity and vaginal transformation zone in a 24-year-old patient with no history of DES exposure. Vaginal acetowhitening represents an area of adenosis found in 3% to 4% of women.

EPIDEMIOLOGY AND RISK FACTORS OF VAGINAL INTRAEPITHELIAL NEOPLASIA AND VAGINAL CANCER

Compared with cervical cancer (8.9/100,000 women), *vaginal neoplasms are rare (0.7/100,000 women),[4]constituting 0.3% of incident cancers and 0.3% of cancer deaths among U.S. women.[5]* The 5-year relative survival rate is 43.8% with the excess occurring in older women.[4] It is reported that only 289 of 30,898 gynecologic cancers (0.9%) are actually primary in the vagina.[6]*History of a prior cervical cancer or cervical intraepithelial neoplasia (CIN), grade 3 (CIN 3) are important risk factors for the development of vaginal cancer.[4,7,8]*

The association between vaginal intraepithelial neoplasia (VaIN) and cervical cancer and precancer is the relationship of both with high-risk human papillomavirus (HPV) that resides throughout the lower genital tract, resulting in a second neoplasm in the vagina or vulva.[9] *HPV appears to be a necessary factor for development of VaIN, just as it is for development of CIN and cervical cancer.* Viral integration sites of HPV types 16 and 18 in women who had a history of anogenital lesions and subsequent development of high-grade vaginal or vulvar lesions were studied. Identical HPV integration loci in the cervical samples and in the vulvar and vaginal samples were found, strongly suggesting that high-grade intraepithelial lesions of the lower gential tract arise from monoclonal lesions of transformed cervical cell populations, rather than de novo.[10] In fact, using the site of HPV deoxyribonucleic acid (DNA) integration as a marker of clonality, identical

HPV DNA integration loci are found in tissue from the initial cervical cancer and CIN 3 and the later-developing VaIN and vaginal cancer.[10] It is also postulated that microscopic foci of malignant cells can be seeded into the vagina at the time of surgery for CIN 3. It is unclear how the CIN 3 migrates to the vagina.[9] Whether the cells disseminate or are actually transplanted is unknown. Some women with primary vaginal cancer have no prior history of CIN 3 or cervical cancer.

In one of the few population-based studies, women with vaginal cancer reported 5 or more lifetime sexual partners (odds ratio [OR] = 3.1) and an earlier age at first coitus (OR = 2.0).[8] Current smoking was reported as a strong risk factor for vaginal cancer (OR = 2.1), was independent of the number of cigarettes smoked, and was highest among women who have smoked for longer than 30 years.[8] In another hospital-based case-control study, the relationship between smoking and vaginal cancer was not significant.[7] More than 50% of women with vaginal neoplasia have had a previous hysterectomy compared with 25% of control subjects, representing a nearly fourfold risk. In this population-based study, the excess risk was seen in women with no history of anogenital cancer.[8] Thirty percent of women with invasive vaginal cancer had a prior anogenital cancer, compared with 2% of controls. Only 23% reported prior cervical disease (OR = 16.0), and in a third of these women, more than 15 years had elapsed since cervical disease diagnosis. Because of the methodology used in the study, the data on hysterectomy may be invalid and should be interpreted with caution. One small study found genetic susceptibility as one factor contributing to progression of anogenital cancer.[11] Additional studies are needed before genetics can be considered in causality.

The true incidence of VaIN is difficult to assess.[12] Because women with VaIN are usually asymptomatic, and because the majority of cases are found after an abnormal Papanicolaou (Pap) smear, the frequency can be related to the prevalence of cytologic screening in a population. The incidence of VaIN is reported to be 0.2 to 0.3 per 100,000 women.[6] With increased cytologic screening, the condition may be more readily diagnosed and found to be more prevalent.[12] *VaIN is reported with 100 times lesser frequency than CIN.[13]*

The reported mean age of VaIN ranges from 35 to 55 years of age.[14,15] There is disagreement as to whether the grade of VaIN increases with a woman's age.[14,15] Women diagnosed with VaIN appear to be older than those diagnosed with CIN.[16]

The etiology of VaIN has not been conclusively determined, but it appears that exposure to HPV is the most likely predisposing factor. The precise relationship between HPV and VaIN may involve a multistep process associated with cofactors such as sexual activity, smoking, history of other sexually transmitted diseases (STDs), and a history of HPV-associated disease in sites other than the vagina. The demographic features are similar among women with CIN and VaIN.[14]

Women with vaginal cancer (44%) and VaIN (44%) demonstrate antibodies to HPV DNA types 16 and 18.[8] In this population-based study, women who were HPV DNA positive did not differ from controls by number of sexual partners or smoking status, but they tended to be older. These numbers may seem low because the majority of vaginal cancers and VaIN follow previous cervical cancer or CIN. It is notable that not all women mount an antibody response to HPV, the response may wane over time, and the antibody test may have been too insensitive in some cases. Furthermore, a test for HPV DNA was not available for this study. *Compared with CIN development, the development of VaIN following HPV infection may require a greater period of time and may occur less frequently because of the different type of epithelium from which VaIN arises.*

The presence of HPV in the vagina of women following hysterectomy has been associated with an increase in VaIN.[17] If CIN and VaIN share a common etiology, it would explain reports that describe 36% to 48% of women with VaIN as having concurrent CIN.[18,19] Approximately 51% to 62% of women with VaIN have been treated for CIN, and as many as 25% have undergone hysterectomies for CIN as well. Almost 75% of women with VaIN have preceding or coexisting squamous carcinomas of the cervix or vulva.[20–24] Despite these figures, VaIN occurs in less than 1% of women who have undergone hysterectomy for CIN in a 10-year follow-up period.[24]

NATURAL HISTORY

Careful evaluation of the progressive potential of the various cervical, vaginal, and vulvar lesions has led to the suggestion that *despite the similarities among CIN, vulvar intraepithelial neoplasia (VIN), and VaIN, these conditions may not be similar in their biological behavior.*[25]

VaIN is categorized into VaIN 1, 2, and 3. In 121 women with VaIN, VaIN 1 was present in 40 (33%), VaIN 2 in 55 (46%), and VaIN 3 in 26 (21%).[14] *VaIN 1 is most likely a benign viral proliferation similar to CIN 1, and VaIN 2 is intermediate in risk, whereas VaIN 3 is a true cancer precursor.* Malignant transformation can occur without treatment or following treatment of VaIN.

The natural history of VaIN has not been clearly defined. *The risk that VaIN will progress to invasive vaginal carcinoma appears to be far lower than the risk for CIN progressing to cervical carcinoma.* Most VaIN lesions are asymptomatic, are not clinically identified, and probably regress spontaneously without treatment. Although VaIN 3 has a greater potential for malignant transformation than VaIN 1, all have the potential to progress.[14,18] In the Aho study, 2 of 23 (9%) of women with VaIN who did not receive treatment for 3 years developed vaginal cancer. In the Dodge study, 2 out of 92 (2%) of women treated for VaIN 1 and 2 subsequently developed vaginal cancer. However, because of the difficulty in detecting VaIN, it is impossible to exclude the possibility that these women had occult VaIN 3. One woman had had a hysterectomy for CIN 3 as well as a history of VIN 3.

Studies indicate that although VaIN seems to regress in some women (Aho et al.,[18] 18 of 23 [78%]; Petrilli et al.,[19] 6 of 12 [50%]), it may persist in others (Aho et al.,[18] 3 of 23

[13%]; Petrilli et al.,[19] 6 of 12 [50%]) or may eventually progress to invasive cancer (Aho et al.,[18] 2 of 23 [9%]; Dodge,[14] 2 of 92 [2%]). Lesions not associated with CIN or VIN showed a higher rate of regression (91%) than those associated with CIN or VIN (67%).[18] Spontaneous regression appears to be more common in women with VaIN 1.[18]

CYTOLOGIC SCREENING

The primary method of detecting VaIN is by cytologic examination of asymptomatic women. *VaIN lesions should be suspected in women with cervical or vulvar neoplasia, lower genital tract condylomata, or abnormal cytologic smears after hysterectomy; in women after pelvic irradiation; or in women with abnormal cytology in the absence of a recognizable cervical lesion.*

The detection of VaIN in a woman with a cervix is usually associated with a concurrent or previous diagnosis of CIN or VIN.[27] In these situations, careful colposcopic examination of the entire lower genital tract must be performed before proceeding to a conization. This is especially important in women in whom an abnormal smear persists after treatment of a cervical lesion.[28] Nwabineli and Monaghan found that 103 of 4147 women (2.5%) treated for CIN by laser had coexisting vaginal abnormalities.

Several studies have examined the effectiveness of Pap smears for post-treatment surveillance. Due to the relative rarity of VaIN, studies that assess disease incidence and detection involve small numbers of patients. In a study of 31 patients with VaIN following hysterectomy, vaginal cytology correctly identified the disease in 83% of cases.[29] Although cytology is useful for detection of VaIN, Cooper et al. demonstrated that cervical cytologic screening is a poor test to detect vaginal recurrence in women who have been treated for uterine cancer. Fourteen percent of recurrent lesions were asymptomatic and detected on cytology, whereas the remaining 86% of lesions were clinically apparent, and Pap smears were not cost-effective.[30]

Despite the fact that most VaIN is found in women who have undergone hysterectomy for CIN 3 or cervical cancer, the necessity for vaginal cytologic screening after hysterectomy for benign disease has been questioned. The prevalence of VaIN after hysterectomy for benign disease has been shown to be between 0.13% and 0.15%.[31] In another study of 581 women following hysterectomy for benign conditions, there were no cases of VaIN 3 or invasive cancer on follow-up cytology. A total of 3.4% showed atypical squamous cells of undetermined significance (ASC-US) or low-grade VaIN.[32]

The American College of Obstetricians and Gynecologists recommends that after confirming the accuracy of the woman's cervical cytology history and operative history, women who have undergone hysterectomy with removal of the cervix for benign indications and who have no prior history of CIN 2 or CIN 3 or worse may discontinue routine cytology testing. Continued routine vaginal cytology screening in these women is not cost-effective and may cause anxiety and over-treatment.

If the history cannot be verified, screening recommendations may need to be modified.[33]

Fetters et al. reviewed the recommendations of major organizations and textbooks of gynecology and performed a MEDLINE computer search for the years 1966 to 1995.[34] They concluded that data do not support screening for vaginal cancer in women following total hysterectomy for benign disease. Women who have had a subtotal hysterectomy and still have a cervix should continue to be screened according to established guidelines. *Women with maternal diethylstilbestrol (DES) exposure or with a history of abnormal cytologic smears or gynecologic malignancy should continue to receive vaginal screening.* The authors concluded that diligence is needed to distinguish between populations at increased risk for vaginal cytologic abnormalities and those with minimal or no risk. Their conclusions were supported by Pearce et al., who reviewed 9610 Pap smears perfomed on women with a hysterectomy for benign indications as much as 19 years previously and found that only 1.1% had any cytologic abnormalities.[31] On biopsy, there was no VaIN 3 or vaginal cancer. The positive predictive value for detecting vaginal cancer was 0%.[31] The prevalence of vaginal dysplasia after hysterectomy for benign disease was between 0.13% and 0.15%. Noller believed that the use of the Pap smear after hysterectomy for benign disease should become an antiquated procedure.[34] Furthermore, from an ethical perspective, Fetters et al. decried the use of unnecessary Pap smears to gain compliance for health maintenance examinations.[36] *A woman should not be asked to return for a vaginal cytologic smear when the underlying motive is to perform a breast examination or to provide another preventive health service.*

The U.S. Preventive Services Task Force (USPSTF) recommends (D recommendation) against routine Pap smear screening in women who have had a total hysterectomy for benign reasons.[36] The USPSTF found fair evidence that the yield of cytologic screening is very low in women after hysterectomy and poor evidence that screening to detect vaginal cancer improves health outcomes. *The USPSTF concludes that potential harms of continued screening after hysterectomy are likely to exceed benefits.* However, since the USPSTF guidelines were issued in 1996, there was no decrease in reported screenings in the subsequent 6-year period, and it is estimated that 45.6% (10 million) of U.S. women are being screened unnecessarily for cervical cancer.[27] *The American Cancer Society recommends that women who have had a total hysterectomy should stop cervical cancer screening unless the surgery was done as treatment for cervical cancer or precancer.*[37]

On the other hand, women with a previous diagnosis of CIN 2,3 who undergo total hysterectomy should continue annual screening until three consecutive negative vaginal cytology test results are achieved. These women can develop recurrent intraepithelial neoplasia or cancer at the vaginal cuff.[13,38] After the three consecutive negative results, routine screening can be discontinued.[33]

The presence of benign glandular cells in vaginal smears of women following hysterectomy has been described and appears to pose no significant risk for subsequent development of vaginal cancer.[39,40]

COLPOSCOPY OF THE VAGINA

Colposcopic examination of the vagina is indicated for the evaluation of abnormal cytology whenever cervical colposcopy is negative or for the evaluation of abnormal cytology after hysterectomy for CIN 2,3 or invasive cervical cancer. Other indications for vaginal colposcopy may include a history of maternal DES exposure, following the identification of gross vaginal lesions by inspection or palpation, suspected VaIN, or for the evaluation of extensive HPV-associated lesions in the vagina.[2]

The goal of the vaginal colposcopy is to identify the presence and extent of preinvasive or invasive vaginal disease and to select appropriate therapy (Table 16-1). *Colposcopic examination of the vagina is more tedious and more technically challenging than colposcopy of the cervix. The large surface area of the vagina, the presence of vaginal rugae, posthysterectomy "dog ears," and multifocal disease increase the technical difficulty of vaginal colposcopy and make this examination potentially lengthy and uncomfortable for the patient. The speculum blades obscure the anterior and posterior walls of the vagina, and colposcopic grading of lesions in the vagina is undefined.*

Vaginal colposcopy is performed in the dorsal lithotomy position. If possible, the buttocks should be raised 5 to 10 degrees. A thorough inspection of the vulvar vestibule is completed before the vaginal examination. An appropriately sized speculum should be chosen and carefully inserted into the vagina. The size of the speculum should be deep enough to view the cranial portion of the vagina but allow easy rotation so that the entire vagina may be visualized.

The vagina is then thoroughly moistened with 5% acetic acid. Because this solution is stronger than the frequently used 3% acetic acid solution, it accentuates the subtle vaginal lesions more rapidly and effectively.[16] It may be necessary to continuously reapply dilute acetic acid during a prolonged examination. The vaginal mucosal folds are inspected for acetowhite changes by rotating and withdrawing the speculum and observing the epithelium as it rolls over the speculum blades during withdrawal of the speculum. The application of half-strength Lugol's iodine to the

Table 16-1 Indications for Vaginal Colposcopy

| Abnormal cytology in a woman |
| With a normal cervix after colposcopy or therapy |
| Without a cervix after hysterectomy |
| In utero DES exposure |
| Gross lesions by inspection or palpation |
| Suspected VaIN or vaginal carcinoma |
| Widespread lower genital tract HPV infection |

DES, Diethylstilbestrol; *VaIN*, vaginal intraepithelial neoplasia; *HPV*, human papillomavirus.

vaginal mucosa after examination for acetowhite changes is frequently helpful in identifying multifocal areas of epithelial change or areas that were previously undetected. *In well-estrogenized women, the normal vaginal epithelium is well glycogenated and will turn a dark mahogany brown color after the application of half-strength Lugol's iodine. Abnormal vaginal epithelium will reject the iodine and appear yellow in color.* Lugol's iodine will dehydrate the vaginal epithelium, and women should be warned of potential discomfort. If the vaginal speculum needs to be withdrawn and reinserted, a thin coating of lubricating jelly on the speculum can ease the process. The use of an iris hook can expose hidden areas by stretching the mucosa and flattening the rugae, thus enhancing the identification of abnormal areas. An iris hook can aid visualization of the epithelium at the vaginal angles or within the "dog ears" of the vaginal cuff in hysterectomized women.

Biopsy sites in the vagina should be selected at the time of colposcopic examination. The ancillary tools that may be helpful in vaginal colposcopy are listed in Table 16-2. The use of diluted Lugol's iodine aids in selecting sites for biopsy, especially when the lesions are multifocal (Figures 16-2 and 16-3). The vaginal epithelium should also be palpated to detect any indurated areas. Cervical punch biopsy instruments are normally used to obtain the sample. It is helpful to elevate the biopsy site with an iris hook or a single-toothed tenaculum to ensure that the stroma is included in the specimen so that invasive cancer can be excluded. *In performing a vaginal biopsy, the clinician must strike a balance between taking a biopsy that is too deep (the vaginal epithelium may be only 1 mm thick, and a deep biopsy may go through the full thickness of the vaginal wall) and taking one that is too superficial and will not exclude invasion.* When vaginal colposcopy with biopsy cannot be obtained in the office with the use of local anesthesia, an evaluation under conscious sedation may become necessary. It is rarely necessary to suture the vagina after a punch biopsy. Bleeding is generally controlled with the application of thickened Monsel's solution (ferric subsulfate) and direct pressure.

VaIN is usually asymptomatic and is usually identified following colposcopy and biopsy for evaluation of an abnormal Pap smear.[14] VaIN is most commonly discovered in women who have a vaginal examination following hysterectomy for CIN 3. Women occasionally complain of abnormal vaginal bleeding or an unusual vaginal discharge, although these symptoms are uncommon.[14] Occasionally, a color change

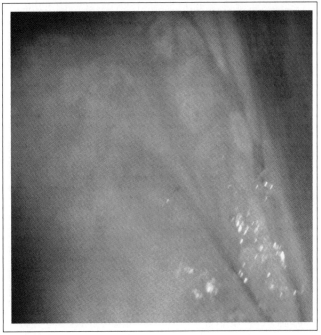

Figure 16-2 Faint, poorly defined, multifocal, grade 1 acetowhite areas in the left anterior vaginal fornix in a patient with persistent high-grade squamous intraepithelial lesion (HSIL) on cervical cytology who had no identifiable cervical lesion. (See next figure.)

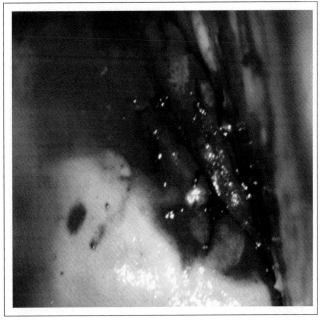

Figure 16-3 Iodine staining with half-strength Lugol's solution defines the nonstaining areas that coincide with the previously noted poorly defined white lesions. Biopsy was reported as VaIN 2.

Table 16-2 Ancillary Tools for Vaginal Colposcopy

Colposcope with variable magnification
Topical anesthesia
5% acetic acid
Skin or iris hook, mirror, and endocervical speculum
Half-strength Lugol's solution
Tischler cervical punch biopsy

of the vaginal epithelium may alert the clinician to an area of abnormal epithelium (Figures 16-4 and 16-5). Nevertheless, identification of VaIN is challenging for the colposcopist because it does not produce a characteristic appearance, like CIN. The colposcopic appearance and histology are more often disparate than in CIN.[41]

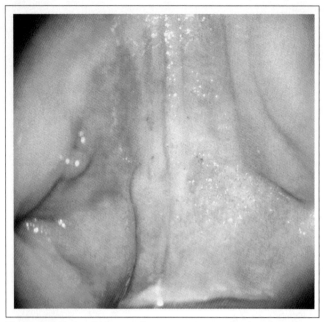

Figure 16-4 The vaginal apex of a woman 10 years after hysterectomy before the application of dilute acetic acid. There is a large erythematous area with foci of vascular prominence. (See next figure.)

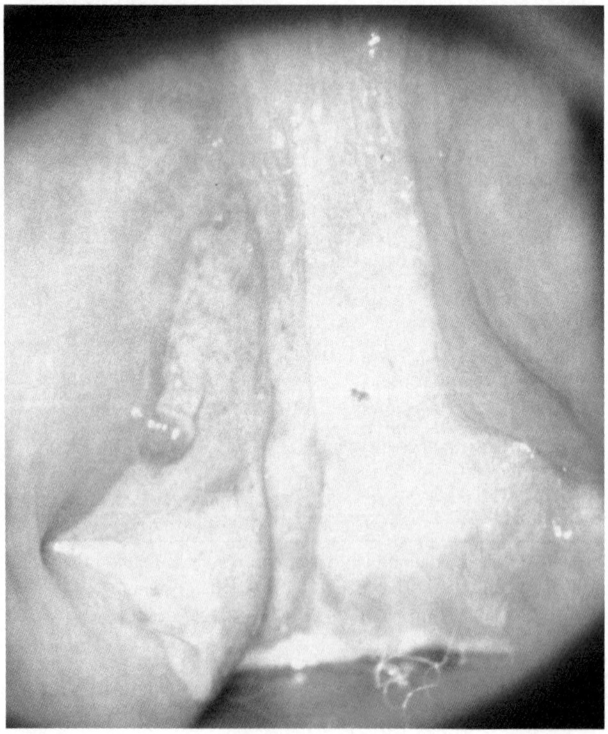

VaIN affects the upper third of the vagina in 78% to 92.4% of cases.[14,16] Fifty percent to 61% of the lesions are multifocal.[14,16] Because the presenting lesions may be located on the anterior or posterior vaginal wall, they may be hidden by the vaginal speculum (Figure 16-6). VaIN may occur in association with vaginal condylomata. VaIN lesions may be leukoplakic (Figure 16-7), erythematous, or ulcerated[42] (Figures 16-8 and 16-9). The most common abnormality detected on colposcopic examination in women with VaIN is acetowhite epithelium (84%).[14] An acetowhite lesion may be either flat or slightly raised and have a sharp or fuzzy border. These lesions may be multifocal and may show a micropapillary surface similar to subclinical condyloma (Figure 16-10). If lesions are present, the surface pattern tends to be irregular, possibly owing to the loose configuration of the vaginal mucosa. Abnormal vessel patterns such as punctation (14%) and mosaic (2%) are much less frequently observed in the vagina than on the cervix (Figures 16-11 and 16-12).

Atrophic changes of the vagina may mask the colposcopic appearance of VaIN. Topical estrogen cream may reverse these changes and allow a more thorough colposcopic examination. The colposcopic examination should be repeated after daily application of topical vaginal estrogen for 3 weeks (Figure 16-13).

Colposcopic patterns of VaIN may reflect findings that are slightly more severe than the histologic diagnosis. Prediction of histology from abnormal colposcopic appearances, especially the lower grades of VaIN, is more difficult in the vagina than on the cervix. Vascular patterns

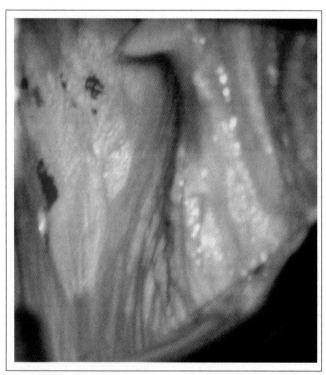

Figure 16-6 Multifocal acetowhite patches in left lateral vaginal fornix (cervix [not seen] is normal). Biopsy was reported as VaIN 2,3.

Figure 16-5 The same area after the application of dilute acetic acid solution. The erythematous region has developed a well-demarcated acetowhite dipping into the "dog ear" at the right apex. Biopsy was reported as VaIN 3.

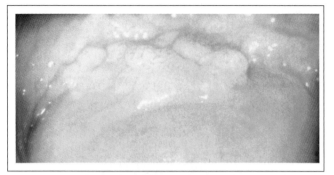

Figure 16-7 Raised white hyperkeratotic area along the anterior fornix. Biopsy was reported as VaIN 1 with "warty" changes.

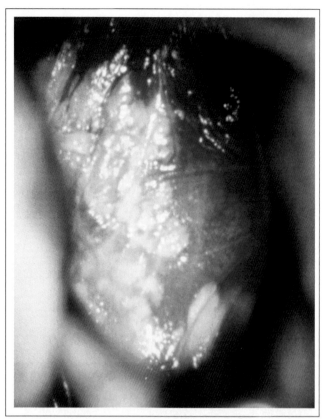

Figure 16-9 Iodine staining with half-strength Lugol's solution clearly defines the large area of atypical vaginal epithelium. Biopsy was reported as VaIN 3.

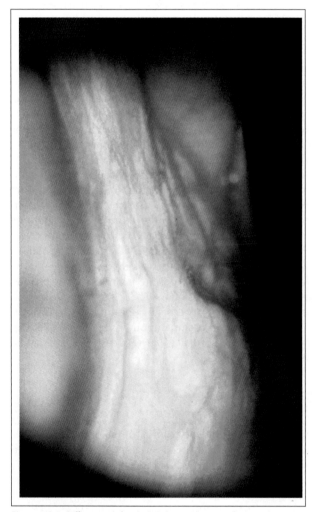

Figure 16-8 Diffuse, multifocal, slightly raised areas of acetowhite seen tangentially along the left upper vaginal sidewall. (See next figure.)

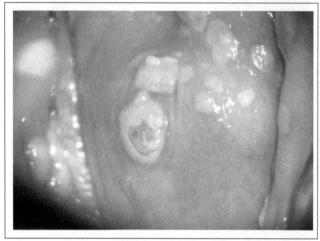

Figure 16-10 The upper vagina of a 29-year-old woman with no known immunocompromise had been treated repeatedly for several years for recurrent cervicovaginal condylomata and recurrent CIN 3 and VaIN 3. Several months following hysterectomy, colposcopy was performed and revealed irregular patchy, high grade acetowhite changes that were multifocal. Biopsy was reported as VaIN 3.

tend to be absent in low-grade (VaIN 1) lesions but present in high-grade (VaIN 3) lesions. Iodine staining may show partial uptake or no staining in low-grade lesions but may be strongly nonstaining in VaIN 3 lesions. *Lesions that are raised, exophytic, or nodular, along with those that exhibit atypical vessels, coarse punctation, or mosaic and ulceration must raise* the suspicion for vaginal carcinoma. Because there is not a strong correlation between vaginal colposcopy and histology, biopsy of all suspicious lesions may be necessary.

The colposcopic appearances of clinical and subclinical HPV lesions are similar to those on the cervix. They may be

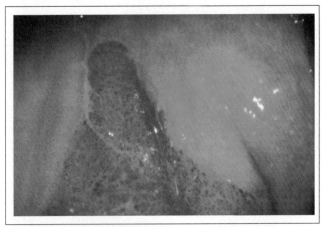

Figure 16-11 Colposcopy of the vagina of a 70-year-old woman. Hysterectomy was done 25 years earlier for uterine myomata. She has had no Pap smear in 15 years. Recent Pap smear was HSIL. The view at high magnification shows a well-defined lesion with coarse punctation.

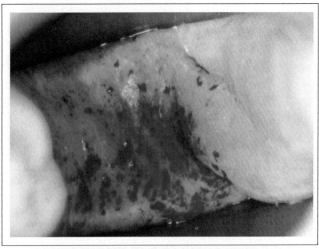

Figure 16-13 Atrophic vaginal epithelium will frequently show areas of ecchymosis and petechial hemorrhage.

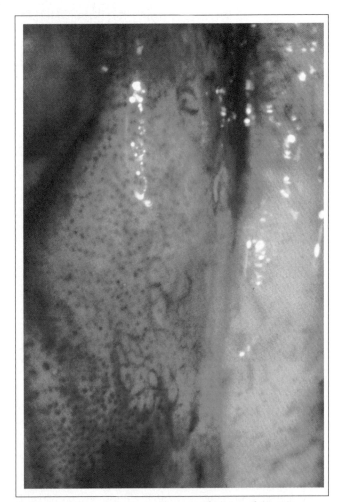

Figure 16-12 The same patient with a magnified view of the right posterior vaginal wall. There is a large area of acetowhite with coarse punctation and mosaic. The biopsy diagnosis was VaIN 3 (CIS).

grossly visible or seen only with the colposcope. They are frequently characterized by the presence of microspikes or exhibit a micropapillary appearance. They are generally keratinized and appear snow white after the application of 5% acetic acid. Flat condylomata may exist as multifocal lesions and be indistinguishable from VaIN, with which they may coexist. It may be difficult to distinguish VaIN 1 and flat condylomata by cytology, colposcopy, and histology.

The colposcopic features of vaginal squamous cancer are similar to those of other lower genital tract squamous carcinomas. Exophytic tumor and true erosions or ulcerations may be present. Examination of the vasculature may reveal atypical corkscrew-like or spaghetti-like vessels similar to those that might be seen on the cervix.

Vaginal lesions that may mimic invasive cancer include traumatic ulcers and erosions such as tampon ulcers and pessary injuries (Figure 16-14), atrophic and postirradiation changes, endometriosis, granulation tissue (Figure 16-15), and inflammatory disorders (Figure 16-16). Biopsy may be necessary for diagnosis.

HISTOLOGY

VaIN is defined as the spectrum of intraepithelial changes beginning with a generally well-differentiated intraepithelial neoplasia, traditionally classified as mild VaIN, and ending with invasive carcinoma.[43] The intraepithelial changes include nuclear pleomorphism, loss of polarity, abnormal mitosis, and loss of differentiation as cells progress from the basement membrane to the surface epithelium and are confined to the squamous epithelium above the basement membrane[43] (Figure 16-17).

Microscopically, the features of VaIN are similar to those of CIN, and similar problems of subjectivity in diagnosis and grading of disease severity exist. Despite this, the traditional grading of CIN has been applied to VaIN. Full-thickness epithelial involvement is termed VaIN 3, whereas VaIN 1 and VaIN 2 denote the presence of cytologic atypia

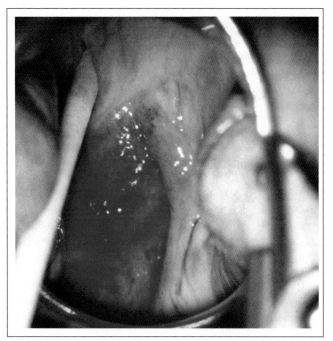

Figure 16-14 Pressure ulcer in the posterior vaginal vault due to the long-standing presence of pessary.

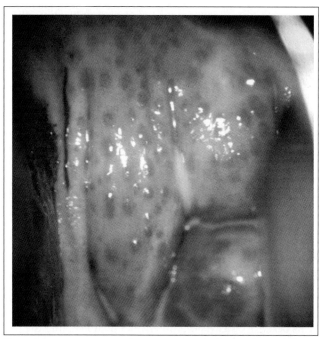

Figure 16-16 In a woman with a severe vaginal infection, the vaginal epithelium erodes in patches, exposing the vascular submucosa. This results in the red patches seen here in a woman with *Trichomonas vaginitis.*

in the lower one third or two thirds of the epithelium, respectively. With regard to treatment and the potential for malignant transformation, Lopes et al. suggested that it may be more useful to simply divide VaIN into low-grade (VaIN 1 and VaIN 2) and high-grade (VaIN 3) lesions.[44]

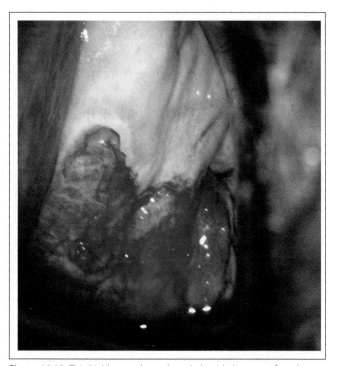

Figure 16-15 This highly vascular and eroded epithelium was found in a woman following surgery with a synthetic mesh to repair vaginal vault prolapse. Biopsies showed granulation tissue. The tissue did not heal or re-epithelialize until the mesh was removed.

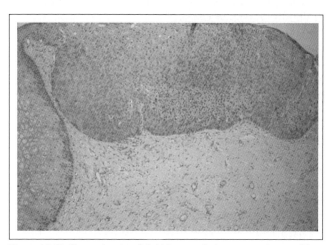

Figure 16-17 Biopsy showing full-thickness cell changes consistent with a diagnosis of VaIN 3.

It has been demonstrated that the cytologic and histologic grading of VaIN is moderately reproducible but also has been noted that the cytologic diagnosis of VaIN 2 is employed infrequently and rarely matches the diagnosis in the corresponding histology.[45] For this reason, Lopes et al. suggested that differentiating VaIN 2 from VaIN 3 is unnecessary. VaIN 3 is considered the true cancer precursor.

MANAGEMENT

The options available for managing VaIN include observation, surgical excision, surgical ablation, radiation, and topical chemotherapy. *Observation without treatment of VaIN may be justified in young women and those with minor-grade lesions.* It may be better to delay aggressive interference and adopt watchful waiting if the possibility exists that the lesion will regress. Conservation of sexual and reproductive function in young woman is of prime concern.

All methods of therapy for VaIN have a reasonably good success rate as long as follow-up is consistent.[45] The treatment options depend on the diagnostic and technical skills of the clinician, the clinician's personal experience, and the equipment available. The treatments are modified and influenced by the size, location, and number of lesions; the age and health status of the patient; and her willingness to comply with follow-up appointments.

Surgical Treatment of Vaginal Intraepithelial Neoplasia

Small and isolated lesions may be sufficiently treated with office biopsy excision as primary treatment, but care must be taken to ensure that the patient will return for follow-up visits because other lesions are frequently noted after the primary excision.[44] Cheng et al. advocate for treatment of VaIN 3 with wide local excision rather than laser ablation due to the possibility of missing an occult area of invasion. Even with wide local excision, 34% of their patients had recurrance of VaIN 3 or invasive cancer.[46]

Vaginectomy is an effective treatment for VaIN 3. It can diagnose occult malignancy in as many as 28% of cases. For lesions in young women that may be somewhat larger but still well demarcated, VaIN has been treated by excising strips of epithelium or performing a partial upper vaginectomy with a small electrosurgical loop electrode. An initial study of five women with VaIN who underwent partial upper vaginectomy indicated lack of morbidity although the amount of vagina excised was not specified.[47] The authors cited the availability of a pathology specimen as an advantage. Women with VaIN have also been treated with partial vaginectomies using loop excision followed by intravaginal 5-fluorouracil cream.[48] With a mean follow-up of 1.8 years, there were no recurrences of VaIN in the 10 hysterectomized women. In this series, one case of invasion was diagnosed. However, a follow-up case report recommends caution and demonstrates that upper vaginectomy with loop excision for VaIN is not without complications including bowel perforation and peritonitis.[49]

Wharton et al. suggested that *if there is any suspicion of invasion or if the patient is older than 40 to 45 years, the treatment of choice is partial upper vaginectomy.*[50] Clearly, excision is warranted when there is a need for extended sampling of VaIN 3 in the upper vagina.[51] It is also used when there is great disparity between a vaginal Pap smear and colposcopic examination of the vagina.[40] Partial vaginectomy, however, will often result in shortening of the vagina, significant blood loss, and need for a skin graft. Cure rates are reported to be as high as 90%. If invasion is found, the patient will require further therapy, usually radiation. *An often-cited advantage of partial vaginectomy is the ability to diagnose occult invasive disease.*

In a recent series of 105 women with VaIN 2,3 who underwent partial upper vaginectomy, all but 1 had undergone hysterectomy for previous disease unrelated to the vagina, and 10 had received radiation therapy.[52] Thirty-four percent of the patients had previously been treated for VaIN. Four patients experienced blood loss > 500 mL, and five patients sustained a cystotomy. Twenty-three patients had negative pathology. Squamous cell cancer was diagnosed in 13 women, 5 of whom had microinvasive disease. The remaining 69 women had VaIN 1-3. On follow-up of 25 months, 88% of the women had no recurrence.

Experienced laser surgeons and colposcopists can also accomplish partial vaginectomy for VaIN with the carbon dioxide laser.[40] This approach has the advantage of allowing the surgeon to work in a smaller space and results in minimal blood loss and less shortening of the vagina. Because it is done under colposcopic visualization, the excision is more precise and allows for better surgical control. No attempt is made to suture or otherwise close the vaginal defect. This approach allows for a functional vagina that will usually undergo re-epithelialization without skin grafting. Unlike with laser vaporization, a histologic specimen is available to ensure that invasion is not present. This procedure is appropriate when the diagnosis cannot be otherwise made by a simpler and less invasive technique.

If invasion is found after surgical excision of VaIN, radiation therapy may be indicated. DeBuben's[53] intracavitary brachytherapy has been used for treatment of both VaIN and early invasive vaginal carcinoma. The intravaginal application of both high-dose and low-dose radiation has been used with excellent therapeutic results.[54-60] The major concerns with this form of therapy are the possibility of radiation-induced cancer and the potential adverse effects on sexual function.[61,62]

Laser Vaporization of Vaginal Intraepithelial Neoplasia

When invasion is not suspected, treatment of VaIN may be performed by laser vaporization of the epithelium. This approach is acceptable only if the lesional areas have been fully visualized and representative areas sampled by adequate biopsy.[63-78] The optimum depth of destruction is 1.5 mm. Although this depth was chosen empirically by early investigators, Benedet et al. carefully studied histology specimens and performed microscopic measurements with a calibrated micrometer to determine the range of epithelial thickness in both involved and uninvolved vaginal tissue.[76] The depth of involvement of dysplastic vaginal epithelium ranged from 0.1 to 1.4 mm. Therapeutic success rates for this form of therapy vary between 63% and 90% after the first treatment with an increase in success rates after multiple treatments. Laser vaporization helps minimize the extent to which therapy may compromise future sexual function.[79] Disadvantages of laser vaporization include the inability to access VaIN lesions extending into vault tunnels or buried in the cuff scar after hysterectomy.[80] Diakomanolis et al. assessed the effectiveness of laser ablation versus upper vaginectomy in the treatment of VaIN. Operator skill level was an important consideration for success of laser treatment. Diakomanolis et al. recommended upper vaginectomy if the VaIN involved the vaginal apex or dog-ear areas, whereas ablation was useful for extensive multifocal VaIN.[81] Laser ablation successfully eliminated VaIN in 70.8% of patients after the first ablation and 79.2% after multiple ablations with a mean follow-up of 26 months.[80] VaIN progressed to invasion in 1 of the 24 patients in the study. There were no prognostic factors that predicted progression or recurrence, suggesting that patients treated with laser vaporization should be followed closely after treatment.

Topical Chemotherapy

Woodruff et al. first reported the use of the topical cytotoxic antimetabolite 5-fluorouracil (5-FU) for the treatment of preinvasive disease of the vagina.[82] They noted successful results in eight of nine treated patients. In 1978 Piver[83] reported on the use of 20% 5-FU, and in 1981 Sillman et al. described the use of 5-FU in chemosurgery.[21] Subsequent reports from several authors indicated cure rates that ranged from 80% to 85%.[84–90]

Most of the reported protocols used 5% 5-FU (1.5–2 g per intravaginal application). The most commonly used regimen consisted of an intravaginal application of 2 g of 5% 5-FU cream for 5 to 7 consecutive nights. A thick application of zinc oxide ointment or petroleum jelly is applied to the introitus and the vulvar skin before insertion of the fluorouracil cream to protect the area from irritation, ulceration, and sloughing. Use of a vaginal tampon does not appear to protect the vulva and may reduce the effectiveness of the fluorouracil. The patient is re-evaluated 12 weeks after initiation of therapy. If the patient still has disease, therapy with 5% 5-FU cream can be repeated once weekly for 10 weeks, or the patient can be treated with laser therapy. Patient compliance is problematic with any 5-FU regimen. Petrilli et al.[26] and Krebs and Helmkamp[26] reported on successive treatments with carbon dioxide laser and topical fluorouracil after a failed first attempt at treatment with fluorouracil.

The side effects of fluorouracil therapy range from minimal to severe. In some cases, the treatments must be discontinued because the side effects are severe. The most common side effects are vaginal burning and dyspareunia.

In a study of long-term sequelae following fluorouracil therapy, Krebs and Helmkamp[91] found that 4 of 25 women developed chemical mucositis 2 to 4 weeks after therapy and 11.4% had acute ulcers. A total of 5.7% of the treated women developed chronic ulcers lasting longer than 6 months (Figure 16-18), and these numbers increased if there was continued prophylactic use of the cream. Most of the patients who developed ulcers were symptomatic, with a serosanguineous or watery discharge and postcoital or irregular bleeding. Only 50% of these ulcers healed without treatment. The development of vaginal adenosis after treatment has also been reported. **Because of the potential adverse events associated with 5-FU therapy, its use should be confined to**

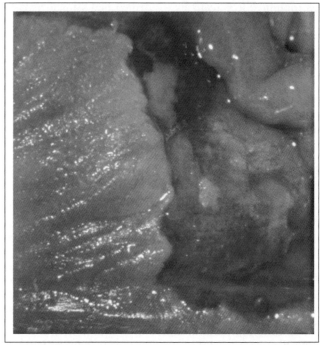

Figure 16-18 An area of denuded epithelium at the vaginal vault. This was noted after the use of intravaginal 5-FU cream and represents a local "burn" of the vaginal mucosa.

treating extensive, widespread, multifocal high-grade VaIN that cannot be treated with other, potentially less morbid modalities.

Other Treatments for Vaginal Intraepithelial Neoplasia

Cryosurgical therapy is not a therapeutic option in the management of VaIN. The imprecise and unpredictable depth of tissue destruction associated with cryosurgery limits its value for a disease process that is frequently multifocal and is most commonly found in the upper vagina, where potential damage to adjacent organs is greater.[92–94]

Isolated descriptions of the use of other topical agents for treatment of VaIN have been reported. A small study of 28 post-hysterectomy patients with various grades of VaIN were treated with 50% trichlooacetic acid (TCA) once a week for 1 to 4 weeks.[95] They had a 71% overall remission rate. All the patients with VaIN 1 resolved, whereas only 53% of those with VaIN 2-3 went into remission. Severity of VaIN was the only significant predictor of persistence/recurrence. The authors suggest that a prospective trial is warranted using different concentrations of TCA.[95]

Local application of imiquimod cream has been studied as an alternative therapy for VaIN 2,3. Imiquimod, an imidazoquinolone amine, is an immune response modifier that stimulates the immune system. Its action mimics the natural response to HPV, resulting in production of cytokines. A small study was conducted on seven women with VaIN 2,3 who had failed other treatments and had multifocal disease.[96] Imiquoid cream 5% was inserted vaginally three times per week for 8 weeks with a mean follow-up period of

18 months. After treatment, 6 women had VaIN 1 or HPV infection. One had persistent VaIN 2 that progressed to VaIN 3. Minor vaginal burning was reported, and no systemic adverse effects were reported. It was possible to successfully apply the cream into the folds of the vagina. Use of imiquimod for treatment of VaIN will have to be assessed in larger trials. The duration of effect is unknown, and the potential for rebound effect that could trigger a flare-up is a concern.

INVASIVE CANCER

The most common invasive cancers of the vagina are metastatic from the endometrium, cervix, or ovary. Squamous cell cancer of the vagina is most often an extension of a squamous cell cancer of the cervix, or it may arise from vulvar cancer or represent secondary invasion from another site. Choriocarcinoma and any intra-abdominal cancer can metastasize to the vagina.

Primary squamous cell cancer of the vagina is rare. Less than 20% of vaginal carcinomas are diagnosed in women younger than 50 years.[97] Peters et al. described six patients with superficial or microinvasive vaginal cancer arising in a field of carcinoma *in situ*, three of whom had no associated cervical lesion.[98] Squamous cell carcinoma is the most common histology type, representing 80% to 92% of all primary vaginal cancers.[97] *The International Federation of Gynecology and Obstetrics (FIGO) criteria state that only cases in which the primary site of growth is in the vagina can be classified as vaginal carcinomas.* A tumor that extends from the vagina to other sites such as the vulva or cervix should not be classified as primary in the vagina.[99] Critics of the FIGO staging for vaginal carcinoma state it is clinical and not surgical staging.

The World Health Organization has published a classification of carcinomas of the vagina[100] (Table 16-3). Squamous cell cancers include keratinizing, nonkeratinizing, verrucous, and warty (condylomatous) types (Figures 16-19 to 16-23). Adenocarcinomas include clear-cell, endometrioid, mucinous, and mesonephric types. Other vaginal cancers include adenosquamous, adenoid cystic, and adenoid basal, as well as carcinoid, small-cell, and undifferentiated types. Woodruff and Parmley described a series of malignant tumors arising in the vagina that are not commonly seen in the lower genital tract.[101] These included sarcoma botryoides, endodermal sinus tumor, malignant melanoma, and tumors of the paravestibular glands—various malignant variants of fibromas and myomas and lymphomas.

Most vaginal cancers are initially asymptomatic but may be associated with vaginal discharge, postcoital staining, or malodor. A high index of suspicion is often required to make an early diagnosis. If colposcopic findings are present, atypical vessels are usually seen.

Vaginal cancer spreads mainly by local and lymphatic invasion. Knowledge of the nodal involvement rates is very limited because most vaginal cancer is treated with primary radiation therapy. Age of the patient, size and site of the lesion, lymph

Table 16-3 Classification of Carcinoma of the Vagina

Squamous cell carcinoma
Keratinizing
Nonkeratinizing
Verrucous
Warty (condylomatous)
Adenocarcinoma
Clear cell
Endometrioid
Mucinous
Endocervical
Intestinal
Mesonephric
Others
Adenosquamous
Adenoid cystic
Adenoid basal
Carcinoid
Small cell
Undifferentiated

Data from Scully RE, Bonfiglio TA, Kurman RJ. Vulva. In: Scully RE (ed). Histological Typing of Female Genital Tract Tumors, ed 2. Berlin: Springer-Verlag, 1994, p 9.

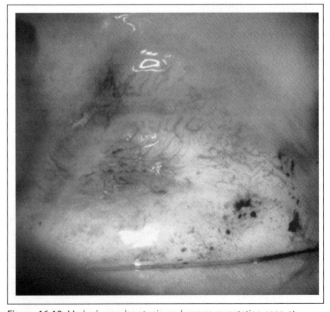

Figure 16-19 Marked vascular atypia and coarse punctation seen at colposcopy. Biopsy revealed early squamous cell carcinoma of the vagina.

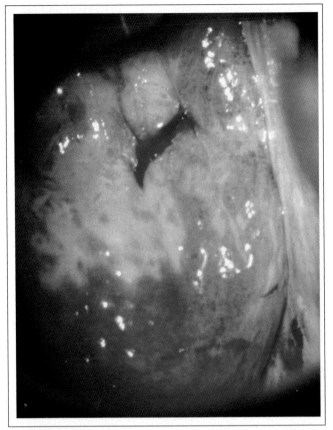

Figure 16-20 Diffuse acetowhitening, mild vascular atypias, and a central ulcer of the vaginal vault. Biopsy reported as early invasive squamous cell carcinoma of the vagina.

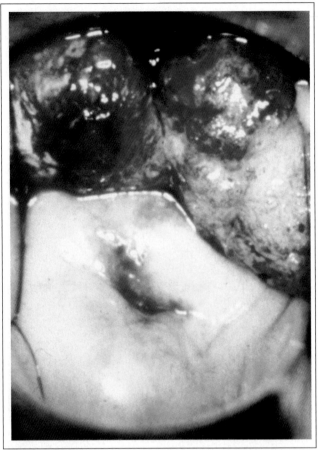

Figure 16-22 Large, bulky mass in the upper vagina with marked atypical vessels in an area of acetowhite in the left anterior vagina. Biopsy reported invasive squamous cell carcinoma.

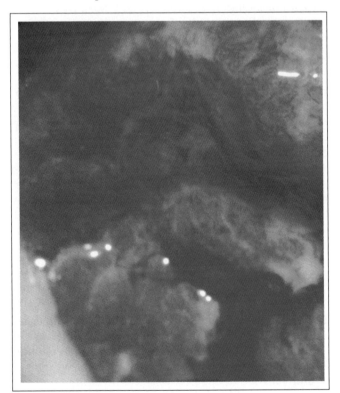

Figure 16-21 Raised, irregular friable area at the vaginal apex. Biopsy revealed invasive squamous cell carcinoma of the vagina.

node status, FIGO stage, and treatment are prognostic factors, with age and size of tumor being the most important.[99] Disease limited to one third of the vagina is associated with better survival.[102] Reported overall 5-year survival rates are 61% (100% for stage 0, 82% for stage 1, 70% for stage 2, 0% for stage 3, and 14% for stage 4). Patients with stage 1 or 2 had a significantly better survival than those with stage 3 or 4 disease (p < 0.05).[103] Numbers in this particular observational study were low (n = 51).

Because of the rarity of primary vaginal cancer, there is no accepted standard treatment. Evidence-based outcome data are lacking. Treatment usually consists of surgery, radiotherapy, or a combination of both.[99] There are little data on conservative surgical therapy that preserves sexual and reproductive function in young women, and larger studies need to validate the safety of conservative therapy.[104] It is assumed that surgical therapy will compromise vaginal function.

All relapses in stages 0 to 2 were related to local failure, suggesting that intensive local therapy followed by radiotherapy may be the most effective treatment. Treatment failure in stages 3 and 4 was because of persistent local disease or new distant metastasis. Conventional radiotherapy may not be effective

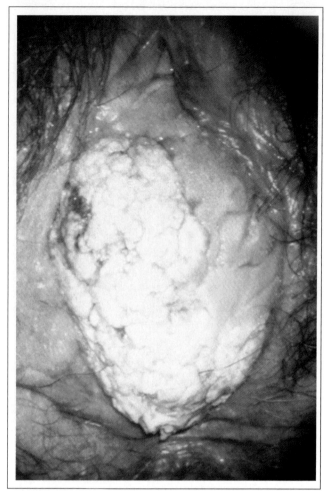

Figure 16-23 Vaginal vault prolapse after prior hysterectomy revealing a thick hyperkeratotic area over the right two thirds of the prolapsed vaginal epithelium. Biopsy revealed invasive squamous cell carcinoma.

as the primary treatment for advanced disease. However, radiotherapy preserves some vaginal function. At least part, if not all, of the vagina will be excised at the time of surgery. For patients with stage 1 and selected stage 2 (minimal extension outside the vaginal wall) vaginal cancer, local tumor control can be achieved with initial surgery followed by selective radiotherapy. For advanced stage 2,3, or 4 vaginal cancer, a combination of brachytherapy and external radiotherapy is the treatment of choice.[99] Treatment failure is a significant concern.

MANAGEMENT SCENARIOS

Scenario 1

Sentinel Pap: ASC-US or low-grade squamous intraepithelial lesion (LSIL)
Colposcopic findings or histologic cell type if a biopsy was done: No squamous intraepithelial lesion (SIL) found on the

cervix, or the patient has had a hysterectomy and no cervix is present. Vaginal biopsy reveals VaIN 1
HPV testing for high-risk (oncogenic) HPV types: Positive if the Pap was ASC-US; not applicable (N/A) if the Pap was LSIL
Satisfactory colposcopy: Either Yes or No
Fertility desires: N/A

This is a patient with VaIN 1. VaIN 1 is a productive viral infection of the vagina (a vaginal wart) that has virtually no premalignant potential. The presence or absence of CIN 1 is not relevant because 2006 guidelines do not call for treatment of women with ASC-US or LSIL cytology or those with CIN 1 in the absence of high-grade CIN regardless of whether the colposcopy is satisfactory or not. Appropriate management of this condition includes observation or, if the condition is extensive or persistent, it may be treated with topical TCA or laser surgery. In women with a compromised immune system, any form of treatment that does not improve immune function is doomed to failure and not warranted. Follow-up should be with cytology and colposcopy to exclude the possibility of occult high grade disease on either the cervix or the vagina.

Scenario 2

Sentinel Pap: ASC-US or LSIL
Colposcopic findings or histologic cell type if a biopsy was done: White epithelium noted on the cervix that extends 3 cm onto the anterior vaginal reflection. Biopsy revealed CIN 3 and VaIN 3
HPV testing for high-risk (oncogenic) HPV types: N/A
Satisfactory colposcopy: Either Yes or No
Fertility desires: Desires future fertility

Although treatment of this woman's cervical and vaginal disease should be done at the same time, the treatment decisions should not affect one another. If the colposcopy is satisfactory, her cervix should be treated with excision or ablation of the transformation zone, and if the colposcopy is unsatisfactory, it should be treated with excision of the transformation zone. Vaginal disease should be treated by surgical or electrosurgical excision or laser ablation of the lesion. Care must be taken to avoid an en block removal of the cervical and vaginal lesions because, at best, this would remove too much cervical and vaginal tissue, and at worst it risks damage to the ureter and other paravaginal structures.

Scenario 3

Sentinel Pap: ASC-US or LSIL
Colposcopic findings or histologic cell type if a biopsy was done: The cervix is flush with the vaginal vault. White epithelium is noted on the cervix, extending 3 cm onto the anterior vaginal reflection. Biopsy revealed CIN 3 and VaIN 3
HPV testing for high-risk (oncogenic) HPV types: N/A
Satisfactory colposcopy: Either Yes or No

Fertility desires: The patient has fibroid-related dysmenorrhea and desires hysterectomy rather than local treatment

If it is feasble to treat the cervix, preferable management of this patient should be identical to Scenario 2. However, if the clinical situation precludes local treatment, use of a simple hysterectomy for treatment of CIN is acceptable. In this case, due to the close proximity of the vagina to the cervix, along with her symptomatic fibroids, a vaginal hysterectomy was considered appropriate. The important point is that if a colposcopy had not been done prior to the hysterectomy, the VaIN 3 would have been missed and might have been imbedded in the dog ears. This can lead to undetected progression of VaIN 3 to invasive cancer.

Scenario 4

Sentinel Pap: High-grade squamous intraepithelial lesion (HSIL)
Colposcopic findings or histologic cell type if a biopsy was done: Normal cervical exam, but there was a 2-cm area of iodine negative epithelium in the upper one third of the vagina that was VaIN 3 on biopsy
HPV testing for high-risk (oncogenic) HPV types: N/A
Satisfactory colposcopy: Either Yes or No
Fertility desires: She is 40 and wants to maintain fertility

HPV testing is not indicated in this scenario because the presence of a HSIL smear warrants colposcopic assessment regardless of HPV status. This scenario also demonstrates the importance of doing a thorough vaginal assessment when faced with abnormal cytology and normal cervical colposcopy. Vaginal lesional cells can shed and be detected on a cervical smear. Vaginal and cervical squamous cells are morphologically identical, so it is prudent for the colposcopist to evaluate the vagina when there is no cervical lesion. Because VaIN 3 is a cancer precursor, treatment is warranted by local ablation or excision. Hysterectomy is not appropriate in a woman desirous of future fertility regardless of her age.

Scenario 5

Sentinel Pap: Any
Colposcopic findings or histologic cell type if a biopsy was done: White epithelium is noted in the middle of the anterior vaginal wall. Biopsy reveals VaIN 3
HPV testing for high-risk (oncogenic) HPV types: N/A
Satisfactory colposcopy: Either Yes or No
Fertility desires: The patient has fibroid-related dysmenorrhea and desires hysterectomy rather than local treatment

The unique feature of this scenario is the location of the vaginal lesion. Even if the patient is to be treated with a hysterectomy, it would not be appropriate to treat the cervix and vagina in one block because this would result in excision of too large a portion of the vagina. Therefore the cervix and vagina should be treated separately, and the decision to perform a hysterectomy should not reflect on the treatment modality used for treatment of the vagina.

Scemario 6

Sentinel Pap: Any
Colposcopic findings or histologic cell type if biopsy was done: History of a hysterectomy for CIN 3, 10 years previously. A friable lesion was noted at the cuff, and biopsy revealed invasive squamous cell cancer
HPV testing for high-risk HPV types: N/A
Fertility desires: N/A

Once invasive cancer is confirmed, treatment should be planned in consultation with a gynecologic oncologist, a radiation oncologist, or both. The patient should undergo a combination of one or more of a radical vaginectomy, radical radiation therapy or chemoradiation as recommended by the consulting specialists.

COUNSELING SCENARIOS

Scenario 1

In women with VaIN 1, there is often a fear or concern about the premalignant potential of the lesion, which prompts overly aggressive therapy. Women with VaIN 1 should be reassured that their lesion has minimal premalignant potential. In fact, although no consensus management guidelines exist for VaIN, conclusions may be drawn from the consensus guidelines for CIN 1. The 2006 Consensus Guidelines for CIN 1 indicated that no consideration should be given to treating CIN 1 unless it has been persistent for at least 2 years. After 2 years, follow-up without treatment is still preferred but treatment is acceptable. With VaIN 1, the risk of progression to invasive cancer is even smaller than would be expected with CIN 1, so the management guidelines should be even more conservative. Both the patient and healthcare provider should take comfort from that natural history, and the woman should be reassured that there is no need to treat her aggressively for a benign viral infection. Treatment in the office with TCA may help speed resolution of these lesions, but aggressive treatment using surgery or laser treatment under general anesthesia is usually not necessary.

Counseling Scenario 2

A 40-year-old woman has an HSIL smear and no cervical lesion is noted on colposcopic biopsy, but she does have an extensive VaIN 3 lesion of the upper one third of her vagina. She is concerned about the need for a hysterectomy. This woman can be informed that in most cases the VaIN 3 can be effectively treated either by local excision or by CO_2 laser-directed vaginectomy with preservation of vaginal tube integrity. In fact, the use of hysterectomy to treat this lesion is likely to result in shortening of the vaginal tube and may cause subsequent coital difficulty. Depending on the location and extent of the vaginal lesion, it may be advisable to treat the lesion first and make the decision for hysterectomy independently of the diagnosis of VaIN.

REFERENCES

1. Platzer W, Poisel S, Hafez ESE. Functional anatomy of the human vagina. In: Hafez ESE, Evans TN (eds). The Human Vagina. London: Elsevier, 1978, pp 41–53.
2. Davis GD. Colposcopic examination of the vagina. Obstet Gynecol Clin North Am 1993;20:217–229.
3. Coppleson M, Pixley E, Reid B. The vagina. In: Coppleson MC, Pixley E (eds). Colposcopy, ed 3. New York: Charles C Thomas, 1985, pp 403–434.
4. National Cancer Institute. Surveillance, epidemiology and End Results (SEER) Program. SEER Stat Database: Cancer Statistics Branch, released April 2005. Available at www.seer.cancer.gov; accessed March 2007.
5. Jemal A, Murray T, Ward E, et al. Cancer statistics, 2005. CA Cancer J Clin 2005;55:10–30.
6. Beller U, Maisonnueve P, Benedet JL, et al. Carcinoma of the vagina. Int J Gynaecol Obstet 2003;83(Suppl 1):27–39.
7. Brinton LA, Nasca PC, Mallin K, et al. Case-control study of in situ and invasive carcinoma of the vagina. Gynecol Oncol 1990;38:49–54.
8. Daling JR, Madeleine MM, Schwartz SM, et al. A population-based study of squamous cell vaginal cancer: HPV and cofactors. Gynecol Oncol 2002;84:263–270.
9. Feng Q, Kiviat NB. New and surprising insights into pathogenesis of multicentric squamous cancers in the female lower genital tract. J Natl Cancer Inst 2005;97:1798–1799.
10. Vinokurova S, Wentzensen N, Einenkel J, et al. Clonal history of papillomavirus-induced dysplasia in the female lower genital tract. J Natl Cancer Inst 2005;97:1816–1821.
11. Magnusson PKE, Sparen P, Gyllensten UB. Genetic link to cervical tumors. Nature 1999;400:29–30.
12. Lopes A, Monaghan JM, Roberston G. Vaginal intraepithelial neoplasia. In: Luesley D, Jordan J, Richart RM (eds). Intraepithelial Neoplasia of the Lower Genital Tract. Edinburgh: Churchill Livingstone, 1995, pp 169–176.
13. Sillman FH, Fruchter RG, Chen YS, et al. Vaginal intraepithelial neoplasia: risk factors for persistence, recurrence and invasion and its management. Am J Obstet Gynecol 1997;176:93–99.
14. Dodge JA, Eltabbakh GH, Mount SL, et al. Clinical features and risk of recurrence among patients with vaginal intraepithelial neoplasia. Gynecol Oncol 2001;83:363–369.
15. Benedet JL, Sanders BH. Carcinoma in situ of the vagina. Am J Obstet Gynecol 1984;148:695–700.
16. Audet-Lapointe P, Body G, Vauclair R, et al. Vaginal intraepithelial neoplasia. Gynec Oncol 1990;36:232–239.
17. Schneider A, de Villiers EM, Schneider V. Multifocal squamous neoplasia of the female genital tract: significance of human papillomavirus infection of the vagina after hysterectomy. Obstet Gynecol 1987;70:294–298.
18. Aho M, Vesterinen E, Meyer B, et al. Natural history of vaginal intraepithelial neoplasia. Cancer 1991;68:195–197.
19. Mao CC, Chao KC, Lian YC, et al. Vaginal intraepithelial neoplasia: diagnosis and management. Chin Med J (Taipei) 1990;46:35–42.
20. Lenehan PM, Meffe F, Lickrish GM. Vaginal intraepithelial neoplasia: biologic aspects and management. Obstet Gynecol 1986;68:333–337.
21. Sillman FH, Sedlis A, Boyce JG. A review of lower genital intraepithelial neoplasia and the use of topical 5-fluorouracil. Obstet Gynecol Surv 1985;40:190–220.
22. Benedet JL, Sanders BH. Carcinoma in situ of the vagina. Am J Obstet Gynecol 1984;148:695–700.
23. Kanbour AI, Klionsky B, Murphy AI. Carcinoma of the vagina following cervical cancer. Cancer 1974;34:1838–1841.
24. Gemmell J, Holmes DM, Duncan ID. How frequently need vaginal smears be taken after hysterectomy for cervical intraepithelial neoplasia? Br J Obstet Gynecol 1990;97:58–61.
25. Jenkins D. The pathology of lower genital tract premalignancy. Clinical Practice of Gynecology 1990;2:51–85.
26. Petrilli ES, Townsend DE, Morrow CP, et al. Vaginal intraepithelial neoplasia: biologic aspects and treatment with topical 5-fluorouracil and the carbon dioxide laser. Am J Obstet Gynecol 1980;138:321–328.
27. Sirovich BE, Welch HG. Cervical cancer screening among women without a cervix. J Am Med Assoc 2004;291:2990–2993.
28. Nwabineli NJ, Monaghan JM. Vaginal epithelial abnormalities in patients with CIN: clinical and pathological features and management. Brit J Obstet Gynecol 1991;98:25–29.
29. Davila RM, Miranda MC. Vaginal intraepithelial neoplasia and the Pap smear. Acta Cytol 2000;44:137–140.
30. Cooper AL, Dornfeld-Finke JM, Banks HW, et al. Is cytologic screening an effective surveillance method for detection of vaginal recurrence of uterine cancer? Obstet Gynecol 2006;107:71–76.
31. Pearce KF, Haefner HK, Sarwar SF, et al. Cytopathological findings on vaginal Papanicolaou smears after hysterectomy for benign gynecologic disease. N Engl J Med 1996;335:1559–1562.
32. Farghaly H, Bourgeois D, Houser P, et al. Routine vaginal Pap test is not useful in women status-posthysterectomy for benign disease. Diagn Cytopathol 2006;34:640–643.
33. American College of Obstetricians and Gynecologists. ACOG Practice Bulletin, No.45. Cervical cytology screening. Obstet Gynecol 2003;102:417–427.
34. Fetters MD, Fischer G, Reed BD. Effectiveness of vaginal Papanicolaou smear screening after total hysterectomy for benign disease. J Am Med Assoc 1996;275:940–947.
35. Noller KL. Screening for vaginal cancer. N Engl J Med 1996;335:1599–1600.
36. www.ahcpr.gov/clinic/uspstf/uspscerv.htm. Accessed February 2008.
37. American Cancer Society. www.cancer.org. Accessed 2007.
38. Kalogirou D, Antoniou G, Karakitsos P, et al. Vaginal intraepithelial neoplasia (VaIN) following hysterectomy in patients treated for carcinoma in situ of the cervix. Eur J Gynaecol Oncol 1997;18:188–191.
39. Ponder TB, Easley KO, Davila RM. Glandular cells in vaginal smears from posthysterectomy patients. Acta Cytol 1997;41:1701–1704.
40. Ramirez PE, Valente PT. Paradoxical glandular cells in vaginal cuff cytology: metaplasia versus neoplasia. Acta Cytol 1995;39:1980.
41. Julian TM, O'Connell BJ, Gosewehr JA. Indications, techniques, and advantages of partial laser vaginectomy. Obstet Gynecol 1992;80:140–143.
42. Rhodes-Morris HE. Treatment of vulvar intraepithelial neoplasia and vaginal intraepithelial neoplasia. Clin Consult Obstet Gynecol 1994;6:44–53.
43. Ferenczy A, Wright TC. Anatomy and histology of the cervix. In: Kurman RJ (ed). Blaustein's Pathology of the Female Genital Tract, ed 4. New York: Springer-Verlag, 1994, p 185.
44. Townsend DE. Intraepithelial neoplasia of the vagina. In: Coppleson M (ed). Gynecologic Oncology. Edinburgh: Churchill Livingstone, 1992, pp 493–499.

45. Sherman ME, Paull G. Reproducibility of pathologic diagnosis and correlation of smears and biopsies. Acta Cytol 1993;37:699–704.

46. Cheng D, Ng TY, Ngan HY, et al. Wide local excision (WLE) for vaginal intraepithelial neoplasia (VaIN). Acta Obstet Gynecol Scand 1999;78:648–652.

47. Patsner B. Treatment of vaginal dysplasia with loop excision: report of five cases. Am J Obstet Gynecol 1993;169:179–180.

48. Fannning J, Manahan KJ, McLean SA. Loop electrosurgical excision procedure for partial upper vaginectomy. Am J Obstet Gynecol 1999;181:1382–1385.

49. Powell JL, Asberry DS. Treatment of vaginal dysplasia: Just a simple loop electrosurgical excision procedure? Am J Obstet Gynecol 2000;182:731–732.

50. Wharton JT, Tortolero-Luna G, Linares AC, et al. Vaginal intraepithelial neoplasia and vaginal cancer. Obstet Gynecol Clin North Am 1996;23:325–345.

51. Hoffman MS, De Cesare SL, Roberts WS, et al. Upper vaginectomy for in situ and occult, superficially invasive carcinoma of the vagina. Am J Obstet Gynecol 1992;166:30–33.

52. Indermaur MD, Martino MA, Fiorica JV, et al. Upper vaginectomy for the treatment of vaginal intraepithial neoplasia. Am J Obstet Gynecol 2005;193:577–581.

53. DeBuben I. Radium in the treatment of cancer of the vagina. Surg Gynecol Obstet 1931;52:844–886.

54. Brown GR, Fletcher GH, Rutledge FN. Irradiation of "in-situ" and invasive squamous cell carcinomas of the vagina. Cancer 1971;28:1278–1283.

55. Usherwood MM. Management of vaginal carcinoma after hysterectomy. Am J Obstet Gynecol 1975;122:352–354.

56. Woodman CB, Mould JJ, Jordan JA. Radiotherapy in the management of vaginal intraepithelial neoplasia after hysterectomy. Br J Obstet Gynecol 1988;95:976–979.

57. Oliver JA Jr. Severe dysplasia and carcinoma in situ of the vagina. Am J Obstet Gynecol 1979;134:133–137.

58. Stock RG, Mychalczak B, Armstrong JG, et al. The importance of brachytherapy technique in the management of primary carcinoma of the vagina. J Radiat Oncol Biol Phys 1992;24:747–753.

59. MacLeod C, Fowler A, Dalrymple C, et al. High-dose-rate brachytherapy in the management of high-grade intraepithelial neoplasia of the vagina. Gynec Oncol 1997;65:74–77.

60. Ogino I. High-dose-rate intracavitary brachytherapy in the management of cervical and vaginal intraepithelial neoplasia. Int J Radiat Oncol Biol Phys 1998;40:881–887.

61. Barrie JR, Brunschwig A. Late second cancers after apparent successful initial radiation therapy. Am J Roentgenol Ther Nucl Med 1970;108:109–112.

62. Boice JD Jr, Day NE, Andersen A. Second cancers following treatment for cervical cancer. J Natl Cancer Inst 1985;74:955–975.

63. Stafl A, Wilkinson EJ, Mattingly RF. Laser treatment of cervical and vaginal intraepithelial neoplasia. Am J Obstet Gynecol 1977;128:128–136.

64. Capen CV, Masterson BJ, Magrina JF, et al. Laser therapy of vaginal intraepithelial neoplasia. Am J Obstet Gynecol 1982;142:973–976.

65. Townsend DE, Levine RU, Crum CP, et al. Treatment of vaginal carcinoma in situ with the carbon dioxide laser. Am J Obstet Gynecol 1982;143:565–568.

66. Jobson VW, Homesley HD: Treatment of vaginal intraepithelial neoplasia with the carbon dioxide laser. Obstet Gynecol 1983;62:90–93.

67. Stein S. Carbon dioxide laser surgery of the cervix, vagina and vulva. Surg Clin North Am 1984;885–897.

68. Woodman CB, Jordan JA, Wade-Evans T. The management of VaIN after hysterectomy. Br J Obstet Gynecol 1984;91:707–711.

69. Curtin JP, Twiggs LB, Julian TM. Treatment of vaginal intraepithelial neoplasia with the carbon dioxide laser. J Reprod Med 1985;30:942–944.

70. Stuart GC, Flagler EA, Nation JG, et al. Laser vaporization of vaginal intraepithelial neoplasia. Am J Obstet Gynecol 1988;158:240–243.

71. Sherman AI. Laser therapy for vaginal intraepithelial neoplasia after hysterectomy. J Reprod Med 1990;35:941–944.

72. Jobson VW, Campion MJ. Vaginal laser surgery. Obstet Gynecol Clin North Am 1991;18:511–524.

73. Hoffman MS, DeCesare SL. Laser vaporization of grade 3 vaginal intraepithelial neoplasia. Am J Obstet Gynecol 1991;165:1342–1344.

74. Volante R, Pasero L, Saraceno L, et al. Carbon dioxide laser surgery in colposcopy for cervicovaginal intraepithelial neoplasia treatment. Ten years experience and failure analysis. Eur J Gynaecol Oncol 1992;13(1 Suppl):78–81.

75. Diakomanolis E, Rodolakis A, Sakellaropoulos G, et al. Conservative management of vaginal intraepithelial neoplasia (VaIN) by carbon dioxide laser. Eur J Gynaecol Oncol 1996;17:389–392.

76. Benedet JL, Wilson PS, Matisic JP. Epidermal thickness measurements in VaIN. A basis for optimal CO_2 laser vaporization. J Reprod Med 1992;37:809–812.

77. Spitzer M, Krumholz BA, Seltzer VL. Fevers in patients undergoing vaginal laser surgery. Obstet Gynecol 1988;71:480–481.

78. Sedlacek TV, Riva JM, Magen AB, et al. Vaginal and vulvar adenosis. An unsuspected side effect of carbon dioxide laser vaporization. J Reprod Med 1990;35:995–1001.

79. Campagnutta E, Parin A, DePiero G, et al. Treatment of vaginal intraepithelial neoplasia with the carbon dioxide laser. Clin Exp Obstet Gynecol 1999;26:127–130.

80. Yalcin OT, Rutherford TJ, Chambers SK, et al. Vaginal intraepithelial neoplasia; treatment by carbon dioxide laser and risk factors for failure. Eur J Obstet Gynecol 2003;106:64–68.

81. Diakomanolis E, Rodalakis A, Boulgaris Z, et al. Treatment of vaginal intraepithelial neoplasia with laser ablation and uupper vaginectomy. Gynecol Obstet Invest 2002;54:17–20.

82. Woodruff JD, Parmley TH, Julian CG. Topical 5-fluorouracil in the treatment of vaginal CIS. Gynec Oncol 1975;3:124–132.

83. Piver MS, Barlow JJ, Tsukada Y, et al. Postirradiation squamous cell carcinoma in situ of the vagina: treatment by topical 20 percent 5-fluorouracil cream. Am J Obstet Gynecol 1979;135:377–380.

84. Ballon SC, Roberts JA, Lagasse LD. Topical 5-fluorouracil in the treatment of intraepithelial neoplasia of the vagina. Obstet Gynecol 1979;54:163–166.

85. Stokes JM, Sworn MJ, Hawthorne JH. A new regimen for the treatment of vaginal carcinoma in situ using 5-fluorouracil. Br J Obstet Gynecol 1980;87:920–921.

86. Bowen-Simpkins P, Hull MG. Intraepithelial vaginal neoplasia following immunosuppressive therapy treated with topical 5-FU. Obstet Gynecol 1975;43:360–362.

87. Daly JW, Ellis GF. Treatment of vaginal dysplasia and carcinoma in situ with topical 5-fluorouracil. Obstet Gynecol 1980;55:350–352.

88. Pride GL, Chuprevich TW. Topical 5-fluorouracil treatment of transformation zone intraepithelial neoplasia of cervix and vagina. Obstet Gynecol 1982;60:467–472.

89. Caglar H, Hertzog RW, Hreshchyshyn MM. Topical 5-fluorouracil treatment of vaginal intraepithelial neoplasia. Obstet Gynecol 1981;58:580–583.

90. Krebs HB. Treatment of VaIN with laser and topical 5-flourouracil. Obstet Gynecol 1989;73:657–660.

91. Krebs HB, Helmkamp F. Chronic ulceration following topical therapy with 5-fluorouracil for vaginal human papillomavirus-associated lesions. Obstet Gynecol 1991;78:205–208.

92. Adducci J. Carcinoma in situ of the vagina. Treatment by combined excision and cryosurgery. Geriatrics 1972;121–123.

93. Jobson VW. Cryotherapy and laser treatment for intraepithelial neoplasia of the cervix, vagina and vulva. Oncology 1991;5:69–72, 77; discussion, 79–81, 84.

94. Kirwan PH, Smith IR, Naftalin NJ. A study of cryosurgery and the carbon dioxide laser in treatment of CIS of the uterine cervix. Gynecol Oncol 1985;22:195–200.

95. Lin H, Huang EY, Chang HY, et al. Therapeutic effect of topical applications of trichloroacetic acid for vaginal intraepithelial neoplasis after hysterectomy. Jpn J Clin Oncol 2005;35:651–654.

96. Haidopoulos D, Diakomanolis E, Rodolakis Z, et al. Can local application of imiquimod cream be an alternative mode of therapy for patients with high-grade intraepithelial lesions of the vagina? Int J Gynecol Cancer 2005;15:898–902.

97. Hellman K, Silfversward C, Nilsson B, et al. Primary carcinoma of the vagina: factors influencing the age at diagnosis. The Radiumhemmet series 1956–1996. Int J Gynecol Cancer 2004;14:491–501.

98. Peters WA 3rd, Kumar NB, Morley GW. Microinvasive carcinoma of the vagina: a distinct clinical entity? Am J Obstet Gynecol 1985;153:505–507.

99. Tjalma WAA, Monaghan JM, Lopes AB, et al. The role of surgery in invasive squamous carcinoma of the vagina. Gynecol Oncol 2001;81:360–365.

100. Scully RE, Bonfiglio TA, Kurman RJ. Vulva. In: Scully RE (ed). Histological Typing of Female Genital Tract Tumors, ed 2. Berlin: Springer-Verlag, 1994, p 9.

101. Woodruff JFD, Parmley TH. Vaginal tumors, benign and malignant. In: Hafez ESE, Evans TN (eds). The Human Vagina. Amsterdam: North-Holland, 1978, pp 371–381.

102. Stock RG, Chen AS, Seski J. A 30-year experience in the management of primary carcinoma of the vagina: analysis of prognostic factors and treatment modalities. Gynecol Oncol 1995;56:45–52.

103. Tabata T, Takeshima N, Nishida H, et al. Treatment failure in vaginal cancer. Gynecol Oncol 2002;84:309–314.

104. Cutillo G, Cignini P, Gianbeppi G, et al. Conservative treatment of reproductive and sexual function in young women with squamous carcinoma of the vagina. Gynecol Oncol 2006;103:234–237.

CASE STUDY 1 QUESTIONS

A 48-year-old woman with a history of a simple hysterectomy for microinvasive cervical cancer presents for evaluation of HSIL cytology of the vaginal cuff.

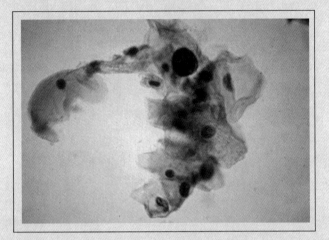

a. This is her cytology. What do you see?

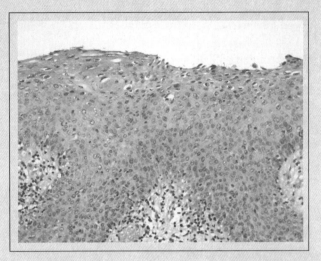

c. This is the histology from the biopsy. What is your diagnosis?

d. Based upon this diagnosis, what treatment is warranted?

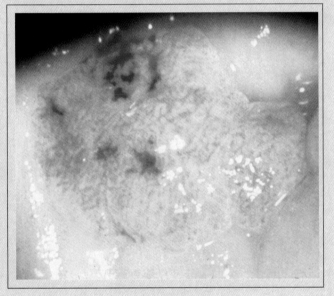

b. This is her vaginal cuff after the application of 5% acetic acid. What do you see?

CASE STUDY 1 ANSWERS

a. The vaginal cytology shows nuclear enlargement and hyperchromasia, consistent with HSIL of the vagina.

b. Raised papillary area of dense white epithelium of the vaginal vault 6 months after hysterectomy. This area also shows mosaic and punctation. Biopsy reported as VaIN 3.

c. Histology revealed VaIN 3 with full thickness nuclear atypia.

d. Although treatment with laser ablation or excision is an option, due to the concerning nature of the colposcopic finding, she will be treated with a partial vaginectomy to ensure there is no hidden focus of invasive disease.

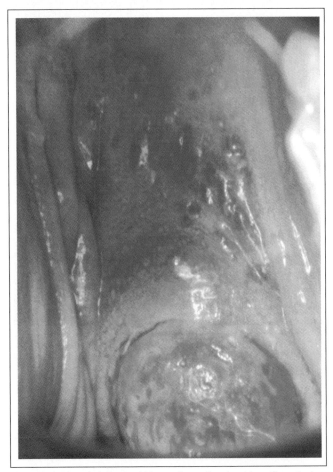

Plate 16-1 Cervical deformity (ridge and pseudopolypoid configuration) with extensive vaginal transformation zone in a DES-exposed woman.

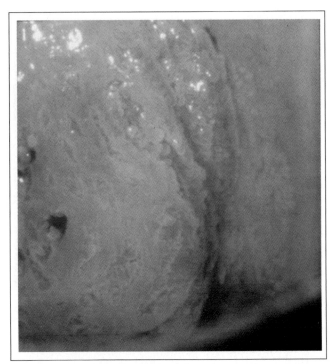

Plate 16-2 Extensive cervicovaginal transformation zone demonstrating crypts, folds, gland openings, and "grape-like" villi.

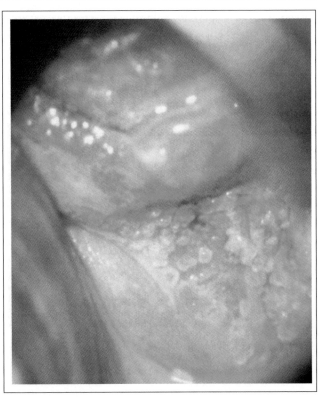

Plate 16-3 Grape-like villi in the posterior vaginal fornix (DES-exposed patient).

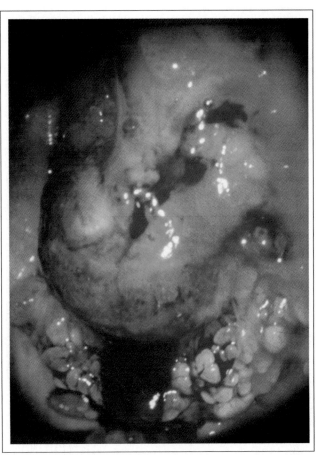

Plate 16-4 Normal cervical transformation zone and exaggerated grape-like villi in the posterior fornix (DES-exposed patient).

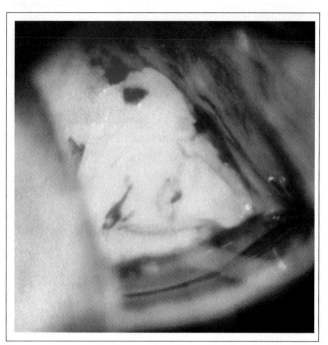

Plate 16-5 One year after hysterectomy, the upper vagina of an 80-year-old woman revealed thick acetowhite and hyperkeratotic areas at the vault of the vagina. Minor vascular atypia was noted. Biopsy was reported as VaIN 3.

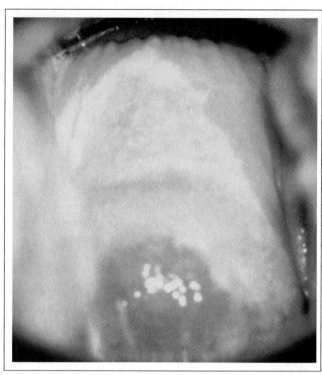

Plate 16-7 Grade 2 acetowhitening of cervix and anterior vaginal fornix reveals a sharp border, slightly raised surface, and irregular mosaic. Biopsies were reported as concurrent CIN 3 and VaIN 3.

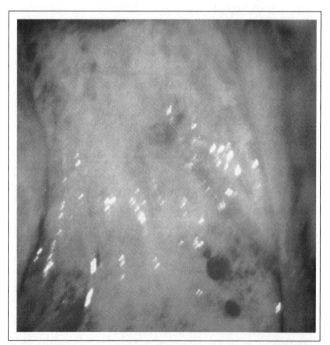

Plate 16-6 Atypical adenosis in the vaginal vault characterized by aceotwhitnening and atypical vessels in a 30-year-old woman who had a radical hysterectomy at age 15 for clear-cell adenocarcinoma of the cervix.

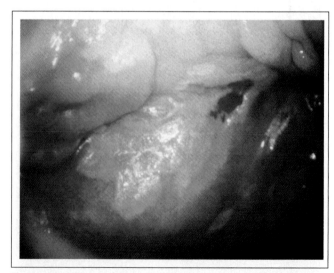

Plate 16-8 Wide area of acetowhite change with well-defined borders at the vaginal vault. There is a small ulcer at the vaginal apex. A few isolated satellite lesions can be seen.

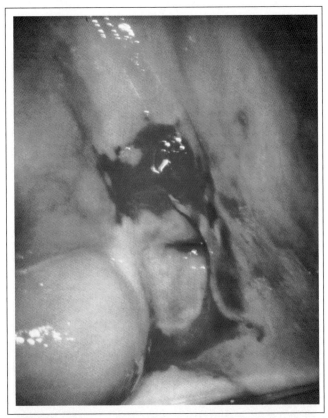

Plate 16-9 Patient previously treated with laser ablation for VaIN 3 returned with HSIL cytology. Colposcopy revealed a focally denuded area mixed with poorly adherent acetowhite epithelium. (See next figure.)

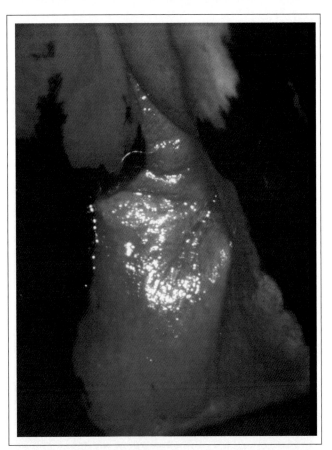

Plate 16-11 Half-strength Lugol's solution may be used to stain normal well-differentiated squamous epithelium so that it can be differentiated from non-staining areas that are abnormal.

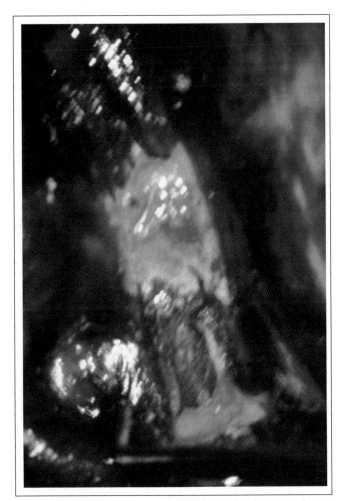

Plate 16-10 Iodine staining with half-strength Lugol's solution reveals non-staining in the denuded areas. Biopsy was reported as VaIN 3.

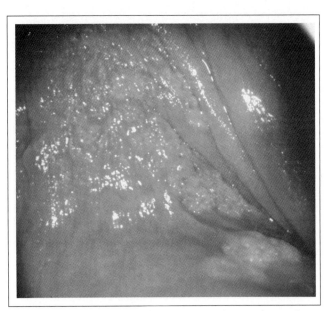

Plate 16-12 The anterior vaginal fornix shows a wide area of acetowhite change with a "warty" surface contour and an isolated "warty" lesion on the anterior portio of the cervix. Biopsies were reported as VaIN 3 and CIN 3.

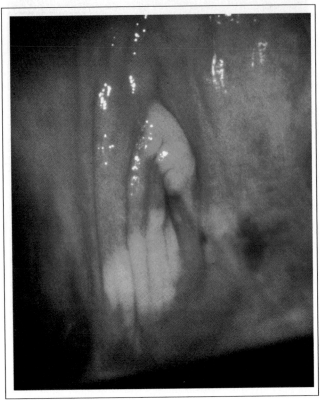

Plate 16-13 Focal high grade acetowhite change at the right upper corner of the vaginal vault near the post-hysterectomy "dog-ear." Biopsy was reported as VaIN 3.

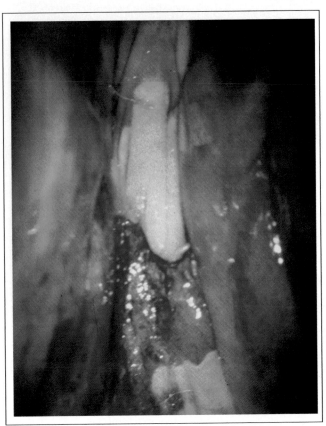

Plate 16-15 The upper vaginal cuff of a 72-year-old woman with a prior hysterectomy noted to have an abnormal Pap smear. Colposcopy revealed two large areas of high grade acetowhite change with peeling edges. Biopsy was reported as VaIN 3.

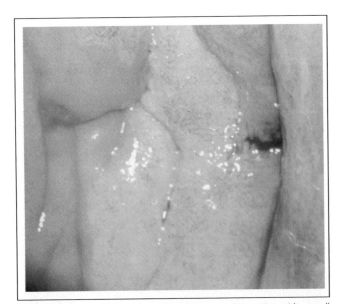

Plate 16-14 The vaginal vault reveals a large acetowhite region with a small focal ulcer. Biopsy was reported as VaIN 3.

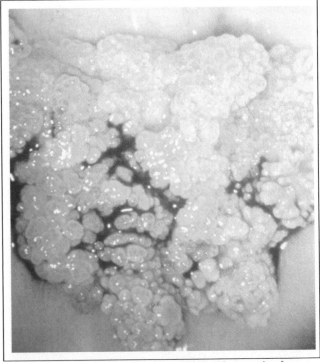

Plate 16-16 Raised papillary area of the vaginal vault 6 months after hysterectomy. Biopsy revealed condyloma acuminata.

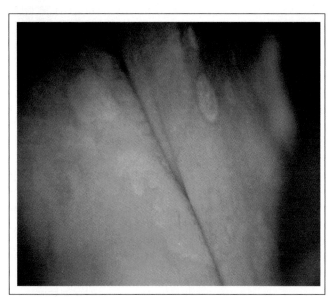

Plate 16-17 Multiple, diffusely arranged, minimally acetowhite areas in the left anterior vaginal fornix. Biopsy was reported as "flat" condyloma.

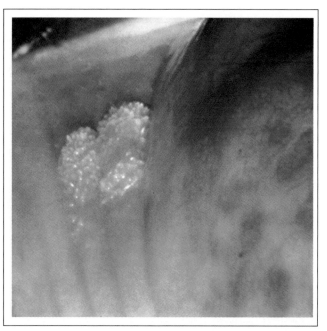

Plate 16-19 Isolated focus of a micropapillary lesion in the right anterior fornix. Biopsy was reported as condyloma acuminata.

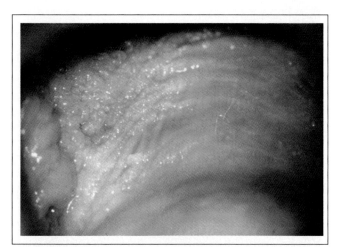

Plate 16-18 Diffuse, raised, irregular areas along the anterior vaginal fornix. The areas are micropapillary and confluent. The biopsy showed condylomata acuminata.

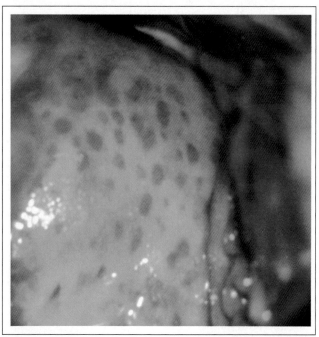

Plate 16-20 Upper vaginal vault, seen with green filter, reveals diffuse pattern of "strawberry" epithelium seen in *T. vaginitis* and other severe vaginal inflammations.

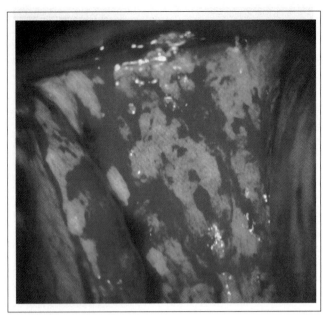

Plate 16-21 Vaginal vault with extensive areas of friable tissue and diffuse areas of atypical vessels. These are seen in the vaginal vault of a 76-year-old woman with vault prolapse and pessary use for several years. Biopsy revealed marked inflammation. Local therapy with topical estrogen cream resulted in a return to normal.

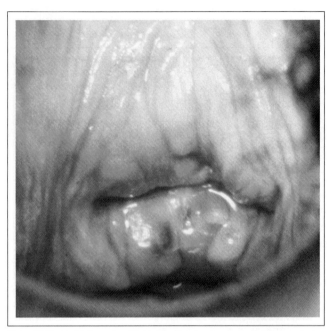

Plate 16-23 Multiple cysts with bluish discoloration noted at the vaginal vault 2 years after hysterectomy for endometriosis. Biopsy revealed endometriosis.

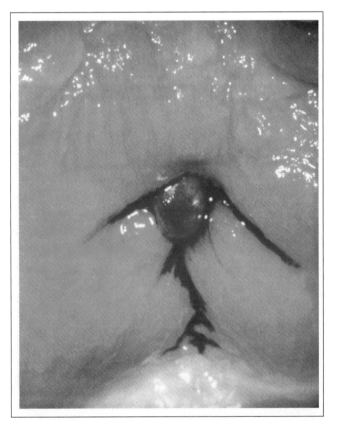

Plate 16-22 A focal red raised area at the upper vagina in a woman 3 months after hysterectomy was an area of granulation tissue.

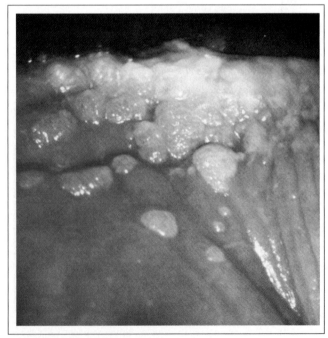

Plate 16-24 Raised vaginal condyloma.

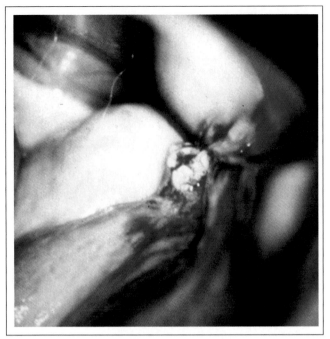

Plate 16-25 A small area of both raised and ulcerated vaginal epithelium. Squamous cell cancer was identified on biopsy.

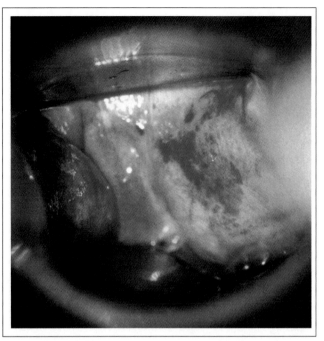

Plate 16-27 The appearance of erosive lichen planus in the vagina is similar to that of marked vaginal atrophy due to estrogen deficiency. This patient is 38 years old and is menstruating, so hypoestrogenic atrophy is unlikely.

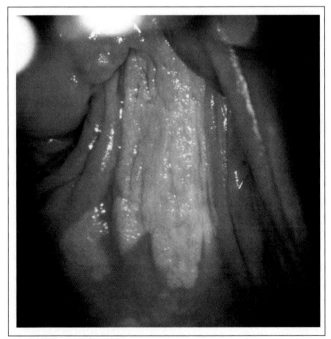

Plate 16-26 An area of flat to slightly raised acetowhite vaginal epithelium. The biopsy showed VaIN l.

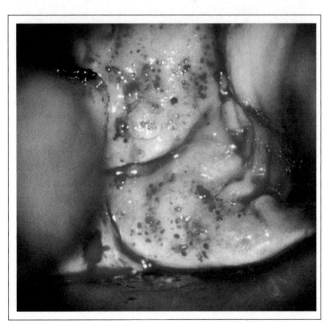

Plate 16-28 This patient was treated with pelvic radiation for a squamous cell cancer. Multiple biopsies of these hemangioma-like lesions showed no recurrence of cancer. The lesions resolved with intensive vaginal estrogen therapy.

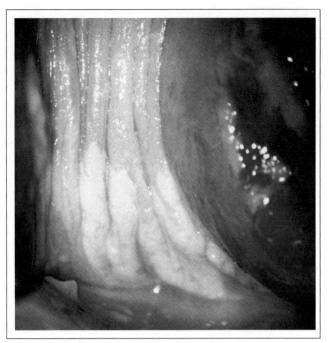

Plate 16-29 Flat, dense acetowhite epithelium. A biopsy showed VaIN 1.

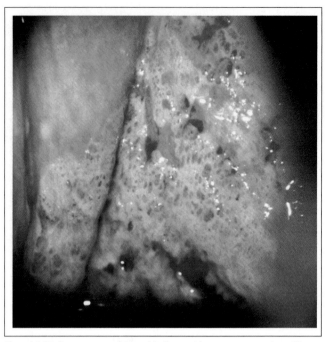

Plate 16-31 Dense acetowhite epithelium with course punctations. Biopsy showed VaIN 3.

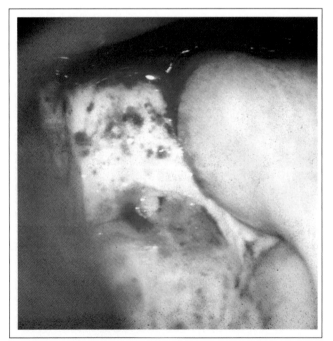

Plate 16-30 Dense acetowhite epithelium with course punctation and ulceration. Biopsy showed VaIN 3, but invasive cancer must be considered, and therefore therapy should be with wide local excision rather than ablation.

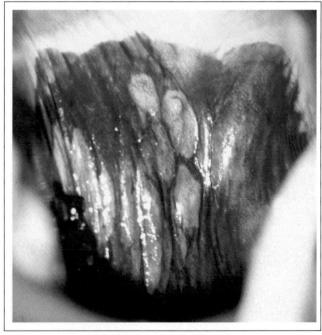

Plate 16-32 Appearance of VaIN after the application of Lugol's iodine. Lugol's-negative patches represent VaIN 1.

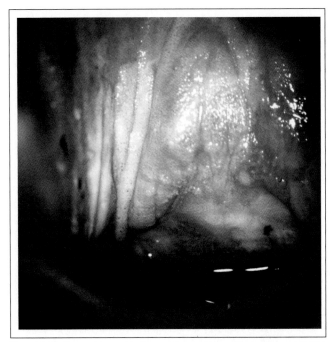

Plate 16-33 Acetowhite epithelium with punctation. Biopsy showed VaIN 1

CHAPTER 17

Non-Neoplastic Epithelial Lesions of the Vulva

Lynette J. Margesson

KEY POINTS

- Hypoestrogenic atrophy results in loss or alteration of epithelial barrier functions, resulting in increased susceptibility to irritation and infection.
- The most frequently misinterpreted vulvar anatomic variations are sebaceous hyperplasia and vulvar papillomatosis.
- *Eczema* and *dermatitis* are synonyms.
- Atopic dermatitis, the most common dermatitis, is a recurrent and very itchy inflammatory dermatosis.
- Lichen simplex chronicus is the end stage of the itch-scratch-itch.
- Vulvar diseases are often caused or worsened by irritant or allergic contact dermatitis. A vulvar complaint, especially any vulvar inflammation that is not responding to treatment, may be from a contact.
- Hygiene practices and lists of all topical products used should be assessed.
- Allergic contact dermatitis results from a frank allergic reaction to small amounts of a chemical.
- Intertrigo is a mechanical inflammatory dermatosis in the skin folds caused by friction, heat, sweating, and occlusion.
- Psoriasis is a common hereditary papulosquamous disease of the skin characterized by well-defined, reddish papules and plaques with adherent, silvery-white scale.
- The etiology of lichen sclerosus is unknown. Various genetic, immunocytologic, autoimmune, hormonal, infectious, and local factors have been suggested. The cause is probably multifactorial and includes genetic and environmental factors.
- On physical examination, lichen sclerosus classically appears as white, atrophic, crinkly papules or plaques. The skin has a shiny, almost cellophane-like sheen. With continued atrophy, there is a gradual effacement and complete disappearance of the clitoris, labia minora, or both.
- The diagnosis of lichen sclerosus is made clinically and confirmed by biopsy.
- Squamous cell carcinoma can develop in 4% to 5% of cases of vulvar lichen sclerosus.
- Topical superpotent steroids are the cornerstone of treatment for lichen sclerosus.
- Lichen planus is a relatively common, inflammatory, lymphocyte-mediated mucocutaneous dermatosis affecting 1% to 2% of the population. The etiology is unknown although evidence suggests it is a disorder of cell-mediated immunity.
- Lichen planus is typically found on the mucous membranes of the mouth or genitalia. In the mouth there are white, lacy, fern-like patterned lesions, but on the vulva usually there are smudgy, white and/or red, often eroded areas.
- The diagnosis of lichen planus is based on the clinical presentation and biopsy. The pathology can be nonspecific. The presence of nonspecific histology must not exclude the diagnosis.

All too commonly, vulvar disorders are missed. They are either not seen or not recognized by medical practitioners. Cursory histories are taken, quick Papanicolaou (Pap) tests are obtained, and the next year's appointment is scheduled. The vulva is hardly seen, and any changes in normal anatomy are missed. Colposcopists have an opportunity to recognize and initiate management of vulvar disease. They are in a unique position to visualize the vulva, magnify areas as needed, and biopsy any questionable lesions.

The examiner must be familiar with variations in the normal vulvar anatomy and with vulvar dermatoses. Women often receive little to no education about their external genitalia. Some practitioners lack education in this area, having had little to no training in skin disease. This chapter will briefly cover the appearance of the normal vulva and the major vulvar dermatoses, with a short review of their management. The focus is on the recognition of these conditions.

NORMAL VULVAR ARCHITECTURE

The vulva is the structure between the thighs bounded laterally by the genitocrural folds, anteriorly by the mons pubis, and posteriorly by the posterior commissure. The main anatomic structures include the mons pubis, labia majora, labia minora, clitoris, vestibule, urethral meatus, hymen, vestibular glands, and Bartholin's glands. *The innermost aspect of the vulva is the vestibule; it encompasses the openings of the urinary tract with the urethral meatus and the vagina with the hymenal ring. It is defined as the part of the vulva that extends from the clitoral frenula, posteriorly to the posterior commissure and laterally to Hart's line, where the nonkeratinized transitional epithelium of the vestibule joins the keratinized squamous epithelium at the base of the medial aspects of the labia minora.* The nonkeratinized squamous epithelium in this area contrasts with the keratinized surface of the labia majora and with skin elsewhere and has greater similarity to the mucous membranes of the oropharynx. This explains the similar changes seen in both areas in conditions such as lichen planus and aphthae. *The lack of a protective keratinized surface in this tissue to act as a barrier explains why it is so easily irritated and infected under certain circumstances, such as incontinence.*

Role of Age and Hormones

The normal appearance of the vulva is variable depending on age and ethnic background. Hormones further modify the size and shape of the labia, hymenal ring, degree of pigmentation, and hair growth. The labia minora vary widely in size, shape, and texture, ranging from small, smooth, and symmetric to asymmetric, long, and notched. There can be considerable variation in the appearance of the hymen, from the normal crescentic appearance to a cribriform or imperforate hymen. *At birth, placental estrogen plumps up the hymen and the vestibule. Through infancy and then childhood, the hymen and the vestibular skin are thinner, leaving the area with a weakened barrier and susceptible to trauma.* In infancy, the labia majora are prominent, the labia minora are small, the vulvar area is hairless, and the hymen is intact. With puberty, hair develops over the labia majora, mons pubis, and perineum, with variable increase in pigmentation of the labia. The labia minora become more prominent, and the vulvar trigone is pink and moist. After menopause, with loss of estrogen, the vulvar vestibule pales, the hair thins and whitens, and the pigmentation fades. The labia majora thin, and the labia minora can exhibit significant atrophy. The clitoris may become more prominent because of the relative increase in androgens. The introitus may be significantly altered, depending on trauma from previous pregnancies and associated weakening of the pelvic floor.[1-4]

Atrophic vulvovaginitis develops with loss of adequate estrogen. Loss of estrogen can result from natural or surgical menopause, antiandrogens, selective estrogen receptor modulators, or ovarian dysfunction. *Relative lack of estrogen also occurs before menarche, during breastfeeding, and postpartum. The result is a thin, relatively dry vulvovaginal epithelium. Epithelial barrier functions are altered, resulting in increased susceptibility to irritation and infection.* Patients may complain of vulvar burning, dysuria, pruritus, tenderness, and dyspareunia. On examination of the vulvar trigone and vagina, the epithelium is pale and thinned and the vaginal folds are smoothed (Figure 17-1). Introital stenosis, petechiae, and fissuring may be present. In severe cases there may be a heavy, malodorous discharge. Treatment involves avoidance of irritants and topical or systemic replacement of estrogen.

Anatomic Variants

The most frequently misinterpreted vulvar anatomic variations are sebaceous hyperplasia and vulvar papillomatosis. The sebaceous glands on the inner aspect of the labia minora in some patients may be very prominent, coalescing into yellow, cobbled plaques (Figure 17-2). They can be confused with neoplasia or rashes. They are harmless glands that cause no symptoms or problems. Reassurance is all that is needed.

Vestibular papillae can develop around the vulvar vestibule in premenopausal women (Figure 17-3). These are tubular to slightly filiform projections that are symmetric,

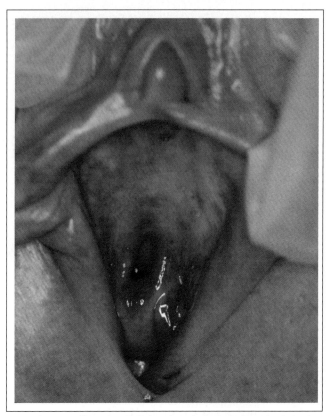

Figure 17-1 Atrophic vulva. Slightly enlarged clitoris with a pale, thin vulvar vestibule related to loss of estrogen.

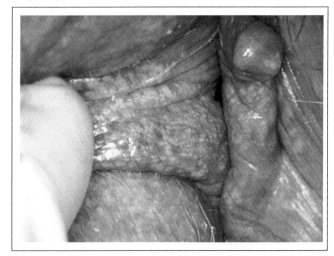

Figure 17-2 On the inner edge of the labia majora are variably sized yellow papules. These are prominent normal sebaceous glands referred to as *sebaceous hyperplasia.*

soft, and completely asymptomatic. They are easily confused with condylomata. Condylomata are firm, often asymmetric, filiform papules that are skin colored to reddish. Colposcopy, palpation, or biopsy will differentiate them. Patient reassurance is all that is needed.

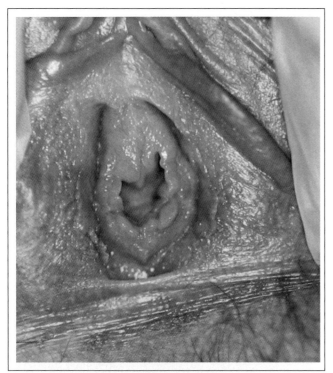

Figure 17-3 Around the hymenal ring on the inner aspect of the vulvar vestibule from 3 to 9 o'clock are skin-colored, filiform, or small tubular papules that are soft and completely asymptomatic.

History and Physical Examination

The clinical evaluation of the patient with vulvar complaints takes time. Many of these patients have chronic symptoms and have had multiple ineffective treatments. It is important to listen patiently to and without judgment of these patients. The history should be accurately documented, noting previous treatments, response to treatment, and so on. The usual menstrual, sexual, and gynecologic history, the use of over-the-counter preparations, and hygiene practices should be noted. *Physically aggressive hygiene practices using "wipes" and washcloths with or without caustic or highly perfumed products may result in marked irritation.*

The most common symptoms of vulvar disease are pruritus and pain, alone or in combination. Pain may be manifested as burning. It is important to further characterize the symptoms by noting menstrual association, interventions that relieve or worsen the symptoms, degree of incapacity, when in the menstrual cycle the symptoms occur, and any tendency toward recurrence.

During the physical examination, the entire lower genital tract should be examined. The absence of any anatomic landmarks such as the labia minora, prepuce, and frenula should be noted. It is important to check for contracture of the clitoral hood or stenosis of the introitus. *Consider looking elsewhere on the body surface to confirm certain diagnoses, such as examining the oral mucosa to diagnose lichen planus or examining the elbows and knees to confirm that a diffuse, red, scaly rash on the vulva is psoriasis.* Proper lighting is imperative. It should be bright without glare. Magnification

should be used as needed. The signs of vulvar disease are erythema, whiteness, lichenification, purpura, crusting, erosions, ulcerations, exudate, discharge, scarring, and loss of architecture. Questionable areas should be biopsied as needed.[5-7]

With an organized approach and directed training and experience, recognizing vulvar disease can be simplified and can be very rewarding for the patient and the practitioner.

ECZEMA

Eczema and dermatitis are synonyms. Eczema, the most common cause of vulvar rashes, is a generic term that comprises atopic dermatitis, primary irritant and allergic contact dermatitis, and lichen simplex chronicus. Atopic individuals have a genetic defect of keratinization and possibly immunomodulation that predisposes them to easily induced primary irritant contact dermatitis, which is then termed *atopic dermatitis.* The same process in non-atopic patients is simply called *primary irritant contact dermatitis.* In both, a type IV allergy is called *allergic contact dermatitis,* which may arise de novo or complicate preexistent disease. The itching that arises is the drive to the scratching that triggers lichen simplex chronicus as an end state.

Eczema is the most common cause of chronic vulvar pruritus. Contact dermatitis is the most common of the vulvar dermatoses/eczemas. Histologically, all show epidermal spongiosis, with or without acanthosis, and perivascular lymphohistiocytic infiltrates in the dermis. Other skin or vulvar conditions can be involved secondarily (e.g., irritated lichen sclerosus, lichen sclerosus with an associated allergic contact dermatitis).

ATOPIC DERMATITIS

Atopic dermatitis, the most common dermatitis, is a recurrent and very itchy inflammatory condition. Atopy affects as many as 20% of the population. It typically occurs in early childhood in children with a family or personal history of one or more of the following atopic conditions: asthma, allergies, hay fever, or hives. *The vulvar area in these patients is more susceptible to contactants, chronic irritation, and the development of lichen simplex chronicus.*

The pathogenesis of atopy has recently been clarified somewhat by the finding that atopic patients have an underlying genetically based defect in keratin formation[9] with a predisposition to skin barrier breakdown. *These patients have a more permeable skin barrier, with increased water loss resulting in chronically dry skin. This dry skin cracks easily and provides an entry for allergens, irritants, and skin pathogens.*[8] *Environmental agents such as soaps and detergents cause more barrier disruption, such that other irritants and pathogens gain entry to the epidermis.*[10] The skin condition develops as a result of this complex interrelationship among genetic, environmental, immunologic, and pharmacologic factors and possibly an immunoregulatory abnormality. With skin barrier dysfunction, ease of penetration of antigens means more Type IV allergic reactions add to the problem and play a role in some patients. This involves the complex interaction of local cytokines, T-helper cells, immunoglobulin E (Ig E), and other skin-directed cell responses. Atopic dermatitis can be exacerbated by fungal, bacterial, parasitic, and viral skin infections, either directly or with superantigens. *Staphylococcus aureus* is the most common infectious agent to exacerbate and maintain atopic dermatitis.[8,11–13]

In atopic patients, the irritation and inflammation trigger cellular and humoral immune responses that lead to the first symptom of atopic dermatitis: itch. This itch precedes the development of the rash itself and thus has been referred to as the "itch that rashes." This readily induced, ongoing inflammation and the altered skin immune response leads to itching, rubbing, and scratching, producing the secondary changes of lichenification, weeping, and secondary infection.[14–16] Typically, atopic patients worsen with exposure to high-pH soaps and cleansers and are irritated by perfumed products and even sanitary napkins. *As in all itchy rashes, heat, humidity, and stress make the itch worse.* Patients then develop an itch-scratch-itch cycle that results in the development of lichen simplex chronicus.

Most atopic patients are recognized during childhood with itchy rashes on the limbs and torso. The vulva in atopic children is seldom involved, but adults may have vulvar eczema. The vulva is probably more commonly affected than is realized. *The symptoms are itching and irritation. With excessive scratching, burning, rawness, and even pain may occur.* There is often a history of a precipitating irritant.

On physical examination, various stages of atopic dermatitis are seen, depending on the chronicity of the condition. The pattern can be subtle with redness and little to no scaling because the area is moist. The area involved includes the labia majora and, variably, the labia minora and less commonly the inner thighs and the gluteal cleft (Figure 17-4). Lichen simplex chronicus is the most common presentation of adult vulvar eczema (see the following discussion).

Treatment is directed at preventing inflammation, itching, and secondary problems. The triggering factors must be removed, the skin must be hydrated, and mid-potency corticosteroids, preferably ointments, are used.

LICHEN SIMPLEX CHRONICUS

Lichen simplex chronicus is the end stage of the itch-scratch-itch cycle. Outdated synonyms for lichen simplex chronicus include "neurodermatitis," "squamous hyperplasia," and "hyperplastic dystrophy." *Intense, chronic pruritus results in repetitive rubbing and scratching. The skin responds by thickening, producing increased skin markings called* lichenification.[17] This lichenified skin develops in previously normal skin. It is the chronic, localized thick and lichenified form of the disorder known variously as *eczema* or *atopic dermatitis*.[18] It does, however, also develop as a common endpoint of several conditions that are chronically scratched (e.g., lichen sclerosus, contact dermatitis).[19]

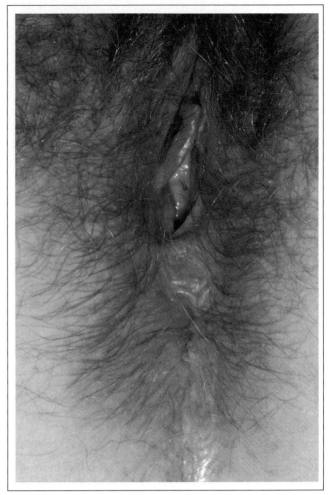

Figure 17-4 Atopic dermatitis. Subacute dermatitis of the vulva and perineum, with mild redness around inferior labia majora, perineum, and perianal area extending to gluteal cleft.

Conditions that may underlie lichen simplex chronicus are listed in Table 17-1. The most important of these are atopic dermatitis, contact dermatitis, and psoriasis.[20]

The pathophysiologic mechanisms in this condition are the same as those in atopic dermatitis (see previous section).[18] There is an altered barrier function,[21] with involvement of allergens, irritants, and skin pathogens along with altered immunoregulatory processes. Stress plays a major role in this condition, and that further deranges epidermal function.[22] *The defining characteristic of lichen simplex chronicus is relentless pruritus that is worse with heat, stress, and menstruation. The patient has often had years of chronic itch.* A tendency to habitual, almost compulsive scratching exists. Typically, she states that "nothing helps." Nocturnal scratching is common. This results in sleep disturbances and ruins the efficacy of daytime treatments.[23] At times, when the vulva is raw, the symptoms change from itch through burning to even frank pain.

On physical examination, the vulvar skin is diffusely thickened with increased skin markings (lichenification). The labia may be enlarged and rugose, with variable edema. The involvement

Table 17-1 Conditions That May Underlie Lichen Simplex Chronicus

Infections
Candidiasis
Dermatophytosis

Dermatoses
Atopic dermatitis
Lichen sclerosus
Lichen planus
Psoriasis

Metabolic Conditions
Diabetes
Iron-deficiency anemia

Neoplasias
Vulvar intraepithelial neoplasia

may be unilateral or bilateral. It may extend widely out onto the labiocrural and inguinal folds. The color is variable with a variety of shades—pink, red, violet, ruddy brown, or grayish black. Hyperpigmentation or hypopigmentation may be present. Scratching results in loss of hair. With continued excoriations, there are open erosions with oozing, fissuring, and honey-colored to serosanguineous crusting[24,25] (Figure 17-5A–C).

The diagnosis is clinical, based upon a thorough history and physical exam. A biopsy may be needed to make the diagnosis and to sort out the underlying conditions listed in Table 17-1, which shows the spectrum of the differential diagnoses.

The aim of treatment is to stop the itch-scratch-itch cycle. To do this one must eliminate irritants and allergens, restore barrier function, reduce the inflammation, stop the itch, and treat secondary problems.[18] To restore barrier function, the skin needs a "soak and seal" routine. This starts with a long soak in a sitz bath or a tub with plain water twice a day. Bathing hydrates the skin and soothes open, excoriated areas. During bathing, the avoidance of all cleansers is preferred. A mild, unscented soap substitute may be used in soiled areas only. After the soak, and after a careful rinse if soap substitutes are used, an ointment must be applied, both as an emollient to seal in the moisture and as a vehicle for medication.[15] After the soak, to control inflammation, a superpotent corticosteroid ointment should be used for a short period of time (4–6 weeks).[26] A short course of oral corticosteroids or intramuscular triamcinolone 1 mL/kg, repeated in 4 to 8 weeks if needed, may be necessary. Intralesional triamcinolone acetonide (3.5–5 mg/mL) can be used for very thickly lichenified areas.[20] Cool, ventilated, loose clothing of natural fibers is best. Fabric softeners should be avoided, and laundry detergents must be free of softeners, perfumes, and dyes. Dry skin must be controlled. Avoid so-called moisturizer lotions, which tend to be drying. Use plain water and a simple humectant such as petrolatum, glycerin, mineral oil, or lanolin. Infection must be treated with an appropriate antibiotic, an anticandidal medication, or both.[13,27] To control the pruritus, antihistamines should be given during the day and at night (e.g., nonsedating cetirizine 20 mL in the morning during the day, doxepin for sedation from 10 to 25 mL up to 30 to 100 mL at night). Nighttime scratching must be stopped; otherwise no recovery will occur. Antidepressants such as fluoxetine or sertraline can also be useful for controlling pruritus. Stress must be addressed. Local cold packs can help.[11,14,16,28,29]

If the condition continues and is difficult to resolve, look for contact dermatitis due to common irritants or (less common) allergies and eliminate superimposed. Allergens should be identified and eliminated (see the following section).[15,30] These patients need a lot of support and ongoing treatment. Relapse is not infrequent.

CONTACT DERMATITIS

Contact dermatitis is an inflammation of the skin resulting from an external agent that acts as an irritant or as an allergen. It is vital to differentiate an irritant from an allergen. It may be acute, subacute, or chronic. On the vulva, the most common contact dermatitis is primary irritant dermatitis.

Primary irritant dermatitis results from repeated exposure to a caustic or physically irritating agent. Anyone exposed to such a product, after enough insult, will react. This is a nonimmunologic reaction. The skin is damaged directly. Examples of such agents are trichloroacetic acid, urine, and feces.[31,32] Many factors such as loss of estrogen, pre-existing atopy or other skin conditions, infection, or trauma any can weaken the epidermal barrier function, making the skin more susceptible to irritant contact dermatitis. With repeated exposure the open skin may be sensitized, resulting in a true allergic contact dermatitis. *Allergic contact dermatitis results from a frank allergic reaction to a low dose of a chemical.* This is a type IV reaction, an immunologic reaction to a sensitizing chemical. Examples are poison ivy, neomycin, and benzocaine.[33]

Vulvar contact dermatitis is a very common and very important complicating factor in patients with persistent vulvar pruritus, irritation, or burning. Patients self-medicate, applying over-the-counter topical products for yeast infection, pain, or itch to open, already irritated skin. Many caregivers are consulted, adding to the list of products. Too commonly patients try to "wash their problem away." The correct diagnosis of a contact dermatitis can be challenging and is often missed.

The clinical complaints are much the same with both irritant and allergic contact dermatitis—varying degrees of itch, burning, and irritation that onset acutely or gradually. With an irritant, there is a history of repeated exposure. The condition often presents as a subacute or chronic problem. It is most common in patients who are obsessive about personal hygiene. Hygiene practices should always be reported in detail. Patients repeatedly and overzealously use "wipes," washcloths, scented cleansers, or soaps with damagingly high pH; therefore history taking in this situation must be as obsessive as the patient's own habits.

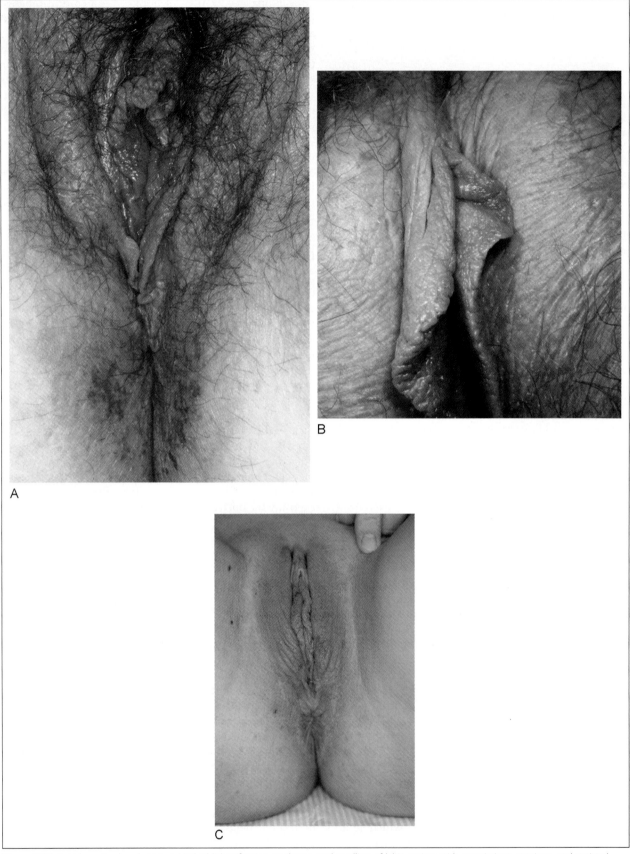

Figure 17-5 A, Lichen simplex chronicus. Marked lichenification, erythema, and swelling of labia majora with excoriations, erosions, and perianal crusting. **B,** Lichen simplex chronicus. Lichenification of medial aspects of the labia majora. **C,** Lichen simplex chronicus with pink to gray lichenification noted around the prepuce of the clitoris, lower labia minora and majora, perineum, and perianal area.

Vulvar hygiene is difficult for elderly patients. These patients commonly have problems with vulvar contact dermatitis owing to incontinence, with complicating factors of obesity, reduced mobility, and chronic use of panty liners. They develop, not infrequently, an irritant "diaper dermatitis."[25] Too often they use panty liners or menstrual pads inappropriately (instead of the proper appliances) for urinary incontinence, such that the vulva is wet and macerated all day long. Medicated "wipes" are used for cleansing and odor control. With the age-related loss of estrogen, the vulvar skin barrier function is further compromised. The result is an irritant contact dermatitis.

The most common causes of irritant contact dermatitis are soaps, cleansers, pads, urine, feces, sweat, vaginal secretions, and face cloths.

Allergic contact dermatitis can be more acute than irritant dermatitis, with sudden onset of symptoms of itching and burning. The patient may be able to identify the offending contactant by this acute onset. The itching is intense, and burning may occur.

On physical examination, the clinical presentation is variable. In a severe acute reaction, there may be erythema, swelling, vesiculation, or even frank bullae. Considerable weeping may be present, with scratching causing the secondary changes of excoriation, or serosanguineous or honey-colored crusting, with or without infection. In subacute reactions, there is less swelling, no vesiculation, and more crusting, dryness, or scaling (Figure 17-6AB). In chronic contact dermatitis, there is a thickening of the skin with increased skin markings (lichenification), induration, erythema, and altered pigmentation (dyspigmentation). These are the same changes seen in lichen simplex chronicus (see previous section).

The diagnosis is made clinically from the history and physical examination. The allergen(s) may be defined by patch testing. Standardized concentrations of known potentially allergenic chemicals are placed on the skin of the back and taped in place for 48 to 72 hours. They are then removed, and the skin is assessed 24 hours later. The 50 antigens in the North American Contact Dermatitis Group are preferred. Most dermatologists can perform these tests.[34] For some chemicals, a "use test" is performed. The patient puts a small amount of the substance on the skin of the inner arm repeatedly for 3 days.

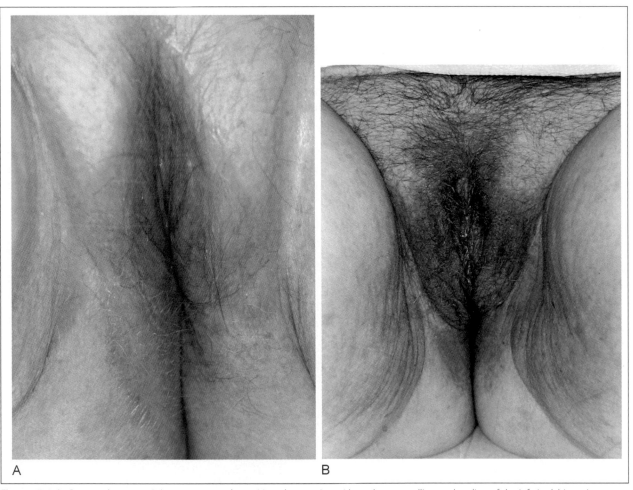

A   B

Figure 17-6 A, Contact dermatitis. Subacute contact dermatitis to benzocaine with erythema, swelling, and scaling of the inferior labia majora extending on the right side of the perineum to the perianal area with minor extension to the right labiocrural fold. **B,** Acute allergic contact dermatitis with redness and swelling due to benzocaine.

The most common allergens in the vulvar area are benzocaine, fragrance, and neomycin. The potential list of allergens is very long, ranging from rubber products to topical steroids.[25] It is very important to realize that the products patients are using may be contributing to their problems (e.g., a nonresponsive lichen sclerosus patient with allergic reaction to bacitracin).[25,35] It is also possible that the patient is having problems with both an irritant and an allergen. Panty liners, soaps, and face cloths are very traumatic to skin. Urine and feces are also very traumatic. Creams may have perfumes or preservatives such as formalin or imidazolidinyl urea, or the steroid molecule itself may be the allergen. The treatment can be the cause.[35–39]

Examples of allergens and irritants in vulvar contact dermatitis are listed in Table 17-2. The differential diagnosis can be very broad and includes eczema, psoriasis, intertrigo, and even bullous pemphigoid. To make a diagnosis, a very specific history is necessary. All products used by the patient must be identified, including medications ingested.[40–42]

The most important treatment is to remove the offending agent or practice and to treat with topical or even systemic corticosteroids and an antihistamine for sedation. Patch testing by a dermatologist may be necessary to define allergens. For severe, acute dermatitis, sitz baths may be necessary, followed by bland zinc oxide ointments and topical or even systemic corticosteroids. Antibiotics are necessary for infection. For subacute or chronic eruptions, a mid- to high-potency corticosteroid ointment can be used, such as triamcinolone 0.1% ointment or even clobetasol 0.05% ointment twice a day for 1 to 2 weeks, plus an antihistamine for sedation.[43–47]

Vulvar diseases rarely stand alone. They are often caused or worsened by irritant or allergic contact dermatitis. Always look for potential allergic contactants when evaluating a vulvar complaint, especially any vulvar inflammation that is not responding to treatment. Always get details of all hygiene practices and lists of all topical products used.

INTERTRIGO

Intertrigo is a mechanical inflammatory dermatosis in the skin folds caused by friction, heat, sweating, and occlusion. This is a very common problem in women with deep skin folds. The skin surfaces of the folds rub together, and this friction and the resulting sweat and heat produce maceration. The resulting weeping, dermatitic skin is very susceptible to secondary infection with yeast and bacteria. Humidity, tight synthetic clothing, and incontinence all make this worse. Obesity significantly compounds the problem. Diabetic patients are particularly susceptible to difficulties.[48] This condition is becoming a common problem for immobile, obese, elderly, and (especially) incontinent women. It commonly complicates and exacerbates psoriasis in the skin folds of the groin.

Clinically, the symptoms of intertrigo are burning, itching, and irritation, with variable malodor in the labiocrural and inguinal folds, under the abdominal pannus, and in the inframammary area. All are areas where skin surfaces chronically rub together. Physical examination reveals maceration, erythema, fissuring, and weeping in these skin folds. There may be scaling around satellite pustules with secondary candidiasis. The surrounding skin may be acutely inflamed and red or chronically hyperpigmented[20] (Figure 17-7).

Table 17-2 Examples of Allergens and Irritants in Vulvar Contact Dermatitis

Allergens
Sexual allergens
   Rubber condoms (thiuram)
   KY jelly (propylene glycol)
   Quinine hydrochloride (spermicide)
   Semen
Metals
   Nickel, chromate
Perfumes
   Balsam of Peru, cinnamates, citronellal in hygiene
   products
Medications
   Anesthetic (benzocaine)
   Antibiotic (neomycin, bacitracin, gentamycin)
   Antiseptics (thimerosal, povidone-iodine)
   Corticosteroids (tixocortol pivalate, triamcinolone
   acetonide)

Irritants
Medications (fluorouracil, podophyllotoxin, trichloroacetic acid)
Heat (hot-water bottles, heating pads)
Solvents
Bleach (sodium hypochlorite)
Alcohol
Sweat, urine, feces
Panty liners, sanitary napkins
Frictional trauma

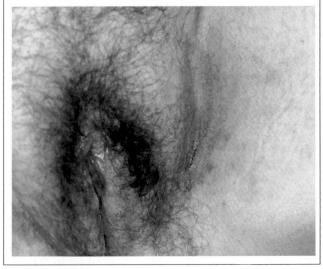

Figure 17-7 Intertrigo. Acute intertrigo with erythema and fissuring in the labiocrural folds in a patient with vulvar lichen planus.

The diagnosis is made clinically. The differential diagnosis includes erythrasma, psoriasis, seborrheic dermatitis, lichen sclerosus, and familial benign pemphigus. *Treatment is directed at controlling the precipitating factors. The friction, sweating, and heat must be controlled.* Tight, synthetic clothing must be replaced with cool, ventilated clothing of natural fibers. The area should be gently cleansed with a mild soap substitute. For simple cases, a plain powder-like cornstarch may be all that is necessary. Efforts should be made to separate the skin folds and keep them from rubbing together. This can be accomplished with cornstarch and strips of soft, thin, cotton laid into the folds to keep apart the skin surfaces. For the rash, a 1% hydrocortisone cream can be used, possibly with an imidazole cream. Tacrolimus 0.1% ointment twice a day has been reported as an effective, nonsteroidal alternative treatment.[49] Iodoquinol combined with 1% hydrocortisone in a cream or aqueous gel base can be of great value, but it may be best to initiate treatment of severe intertrigo with an antibiotic and anti-yeast medication orally for 1 week to control the infectious component.[20,50–52]

PSORIASIS

Psoriasis is a common, chronic, hereditary, papulosquamous disease of the skin characterized by well-defined, reddish papules and plaques with adherent, silvery-white scale. Psoriasis affects about 2% of the population and frequently involves the vulva, where it is often hidden, ignored, or missed. Women may not discuss it with their dermatologist, and at genital examinations their practitioners may not recognize or treat it.

It is characterized on most of the skin surfaces by well-defined, reddish papules and plaques with adherent, silvery-white scale. Typically, it affects the elbows, knees, scalp, and nails. When it is found in the body folds, it is referred to as *inverse psoriasis* or *flexural psoriasis. In folds, it is often a confluent shiny red patch and, as the area is moist, there is little to no scale.*

The etiology of psoriasis seems to be a defective or altered immune response with reactive abnormal epidermal differentiation and hyperproliferation in a genetically predisposed individual. The immune-based inflammatory mechanism is most likely initiated and maintained by dermal T cells. T cells interact with an antigen-presenting cell, with a resulting release of cytokines that induce epidermal proliferation. This in turn activates T cells in a vicious sustained and T cell–mediated, inflammatory loop.[53–55] Both genetic and environmental factors are involved in the pathophysiology. Several putative genetic susceptibility loci have been identified.

Psoriasis is triggered by a variety of environmental factors. Trauma to the skin, whether physical (scratching or rubbing), biological (bacteria or yeast), or chemical (irritating creams, urine, or feces) is important.[13,56] Drugs such as antimalarials, lithium, and beta blockers cause flaring of psoriasis.[57] Stress can play a major factor through the release of substance P. Stress has also been shown to alter epidermal barrier function.[22,58] Pruritus in a setting of

depression or anxiety can promote scratching and exacerbation of psoriasis from trauma—the classic isomorphic response of Koebner. Psoriasis severity fluctuates with hormonal changes. It peaks at puberty and menopause. Alcohol consumption and smoking are triggers. In the vulva, trauma plays the main role.

Clinically, the patient complains of irritation or itching. This symptom may vary from mild to intense. Scratching spreads the condition and makes the surface open and raw, and the patient may then complain of pain and burning. *Symptoms are made worse, as in the eczemas and intertrigo, by stress, heat, humidity, and use of sanitary napkins, tight synthetic clothing, and irritating soaps and lotions.* Many simple topical products burn the sensitive tissue of the vulva.

On physical examination, the picture is variable.[59] Papulosquamous lesions may be dispersed throughout the hairy areas of the mons pubis and labia. These can be thin, scattered, pink lesions of variable size and shape with minor scale (Figure 17-8A,B). Less commonly, there is a thick, confluent plaque that can be seen forming a horseshoe pattern with a more classic, silvery-white, adherent scale involving all of the hairy area. The inverse form occurs in a bilaterally symmetric, linear pattern following the folds of the inguinal crease, labiocrural fold, perineum, and gluteal cleft. In these areas, there is erythema, maceration, and fissuring. The vulvar mucosa is not involved. Secondary changes such as excoriation, crusting, and lichenification plus bacterial and yeast infections may further confuse the presentation. Very rarely, a pustular presentation is seen as part of a generalized pustular psoriasis.[25,58–62]

The diagnosis is clinical. It is important to note a history of previous skin rashes and a family history of psoriasis. *Check other parts of the skin (scalp, ears, elbows, knees, and nails) for psoriatic changes. Finding typical psoriasis elsewhere on the body confirms the diagnosis.* Biopsy is seldom necessary. Differential diagnosis includes candidiasis, lichen simplex chronicus, dermatophyte infection, intertrigo, contact dermatitis, vulvar intraepithelial neoplasia, and extramammary Paget's disease.

Treatment depends on severity and extent of disease. Seldom is psoriasis limited to the vulva; it is usually part of a generalized condition. All efforts should be made to stop inflammation, itching, and secondary infection. All triggering factors must be removed. The same general approach is outlined in the section on atopic dermatitis. Because trauma causes this condition to spread, scratching must stop. Systemic medications may be needed. Infection must be treated.

Specific treatments are topical and systemic. For mild to moderate disease, low- to intermediate-potency topical steroid ointments can be used for 2 weeks and then tapered to intermittent use. A topical vitamin D–derivative ointment can then be alternated with the topical steroid, although at times it can also be irritating. Tacrolimus ointment 0.03% or 0.1%, a topical calcineurin inhibitor, applied twice a day, can be used alone for 2 to 3 weeks or to follow the use of topical steroids as a steroid sparer. It can be irritating. For severe disease, superpotent topical steroid may be necessary for 2 to

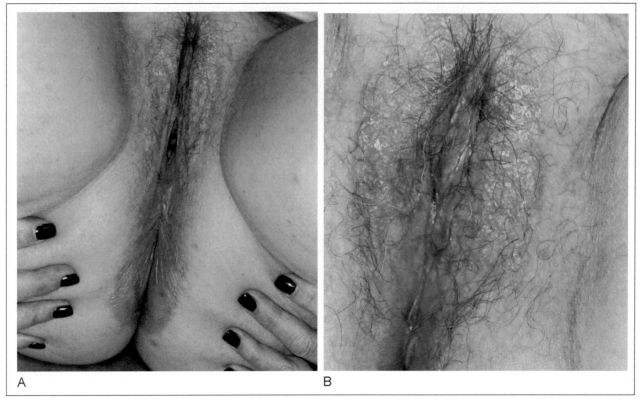

Figure 17-8 A, Psoriasis. A red scaly plaque is noted from the mons pubis, extending to the perineum and perianal excoriation. **B,** Psoriasis. Higher-power view of a red scaly plaque in the hairy areas of the mons pubis and labia majora.

3 weeks; then it too can be alternated with vitamin D–based calcipotriol/calcipotriene ointment 0.005%.[63,64] Long-term use of topical steroids should be avoided. To clear inverse psoriasis, the topical calcineurin inhibitor tacrolimus ointment is sometimes effective in both children and adults and thus avoids or shortens the use of topical corticosteroids.[65,66] In very extensive, recalcitrant psoriasis, systemic therapy may be necessary. Such treatments include methotrexate, acitretin, hydroxyurea, or cyclosporine.[67] Help from a dermatologist is recommended. A full discussion of these other options is beyond the scope of this chapter.[68,69]

LICHEN SCLEROSUS

Lichen sclerosus (LS) is the most common chronic inflammatory vulvar condition seen in vulvar clinics. The skin and genital lesions are white with tissue thinning and scarring. It is variably symptomatic with itching, irritation, or both and, less commonly, pain. It causes progressive vulvar dysfunction and destruction. Excellent reviews are available.[70–74] The prevalence of this condition is difficult to estimate because women may be asymptomatic or may not seek advice about their condition. It is estimated to affect 1:300 to 1:1000 adults and 1:900 children.[75–78] It is a condition most commonly reported in white individuals. The average age of onset is difficult to pinpoint. The majority of patients are ages 40 to 70 years but range from age 6 months to late adulthood.[79,80]

The etiology of LS is unknown. Various genetic, immunocytologic, autoimmune, hormonal, infectious, and local factors have been suggested. The cause is probably multifactorial, with genetic and environmental input. Family history is positive in 22% of patients. There is an association with human leukocyte antigen system (HLA) class II antigens, tissue-specific antibodies, and autoimmune diseases. HLA type 2 antigen DQ-7, -8, and -9 is found in both adult women and children.[79,81–83] A recent report found increased DRB1*12 (DR 12) and investigated the HLA-DR and DQ antigens and their haplotypes in susceptibility and protection from LS.[84] The immunogenetic profile can determine the site of the disorder, degree of scarring, and risk of malignant change.[76] Some work indicates persistent, antigen-driven inflammation.[85,86] Many studies have now focused on immunologic alterations, from cytokines to T cell function.[87,88] Inflammation and altered fibroblast function in the papillary dermis leads to fibrosis of the upper dermis. Several recent studies have identified autoantibodies to glycoprotein extracellular matrix protein 1 (ECM 1) and basement membrane zone antigens.[89,90] This may be associated with a local vasculitis, resulting in a duplication of the basement membrane in the blood vessels. How the autoantibodies cause this microvascular change is being investigated. What starts all this is still unknown. This condition has been linked to autoimmune diseases. As many as 44% of women have various autoantibodies and 40% have thyroid or parietal cell autoantibodies.[91,92] *The autoimmune diseases most often associated with LS are vitiligo, alopecia areata, and thyroid disease. Others include lupus erythematosus, morphea, pernicious anemia, and cicatricial pemphigoid.*[93,94] The relevance of these autoimmune associations is still not clear.

Hormonal factors have been postulated because the onset occurs when endogenous estrogen is low during childhood and menopause. Defective androgen metabolism has been suggested. *Thus far, hormones do not seem to have an etiologic role.*[71] Infection has been linked to lichen sclerosus. The spirochete *Borrelia burgdorferi* has been most often postulated, but it probably is not a causative agent.[95] No other organisms have been found so far.[96] There is no doubt that local factors are important. Any trauma, from scratching to radiation, as in all these vulvar conditions, may trigger LS.[97]

The clinical presentation is varied. Women complain of pruritus or a mixture of pruritus, soreness, irritation, dysuria, and dyspareunia. Too often, there may be few or no symptoms. The patient may complain of late changes of scarring with dyspareunia or even urinary retention. The practitioner may not have noted the loss of normal vulvar architecture or hypopigmentation or may have presumed these structural changes were due to early menopause. *Overall, the most common complaint is pruritus, which may be severe and intractable.* The patient may wake up at night scratching. A little girl may rub herself all day long. *Uncontrollable scratching results in purpura, open excoriations, fissures, and secondary infection with pain, dysuria, and dyspareunia.*[97] *With scratching, the condition flares.* If the anal area is involved, defecation can be difficult, and children often present with chronic constipation. Patients are worse during menses, and sanitary napkins cause further irritation. These patients are predictably frustrated and anxious.

On physical examination, there are classic white, atrophic, crinkly papules and plaques anywhere on the vulva, perineum, or perianal areas. The skin has a shiny, almost cellophane-like sheen. The vulva is involved in 98% of cases, and both vulva and perineum are involved in 48% of cases. Several patterns exist.[92] The typical figure-of-eight pattern is a common generalized pattern involving the periclitoral area, through the interlabial sulcus and labia minora to the perineum, and it extends in a circle perianally. With continued atrophy, there is a gradual effacement and complete disappearance of the clitoris, labia minora, or both (Figure 17-9A). In end-stage disease, the introitus is stenosed, and it may even be completely closed.[98–100] Patchy involvement of the perineum can occur, with just a few scattered white papules or some small white plaques. Other clinical patterns less commonly seen are diffuse erythema with fissures, an overall hypopigmented or vitiliginous pattern, and (rarely) a bullous form. These patterns are not mutually exclusive and can often overlap. Secondary changes are common. *Scratching causes purpura and erosions with excoriations, fissuring, and crusting. Repeated scratching spreads the condition.* The tissue also thickens (lichenification) (see Figure 17-9B). Sometimes

a warty change may occur. Children with LS and torn vulvar tissue, purpura, and scarring are often mistaken for victims of sexual abuse.[101]

As many as 20% of patients have LS elsewhere on the skin. Typically the neck, shoulders, axillae, and breasts are involved. The vagina is spared. Reports of oral LS are rare.[102] *The diagnosis is made clinically and confirmed with biopsy.* The pathology typically shows epidermal atrophy with orthohyperkeratosis and hydropic degeneration of the basal layer. The upper dermis shows edema and homogenization of the collagen; beneath is an inflammatory infiltrate of mononuclear cells.[103]

The differential diagnosis includes vitiligo, lichen planus, postmenopausal atrophy, cicatricial pemphigoid, pemphigus vulgaris, lichen simplex chronicus, sexual abuse (in children), and extramammary Paget's disease.

As a chronically scarring, inflammatory dermatosis, vulvar LS may act as an initiator or promoter of carcinogenesis[85] (see Figure 17-9C). *Squamous cell carcinoma can develop in 4% to 5% of cases of lichen sclerosus.* This association has been well documented.[104,105] Although squamous cell carcinoma is the primary malignancy associated with LS, there are rare reports of associated malignant melanoma and basal cell carcinoma.[106, 107] It has been suggested that the immune dysregulation may permit the development of cancer.[108]

Treatment can result in dramatic improvement. The goal is for controlled maintenance, as no cure is available at present. After a thorough assessment and a good general skin examination are performed to find other involved skin areas, a biopsy should be done to confirm the diagnosis because this is a chronic condition requiring long-term care. In children a biopsy is not always required, as the procedure is too traumatic. Topical treatment starts with avoidance of irritants and a regimen of gentle care (see the section on atopic dermatitis). Infection must be treated. Topical estrogen may be needed for concurrent vulvovaginal atrophy.

Topical steroids are the cornerstone of treatment. A superpotent steroid, clobetasol or halobetasol 0.05% ointment, is used once daily for 2 to 3 months and then intermittently for maintenance one to three times per week.[76,109,110] It is important to show the patient exactly where to apply the ointment and how much to use. A tiny amount of ointment (what can be picked up with the broad end of a toothpick) will cover the vulva with a thin film. A 15-g tube will usually last 12 weeks. For the perianal area, where the skin is thinner, 4 weeks of daily treatment is followed by a decrease to three times per week, then maintenance once or twice a week. If treatment is effective, the fissures, erosions, purpura, and thick white areas will fade, although not all disappear. *The longer the process has been active, the more resistant the skin is to change.* Longer, regular use of the superpotent steroids for as long as 6 months may be needed for postmenopausal patients.[111] By 12 weeks, there is a dramatic improvement, with 77% to 90% of patients seeing remission in symptoms and complete clearance in 23% of cases. Long-term treatment controls but does not cure. Lifetime follow-up is indicated.[112,113] Intermittent superpotent

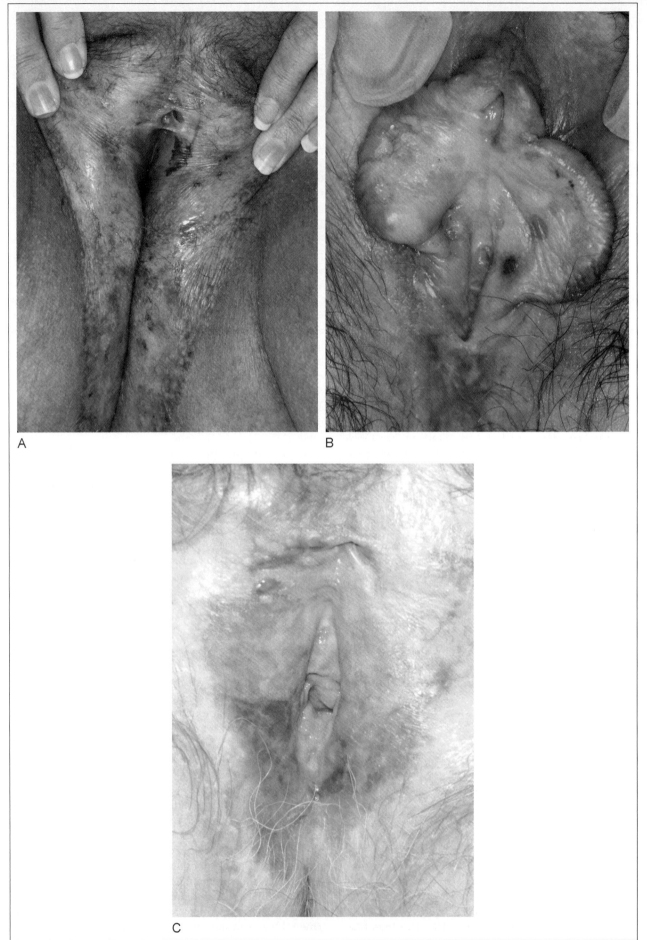

Figure 17-9 A, Lichen sclerosus. Figure-of-eight pattern around the vulva and perianal area with shiny, white, cellophane-like skin; marked purpura; and loss of labia minora and most of the clitoris, along with excoriations, erosions, and crusting. **B,** Swollen, thick, lichenified labia minora with scarring of the clitoris. Very white, shiny color of the inner labia minora and vulvar trigone, with extension of involvement to the edge of the meatus and down through the perineum. One excoriation is noted. **C,** LS with open areas of squamous cell carcinoma. Very scarred vulva with almost complete loss of clitoris; loss of labia minora; open, slightly thickened, linear erosions beside the clitoris; and open erosions around the right side of the vestibule and posterior fossa, with typical white shiny pattern of LS around the whole area.

steroids can be used for maintenance.[114] *Without long-term treatment, 85% of cases will relapse; although controversial, ongoing maintenance treatment once or twice per week is recommended.*[112] Superpotent steroids can be used efficaciously and safely in treating children although they may respond to a mid-potency product.[115,116] Side effects from topical steroids, when used properly, are rare. For very thick, resistant, hypertrophic LS, intralesional triamcinolone can be helpful.[99,117]

Topical testosterone was recommended in the past but is minimally effective and is no longer recommended.[118,119] Retinoids have been used topically and systemically but have too many side effects.[120,121] Topical calcineurin inhibitors (CNIs), pimecrolimus and tacrolimus, have both been used successfully.[122-124] There is debate regarding their safety in a condition with altered immunity and neoplastic potential, as CNIs present possible increased neoplastic risk.[125] Topical steroids work well in this condition and are the mainstay of treatment until further studies answer this controversy.

Other treatments described range from anti-malarials and cyclosporine to photodynamic therapy. These range from antimalarials and cyclosporine to photodynamic therapy.

Surgical management for this condition has been controversial because LS can flare with the irritation of surgery. It is, however, very important for specific patient needs, such as opening fused labia, dissecting free a buried clitoris, or correcting introital stenosis. It is always necessary for malignant disease.[126] Other surgical treatments have been reported, including laser treatment, but their long-term effectiveness is unclear.[127]

These patients need to be followed long term to prevent further scarring and to watch for the small but significant risk of malignancy. Overall, they usually do very well. If treatment is failing, consider whether the diagnosis is correct. Look for an added problem such as contact dermatitis (from overwashing or a reaction to the topical ointment), an infection, or cancer. Poor compliance is common due to fear of topical steroids, inability to use a topical (obesity or arthritis), or poor understanding. Pain may be due to mechanical factors from scarring. A little more practitioner time may be needed to deal with these issues.

LICHEN PLANUS

Lichen planus (LP) is a relatively common, inflammatory, lymphocyte-mediated mucocutaneous dermatosis affecting 1% to 2% of the population. Typically on the mucous membranes of the mouth or genitalia, there are white, lacy, fern-like patterned lesions, but smudgy, white and/or red, often eroded areas usually are found on the vulva. It usually affects the skin and the oral cavity. Twenty-five percent of cases affect mucosa alone, and 57% of women with oral LP have vulvovaginal involvement.[128-130] The incidence of vulvovaginal LP is unknown, as it is poorly recognized by practitioners and even those that treat the mouth or the skin seldom examine the genital

area. Skin LP is characterized by a skin eruption of polygonal, pruritic papules and polyhedral plaques that are often shiny with flat tops and show tiny white striae on the surface (Wickham's striae).

Synonyms for vulvovaginal lichen planus are *erosive lichen planus, desquamative inflammatory vaginitis, vulvovaginal-gingival syndrome,* and *ulcerative lichen planus.* The etiology is unknown, although evidence strongly suggests that it is a disorder of cell-mediated immunity in which an exogenous, antigenic stimulus such as a drug, chemical, or superantigen induces cell-mediated immune response in the epithelium, with infiltration of T cells in a genetically predisposed individual. The release of cytokines alters the keratinocytes, triggering an autoimmune reaction with basal keratinocyte destruction.[131-139] There is a strong association with and family history of autoimmune diseases.[140] HLA DR1 has been found in oral and cutaneous LP, supporting a genetic component. A recent report on HLA typing found a potential association with the DQB1*0201 in cases of the vulvovaginal gingival syndrome of LP.[134,136] In erosive LP, widespread damage has been found to the basement membrane zone (BMZ) of the epidermis. It is suggested that alteration to this zone may make it prone to damage by autoantibodies. Further work has demonstrated weak anti-basement membrane antibodies (perhaps due to BMZ injury), supporting the evidence that LP, whether cutaneous or erosive, is the result of autoimmune, T cell–mediated damage to basal cell keratinocytes.[141]

Various chemicals are known to flare LP, possibly as antigens. The list of drugs is extensive and includes thiazides, nonsteroidal anti-inflammatory drugs, beta blockers, and antimalarials. Environmental metals, from gold in schnapps to mercury in dental fillings, have been implicated. Even some plastics have created problems.[142-144] Infections such as hepatitis B and C and human immunodeficiency virus (HIV) are linked in some cases to LP.[145-149]

The disease has three main patterns that are not mutually exclusive. The classic presentation is itchy polygonal papules and plaques on wrists and ankles. Vulvar involvement without atrophy or scarring can be part of the generalized rash, with papules on the mons and labia. The vulvovaginal-gingival syndrome is an erosive, destructive form involving the mucous membranes of the mouth, vulva, and even conjunctiva and esophagus, with atrophy and scarring. The hypertrophic form is relatively rare, with extensive, thick vulvar scarring and variable hyperkeratosis.[150]

LP of the vulva has been reported and reviewed extensively.[147,151-165] It is part of a wide spectrum of disease involving the skin, oral mucosa, scalp, nails, eyes, esophagus, bladder, nose, larynx, and anus.[129,156] The typical patient is 30 to 60 years old. The symptoms are variable. Soreness, pain, and/or pruritus are most common; however, patients presenting with reticular pattern disease may be asymptomatic. Itching may be mild to moderate in the papular form or severe in the hypertrophic form, but these symptoms are not mutually exclusive. Erosive or ulcerative LP causes burning and pain that can be chronic and very severe. With vaginal erosion, a discharge occurs that can be purulent, malodorous, and copious. More than half of patients report dyspareunia and apareunia.[129,152,159,160,163] This contributes to anger, frustration, and relationship distress that compromise the therapeutic relationship.[150]

On physical examination, the findings vary depending on the overall pattern. *In the majority there is a red, eroded eruption with scalloped, whitish reticulated margins and often a glossy/glazed erythema. In some patients, the pattern may vary over time, from a lacy, reticulated pattern to erosive disease.* Disease in the vulva, vagina, or both may be active simultaneously or at different times. In the classic papulosquamous form, there are small, purple, itchy papules and plaques on the mons pubis, thighs, and labia majora. Reticulated white striae may be seen over the mucous membranes of the vulva, perineum, or perianal area. Scratching spreads this condition, and secondary changes from scratching may occur (Figure 17-10A). In the very hypertrophic form, there is thick, white induration of the vulva with scarring and loss of the labia and clitoral area, as in LS. The introitus may be totally stenosed.

In the erosive form, erosions may be small or large. They may be scattered around the inner labia minora and vulvar trigone. The edges are often white to grayish and scalloped. At the edge of the ulcers, the typical lacy pattern may be seen. The red areas may be a glossy red with a glazed appearance called "glazed erythema." Some areas may have a smudgy gray-white color. There is wide variation and loss of normal architecture (see Figure 17-10B,C). In one series, 70% of women had vaginal involvement.[163] It is difficult to know how many have vaginal disease because many women with vulvar LP do not have a vaginal examination. The vaginal changes include acute inflammation and erosion with heavy, thick, seropurulent discharge. There may be a gray pseudomembrane of coagulated serum over the eroded areas. Synechiae can be seen. Stenosis of the vagina is common. With continued disease, the vagina contracts, is foreshortened, and may close completely. Examining a patient with this condition is very difficult. Stenosis may make routine Pap smears impossible. In chronic, noneroded vaginal LP, there may be only loss of rugae and a residual atrophic lining.[150,166,167]

Signs of LP may first be identified elsewhere on the skin. Seeing these lesions facilitates the diagnosis. In the mouth, a white, lacy pattern on the buccal mucosa and gum margins may be seen. Ulcers and erosions may be present on the tongue and buccal mucosa. Severe involvement of the mouth may result in scarring. The severity of oral involvement does not correlate with genital disease. On the skin, a fine, red, papulosquamous rash or scattered, itchy, purple papules may be seen. The scalp may show a scarring alopecia. Nails will be thinned, with ridging and even diffuse scarring. To make a diagnosis, it is important to look at all these areas. The esophagus can be affected, resulting in narrowing and difficulty swallowing.

The diagnosis of LP is based on the clinical presentation and biopsy. Histopathology typically shows a bandlike lymphocytic infiltrate at the dermoepidermal junction, with a sawtoothed pattern at the rete ridges, acanthosis, hyperkeratosis, and a prominent granular layer.[168] The epithelium may be lost. The basal cells may be disorganized and vacuolated. Plasma cells may be seen.[157,166] Typical changes are not always seen in the mucosal lesions, and thus the pathology can be nonspecific. *The presence of nonspecific histology must not exclude the diagnosis. Immunofluorescence may be needed to differentiate LP from bullous disease.*

The differential diagnosis is mostly between LS and the vesiculobullous diseases, bullous and cicatricial pemphigoid and pemphigus. Behçet's syndrome and lupus erythematosus rarely may present with vulvar ulcers and erosions. Other causes of desquamative vaginitis include genital graft-versus-host disease, severe erythema multiforme, and toxic epidermal necrolysis. *Most of these conditions can be differentiated using the clinical pattern and histopathology.* LS and LP may overlap in the same patient.[169,170] When the vulva is thick and scratched in hypertrophic vulvar LP, lichen simplex chronicus must be considered, although the patient may have both conditions. *Although uncommon, squamous cell carcinoma must be excluded when nonhealing erosions and ulcers are found.*[171-173] The incidence is uncertain but was 2.6% in a recent series.[174,175]

Treatment is challenging. *No single agent is universally effective.* Topical superpotent steroid ointment such as 0.05% clobetasol or halobetasol is used. It may be applied to the vulva or applied intravaginally. Hydrocortisone acetate in a suppository or foam can be effective for vaginal involvement. Systemic steroids may be needed on an emergency basis to prevent destructive vulvovaginal scarring. Specific management of this difficult problem follows.

For all types of vulvar LP, it is important to control symptoms of itching and pain, stop irritation and trauma, and treat infections with bacteria or yeast, as outlined in the sections on atopic dermatitis and psoriasis. Depression and frustration must be addressed.[156] *Topical steroids are still the mainstays of treatment.* A topical superpotent steroid ointment such as 0.05% clobetasol or halobetasol may be applied to the vulva or applied intravaginally. Vaginal involvement may be treated with nightly hydrocortisone acetate in a suppository or foam (25 to 100 mL). Effort is made to avoid steroid atrophy. Systemic corticosteroids are the only medications to promptly and consistently improve erosive LP. Although oral prednisone (40–60 mg/day for 3–6 weeks) can control LP, intramuscular triamcinolone acetonide (1 mg/kg every 4 weeks for 3–4 months) also provides a rapid and effective response and is better tolerated. For limited areas, intralesional triamcinolone acetonide, 5 to 10 mg/mL, may be effective. Vaginal dilators coated with topical steroids can be used to prevent synechiae. Once control is achieved, the use of steroids is tapered.[151,157]

Topical off-label use of calcineurin inhibitors tacrolimus and pimecrolimus has been reported to be useful.[161,176-180] Tacrolimus has been used as a 0.1% ointment or compounded vaginal cream, and pimecrolimus as a 1% cream.[181] Reports of effectiveness, side effects, and safety are mixed. The ointment can cause unacceptable burning. The vaginal preparation can be absorbed, giving low but measurable blood levels. There is also a theoretical risk of squamous

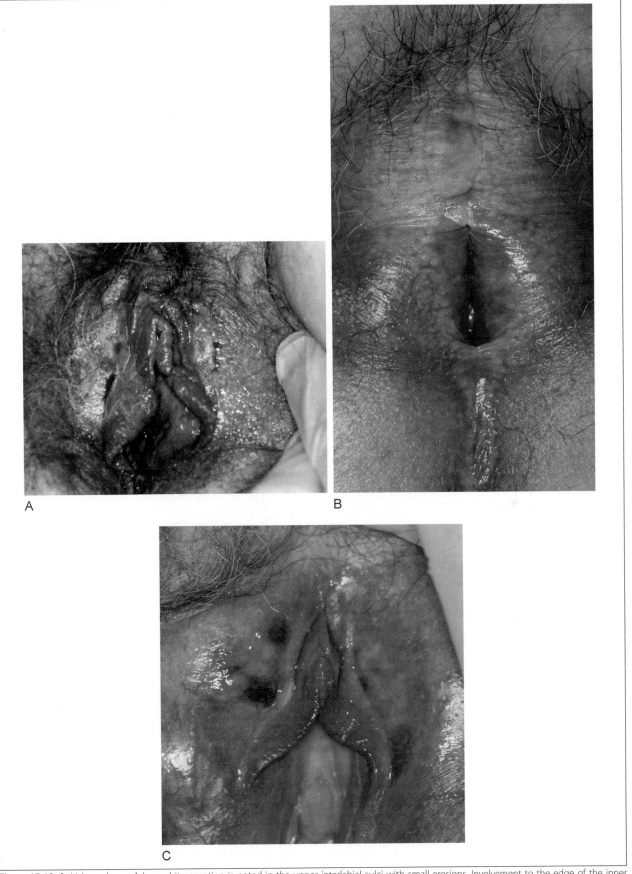

Figure 17-10 **A,** Lichen planus. A lacy white eruption is noted in the upper interlabial sulci with small erosions. Involvement to the edge of the inner and outer labia minora and around the prepuce. **B,** Whitish, scarred vulva with complete loss of the clitoris and labia minora and partial vaginal stenosis. **C,** Periclitoral erosions with surrounding whitish scarred areas with no loss of architecture.

cell carcinoma with LP, and the long-term effect of these modulators on the risk of cancer is unknown.

Many other treatments have been used for this difficult disease. Oral retinoids have been used to control erosive disease, but little has been published on the use of these agents for vulvar disease. In one series they were reported as unhelpful.[136,182–184] Azathioprine has been used effectively as a steroid-sparing agent.[183] Cyclosporine systemically and topically has been used with varying success.[185–188] Methotrexate at 5 to 15 mg per week has been very effective.[189] Griseofulvin and dapsone,[152,163] hydroxychloroquine,[190] and tetracycline with nicotinamide[190,191] are not helpful.[136] Metronidazole has occasionally been used for generalized disease.[193,194] Other treatments have included thalidomide,[195,196] interferon and heparin,[131] tacrolimus, and photodynamic therapy. Recently mycophenolate mofetil and etanercept have been tried, but it is too soon to know whether these are effective. In the review by Petruzzi, many of the treatments are summarized and an algorithm of treatment is suggested.[161]

Surgery may be necessary for vaginal synechiae and for some cases of stenosis. There is always the potential for rebound flare of LP after surgery, and the immediate postoperative use of topical superpotent or systemic steroids may be necessary.

The prognosis is variable and notoriously unpredictable. LP can remit for years, leaving only some scarring. In one series, 38% of patients with vulvar LP had complete resolution, 30% had significant resolution, and the rest had ongoing problems. In another series of patients with erosive LP, 9% had complete remission and 58% became asymptomatic.[174] *Because no single treatment is universally successful, treatments may have to be combined and regularly reassessed to find a safe and effective program.*

MANAGEMENT SCENARIOS

Scenario 1

A 26-year-old woman presents with intense, intractable, vulvar and perineal pruritus for 3 years. She wakes up scratching at night. Nothing helps. She has seen several practitioners, and the topicals preparations she was offered all caused burning. On examination, she is a healthy-appearing, fair-skinned, Caucasian woman with a rash confined to the vulva, perineum, and perianal area.

Clinical picture: Figure 17-11
What to look for in the picture?

- Any loss of architecture
- Color of the skin
- Texture of the skin: thick, thin, and so on
- Secondary changes, such as from scratching or infection

What to ask?

- Is she or is anyone in her immediate family atopic?
- Does anyone in her immediate family have allergies, hay fever, asthma, hives, or eczema?

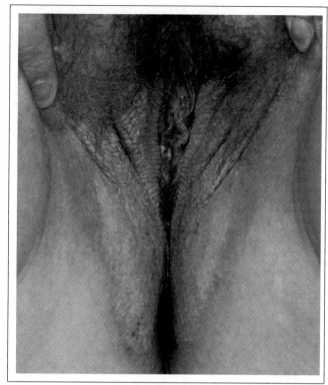

Figure 17-11 Scenario 1.

- What are her personal hygiene habits?
  - Which type of soap or detergent does she use?
  - Does she use her hands or a face cloth or wipes for cleansing?
  - Frequency of cleansing?
- What type of sanitary napkin is used; any regular use of panty liners?
- What does she put on her skin? Be sure to get the entire list of everything she uses.

Diagnostic steps:

- Careful and detailed history
- Physical examination showing the typical lichenified vulva—this is a clinical diagnosis
- Culture bacteria and yeast

Diagnosis: Lichen simplex chronicus (the itch-scratch-itch disease) with secondary infection from scratching and contact dermatitis.

Tip: This type of patient experiences relentless pruritus and is constantly scratching. As she continues to scratch, the skin thickens. It is typically made worse by heat, humidity, stress, and irritants. It is most commonly found in patients with atopic dermatitis, sometimes psoriasis, LS, and rarely vulvar intraepithelial neoplasia. In all these cases there is more than one problem, and it is almost always a combination of a dermatosis, contactants, and infection. These patients are constantly rubbing, scratching, and otherwise irritating their vulvar skin. Many topical products are caustic. As patients scratch, the skin breaks down and becomes infected, and the infection causes further flares.

What to do?

The skin in these women is so scratched, open, and irritated that all topical products will burn. Therefore it is wise to start with oral treatments and bland topical skin therapy such as plain water soaks and topical plain petrolatum for 2 to 3 days before adding active topical agents.

- Stop the itch-scratch-itch cycle.
- Stop all irritants: no soaps.
- Soothe the skin with soaks to seal in moisture with sitz baths or soaks in the tub for 10 minutes twice per day.

1. Reduce inflammation with superpotent steroids; clobetasol or halobetasol 0.05% ointment bid for 2 weeks, *then* once a day for 2 weeks, *then* M-W-F for 2 weeks using plain Vaseline on the alternate days.
   - If it is very severe, consider a brief burst and taper of systemic steroids.
2. Control infection:
   - Cefadroxil 500 mg bid for 7 days
   - Fluconazole 150 mg repeated 1 week later to make sure there is no candida
3. Sedation:
   - Doxepin or hydroxyzine 10 to 25 mg at night at 6 to 7 PM so that it will be out of her system when she wakes up in the morning and she will not be sleepy
   - Fluoxetine 20 mg in the morning if needed
4. Review and re-review topical products. Patients often restart irritating soaps, wipes, panty liners, and others.

Scenario 2

A 45-year-old Caucasian woman gradually developed vulvar itching and burning more than 2 years ago. She was initially treated for a yeast infection with imidazole creams and then with oral fluconazole but with no response. She was believed to be premenopausal. The vulva appeared atrophic. The burning became worse, and she now has significant dyspareunia.

On examination she is a healthy 45-year-old woman with brown hair. This examination is limited to the vulva.

Clinical picture: Figure 17-12A,B

What to look for in the picture?

- Any loss of architecture
- Color of the skin
- Texture of the skin
- Any unique markings
- Any other areas of involvement

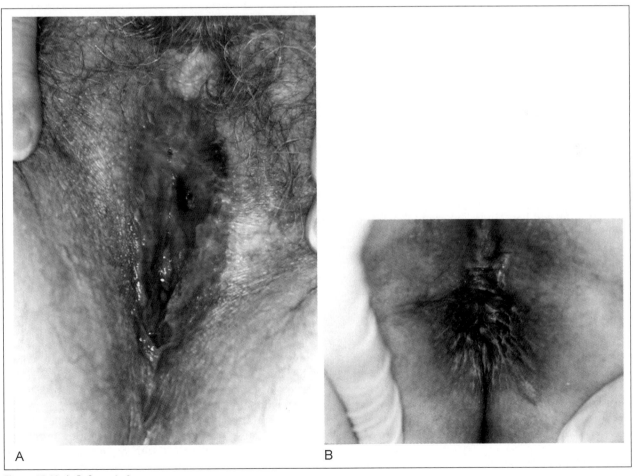

A

B

Figure 17-12 A, B, Scenario 2.

Where else to look?

- Skin elsewhere on the body
- Anal area
- Oral mucosa
- Scalp

See picture of perianal area (Figure 17-12b). What to ask?

- What else did she use to treat the problem?
- Does she have any complaints in the oral cavity?
- What are her hygiene habits? Identity any factors that could be making her worse—see Scenario 1.

Diagnostic steps:

- Careful and detailed history
- Thorough examination of the vulva, vagina, perineum, perianal area, oral cavity, and skin
- Skin biopsy for hematoxylin and eosin stain and immunofluorescence

Diagnosis: LP of the vulva, perineum, and perianal area. Note the obvious lacy LP white pattern found on the perianal area. On the vulva, one also sees a glazed erythema, loss of the normal architecture, and a gray scalloped edge around the vulvar trigone. This pattern is so classic, especially perianally, that a biopsy is not needed in this case.

LP is a chronic inflammatory cutaneous eruption in the vulvar area.

The differential diagnosis is LS and cicatricial pemphigoid, but none of these give the lacy pattern that is seen here.

Tips:

- Vaginal involvement rules out LS.
- Erosions are present in 60% to 90% of cases of vulvar LP, and it can involve the vagina in 60% of cases. Women with vaginal involvement will have a desquamative inflammatory vaginitis-like clinical pattern with erosions, synechiae, stenosis, shortening, dyspareunia, and a mucopurulent discharge.
- Look for oral involvement. Sixty percent of patients with erosive vulvar LP will have disease in the oral cavity. It can help confirm the diagnosis.
- Consider lichenoid drug eruption. It can be precipitated by drugs such as thiazides and nonsteroidal anti-inflammatory drugs (NSAIDs).

What to do?

- Confirm the diagnosis with a biopsy.
- Stop irritants and scratching (further trauma).
- Stop any suspect drugs.
- Control infection.
- Educate the patient.
- Control inflammation with clobetasol or halobetasol 0.05% ointment once to twice per day.
- Intralesional vulvar and systemic corticosteroids may be needed.
- Topical tacrolimus 0.1% ointment bid can be used as a steroid sparer but can burn.

For severe LP:

1. Systemic corticosteroids starting at higher dosages (e.g., prednisone 40–60 mg daily given as one dose in the morning with food) and then decreasing or triamcinolone acetonide 40 mg/mL, 1 mg/kg IM every 4 weeks for three doses given into the anterior thigh.
2. Intravaginal corticosteroids: hydrocortisone acetate, 25- to 100-mg suppositories nightly for 2 weeks and taper.
3. If the patient is not responding, consider oral cyclosporine 4 to 5 mg/kg for 3 to 4 months or methotrexate 5 to 15 mg weekly. Other considerations: hydroxychloroquine, azathioprine, and etanercept.

These patients often respond well with time. LP can go into remission and relapse intermittently. These patients require long-term follow-up. There is a 3% to 5% risk of associated squamous cell carcinoma of the vulva. If the patient is not responding or doing poorly or if there is any papular change, repeat the biopsy.

Scenario 3

A 35-year-old woman presents with 1 to 2 years of vulvar itching. She is scratching a fair amount at night. She has used over-the-counter antifungal medications. She has been treated with short courses of topical corticosteroids without success and is frustrated.

Clinical picture: Figure 17-13

What to look for in the picture?

- Any loss of architecture
- Texture of the skin
- Color of the skin
- Any secondary changes—scratching or infection

What to ask?

- Does she have this rash anywhere else on the body?
- Is there a personal or family history of thyroid disease or any other autoimmune disease?
- Find out details about hygiene habits (see previous scenarios).

Diagnostic steps

- Thorough examination of the vulva, perineum, and perianal area
- Biopsy for pathology

Diagnosis: Lichen sclerosus

This shows a fairly typical picture with the very white, shiny pattern; purpura; flattening of the normal vulvar architecture; and loss of the labia minora. Involvement extends to the perianal area but does not demonstrate the classic figure-of-eight pattern.

Differential diagnosis: LP is not as shiny white; vitiligo does not cause scarring; and lichen simplex chronicus would be thicker and grayer with no scarring. Cicatricial pemphigoid can cause whiteness and scarring, but it is rare and can be ruled out with a biopsy.

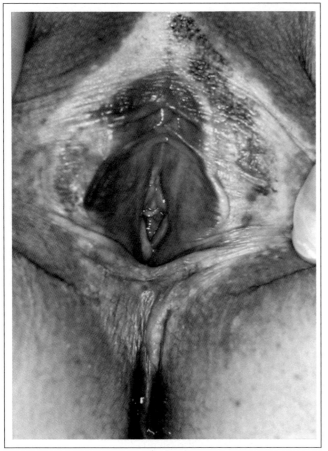

Figure 17-13 Scenario 3.

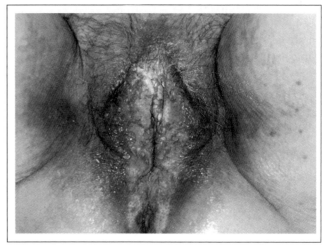

Figure 17-14 Scenario 4.

function. She had a slightly itchy vulva for many years. Her only treatment has been Vagisil, an anti-itch cream.

Clinical picture: Figure 17-14

What to look for in the picture?

- Pattern of the eruption: Is it limited to the vulva?
- Color(s) of the skin (around the periclitoral area is white ointment, not part of the eruption)
- Any ulcers or erosions?

What to ask?

- What are her hygiene habits?
- What is she using for cleansing and how?
- What is she putting on her skin?
- What are the products she is using and how often a day?
- Does she have problems with urinary incontinence?
- Is she using panty liners?
- Is there a family history of hypothyroidism?

Diagnostic steps:

- Careful and detailed history
- Physical exam; outline of the eruption; what areas are involved? Does this woman have one or multiple causes of her symptoms?
- Would a biopsy or biopsies be helpful?

Diagnosis: Severe ulcerative contact dermatitis, a primary irritant dermatitis due to chronic use of a benzocaine-containing cream in an elderly woman with previously unrecognized LS.

Tip: This elderly woman has a caustically burned vulva from the topical product she has been putting on, by history, 6 to 8 times per day. She was not biopsied. A biopsy of the red area should have been performed, which would have showed contact dermatitis on histopathology. The white area where she has the LS may have showed a mixed pattern on pathology because of a combination of contact dermatitis and LS. Patch testing, a full screen, inducing topical Vagisil did not show any positive reactions, confirming a severe irritant contact dermatitis. She has had LS for many years, but

What to do?

- Perform a biopsy to confirm the diagnosis.
- Stop irritants.
- Control infection.
- Educate.
- Treat with superpotent steroids: clobetasol or halobetasol 0.05% ointment daily in a thin invisible film for 12 weeks and then maintenance 1 to 3 times per week indefinitely.
- Treat any secondary infection, particularly yeast infection.
- Stop scratching, as it will flare the condition.
- If needed, use sedation as for the lichen simplex chronicus in Scenario 1.
- If very thick, consider intralesional triamcinolone, 10 mg/mL, injected using a 30-gauge needle just under the skin. It is best to use a topical anesthetic ointment for 20 to 30 minutes under occlusion before the injection.
- Long-term follow-up is forever.

If the patient is not responding, reassess and rebiopsy to rule out squamous cell carcinoma or contact dermatitis.

Scenario 4

A 66-year-old postmenopausal woman presented with a severely painful, raw vulva that has been worsening for 6 weeks. She is up all night pacing and crying and cannot it went unrecognized. The Vagisil she used is a cream commonly used for vulvar discomfort. It can cause either an allergic contact dermatitis due to benzocaine or an irritant/caustic reaction. The diagnosis is made on history and confirmed by the pattern seen on the vulva. It should be determined whether hygiene habits such as the use of soaps, wipes, and sanitary napkins are making the condition worse. Vulvar contact dermatitis is common, and it complicates all vulvar conditions. Irritant contact is the most frequent type.

What to do?

This woman needs relief of the burning and irritation and rest. As she was elderly, so incapacitated, and living alone, she was hospitalized for the first 48 hours.

- Stop the burning and irritation; use sedation.
- Doxepin 10 to 25 mg in the evening or 10 to 20 mg bid, depending on tolerance. This is appropriate in hospital, but on discharge it was ordered for nighttime sedation only.
- Sitz baths or saline compresses for 5 to 10 minutes, 4 times per day for the first 2 days, then 1 to 2 times per day.
- Cool gel packs as needed (use a gel soft picnic pack). This is kept in a self-sealing plastic bag kept cool (not frozen) in the refrigerator. It can be applied directly onto the skin or wrapped in a thin cotton cloth and applied directly as needed and then washed and returned to the plastic bag and replaced in the refrigerator. Avoid frozen packs because they cause more damage.

1. Reduce inflammation with superpotent steroids.
   a. Clobetasol or halobetasol 0.05% ointment applied bid for 1 week, then once daily, continuing as for LS (see previous scenario).
   b. Topical petrolatum after the other plain water soaks in the first few days.
   c. Systemic corticosteroids; begin with 1 mg/kg per day in divided doses, twice daily for the first 4 to 5 days and then once daily for another week. The total duration of treatment is dependent on the response.
2. Support, education, and long-term follow-up are very important in this case.

Scenario 5

A 34-year-old woman presents with a 2-year history of an itchy, burning vulvar eruption. She has been treated on a number of occasions for yeast and bacterial vaginosis. Her main complaint was burning and irritation in the "skin splits," entry dyspareunia, and painful recurrent perineal lesions. On history she admits to washing two to three times per day with potentially caustic soaps or using "wipes." She frequently wears a panty liner because of a chronic discharge. She has been on tetracycline for rosacea but not recently.

Clinical picture: Figure 17-15

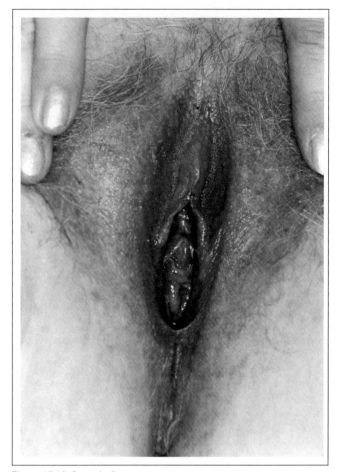

Figure 17-15 Scenario 5.

What to look for in the picture?

- Any loss of architecture
- Color of the skin
- Pattern of the eruption

What to ask?

- Have past examinations during her regular checkups noted any vulvar changes?
- Does she have any skin rashes anywhere else on the body?
- Is there a personal or family history of thyroid disease or other autoimmune disease?
- What are her hygiene habits? (See previous scenarios.)

Diagnostic steps:

- Good clinical exam of the vulva, perineum, and perianal area
- Vaginal exam and wet prep
- Biopsy for pathology
- Culture of fissures for yeast and bacteria

Diagnosis: Lichen sclerosus with associated fissuring from irritation and secondary candidiasis; contact dermatitis: irritant, from hygiene practices.

This shows a confusing picture of a very red vulva with little architectural change and no frank white areas. There is swelling around the clitoral area and upper interlabial sulcus, notably small labia minora, and fissuring in the perineum extending to the perianal area.

Fissuring associated with *Candida* is classically in the interlabial folds and sometimes involves the posterior fourchette. Fissuring associated with LS is also typically found in the interlabial folds. Any skin disease can cause skinfold fissures, especially if there is any rubbing or scratching. The posterior fourchette area is a common site of traumatic splitting, and in this case the LS predisposes to that fissuring found in that area.

What to do?

- Biopsy to confirm the diagnosis
- Stop all irritants, soaps, wipes and pads, and so on
- Control infection with oral fluconazole
- Educate
- Topical superpotent steroid ointment (see Scenario 3)
- Long-term follow-up

REFERENCES

1. DiSaia DJ. Clinical anatomy of the female genital tract. In: Scott JR (ed). Danforth's Obstetrics and Gynecology, ed 7. Philadelphia: Lippincott, 1994, pp 1–8.
2. Lynch PJ, Edwards L. Anatomy. In: Lynch PJ, Edwards L (eds). Genital Dermatology. New York: Churchill Livingston, 1994, pp 1–3.
3. Margesson LJ. Normal anatomy of the vulva. In: Fisher BK, Margesson LJ (eds). Genital Skin Disorders—Diagnosis and Treatment, ed 1. St Louis: Mosby, 1998 pp 99–107.
4. McLean JM. Anatomy and physiology of the vulva. In: Ridley CM, Neill SM (eds). The Vulva, ed 2. London: Blackwell Science, 1999, pp 37–63.
5. Lynch PJ, Edwards L. Diagnostic procedures. In: Lynch PJ, Edwards L (eds). Genital Dermatology. New York: Churchill Livingston, 1994, pp 7–8.
6. Margesson LJ. Appendix B. Clinical evaluation of vulvar patients. In: Fisher BK, Margesson LJ (eds). Genital Skin Disorders—Diagnosis and Treatment. St Louis: Mosby, 1998, pp 235–236.
7. Turner ML, Marinoff SC. General principles in the diagnosis and treatment of vulvar diseases. Dermatol Clin 1992;10: 275–281.
8. Leung DY, Soter NA. Cellular and immunologic mechanisms in atopic dermatitis. J Am Acad Dermatol 2001;44(1 Suppl): S1–S12.
9. Irvine AD, McLean WH. Breaking the (un)sound barrier: filaggrin is a major gene for atopic dermatitis. J Invest Dermatol 2006;126:1200–1202.
10. Cork MJ, Robinson DA, Vasilopoulos Y, et al. New perspectives on epidermal barrier dysfunction in atopic dermatitis: gene-environment interactions. J Allergy Clin Immunol 2006;118:3–21.
11. Abeck D, Mempel M. Staphylococcus aureus colonization in atopic dermatitis and its therapeutic implications. Br J Dermatol 1998;139(Suppl 53):13–16.
12. Bunikowski R, Mielke ME, Skarabis H, et al. Evidence for a disease-promoting effect of *Staphylococcus aureus*-derived exotoxins in atopic dermatitis. J Allergy Clin Immunol 2000;105:814–819.
13. Saloga J, Knop J. Superantigens in skin diseases. Eur J Dermatol 1999;9:586–590.
14. Tofte SJ, Hanifin JM. Current management and therapy of atopic dermatitis. J Am Acad Dermatol 2001;44(1 Suppl): S13–S16.
15. Ball SB, Wojnarowska F. Vulvar dermatoses: lichen sclerosus, lichen planus, and vulval dermatitis/lichen simplex chronicus. Semin Cutan Med Surg 1998;17:182–188.
16. Hanifin JM, Tofte SJ. Patient education in the long-term management of atopic dermatitis. Dermatol Nurs 1999;11: 284–289.
17. Ridley CM, Neill SM. Non-infective cutaneous conditions of the vulva. In: Ridley CM, Neill SM (eds). The Vulva, ed 2. London: Blackwell Science, 1999, pp 151–152.
18. Lynch PJ. Lichen simplex chronicus (atopic/neurodermatitis) of the anogenital region. Dermatol Ther 2004;17:8–19.
19. Virgili A, Corazza M, Bacilieri S, et al. Contact sensitivity in vulval lichen simplex chronicus. Contact Dermatitis 1997; 37:296–297.
20. Margesson LJ. Inflammatory diseases of the vulva. In: Fisher BK, Margesson LJ (eds). Genital Skin Disorders—Diagnosis and Treatment. St Louis: Mosby, 1998, p 164.
21. Cork MJ, Robinson D, Vasilopoulos Y, et al. Predisposition to sensitive skin and atopic eczema. Community Pract 2005;78:440–442.
22. Garg A, Chren MM, Sands LP, et al. Psychological stress perturbs epidermal permeability barrier homeostasis: implications for the pathogenesis of stress-associated skin disorders. Arch Dermatol 2001;137:53–59.
23. Koca R, Altin R, Konuk N, et al. Sleep disturbance in patients with lichen simplex chronicus and its relationship to nocturnal scratching: a case control study. South Med J 2006;99: 482–485.
24. Lynch PJ, Edwards L. Red plaques with erythematous features. In: Lynch PJ, Edwards L (eds). Genital Dermatology. New York: Churchill Livingstone, 1994, pp 27–34.
25. Pincus SH. Vulvar dermatoses and pruritus vulvae. Dermatol Clin 1992;10:297–308.
26. Brunner N, Yawalkar S. A double-blind, multicenter, parallel-group trial with 0.05% halobetasol propionate ointment versus 0.1% diflucortolone valerate ointment in patients with severe, chronic atopic dermatitis or lichen simplex chronicus. J Am Acad Dermatol 1991;25:1160–1163.
27. Veien NK. The clinician's choice of antibiotics in the treatment of bacterial skin infection. Br J Dermatol 1998;139(Suppl 53): 30–36.
28. Hanifin JM, Chan S. Biochemical and immunologic mechanisms in atopic dermatitis: new targets for emerging therapies. J Am Acad Dermatol 1999;41:72–77.
29. Margesson LJ. Inflammatory diseases of the vulva. In: Fisher BK, Margesson LJ (eds). Genital Skin Disorders—Diagnosis and Treatment. St Louis: Mosby, 1998, pp 154–155.
30. Virgili A, Bacilieri S, Corazza M. Evaluation of contact sensitization in vulvar lichen simplex chronicus. A proposal for a battery of selected allergens. J Reprod Med 2003;48: 33–36.
31. Denig NI, Hoke AW, Maibach HI. Irritant contact dermatitis. Clues to causes, clinical characteristics, and control. Postgrad Med 1998;103:199–208, 212.

32. Margesson LJ. Inflammatory diseases of the vulva. In: Fisher BK, Margesson LJ (eds). Genital Skin Disorders—Diagnosis and Treatment. St Louis: Mosby, 1998, pp 155–157.

33. Lynch PJ, Edwards L. Geriatric problems. In: Lynch PJ, Edwards L (eds). Genital Dermatology. New York: Churchill Livingstone. 1994, pp 265–266.

34. Rietschel RL, Fowler JF (eds). Fisher's Contact Dermatitis. Philadelphia: Lippincott, Williams and Wilkins, 2001, pp 9–26.

35. Corazza M, Mantovani L, Maranini C, et al. Contact sensitization to corticosteroids: increased risk in long term dermatoses. Eur J Dermatol 2000;10:533–535.

36. Eason EL, Feldman P. Contact dermatitis associated with the use of Always sanitary napkins. CMAJ 1996;154:1173–176.

37. Lewis FM, Shah M, Gawkrodger DJ. Contact sensitivity in pruritus vulvae: patch test results and clinical outcome. Am J Contact Dermat 1997;8:137–140.

38. Sterry W, Schmoll M. Contact urticaria and dermatitis from self-adhesive pads. Contact Dermatitis 1985;13:284–285.

39. Virgili A, Corazza M, Califano A. Diaper dermatitis in an adult. A case of erythema papuloerosive of Sevestre and Jacquet. J Reprod Med 1998;43:949–951.

40. Bauer A, Geier J, Elsner P. Allergic contact dermatitis in patients with anogenital complaints. J Reprod Med 2000;45:649–654.

41. Gaffoor PM. Sexually induced dermatoses. Cutis 1996;57:252–254.

42. Sonnex C. Sexual hypersensitivity. Br J Hosp Med 1988;39:40–49.

43. Bauer A, Rodiger C, Greif C, et al. Vulvar dermatoses—irritant and allergic contact dermatitis of the vulva. Dermatology 2005;210:143–149.

44. Farage MA. Vulvar susceptibility to contact irritants and allergens: a review. Arch Gynecol Obstet 2005;272:167–172.

45. Margesson LJ. Inflammatory diseases of the vulva. In: Fisher BK, Margesson LJ (eds). Genital Skin Disorders—Diagnosis and Treatment. St Louis: Mosby, 1998, pp 155–157.

46. Margesson LJ. Contact dermatitis of the vulva. Dermatol Ther 2004;17:20–27.

47. Nardelli A, Degreef H, Goossens A. Contact allergic reactions of the vulva: a 14-year review. Dermatitis 2004;15:131–136.

48. Yosipovitch G, Tur E, Cohen O, et al. Skin surface pH in intertriginous areas in NIDDM patients. Possible correlation to candidal intertrigo. Diabetes Care 1993;16:560–563.

49. Chapman MS, Brown JM, Linowski GJ. 0.1% tacrolimus ointment for the treatment of intertrigo. Arch Dermatol 2005;141:787.

50. Guitart J, Woodley DT. Intertrigo: a practical approach. Compr Ther 1994;20:402–409.

51. Hedley K, Tooley P, Williams H. Problems with clinical trials in general practice—a double-blind comparison of cream containing miconazole and hydrocortisone with hydrocortisone alone in the treatment of intertrigo. Br J Clin Pract 1990;44:131–135.

52. Janniger CK, Schwartz RA, Szepietowski JC, et al. Intertrigo and common secondary skin infections. Am Fam Physician 2005;72:833–838.

53. Krueger G, Ellis CN. Psoriasis—recent advances in understanding its pathogenesis and treatment. J Am Acad Dermatol 2005;53(1 Suppl 1):S94–S100.

54. Ortonne JP. Recent developments in the understanding of the pathogenesis of psoriasis. Br J Dermatol 1999;140(Suppl 54): 1–7.

55. Terui T, Ozawa M, Tagami H. Role of neutrophils in induction of acute inflammation in T cell–mediated immune dermatosis, psoriasis: a neutrophil-associated inflammation-boosting loop. Exp Dermatol 2000;9:1–10.

56. Rasmussen JE. The relationship between infection with group A beta hemolytic streptococci and the development of psoriasis. Pediatr Infect Dis J 2000;19:153–154.

57. Wolf R, Ruocco V. Triggered psoriasis. Adv Exp Med Biol 1999;455:221–225.

58. Farber EM, Nall L. Psoriasis: a stress-related disease. Cutis 1993;51:322–326.

59. Drew GS. Psoriasis. Prim Care 2000;27:385–406.

60. Lynch PJ, Edwards L. Red plaques with papulosquamous features. In: Lynch PJ, Edwards L (eds). Genital Dermatology. New York: Churchill Livingstone, 1994, pp 57–61.

61. Margesson LJ. Inflammatory diseases of the vulva. In: Fisher BK, Margesson LJ (eds). Genital Skin Disorders—Diagnosis and Treatment. St Louis: Mosby, 1998, pp 167–169.

62. Weinrauch L, Katz M. Psoriasis vulgaris of labium majus. Cutis 1986;38:333–334.

63. Fogh K, Kragballe K. Recent developments in vitamin D analogs. Curr Pharm Des 2000;6:961–972.

64. Smith KC, Lebwohl M. Topical antipsoriatics. Skin Therapy Lett 2000;5:1–2.

65. Scheinfeld N. The use of topical tacrolimus and pimecrolimus to treat psoriasis: a review. Dermatol Online J 2004;10:3.

66. Steele JA, Choi C, Kwong PC. Topical tacrolimus in the treatment of inverse psoriasis in children. J Am Acad Dermatol 2005;53:713–716.

67. Lebwohl M. A clinician's paradigm in the treatment of psoriasis. J Am Acad Dermatol 2005;53(1 Suppl 1):S59–S69.

68. Ashcroft DM, Li Wan PA, Griffiths CE. Therapeutic strategies for psoriasis. J Clin Pharm Ther 2000;25:1–10.

69. Koo JY. Current consensus and update on psoriasis therapy: a perspective from the U.S. J Dermatol 1999;26:723–733.

70. Funaro D. Lichen sclerosus: a review and practical approach. Dermatol Ther 2004;17:28–37.

71. Smith YR, Haefner HK. Vulvar lichen sclerosus: pathophysiology and treatment. Am J Clin Dermatol 2004;5:105–125.

72. Tasker GL, Wojnarowska F. Lichen sclerosus. Clin Exp Dermatol 2003;28:128–133.

73. Val I, Almeida G. An overview of lichen sclerosus. Clin Obstet Gynecol 2005;48:808–817.

74. Yesudian PD, Sugunendran H, Bates CM, et al. Lichen sclerosus. Int J STD AIDS 2005;16:465–473, test.

75. Powell J, Wojnarowska F. Childhood vulvar lichen sclerosus: an increasingly common problem. J Am Acad Dermatol 2001;44:803–806.

76. Powell JJ, Wojnarowska F. Lichen sclerosus. Lancet 1999;353: 1777–1783.

77. Wakelin SH, Marren P. Lichen sclerosus in women. Clin Dermatol 1997;15:155–169.

78. Wallace HJ. Lichen sclerosus et atrophicus. Trans St Johns Hosp Dermatol Soc 1971;57:9–30.

79. Ridley CM. Genital lichen sclerosus (lichen sclerosus et atrophicus) in childhood and adolescence. J R Soc Med 1993;86: 69–75.

80. Thomas RH, Ridley CM, McGibbon DH, et al. Anogenital lichen sclerosus in women. J R Soc Med 1996;89:694–698.

81. Cox NH, Mitchell JN, Morley WN. Lichen sclerosus et atrophicus in non-identical female twins. Br J Dermatol 1986; 115:743.

82. Powell J, Wojnarowska F, Winsey S, et al. Lichen sclerosus premenarche: autoimmunity and immunogenetics. Br J Dermatol 2000;142:481–484.

83. Sahn EE, Bluestein EL, Oliva S. Familial lichen sclerosus et atrophicus in childhood. Pediatr Dermatol 1994;11:160–163.

84. Gao XH, Barnardo MC, Winsey S, et al. The association between HLA DR, DQ antigens, and vulval lichen sclerosus in the UK: HLA DRB112 and its associated DRB112/DQB10301/04/09/010 haplotype confers susceptibility to vulval lichen sclerosus, and HLA DRB10301/04 and its associated DRB10301/04/DQB10201/02/03 haplotype protects from vulval lichen sclerosus. J Invest Dermatol 2005;125: 895–899.

85. Carlson JA, Grabowski R, Chichester P, et al. Comparative immunophenotypic study of lichen sclerosus: epidermotropic CD57+ lymphocytes are numerous—implications for pathogenesis. Am J Dermatopathol 2000;22:7–16.

86. Lukowsky A, Muche JM, Sterry W, et al. Detection of expanded T cell clones in skin biopsy samples of patients with lichen sclerosus et atrophicus by T cell receptor-gamma polymerase chain reaction assays. J Invest Dermatol 2000; 115:254–259.

87. Regauer S. Immune dysregulation in lichen sclerosus. Eur J Cell Biol 2005;84:273–277.

88. Tchorzewski H, Rotsztejn H, Banasik M, et al. The involvement of immunoregulatory T cells in the pathogenesis of lichen sclerosus. Med Sci Monit 2005;11:CR39–CR43.

89. Howard A, Dean D, Cooper S, et al. Circulating basement membrane zone antibodies are found in lichen sclerosus of the vulva. Australas J Dermatol 2004;45:12–15.

90. Oyama N, Chan I, Neill SM, et al. Autoantibodies to extracellular matrix protein 1 in lichen sclerosus. Lancet 2003;362: 118–123.

91. Meyrick Thomas RH, Ridley CM, Black MM. The association of lichen sclerosus et atrophicus and autoimmune-related disease in males. Br J Dermatol 1983;109:661–664.

92. Meyrick Thomas RH, Ridley CM, McGibbon DH, et al. Lichen sclerosus et atrophicus and autoimmunity—a study of 350 women. Br J Dermatol 1988;118:41–46.

93. Harrington CI, Dunsmore IR. An investigation into the incidence of auto-immune disorders in patients with lichen sclerosus and atrophicus. Br J Dermatol 1981;104:563–566.

94. Meffert JJ, Davis BM, Grimwood RE. Lichen sclerosus. J Am Acad Dermatol 1995;32:393–416.

95. Weide B, Walz T, Garbe C. Is morphoea caused by *Borrelia burgdorferi*? A review. Br J Dermatol 2000;142:636–644.

96. Farrell AM, Millard PR, Schomberg KH, et al. An infective aetiology for vulval lichen sclerosus re-addressed. Clin Exp Dermatol 1999;24:479–483.

97. Todd P, Halpern S, Kirby J, Pembroke A. Lichen sclerosus and the Kobner phenomenon. Clin Exp Dermatol 1994;19: 262–263.

98. Lynch PJ, Edwards L. White patches and plaques. In: Lynch PJ, Edwards L (eds). Genital Dermatology. New York: Churchill Livingstone, 1994, pp 149–158.

99. Margesson LJ. Pigmentary changes of the vulva. In: Fisher BK Margesson LJ (eds). Genital Skin Disorders—Diagnosis and Treatment. St Louis: Mosby, 1998, pp 189-193.

100. Ridley CM, Neill SM. Non-infective cutaneous conditions of the vulva. In: Ridley CM, Neill SM (eds). The Vulva, ed 2. London: Blackwell Science, 1999, pp 154–164.

101. Warrington SA, de San LC. Lichen sclerosus et atrophicus and sexual abuse. Arch Dis Child 1996;75:512–516.

102. Schulten EA, Starink TM, van der Waal I. Lichen sclerosus et atrophicus involving the oral mucosa: report of two cases. J Oral Pathol Med 1993;22:374–377.

103. Jaworsky C. Connective tissue diseases. In: Elder D, Elenitsas R, Jaworsky C, et al (eds). Lever's Histopathology of the Skin, ed 8. Philadelphia: Lippincott-Raven, 1997, pp 281–282.

104. Derrick EK, Ridley CM, Kobza-Black A, et al. A clinical study of 23 cases of female anogenital carcinoma. Br J Dermatol 2000;143:1217–1223.

105. Scurry JP, Vanin K. Vulvar squamous cell carcinoma and lichen sclerosus. Australas J Dermatol 1997;38(Suppl 1): S20–S25.

106. Hassanein AM, Mrstik ME, Hardt NS, et al. Malignant melanoma associated with lichen sclerosus in the vulva of a 10-year-old. Pediatr Dermatol 2004;21:473–476.

107. Wechter ME, Gruber SB, Haefner HK, et al. Vulvar melanoma: a report of 20 cases and review of the literature. J Am Acad Dermatol 2004;50:554–562.

108. Regauer S, Reich O, Beham-Schmid C. Monoclonal gamma-T-cell receptor rearrangement in vulvar lichen sclerosus and squamous cell carcinomas. Am J Pathol 2002;160:1035–1045.

109. Dalziel KL, Millard PR, Wojnarowska F. The treatment of vulval lichen sclerosus with a very potent topical steroid (clobetasol propionate 0.05%) cream. Br J Dermatol 1991;124: 461–464.

110. Lorenz B, Kaufman RH, Kutzner SK. Lichen sclerosus. Therapy with clobetasol propionate. J Reprod Med 1998;43: 790–794.

111. Diakomanolis ES, Haidopoulos D, Syndos M, et al. Vulvar lichen sclerosus in postmenopausal women: a comparative study for treating advanced disease with clobetasol propionate 0.05%. Eur J Gynaecol Oncol 2002; 23:519–522.

112. Cooper SM, Gao XH, Powell JJ, et al. Does treatment of vulvar lichen sclerosus influence its prognosis? Arch Dermatol 2004;140:702–706.

113. Renaud-Vilmer C, Cavelier-Balloy B, Porcher R, et al. Vulvar lichen sclerosus: effect of long-term topical application of a potent steroid on the course of the disease. Arch Dermatol 2004;140:709–712.

114. Sinha P, Sorinola O, Luesley DM. Lichen sclerosus of the vulva. Long-term steroid maintenance therapy. J Reprod Med 1999;44:621–624.

115. Fischer G, Rogers M. Treatment of childhood vulvar lichen sclerosus with potent topical corticosteroid. Pediatr Dermatol 1997;14:235–238.

116. Garzon MC, Paller AS. Ultrapotent topical corticosteroid treatment of childhood genital lichen sclerosus. Arch Dermatol 1999;135:525–528.

117. Mazdisnian F, Degregorio F, Mazdisnian F, et al. Intralesional injection of triamcinolone in the treatment of lichen sclerosus. J Reprod Med 1999;44:332–334.

118. Bornstein J, Heifetz S, Kellner Y, et al. Clobetasol dipropionate 0.05% versus testosterone propionate 2% topical application for severe vulvar lichen sclerosus. Am J Obstet Gynecol 1998;178:80–84.

119. Paslin D. Androgens in the topical treatment of lichen sclerosus. Int J Dermatol 1996;35:298–301.

120. Bousema MT, Romppanen U, Geiger JM, et al. Acitretin in the treatment of severe lichen sclerosus et atrophicus of the vulva: a double-blind, placebo-controlled study. J Am Acad Dermatol 1994;30:225–231.

121. Virgili A, Corazza M, Bianchi A, et al. Open study of topical 0.025% tretinoin in the treatment of vulvar lichen sclerosus. One year of therapy. J Reprod Med 1995;40:614–618.

122. Assmann T, Becker-Wegerich P, Grewe M, et al. Tacrolimus ointment for the treatment of vulvar lichen sclerosus. J Am Acad Dermatol 2003;48:935–937.

123. Bohm M, Frieling U, Luger TA, et al. Successful treatment of anogenital lichen sclerosus with topical tacrolimus. Arch Dermatol 2003;139:922–924.

124. Boms S, Gambichler T, Freitag M, et al. Pimecrolimus 1% cream for anogenital lichen sclerosus in childhood. BMC Dermatol 2004;4:14.

125. Bunker CB, Neill S, Staughton RC. Topical tacrolimus, genital lichen sclerosus, and risk of squamous cell carcinoma. Arch Dermatol 2004;140:1169.

126. Abramov Y, Elchalal U, Abramov D, et al. Surgical treatment of vulvar lichen sclerosus: a review. Obstet Gynecol Surv 1996;51:193–199.

127. Kartamaa M, Reitamo S. Treatment of lichen sclerosus with carbon dioxide laser vaporization. Br J Dermatol 1997;136: 356–359.

128. Bhattacharya M, Kaur I, Kumar B. Lichen planus: a clinical and epidemiological study. J Dermatol 2000;27:576–582.

129. Eisen D. The evaluation of cutaneous, genital, scalp, nail, esophageal, and ocular involvement in patients with oral lichen planus. Oral Surg Oral Med Oral Pathol Oral Radiol Endod 1999;88:431–436.

130. Bella Fiore P, DiFede O, Cabibi D, et al. Prevalence of Vulval Lichen Planus and A Cohort of Women with Oral Lichen Planus: An Interdisciplinary Study. Br J Dermatol 2006;155:994–998.

131. Boyd AS. New and emerging therapies for lichenoid dermatoses. Dermatol Clin 2000;18:21–29, vii.

132. Chaiyarit P, Kafrawy AH, Miles DA, et al. Oral lichen planus: an immunohistochemical study of heat shock proteins (HSPs) and cytokeratins (CKs) and a unifying hypothesis of pathogenesis. J Oral Pathol Med 1999;28: 210–215.

133. DeRossi SS, Ciarrocca KN. Lichen planus, lichenoid drug reactions, and lichenoid mucositis. Dent Clin North Am 2005;49:77–89, viii.

134. La NG, Cottoni F, Mulargia M, et al. HLA antigen distribution in different clinical subgroups demonstrates genetic heterogeneity in lichen planus. Br J Dermatol 1995;132: 897–900.

135. Ognjenovic M, Karelovic D, Mikelic M, et al. Oral lichen planus and HLA B. Coll Antropol 1998;(22 Suppl):93–96.

136. Setterfield JF, Neill S, Shirlaw PJ, et al. The vulvovaginal gingival syndrome: a severe subgroup of lichen planus with characteristic clinical features and a novel association with the class II HLA DQB1*0201 allele. J Am Acad Dermatol 2006;55:98–113.

137. Sugerman PB, Satterwhite K, Bigby M. Autocytotoxic T-cell clones in lichen planus. Br J Dermatol 2000;142:449–456.

138. Sugerman PB, Savage NW, Walsh LJ, et al. The pathogenesis of oral lichen planus. Crit Rev Oral Biol Med 2002;13: 350–365.

139. Thornhill MH. Immune mechanisms in oral lichen planus. Acta Odontol Scand 2001;59:174–177.

140. Singal A. Familial mucosal lichen planus in three successive generations. Int J Dermatol 2005;44:81–82.

141. Cooper SM, Prenter A, Allen J, et al. The basement membrane zone and dermal extracellular matrix in erosive lichen planus of the vulva: an immunohistochemical study demonstrating altered expression of hemidesmosome components and anchoring fibrils. Clin Exp Dermatol 2005; 30:277–281.

142. Laine J, Kalimo K, Happonen RP. Contact allergy to dental restorative materials in patients with oral lichenoid lesions. Contact Dermatitis 1997;36:141–146.

143. Russell MA, King LE Jr, Boyd AS. Lichen planus after consumption of a gold-containing liquor. N Engl J Med 1996; 334:603.

144. Yiannias JA, el-Azhary RA, Hand JH, et al. Relevant contact sensitivities in patients with the diagnosis of oral lichen planus. J Am Acad Dermatol 2000;42:177–182.

145. Chuang TY, Stitle L, Brashear R, et al. Hepatitis C virus and lichen planus: a case-control study of 340 patients. J Am Acad Dermatol 1999;41:787–789.

146. Fitzgerald E, Purcell SM, Goldman HM. Photodistributed hypertrophic lichen planus in association with acquired immunodeficiency syndrome: a distinct entity. Cutis 1995;55: 109–111.

147. Kirtschig G, Wakelin SH, Wojnarowska F. Mucosal vulval lichen planus: outcome, clinical and laboratory features. J Eur Acad Dermatol Venereol 2005;19:301–307.

148. Sanchez-Perez J, De Castro M, Buezo GF, et al. Lichen planus and hepatitis C virus: prevalence and clinical presentation of patients with lichen planus and hepatitis C virus infection. Br J Dermatol 1996;134:715–719.

149. Sanchez-Perez J, Moreno-Otero R, Borque MJ, et al. Lichen planus and hepatitis C virus infection: a clinical and virologic study. Acta Derm Venereol 1998;78:305–306.

150. Margesson LJ. Inflammatory diseases of the vulva. In: Fisher BK, Margesson LJ (eds). Genital Skin Disorders—Diagnosis and Treatment. St Louis: Mosby, 1998, pp 169–172.

151. Bermejo A, Bermejo MD, Roman P, et al. Lichen planus with simultaneous involvement of the oral cavity and genitalia. Oral Surg Oral Med Oral Pathol 1990;69:209–216.

152. Edwards L. Vulvar lichen planus. Arch Dermatol 1989;125: 1677–1680.

153. Eisen D. The vulvovaginal-gingival syndrome of lichen planus. The clinical characteristics of 22 patients. Arch Dermatol 1994;130:1379–1382.

154. Goldstein AT, Metz A. Vulvar lichen planus. Clin Obstet Gynecol 2005;48:818–823.

155. Lewis FM, Shah M, Harrington CI. Vulval involvement in lichen planus: a study of 37 women. Br J Dermatol 1996; 135:89–91.

156. Lewis FM. Vulval lichen planus. Br J Dermatol 1998;138: 569–575.

157. Mann MS, Kaufman RH. Erosive lichen planus of the vulva. Clin Obstet Gynecol 1991;34:605–613.

158. Moyal-Barracco M, Edwards L. Diagnosis and therapy of anogenital lichen planus. Dermatol Ther 2004;17:38–46.

159. Oates JK, Rowen D. Desquamative inflammatory vaginitis. A review. Genitourin Med 1990;66:275–279.

160. Pelisse M. The vulvo-vaginal-gingival syndrome. A new form of erosive lichen planus. Int J Dermatol 1989;28: 381–384.

161. Petruzzi M, De BM, Carriero C, et al. Oro-vaginal-vulvar lichen planus: report of two new cases. Maturitas 2005;50: 140–150.

162. Ramer MA, Altchek A, Deligdisch L, et al. Lichen planus and the vulvovaginal-gingival syndrome. J Periodontol 2003;74: 1385–1393.

163. Ridley CM. Chronic erosive vulval disease. Clin Exp Dermatol 1990;15:245–252.

164. Rogers RS III, Eisen D. Erosive oral lichen planus with genital lesions: the vulvovaginal-gingival syndrome and the peno-gingival syndrome. Dermatol Clin 2003;21:91, vii.

165. Soper DE, Patterson JW, Hurt WG, et al. Lichen planus of the vulva. Obstet Gynecol 1988;72:74–76.

166. Lynch PJ, Edwards L. Red plaques with papulosquamous features. In: Lynch PJ, Edwards L (eds). Genital Dermatology. New York: Churchill Livingstone, 1994, pp 63–72.

167. Ridley CM, Neill SM. Non-infective cutaneous conditions of the vulva. In: Ridley CM, Neill SM (eds). The Vulva, ed 2. London: Blackwell Science, 1999, pp 104–107.

168. Toussaint S, Kamino H. Non-infectious, erythematous, papular and squamous diseases. In: Elder D, Elenitsas R, Jaworsky C, et al (eds). Lever's Histopathology of the Skin, ed 8. Philadelphia: Lippincott-Raven, 1997, pp 166–172.

169. Connelly MG, Winkelmann RK. Coexistence of lichen sclerosus, morphea, and lichen planus. Report of four cases and review of the literature. J Am Acad Dermatol 1985;12: 844–851.

170. Marren P, Millard P, Chia Y, et al. Mucosal lichen sclerosus/lichen planus overlap syndromes. Br J Dermatol 1994;131: 118–123.

171. Dwyer CM, Kerr RE, Millan DW. Squamous carcinoma following lichen planus of the vulva. Clin Exp Dermatol 1995;20: 171–172.

172. Franck JM, Young AW Jr. Squamous cell carcinoma in situ arising within lichen planus of the vulva. Dermatol Surg 1995;21:890–894.

173. Lewis FM, Harrington CI. Squamous cell carcinoma arising in vulval lichen planus. Br J Dermatol 1994;131:703–705.

174. Cooper SM, Wojnarowska F. Influence of treatment of erosive lichen planus of the vulva on its prognosis. Arch Dermatol 2006;142:289–294.

175. Zaki I, Dalziel KL, Solomonsz FA, et al. The under-reporting of skin disease in association with squamous cell carcinoma of the vulva. Clin Exp Dermatol 1996;21:334–337.

176. Byrd JA, Davis MD, Rogers RS III. Recalcitrant symptomatic vulvar lichen planus: response to topical tacrolimus. Arch Dermatol 2004;140:715–720.

177. Jensen JT, Bird M, Leclair CM. Patient satisfaction after the treatment of vulvovaginal erosive lichen planus with topical clobetasol and tacrolimus: a survey study. Am J Obstet Gynecol 2004;190:1759–1763.

178. Kirtschig G, Van Der Meulen AJ, Ion Lipan JW, et al. Successful treatment of erosive vulvovaginal lichen planus with topical tacrolimus. Br J Dermatol 2002;147:625–626.

179. Lotery HE, Galask RP. Erosive lichen planus of the vulva and vagina. Obstet Gynecol 2003;101:1121–1125.

180. Vente C, Reich K, Rupprecht R, et al. Erosive mucosal lichen planus: response to topical treatment with tacrolimus. Br J Dermatol 1999;140:338–342.

181. Lonsdale-Eccles AA, Velangi S. Topical pimecrolimus in the treatment of genital lichen planus: a prospective case series. Br J Dermatol 2005;153:390–394.

182. Laurberg G, Geiger JM, Hjorth N, et al. Treatment of lichen planus with acitretin. A double-blind, placebo-controlled study in 65 patients. J Am Acad Dermatol 1991;24:434–437.

183. Lear JT, English JS. Erosive and generalized lichen planus responsive to azathioprine. Clin Exp Dermatol 1996;21:56–57.

184. Woo TY. Systemic isotretinoin treatment of oral and cutaneous lichen planus. Cutis 1985;35:385–391, 393.

185. Becherel PA, Chosidow O, Boisnic S, et al. Topical cyclosporine in the treatment of oral and vulvar erosive lichen planus: a blood level monitoring study. Arch Dermatol 1995;131: 495–496.

186. Borrego L, Ruiz-Rodriguez R, de Ortiz FJ, et al. Vulvar lichen planus treated with topical cyclosporine. Arch Dermatol 1993;129:794.

187. Jemec GB, Baadsgaard O. Effect of cyclosporine on genital psoriasis and lichen planus. J Am Acad Dermatol 1993;29: 1048–1049.

188. Pigatto PD, Chiappino G, Bigardi A, et al. Cyclosporin A for treatment of severe lichen planus. Br J Dermatol 1990;122: 121–123.

189. Nylander LE, Wahlin YB, Hofer PA. Methotrexate supplemented with steroid ointments for the treatment of severe erosive lichen ruber. Acta Derm Venereol 2002;82:63–64.

190. Eisen D. Hydroxychloroquine sulfate (Plaquenil) improves oral lichen planus: an open trial. J Am Acad Dermatol 1993;28:609–612.

191. Poskitt L, Wojnarowska F. Minimizing cicatricial pemphigoid orodynia with minocycline. Br J Dermatol 1995;132: 784–789.

192. Sawai T, Kitazawa K, Danno K, et al. Pemphigus vegetans with oesophageal involvement: successful treatment with minocycline and nicotinamide. Br J Dermatol 1995;132: 668–670.

193. Buyuk AY, Kavala M. Oral metronidazole treatment of lichen planus. J Am Acad Dermatol 2000;43:260–262.

194. Wahba-Yahav AV. Idiopathic lichen planus: treatment with metronidazole. J Am Acad Dermatol 1995;33:301–302.

195. Camisa C, Popovsky JL. Effective treatment of oral erosive lichen planus with thalidomide. Arch Dermatol 2000;136: 1442–1443.

196. Popovsky JL, Camisa C. New and emerging therapies for diseases of the oral cavity. Dermatol Clin 2000;18:113–125.

CHAPTER 18

Vulvar Intraepithelial Neoplasia

Alex Ferenczy

KEY POINTS

- Current terminology divides vulvar intraepithelial neoplasia (VIN) into: human papillomavirus (HPV)-related, usually poorly differentiated basalo-warty type (formerly VIN grade 2,3), and HPV-unrelated, differentiated type.
- VIN 1 is no longer included in the terminology because it corresponds to flat condyloma.
- HPV-related VIN is more frequent than the HPV-unrelated form. It occurs in younger women and carries the risk factors that are typical of high-risk (oncogenic) cervical HPV infections.
- HPV-unrelated lesions are associated with vulvar dermatoses (squamous cell hyperplasia, lichen sclerosus) and occur in elderly women with a long-term history of itch-scratch cycles.
- Both HPV-related and unrelated VIN have the potential to develop into invasive squamous cell cancer; those developing in the elderly are histologically well-differentiated, keratinizing type; are discovered at an advanced stage; and have significantly poorer survival rates than their histologically poorly differentiated counterparts that originate from HPV-related VIN.
- A multitude of medical and surgical therapies are available for symptomatic, HPV-related VIN, all of which are associated with high rates of recurrence and necessitate multiple attempts to achieve cure.
- The ideal treatment of HPV-unrelated VIN simplex is the use of topical high-potency steroids that treat the underlying vulvar dermatosis and avoids the itch-scratch cycles.
- Prophylactic vaccination with HPV 16, 18 types containing VLP-L1 vaccines will likely prevent the majority of HPV-related VIN lesions.
- HPV-unrelated VIN is best prevented by treating the underlying dermatosis with topical high-potency steroids and genital hygiene.

Since the first report in 1922 of "squamous cell carcinoma *in situ*" of the vulva by French authors Hudelo, Boulanger-Pilet, and Cailliau, the disease has become of increasing clinical, pathologic, therapeutic, and investigative interest.[1] During the past few years, its histologic classification and nomenclature have undergone evolutionary change, and our understanding of its pathogenic development and its relationship with human papillomavirus infection (HPV), as well as our therapeutic approach, have changed dramatically.

In 1987 the Committee on Nomenclature of the International Society for the Study of Vulvar Disease (ISSVD) and the Committee on Histological Classification of Vulvar Tumors and Dystrophies of the International Society of Gynecological Pathologists recommended the use of the unifying generic term *squamous intraepithelial neoplasia of the vulva* or *vulvar intraepithelial neoplasia* (VIN).[2] Accordingly, VIN has replaced a myriad of traditional and often confusing terms such as *leukoplakia, Bowen's disease, Bowenoid papulosis, Bowenoid dysplasia, Bowenoid atypia, erythroplasia of Queyrat, carcinoma simplex, squamous cell carcinoma in situ,* and *hyperplastic dystrophy with severe atypia*. By definition, VIN must be made of neoplastic cells confined to the boundaries of the squamous epithelium. It may regress either spontaneously or after incomplete surgical removal, persist, or progress to invasive carcinoma if untreated.

The Committee on Histological Classification of Vulvar Tumors and Dystrophies and the Committee on Nomenclature of the ISSVD further recommended grading VIN into 1 (mild dysplasia), 2 (moderate dysplasia) and 3 (severe dysplasia to carcinoma *in situ*).[3] *The recommended grading of VIN was based solely on the height of the cellular abnormalities within the squamous epithelium;* in other words; VIN is graded 1 if only the lower third is involved, graded 2 if the lower half is affected, and graded 3 if it contains abnormal cells in the lower two thirds to the full thickness of the epithelium. This grading system has been extrapolated from that applied to the nonkeratinizing squamous epithelium of the cervix.

Unfortunately, there are several problems with extrapolating the grading VIN from its cervical counterpart. First, the vulvar skin is morphologically different from its cervical counterpart in both health and disease. Second, cancer pathogenesis in the vulva is different from that of the cervix. Third, our current understanding of cervical intraepithelial neoplasia (CIN) is more compatible with a two-grade classification system (low- and high-grade CIN)[4] than a three-grade continuum. At best, *VIN could be classified as low and high grade. However, there has been no compelling epidemiologic, pathologic, and virologic evidence to support either the existence or relationship of low-grade to high-grade VIN.* Indeed, although the natural history of the so-called VIN 3 lesion is relatively well known, that of VIN 1 is not. Virtually all studies on the clinical, biological, and morphologic characteristics of VIN have focused on VIN 3. *Not a single scientific publication in the literature describes the natural history of VIN 1 (and for that matter, VIN 2) as being part of a VIN 1–3 "continuum."* Histologically, VIN 1 is a flat condyloma with or without koilocytosis, and colposcopically the lesion often presents as multifocal, slightly elevated acetowhite lesions (Figures 18-1 and 18-2). Such lesions are devoid of nuclear aneuploidy and abnormal mitotic figures that characterize VIN 2,3 lesions. In one study, HPV tracing with polymerase chain reaction technology showed low-risk HPV in 22 of 33 (67%) of VIN 1 lesions, mainly 6 or 11 (42%), and the remainder contained high-risk types.[5] However, only 6% have HPV 16 as compared with 10.1% of high-risk HPV types found in VIN 3, of which 91% are of the HPV 16 type. Also, VIN 1 more frequently contains multiple HPV types (21%), as opposed to only 12% in VIN 3.

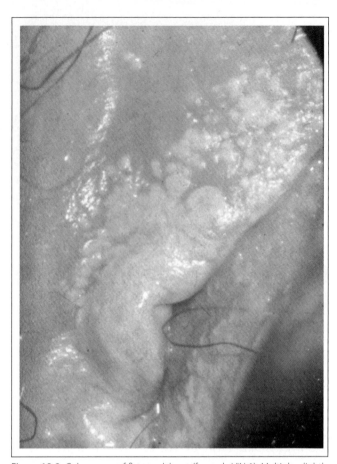

Figure 18-2 Colposcopy of flat condyloma (formerly VIN 1). Multiple, slightly elevated, acetowhite lesions are located on the labia minora. HPV genotyping of one of the lesions revealed type 6.

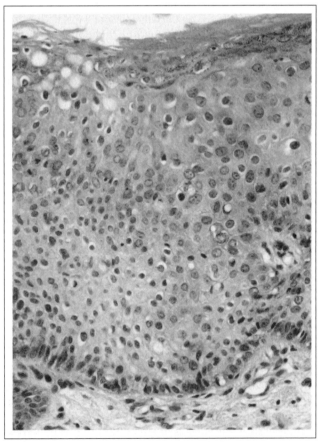

Figure 18-1 Histology of flat condyloma (formerly VIN 1). The lesion is acanthotic and contains occasional mildly atypical cells and surface hyperkeratosis.

The findings indicate that flat lesions designated as VIN 1 are distinct from VIN 3 with respect to their viral content, arguing against their potential to progress to VIN 3. Although occasional reports refer to VIN 1 as pre-existing (4 cases) or associated with invasive squamous cell carcinoma of the vulva, they invariably refer to women with a median age of 71 years old.[6] As will be shown later in this chapter, such women share no clinical, demographic, or morphologic similarities to their younger counterparts who have typical, HPV-related VIN lesions. At best, VIN 1 is a risk indicator for developing VIN 2,3.

The drawback of the artificial creation of the VIN 1,2,3 classification scheme forces pathologists to make a VIN 1 diagnosis whenever they come across vulvar specimens that contain atypical cells in the lower third of an otherwise normal or hyperplastic squamous epithelium. Such alterations can be seen in a variety of dermatologic conditions, most of which have no relationship to vulvar squamous cell neoplasia (Table 18-1). In a review process by expert pathologists, 10% of VIN 1 diagnosed by a commercial laboratory was downgraded to negative.[7] The clinical implication of diagnosing VIN 1 as being part of the traditional VIN 1–3 continuum is twofold: (1) patients are wrongfully told they may have a sexually transmitted disease, which in turn may lead to psychosexual distress; and

Table 18-1 Vulvar Conditions Referred to as Vulvar Intraepithelial Neoplasia 1

Squamous epithelial hyperplasia
Lichen simplex chronicus
Lichen sclerosus
Hyperplastic dystrophy with atypia
Lichen sclerosus/squamous cell hyperplasia with atypia of repair
Lichen planus
Psoriasis
Seborrheic keratosis
Candidiasis
Micropapillomatosis labialis
Seborrheic/contact dermatitis
Flat/papular condylomata
Acuminate condylomata
Keratosis
Vulvar vestibulitis

(2) they may be inappropriately treated, often using ablative and/or excisional methods. For example, a young patient with labial micropapillomatosis or vulvovaginitis due to candidiasis diagnosed as VIN 1 may be inappropriately treated with ablative or even excisional techniques. The worst-case scenario is when young women are subjected to topical 5% 5-FU (Efudex) cream treatment for so-called VIN 1. This may result in adverse events such as severe burning pain associated with extensive epithelial erosions and ulcerations, which, if untreated, may result in scarring and kraurosis vulvae based on personal observations.

Disease classifications are meaningful if they are related to pathogenesis, are diagnostically reproducible, and have implications for management. *According to the currently accumulated data, the ISSVD rightly proposed abolishing the three-tiered grading of HPV-related, basalo-warty VIN, deleting VIN 1 and combing VIN 2 and 3 into VIN.*[8] As a result, *there are now two vulvar cancer precursors based on their morphologic manifestations, clinical characteristics, and HPV content.*[9] One is the so-called HPV-related, basalo-warty VIN referred to as usual type (VIN-u), and the other is the HPV-unrelated VIN 3 differentiated type or VIN-d. VIN-u is characterized histologically by an abnormal epithelial growth exhibiting lack of or impaired cell maturation throughout the epithelium, nuclear aneuploidy, and abnormal mitotic figures. When the lesion is made of a uniform, undifferentiated basal cell–type population, the lesion is referred to as "basaloid" VIN, whereas when it contains highly pleomorphic cell population with individual cell keratinization, multinucleation, and warty/verrucous and hyperkeratinized surface pattern, the lesion is classified as "warty" VIN[7]

(Figures 18-3 and 18-4). In most cases, the two patterns coexist. *From a clinical viewpoint it is not important to distinguish between these two forms of VIN because both are produced by high-risk HPV DNA types 16 and 18* and, less frequently, by other high-oncogenic-risk HPV DNA variants such as 33, 35, 51, 52, and 68.[5,10] *VIN-u tends to occur in younger women (mean age 30 years) and, in most cases, is associated with the same demographic, behavioral patterns, and high-risk HPV positivity rates seen in women with high-grade CIN.* History of multiple sex partners and early onset of sexual activity is typical of these women. Immunosuppression and smoking may be greater risk factors for VIN than for CIN. For example, immunosuppressed women who are human immunodeficiency virus (HIV) positive, those with organ transplants, and those with aplastic (Fanconi) anemia carry a 16-, 100-, and 4000-fold relative risk for developing vulvar neoplasia, repectively.[11,12] *VIN is associated with smoking in 50% to 80% of cases, with an odds ratio (OR) of 8.3.*[13] As in the cervical cancer model, it is likely that high-risk HPV must be integrated into the host cell genome for progression of VIN to invasion. In one study, integration of HPV 16 and 18 DNA into host-cell chromosomes was observed in 30% of 21 HPV 16/18–positive VIN cases.[10] In one case-controlled study, HPV-16 seropositivity was associated with a 3.6- to 13-fold higher relative risk for developing VIN compared with HPV 16–seronegative women.[14]

The most common symptoms of VIN-u are pruritus and burning discomfort, which occur in about 50% of cases. *The definite diagnosis is made by histology.* Although colposcopy does not add much to the clinical impression, it helps to better define the limits of the lesion and can pinpoint small satellite and multifocal lesions that can escape naked-eye examination (Figure 18-5). Also, foci of possible early invasion can be detected. In such cases, if the lesional area is not hyperkeratinized, it contains abnormal vessels that are either growing horizontally or present as irregularly irregular, coarse mosaic and/or punctation patterns (see Figure 18-5). *In addition, because VIN-u is often associated with high-grade CIN, colposcopy of the cervix is mandatory in these women.* Typically, basalo-warty VIN tends to be multifocal and multicentric with involvement of the perianal skin and cervical epithelium in approximately 50% of cases. A recent meta-analysis of 3322 cases of VIN 3 found only 1.2% regression rates, 41% of which occurred during or soon after delivery.[15]

PROGRESSION TO INVASION

The progressive potential of VIN-u is controversial (Figures 18-6 and 18-7). According to some researchers, 80% of never-treated VIN progresses to invasion.[16] Fortunately, in the majority of such cases (70%), dermal invasion does not exceed 1 mm deep (Stage IA), the lymph nodes are negative, and mortality is rare. However, *a meta-analysis of 3322 cases of VIN 3 found only 215 (6.4%) of lesions progressed to cancer irrespective of their treatment history.*[18–20] The author shares the same experience of relatively low rates

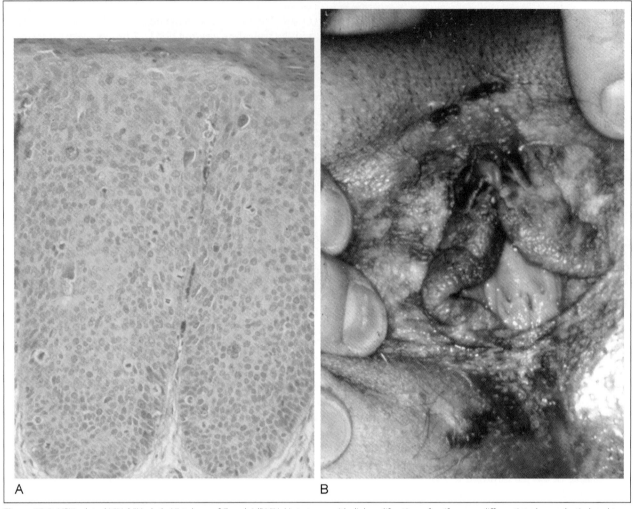

Figure 18-3 HPV-related VIN (VIN-u). **A,** Histology of "basaloid" VIN. Note transepithelial proliferation of uniform, undifferentiated, neoplastic basal-type cells containing numerous mitotic figures. **B,** Clinical appearance of "pigmented" basaloid VIN involving mainly the nonhairy skin of the vulva. Thickened, whitish, brownish epithelium with satellite lesions on pubis.

of progression.[17] One explanation for this discrepancy may be histologic misclassification of pseudoinvasion on tangentially-sectioned slides. Indeed, in such cases, the exuberant, interbranching rete pegs typical of VIN-u may be mistaken for invasion (Figure 18-8). Immunosuppression has been suggested to be a risk factor for progression of VIN-u to invasive vulvar cancer.[11,18,19]

MANAGING HUMAN PAPILLOMAVIRUS–RELATED VULVAR INTRAEPITHELIAL NEOPLASIA

Several options exist for the treatment of VIN-u. Unfortunately, none provide guarantee for cure. In fact, treating VIN is frustrating to both the patient and healthcare provider, as all treatment modalities are associated with high failure and recurrence rates. As a result, most treatment methods are repeated an average of five times before the

clinician decides whether to continue therapy or simply follow the patient at regular intervals without further treatment. *The two major reasons for high failure or recurrence rates after treatment are failure to include all satellite lesions in the treatment field and re-activation of latent HPV DNA in vulvar skin adjacent or at a distance to lesional epithelium.*[13] However, it is noteworthy that therapy is not mandatory in asymptomatic and compliant patients.[17] Those who are symptomatic or request treatment are offered topical medical therapies, surgical interventions, or both. Of course, conservative therapy cannot be undertaken without ruling out invasion through multiple or extended biopsies and should not be offered to a patient who is not reliable to return for long-term follow-up.

Medical Therapies

All medical therapies are off-label use or experimental (Table 18-2). *Five percent 5-FU (Efudex) cream* is a pyrimidine analogue that inhibits DNA synthesis. It was used extensively through

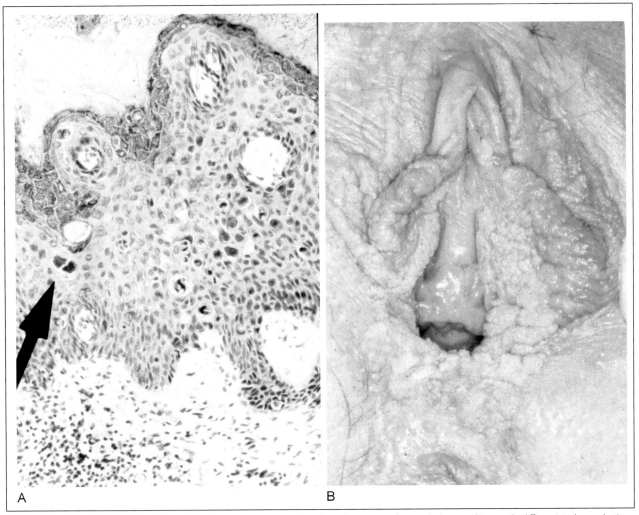

Figure 18-4 HPV-related VIN (VIN-u). **A,** Histology of "warty" VIN. Papillary, hyperkeratotic surface and pleomorphic, poorly differentiated, neoplastic squamous cells. *Arrow* points to a "corps rond," and there are several abnormal mitotic figures *(lower middle)*. **B,** The entire nonhairy skin of labia minora is replaced by confluent, hyperkeratotic, warty lesions resembling condylomata acuminata. Biopsy, however, showed warty VIN shown in **A**.

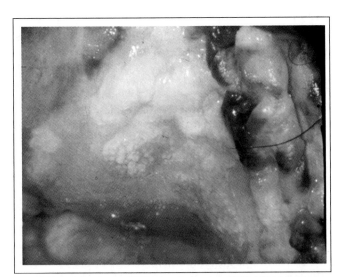

Figure 18-5 Colposcopy of HPV-related, pigmented VIN (VIN-u). Following application of 3–5% acetic acid solution, the true extent of lesional epithelium is visualized in the introitus.

the 1980s in the form of 5% cream.[21] However, treatment regimens have not been standardized, no randomized controlled trials have ever been published, and cure rates have varied from 20% to 80% with an average of 40%. Adverse events can be devastating and include painful erosions with delayed (up to years) healing and, eventually, extensive scarring of the vulvar skin and introitus, occasionally leading to kraurosis vulvae. *5-FU has been largely abandoned as a treatment option.*

Bleomycin and *dinitrochlorobenzene* have been tried in rare, desperate cases with severe side effects including tissue necrosis. Neither is used or recommended for treating VIN.

Photodynamic therapy (PDT) uses either systemic or topical application of a photosensitizing molecule such as 5-aminolevulinic acid (5-AA). This accumulates preferentially in neoplastic cells. With appropriate illumination, 5-AA is converted to protoporphyrin IX, which in turn produces oxygen-induced cell necrosis and some degree of immunomodulation. PDT response rates in uncontrolled

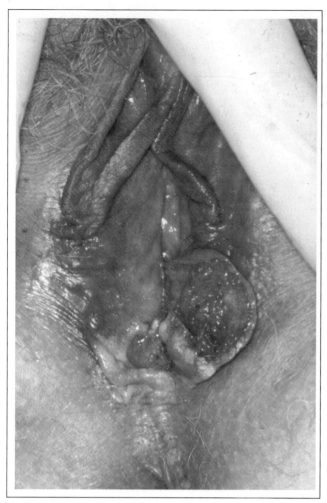

Figure 18-6 Basalo-warty VIN (VIN-u) and invasive carcinoma. A 37-year-old woman who has been a heavy smoker for the past 20 years has an indurated ulcer in the posterior left labia minora. Wide excision showed an invasive, nonkeratinizing squamous cell carcinoma with 5 mm of dermal invasion.

studies range from 0% to 70%, and recurrences occur approximately in 50% of cases.[22–25]

Retinoids stimulate cell differentiation and secretion of transforming growth factor. There are only a few reports on topical application of retinoic acid, none of which were randomized, and most are combined with interferons or cidofovir, precluding determination of which (if any) of the compounds are actually successful.[26,27]

Interferons (IFNs) have antiviral, antiproliferative, and antiangiogenic effects. They can be applied topically subcutaneously (Intron-A). In one prospective, randomized, double-blind crossover study, 14 of 18 (77%) patients demonstrated a partial response to IFN versus a control group using 1% nonoxynol-9 gel. In the same study, however, two cases of invasive carcinoma were discovered, presumably because of the failure to rule out invasive disease prior to enrollment.[28]

Imiquimod 5% cream is a powerful immune system modulator that induces multiple proinflammatory cytokines including IFNs, tumor necrosis factor (TNF), and interleukins. Imiquimod successfully treats external genital warts

(EGWs).[29] Several studies have been published on treatment results with self-applied imiquimod (Aldara) for VIN.[30–35] As with other topical medical therapies, complete response rates vary between 13% and 100%, and partial response rates are between 30% and 50%. However, the number of cases in each study was small and studies were uncontrolled with variable lengths of follow-up. The main problem with 5% imiquimod self-therapy is limited compliance with long-term (16-week) therapy because of severe burning discomfort. In the experience of the author and that of others,[33] most patients tolerate only a once-weekly dose; this is particularly true for patients with fair complexions. Admittedly, a well-designed, multicenter, randomized controlled trial on a large number of patients with VIN-u is needed prior to recommending this form of treatment, as opposed to physician-administered therapy.

Cidofovir is an acyclic nucleotide phosphonate derivative with broad-spectrum antiviral (DNA) activity. It is the only topical, specifically antiviral product currently available for treating precancerous or condylomatous lesions of the lower genital tract and upper aerodigestive tract (respiratory papillomatosis). Unfortunately, cidofovir is very expensive and is difficult to obtain for treating cutaneous lesions. Cidofovir-treated lesional areas undergo necrosis without alterations of normal, adjacent skin, and as with imiquimod, pain limits compliance. In one pilot study of 12 patients, topical self-application of 1% cidofovir gel every other day for as long as 16 weeks resulted in disease clearance in four of eight patients, but the other four failed to respond or their latent HPV persisted. One of the four patients was discovered to have invasive cancer.[36]

The *phytochemical indol-3-carbinol (I3C)* is found abundantly in cruciferous vegetables such as broccoli and cabbage. It promotes cell death by stimulating apoptosis (individual cell death) and inhibits estrogen-promoted growth. I3C and particularly its metabolite diindolymethane (DIM) prevent the development of cervical cancer in HPV-16 transgenic mice.[37] It is mainly used in patients with juvenile onset of recurrent respiratory papillomatosis. Administration is 200 mg orally daily for 6 months.[38] There have been anecdotal reports of I3C use in a few patients with VIN.

Surgical Therapies

Surgical therapies are presented in Table 18-3. The most often used modalities for a lesion of limited size are CO_2 laser vaporization and local wide excision. Other modalities that are generally successful but used less often are electroexcision, fulguration, or both.[39] For extensive lesions, skinning vulvectomy with or without skin graft and even simple vulvectomy are performed.[17] Cryotherapy and diathermy ablation or excision are seldom used. Recurrence rates range from 12% to a more realistic 50%, irrespective of treatment modality used.[19,40–42] Most lesions that recur will do so within 3 months after treatment. *Recurrences are still reported in 17% of patients in whom surgical excisional specimens were reported negative compared with 47% with positive margins,[15] so negative surgical margins are no guarantee of cure.*

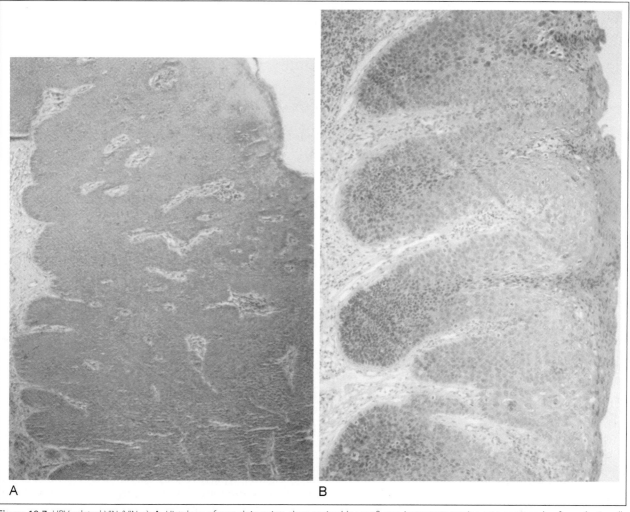

Figure 18-7 HPV-related VIN (VIN-u). **A,** Histology of pseudoinvasion characterized by confluent, interanastomosing rete pegs made of neoplastic cells mimicking early invasive cancer. **B,** Following reorientation of the specimen in the laboratory, the intraepithelial nature of the lesion is obvious.

An alternative to surgical procedures under general anesthesia for extensive, confluent VIN-u is to use either CO_2 *laser vaporization or electrofulguration to ablate one quadrant at a time under local anesthesia* (see Figure 18-8). Once healing has occurred (generally by 8 weeks), a second quadrant is treated until the entire lesion is removed. Curiously, if all surgical lines have been carefully included in the treatment field, the treated area is repaired by normal epithelium. In the experience of the author, complete response rates on the order of 75% have been obtained in 20 patients with an average follow-up of 3 years.[39] In those with early recurrences, *rescue* therapy with 5% imiquimod home therapy is given with approximately 50% complete response rates (personal observation). However, follow-up is too short for generalized recommendations.

Therapeutic Human Papillomavirus Vaccines

As suggested previously, one of the prerequisites for HPV-related squamous cell carcinogenesis is viral integration into the host cell chromosomes. This in turn is followed by destruction of normal growth control mechanisms via inhibition of tumor suppressor genes p53 and Rb protein by viral oncogenes E6 and E7, respectively. Therefore therapeutic vaccines must be manufactured to elicit cell-mediated immunity to HPV E6 and/or E7 oncogenes. One of the therapeutic vaccine candidates uses fused, recombinant vaccinia virus HPV 16/18-E7. A phase II study showed 50% or more reduction of disease in 8 of 12 patients, whose viral load either decreased or cleared.[43] In another study, HPV 16/18 E6/E7 containing vaccine delivered by skin abrasion produced complete response in 1 of 12 patients and decreased lesion size in 10 of 12 patients. However, improvement of symptoms did not occur.[44] In a nonrandomized, phase II, prime-boost vaccine trial using three doses of a recombinant fusion protein containing HPV 16, E6/E7/L2 (TA-CIN), followed by one dose of vaccinia virus producing HPV 16 and 18 E6/E7 (TA-HPV), one complete response and five partial responses were seen in 27 women with HPV-related VIN.[45] Admittedly, much more refinement in therapeutic vaccine

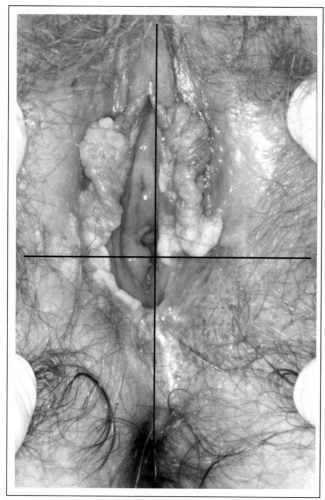

Figure 18-8 Vulvar "quadrectomization." Only one quadrant of this HPV-related lesion is ablated at a time under local anesthesia. Following healing of the treated area, another quadrant is ablated until all four quadrants have been treated. This approach prevents treatment under general anesthesia and excessive postoperative discomfort.

Table 18-2 Medical Treatments for HPV–Related VIN

5% 5-Fluorouracil cream
Retinoids
Bleomycin
Dinitrochlorobenzene
Photodynamic therapy
Interferons
Imiquimod 5% cream
Cidofovir 1%
Indol-3-carbinol
HPV vaccines

HPV, Human papillomavirus; *VIN,* vulvar intraepithelial neoplasia

Table 18-3 Surgical Therapies

Wide excision
Simple vulvectomy
Skinning vulvectomy with or without skin graft
Laser vaporization/excision
Electroexcision/fulguration
Cryotherapy

research is needed to consider this theoretically highly attractive method of therapy as the solution for treatment of VIN-u. In the interim, a number of large, randomized, controlled trials have been completed with prophylactic HPV vaccines containing types 6/11/16/18 L1 VLP given intramuscularly in three doses in women aged 15 to 26 years.[46] *Compared with the placebo group, the vaccine group demonstrated 100% efficacy in preventing VIN 2,3, even in those patients who violated the protocol (intent to treat).* Therefore it is likely that, ultimately, universal vaccination will hold greater promise than treatment in the prevention of VIN.

HUMAN PAPILLOMAVIRUS–UNRELATED, DIFFERENTIATED VULVAR INTRAEPITHELIAL NEOPLASIA (VIN-d)

The HPV-unrelated, differentiated VIN simplex lesion contains nuclear atypia involving only the lower third or sometimes even only the basal cell layer of the squamous epithelium. The cytonuclear atypia seen in such lesions is similar to that seen in repair-related atypia. The upper two thirds of the epithelium contains no abnormal cellular features (Figure 18-9, *A* and *B*). Because of its extremely well-differentiated morphologic presentation, the term *simplex* has been suggested by some and *differentiated* by others.[47–52] Similar alterations are observed in the epithelium of well-differentiated, keratinizing squamous cell carcinomas of the oral cavity and particularly in lip carcinomas. In most instances, the diagnosis is made *incidentally* when it is associated with invasive disease and when histologic continuity within atypical basal cells and foci of invasion is demonstrated (Figure 18-10, *A* and *B*).

Unlike its HPV-related counterpart, VIN-d simplex occurs in older women, most of whom are older than 70 years and lack the behavioral and demographic risk factors of those observed with basaloid and warty forms of cancer.[48,50,53] Also, VIN-d tends to be unifocal and unicentric and is unrelated to HPV infection. Rather, its pathogenic background may be related to *chronic itch-scratch cycles that are associated with squamous cell hyperplasia (lichen simplex chronicus) and lichen sclerosus.*[54] Release of unidentified carcinogenic agents together with the local environment of the chronically irritated and inflamed skin may play a major role in the

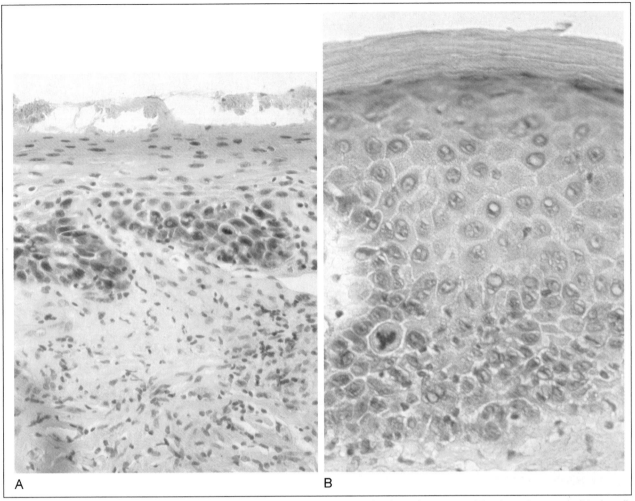

Figure 18-9 HPV-unrelated differentiated VIN (VIN-d). **A,** Histology showing that, other than hyperchromatic nuclei and prominent nucleoli in the cells of the basal/parabasal layers, cohesion and cellular organization are intact, as is cellular differentiation in the upper layers. **B,** High-magnification photomicrograph of an abnormal, tripolar mitotic figure in one of the neoplastic parabasal cells *(lower left).*

development of intraepithelial and ultimately invasive, well-differentiated, keratinizing squamous cell carcinoma of the vulva in the elderly.[55] It has been suggested that an alteration in the p53 tumor suppressor gene may be key in the pathogenesis of VIN-d and progression to invasive carcinoma.[56] In VIN-d, overexpression of p53 can be demonstrated by immunohistochemistry in a transepithelial distribution, whereas it is confined to the lower third of the epithelium in the adjacent lichen simplex chronicus or lichen sclerosus (Figure 18-11, *A* and *B*). The findings can also be used to distinguish between the two conditions in routine diagnostic pathology. *Of note, women with symptomatic lichen simplex chronicus or lichen sclerosus who are treated with high-potency topical corticosteroids rarely, if ever, progress to invasive squamous cell carcinoma.*[54] On the other hand, about 80% of the invasive squamous cell carcinomas in the elderly are associated with untreated, long-standing, symptomatic lichen simplex chronicus/squamous cell hyperplasia/lichen sclerosus[57] (see Figure 18-10, *A*).

If it is true that invasive squamous cell carcinomas of the vulva have two different pathogenic characteristics, then logically the nomenclature should reflect their distinctive features. Consequently, it is time to consider a revision of the current classification of vulvar cancer precursors (Table 18-4). The advantage of the proposed classification is that it is based on morphology and currently emerging clinical and virologic data with respect to the two pathogenic origins and pathways of squamous cell cancers and their precursors of the vulvar skin. Furthermore, the classification can be related to management schemes. It appears that treating rather than following women with vulvar cancer precursors is the appropriate approach. This is likely to reduce the risk of progression to invasion. *The basaloid and warty forms are best treated with ablative and/or excisional techniques, whereas the precursors of the VIN-d variant, squamous cell hyperplasia, and lichen sclerosus seem to respond well to topical application of potent corticosteroid preparations* or topical pro-apoptotic, nonsteroidal anti-inflammatory products

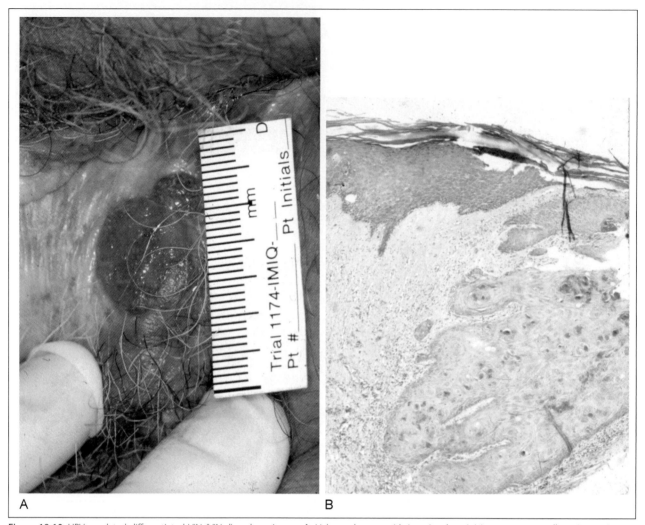

Figure 18-10 HPV-unrelated differentiated VIN (VIN-d) and carcinoma. **A,** Lichen sclerosus with invasive, keratinizing squamous cell carcinoma in a 73-year-old woman. **B,** Histology of HPV-unrelated VIN-d *(left)* adjacent to well-differentiated, keratinizing squamous cells.

such as 0.1% tacrolimus. Future therapeutics for the basaloid/warty VIN lesions may include immune response modifiers such as topical 5% imiquimod or specific antiviral preparations targeting the putative HPV DNA. There is great interest in the efficacy results of the recently Food and Drug Administration–approved prophylactic HPV vaccine 6/11/16/18 L1-VLP (Gardasil), which shows 100% effectiveness in preventing HPV-related VIN in young adult women aged 15 to 26 years.[46]

It is critical to correlate clinical symptoms and signs with histology prior to embarking on any form of therapy. If clinicians are not experienced in this area, referral of patients to colleagues with expertise in gynecologic dermatology may be helpful. The clinical behavior of invasive carcinoma developing from HPV-unrelated versus HPV-related VIN is also different. *The former tends to present with deep invasion and advanced clinical stage including lymph node metastasis (40% stage III), and 5-year survival rates are between 25% and 50% in women with stage III-IV disease. On the other hand, HPV-related invasive cancers tend to be diagnosed in their early stages, I and II, and survival rates are excellent.* Overall, the difference

in prognosis is due at least partly to the fact that women with VIN-u are much younger and seek medical attention much earlier than their elderly counterparts with VIN-d.

SUMMARY

According to current concepts, there are two forms of vulvar cancer precursors: HPV-related VIN-u and HPV-unrelated VIN-d. The former manifests morphologically either as basaloid, warty, or a mixture of both. It occurs in younger women, and both histologic types are caused by high-risk (oncogenic) HPV types, mainly type 16. VIN-u is the precursor of nonkeratinizing basaloid and warty squamous cell carcinomas of the vulvar skin. VIN-d is referred to as *differentiated VIN (VIN-d)*. It occurs in elderly women and evolves from long-standing, symptomatic vulvar dermatoses such as squamous cell hyperplasia or lichen sclerosus. It is the precursor of well-differentiated, keratinizing squamous cell carcinoma of the vulva. It is no longer necessary to subdivide morphologically HPV-related VIN-u into low-

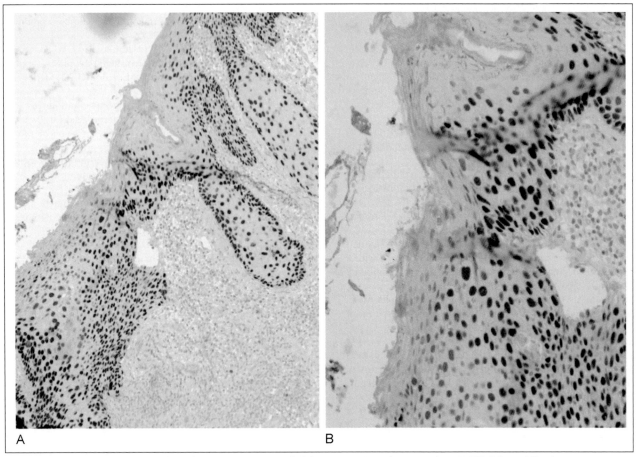

Figure 18-11 *HPV-unrelated VIN (VIN-d).* **A,** There is strong, transepithelial immunostaining for mutated p53 in VIN-d *(lower left),* whereas immunostaining is limited to the basal/parabasal layer of adjacent squamous cell hyperplasia without atypia *(upper right).* **B,** Detailed view of junctional area between VIN-d and squamous cell hyperplasia.

Table 18-4 Proposed Classification of Vulvar Squamous Cell Carcinoma Precursors

HPV-Related VIN-u
undifferentiated, usual type
Basaloid
Warty
Mixed, basalo-warty
HPV-Unrelated VIN-d
differentiated-type

HPV, Human papillomavirus; *VIN,* vulvar intraepithelial neoplasia.

grade (VIN 1) and high-grade (VIN 2,3) types. VIN 1 is a flat condyloma, and although nearly 50% contain high-risk (oncogenic) HPV types, only a minority contains HPV type 16 as opposed to high-grade VIN, which carries HPV 16 in more than 90% of the cases. VIN 1 is not considered to precede high-grade VIN but may indicate risk for developing VIN-u. Molecular and genetic studies are needed to shed further insight into the natural history of the two types of vulvar cancer precursors, including diagnosis, therapy, and particularly the role of prophylactic HPV vaccines in the prevention of vulvar cancer precursors.

REFERENCES

1. Hudelo M, Boulanger-Pilet M, Cailliau M. Erythrokératodermie verruqueuse en nappes symétriques et progressives congénitales. Bull Soc Fr Dermatol Syphiligr 1922;29:45.
2. Colgan TJ. Vulvar intraepithelial neoplasia: a synopsis of recent developments. J Lower Genital Tract Dis 1998;2:31–36.
3. Report of the Committee on Terminology of the International Society for the Study of Vulvar Disease. New nomenclature for vulvar disease. J Reprod Med 1990;35:483–484.
4. Wright TC, Kurman RJ, Ferenczy A. Precancerous lesions of the cervix. In: Kurman RJ (ed). Blaustein's Pathology of the Female Genital Tract, ed 4. New York: Springer-Verlag, 1994, pp 229–277.
5. Srodon M, Kurman RJ, Baber GB, et al. The distribution of low and high risk HPV types in vulvar intraepithelial neoplasia. Mod Pathol 2005;18:205A.
6. Kagie MJ, Kenter GG, Hermans J, et al. The relevance of various vulvar epithelial changes in the early detection of squamous cell carcinoma of the vulva. Int J Gynecol Cancer 1997;7: 50–57.
7. Liau KL, Ronnett B, Ferenczy A, et al. Diagnosis of vulvar and vaginal squamous intraepithelial lesions and condylomata acuminata correlated with HPV 6/11 detection: comparison between a commercial central laboratory and an expert pathology panel. Proceedings of the 23rd International Papillomavirus

Conference & Clinical Workshop, September 1–7, 2006, Prague. Prague: Institute of Hematology and Blood Transfusion, 2006, p 54.

8. Sideri M, Jones RW, Wilkinson EJ. Squamous vulvar intraepithelial neoplasia: 2004 modified terminology, ISSVD Vulvar Oncology Subcommittee. J Reprod Med 2005;50:807–810.

9. Scurry J, Campion M, Scurry B, et al. Pathologic audit of 164 consecutive cases of vulvar intraepithelial neoplasia. Int J Gynecol Pathol 2006;25:176–181.

10. Hillemanns P, Wang X. Integration of HPV-16 and HPV-18 DNA in vulvar intraepithelial neoplasia. Gynecol Oncol 2006;100: 276–282.

11. Korn AP, Abercrombie PD, Foster A. Vulvar intraepithelial neoplasia in women infected with human immunodeficiency virus-1. Gynecol Oncol 1996;61:384–386.

12. Rosenberg PS, Greene MH, Alter BP. Cancer incidence in persons with Fanconi anemia. Blood 2003;101:822–826.

13. Goffin F, Mayrand M-H, Gauthier P, et al. High-risk human papillomavirus infection of the genital tract of women with a previous history or recurrent high-grade vulvar intraepithelial neoplasia. J Med Virol 2006;78:814–819.

14. Hildesheim A, Han CL, Brinton LA, et al. Human papillomavirus type 16 and risk of preinvasive and invasive vulvar cancer: results from a seroepidemiological case-control study. Obstet Gynecol 1997;90:748–754.

15. van Seters M, van Beurden M, Craen AJ. Is the assumed natural history of vulvar intraepithelial neoplasia III based on enough evidence? A systematic review of 3322 published patients. Gynecol Oncol 2005;97:645–651.

16. Jones RW, Rowan DM. Vulvar intraepithelial neoplasia III: a clinical study of the outcome in 113 cases with relation to the later development of invasive vulvar carcinoma. Obstet Gynecol 1994;84:741–745.

17. Todd RW, Luesley DM. Medical management of vulvar intraepithelial neoplasia. J Lower Genital Tract Dis 2005;9: 206–212.

18. Ferenczy A, Coutlée F, Franco EL, et al. Human papillomavirus and HIV coinfection and the risk of neoplasias of the lower genital tract: a review of recent developments. CMAJ 2003;169: 431–434.

19. Herod JJ, Shafi MI, Rollason TP, et al. Vulval intraepithelial neoplasia: long term follow up of treated and untreated women. Br J Obstet Gynecol 1996;103:446–452.

20. Crum CP. Carcinoma of the vulva: epidemiology and pathogenesis. Obstet Gynecol 1992;79:448–454.

21. Sillman FH, Sedlis A, Boyce JG. A review of lower genital intraepithelial neoplasia and the use of topical 5-fluorouracil. Obstet Gynecol Surv 1985;40:190–192.

22. Abdel-Hady ES, Martin-Hirsch P, Duggan-Keen M, et al. Immunological and viral factors associated with the response of vulval intraepithelial neoplasia to photodynamic therapy. Cancer Res 2001;61:192–196.

23. Kurwa HA, Barlow RJ, Neill S. Single-episode photodynamic therapy and vulval intraepithelial neoplasia type III resistant to conventional therapy. Br J Dermatol 2000;143:1040–1042.

24. Martin-Hirsch PL, Whitehurst C, Buckley CH, et al. Photodynamic treatment for lower genital tract intraepithelial neoplasia. Lancet 1998;351:1403.

25. Hillemans P, Wang X, Staehle S, et al. Evaluation of different treatment modalities for vulvar intraepithelial neoplasia (VIN): CO_2 laser vaporization, photodynamic therapy, excision and vulvectomy. Gynecol Oncol 2006;100:271–275.

26. Snoeck R, Noel JC, Muller C, et al. Cidofovir, a new approach for the treatment of cervix intraepithelial neoplasia grade III (CIN III). J Med Virol 2000;60:205–209.

27. Koonsaeng S, Verschraegen C, Freedman R, et al. Successful treatment of recurrent vulvar intraepithelial neoplasia resistent to interferon and isotretinoin with cidofovir. J Med Virol 2001;64:195–198.

28. Spirtos NM, Smith LH, Teng NN. Prospective randomized trial of topical alpha-interferon (alpha-interferon gels) for the treatment of vulvar intraepithelial neoplasia III. Gynecol Oncol 1990;37:34–38.

29. Edwards L, Ferenczy A, Eron L, et al. Self-administered topical 5% Imiquimod cream for external anogenital warts. Arch Dermatol 1998;134:25–30.

30. Davis G, Wentworth J, Richard L. Self-administered topical imiquimod treatment of vulvar intraepithelial neoplasia: a report of four cases. J Reprod Med 2000;45:619–623.

31. Diaz-Arrastia C, Arany I, Robazetti SC, et al. Clinical and molecular responses in high-grade intraepithelial neoplasia treated with topical imiquimod 5%. Clin Cancer Res 2001;7: 3031–3033.

32. Jayne CJ, Kaufman RH. Treatment of vulvar intraepithelial neoplasia 2/3 with imiquimod. J Reprod Med 2002;47:395–398.

33. Todd RW, Etherington LL, Luesley DM. The effects of 5% imiquimod cream on high-grade vulval intraepithelial neoplasia. Gynecol Oncol 2002;85:67–70.

34. van Seters M, Fons G, van Beurden M. Imiquimod in the treatment of multifocal vulvar intraepithelial neoplasia 2/3: results of a pilot study. J Reprod Med 2002;47:701–705.

35. Le T, Hicks W, Menard C, et al. Preliminary results of 5% imiquimod cream in the primary treatment of vulvar intraepithelial neoplasia grade 2/3. Am J Obstet Gynecol 2006;194: 377–380.

36. Tristram A, Fiander A. Clinical responses to Cidofovir applied topically to women with high grade vulval intraepithelial neoplasia. Gynecol Oncol 2005;99:652–655.

37. Jin L, Qi M, Chen DZ, et al. Indole-3-carbinol prevents cervical cancer in human papillomavirus type 16 (HPV 16) transgenic mice. Cancer Res 1999;59:3991–3997.

38. Auborn KJ. Therapy for recurrent respiratory papillomatosis. Antiviral Therapy 2002;7:1–9.

39. Ferenczy A, Wright TC Jr, Richart RM. Comparison of CO_2 laser surgery and loop electrosurgical excision/fulguration procedure (LEEP) for the treatment of vulvar intraepithelial neoplasia (VIN). Int J Gynecol Cancer 1994;4:22–28.

40. Vlastos AT, Levy L, Malpica A, et al. Loop electrosurgical excision procedure in vulvar intraepithelial neoplasia treatment. J Lower Genital Tract Dis 2002;6:232–238.

41. Wendling J, Saiag P, Berville-Levy S, et al. Treatment of undifferentiated vulvar intraepithelial neoplasia with 5% imiquimod cream: a prospective study of 12 cases. Arch Dermatol 2004;140;1220–1224.

42. Ait Menguellet S, Collinet P, Debarge VH, et al. Management of multicentric lesions of the lower genital tract. Eur J Obstet Gynecol Reprod Biol 2007;132:116–120.

43. Davidson EJ, Boswell CM, Sell P, et al. Immunological and clinical responses in women with vulval intraepithelial neoplasia vaccinated with a vaccinia virus encoding human papillomavirus 16/18 oncoproteins. Cancer Res 2003;63: 6032–6041.

44. Baldwin PJ, van der Burg SH, Boswell CM, et al. Vaccinia-expressed human papillomavirus 16 and 18 E6 and E7 as a

therapeutic vaccination for vulval and vaginal intraepithelial neoplasia. Clin Cancer Res 2003;9:5205–5213.

45. Fiander AN, Tristram AJ, Davidson EJ, et al. Prime-boost vaccination strategy in women with high-grade, noncervical anogenital intraepithelial neoplasia: clinical results from a multicenter phase II trial. Int J Cancer 2006;16:1075–1081.

46. Villa LL, Costa RLR, Petta CA, et al. Prophylactic quadrivalent human papillomavirus (types 6, 11, 16, 18) l1 virus-like particle vaccine in young women: a randomized, double-blind, placebo-controlled, multicentre phase II efficacy trial. Lancet Oncol 2005;6:271–278.

47. Kurman RJ, Toki T, Schiffman MH. Basaloid and warty carcinoma of the vulva. Am J Surg Pathol 1993;17:133–145.

48. Brinton LA, Nasca PC, Mallin K, et al. Case-control study of cancer of the vulva. Obstet Gynecol 1990;75:863–866.

49. Karram M, Tabor B, Smotkin D, et al. Detection of human papillomavirus deoxyribonucleic acid from vulvar dystrophies and vulvar intraepithelial neoplastic lesions. Am J Obstet Gynecol 1988;159:22–23.

50. Hording U, Junge J, Daugaard S, et al. Vulvar squamous cell carcinoma and papillomaviruses: indications for two different etiologies. Gynecol Oncol 1994;52:241–246.

51. Scurry J, Vanin K, Ostor A. Comparison of histological features of vulvar lichen sclerosis with and without adjacent squamous cell carcinoma. Int J Gynecol Cancer 1997;7:392–399.

52. Leibowitch M, Neill S, Pelisse M. The epithelial changes associated with squamous cell carcinoma of the vulva: a review of the clinical, histological and viral findings in 78 women. Br J Obstet Gynaecol 1990;97:1135–1139.

53. Trimble CL, Hildesheim A, Brinton LA, et al. Heterogeneous etiology of squamous carcinoma of the vulva. Obstet Gynecol 1996;87:59–64.

54. Scurry J. Does lichen sclerosus play a central role in the pathogenesis of human papillomavirus negative vulvar squamous cell carcinoma? The itch-scratch-lichen sclerosus hypothesis. Int J Gynecol Cancer 1999;9:89–97.

55. zur Hausen H. Human genital cancer: synergism between two virus infections or synergism between a virus infection and initiating events. Lancet 1982;2:1370–1372.

56. Yang B, Hart WR. Vulvar intraepithelial neoplasia of the simplex (differentiated) type: a clinicopathologic study including analysis of HPV and p53 expression. Am J Surg Pathol 2000;24:429–441.

57. Zaino RJ, Husseinzadeh N, Hahhas W, et al. Epithelial alteratons in prximity to invasive squamous carcinoma of the vulva. Int J Gynecol Pathol 1982;1:173–184.

CHAPTER 19

External Genital Condyloma

Alex Ferenczy

KEY POINTS

- The lifetime risk of developing external genital warts (EGWs) is 10%.
- The vast majority of EGWs as well as recurrent respiratory papillomatoses are caused by human papillomavirus (HPV) types 6 and 11.
- Although most EGWs are sexually transmitted, those affecting the upper respiratory tract in children are acquired while passing through the birth canal of mothers with EGWs.
- When EGWs present atypically or are resistant to therapy, biopsy is indicated to rule out precancer/cancer or condylomata mimics.
- There are no evidence-based data to suggest that a given type of therapy for EGWs is superior to another.
- Therapy should be based on a mutual decision between the healthcare provider and the patient following an informed consent.
- Both provider-administered and patient-administered therapies can be used as either first-line or second-line therapies, depending on the patient's preference, provider's experience, and number and location of EGWs.
- In general, multiple therapeutic sessions with a single form or multiple forms of therapy are required to achieve complete clearance of EGWs.
- In new relationships or in couples who are not monogamous, constant and correct use of latex condoms will reduce but not eliminate the risk of HPV transmission and the development of EGWs.
- Mass and universal prophylactic HPV vaccination programs with HPV types 6/11–containing vaccines are likely to significantly reduce the burden of disease in at-risk populations.

EPIDEMIOLOGY

Most studies on prevalence and incidence of external genital warts (EGWs) have been conducted in selected populations such as women attending colposcopy clinics or those attending university sexually transmitted infection (STI) clinics. Until recently, the general population has not been extensively studied. Earlier estimates showed approximately 1% of sexually active populations in the United States have EGWs.[1] The prevalence of EGWs in university students was 1.5%, whereas in a health maintenance organization in Washington State, it was 0.8% in women aged 21 to 29 years and 0.6% in those aged 30 to 39 years. Understandably, in those who attend STI clinics, the prevalence of EGWs is the highest, ranging from 4% to 13%, with both men and women having similar rates. In four Nordic countries—Denmark, Iceland, Norway, and Sweden—a random sample of 70,000 women between the ages of 18 and 45 years who completed self-administered questionnaires found a 10.6% lifetime prevalence of EGWs.[2] The history of EGWs correlated with the number of sexual partners, STIs, use of oral contraceptives, and use of condoms, as well as smoking and level of education.

The cumulative incidence of EGWs in a cohort of 898 Norwegian females aged 16 to 24 years was 10.7% at 48 months of follow-up.[3] Approximately 22% of women with HPV types 6 or 11 developed EGWs. Among those with HPV types 6 or 11 and 16 or 18, 29% developed EGWs within 4 years of follow-up. The relative risk for developing EGWs has been estimated to be five times higher in HPV-positive versus HPV-negative women.

TRANSMISSION/ACQUISITION

The vast majority of HPV infections, including EGWs, are sexually transmitted either via intercourse or, less frequently, through genital skin-to-skin contact without penetrative sex.[4] This explains why self-declared virgins may still be found with EGWs. In addition, such individuals test HPV negative in their vaginal and cervical samples, supporting the concept of direct skin-to-skin contact for HPV transmission and acquisition. In one of the rare prospective studies carried out in the 1950s, 60% of women whose male partners returned from the Korean War with EGWs developed genital warts.[5] In the Oriel et al. study, periods of incubation of EGWs ranged from 3 weeks to 18 months with an average of 3 months, whereas most lesions in children develop between 1 and 20 months.[6] In rare instances, auto-inoculation from one site to another or heteroinoculation may be the mechanism of transmission. For example, in heterosexual individuals with perianal condylomata, approximately one half to two thirds of intra-anal lesions are believed to be the result of HPV "transferred" by anodigital insertions rather than receptive intercourse.[7] Oral and laryngeal warts may rarely occur in adults practicing frequent oral sex and in children 2 to 5 years old delivered by mothers with vaginal warts, respectively.[8] Although anogenital warts in children can be acquired at any age as a result of sexual abuse, the majority of them are a result of nonsexual vertical or horizontal transmission of HPV.[8] Children may also develop nongenital verruca vulgaris in their perianal and/or vulvar skin caused by HPV type 2 from their own finger warts or from those found on their parents' or guardians' hands.[6] Typically, the lesions are found at some distance from the pigmented, perianal squamous epithelium.

CLINICAL SIGNIFICANCE AND VIRAL CORRELATES

As mentioned previously, the vast majority (90%) of EGWs are caused by low-risk HPV type 6 and, less often, type 11. Recent epidemiologic viral correlation studies showed geographic variations in HPV 6/11/prevalence of EGWs.[9] Although in the United States 95% of EGWs are caused by HPV 6/11, in Latin America the rate is only 75%. The reason(s) for the differences is not clear. Typically, HPV type 6 and 11 have almost no potential for viral integration into host cell DNA and, consequently, carcinogenic transformation of 6/11-positive EGWs is a very rare phenomenon.[1] The very rare, well-differentiated verrucous squamous cell carcinoma of the external anogenital skin (formerly giant condyloma of Buschke-Lowenstein) has been found to carry HPV type 6, subtype 6b. In immunocompetent individuals, histologically-verified EGWs have little, if any, cancer potential. Furthermore, despite the fact that there is an increased association of EGWs and anogenital precancer and cancer in individuals with cell-mediated immunosuppression, the carcinogenic transformation of EGWs is not increased.[10,11] These patients, such as those with lymphoproliferative disorders, organ transplants, acquired immune deficiency syndrome (AIDS), and aplastic (Fanconi) anemia are prone to multiple low- and high-risk types of HPV infections.[12,13] In such patients, development of invasive squamous cell cancers from preinvasive lesional epithelium as a result of high-oncogenic-risk HPV types occurs alongside the development of EGWs as a result of low-risk HPV infection. The approximately fourfold relative risk of cervical cancer in patients with EGWs is explained by susceptibility of these individuals to be infected by high-oncogenic-risk HPV types.[13]

From a practical point of view, the main significance of EGWs is that they are cosmetically and psychosexually unacceptable and are a source of infection to new sexual partners and, as previously mentioned, rarely to the neonate.

CLINICAL EVALUATION

Condylomata acuminata are sessile, papular, papillary, cauliflower-type lesions with warty or verrucous surfaces. They are found mainly on the nonhairy skin of the external genitals (Figures 19-1 and 19-2). Those that develop in mucosal surfaces (e.g., introitus, anal canal, inner surface of prepuce, meatus, upper respiratory tract, conjunctiva) are soft and whitish to pink in color, and each papillae has a double-looped feeding capillary (Figure 19-3). Surface keratinization is moderate to absent. Condylomata of the hairy genital skin tend to be firm with often a prominent layer of surface keratinization (hyperkeratosis) (Figure 19-4). Acuminate condylomata should be distinguished from their mimics (Table 19-1).

Micropapillomatosis labialis (MPL) is one of the conditions most often confused for condylomata acuminata. Unlike acuminate condyloma in which multiple papillae converge toward a single base, in MPL each fingerlike papillomatous projection has its own base (Figure 19-5). Most patients with MPL have no symptoms or have a history of recurrent candidiasis, *Trichomonas*, or *Chlamydia* infections. HPV is no more prevalent in the epithelium of MPL than in normal labial epithelium.[14,15] The condition is regarded as an exaggerated variant of an otherwise physiologic vulvar skin.

A somewhat analogous condition called *pearly penile papules* is seen in one third of male penises. Pearly penile papules develop after puberty and consist of small papules arranged in linear fashion along the corona glandis and on each side of the frenulum. Ferenczy et al. failed to detect HPV deoxyribonucleic acid (DNA) by polymerase chain reaction technology in any of the 13 cases of pearly penile papules studied.[16]

Molluscum contagiosum (MC) presents as multiple papules with often depressed centers (umbilication), covered by a yellowish membrane. On microscopy, the depression can be seen to be filled with pox virus particles (Figure 19-6). MC tends to aggregate in the pubic and thigh regions; however, it can involve the external anogenital skin as well and be associated with classic condylomata acuminata.

Pigmented mole(s) of the intradermal type and skin tags (acrochordon) are warty variants of vulvar intraepithelial neoplasia (Figure 19-7) and verrucous carcinoma (Figure 19-8) and are not infrequently mistaken for acuminate condylomata. Another condyloma mimic is secondary syphilis or condylomata lata. Unlike the warty surface of condyloma acuminatum, condyloma latum has a shiny, smooth surface and a sharp, demarcated contour (Figure 19-9).

HPV infections are often multicentric, and about one third of individuals with EGWs also have HPV-related changes on the cervix and, less often, in the vagina and urethral meatus.[17] Most cervical lesions are low-grade cervical intraepithelial lesions (CIN 1). High-grade CIN 2,3 is found only in 2% of women, typically in those 25 years or older.[17] Therefore in practices where colposcopy is readily available,

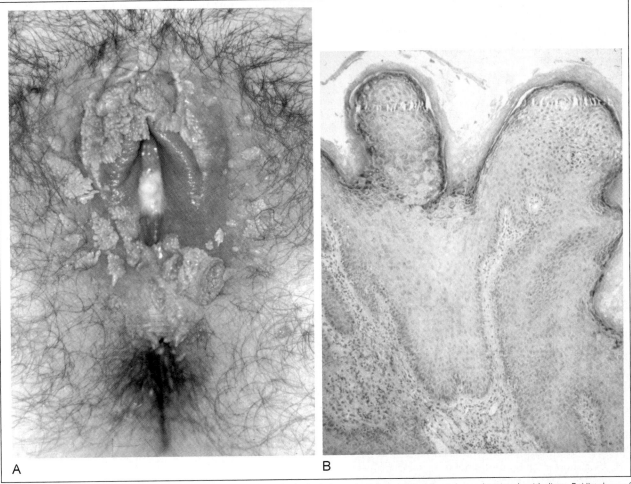

Figure 19-1 Condylomata acuminata. **A,** Multiple lesions involving both the hairy and nonhairy skin of the vulva and perianal epithelium. **B,** Histology of condyloma acuminatum. Papillary growth pattern with club-shaped papillae and surface keratinization as well as elongated (acanthotic) rete pegs extending to the base of the lesion. (**A,** From Ferenczy A. External genital human papillomavirus infections. Curr Obstet Gynaecol 1995;5:98–106.)

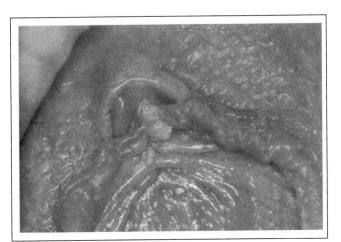

Figure 19-2 Condylomata acuminata. Lesions seen on the clitoris and subclitoral mucous membrane of the labia minora. (From Richart RM, Ferenczy A, Meisels A, et al. Condyloma virus and cervical cancer—how strong a link? Contemp Ob Gyn 1984;23:210–224.)

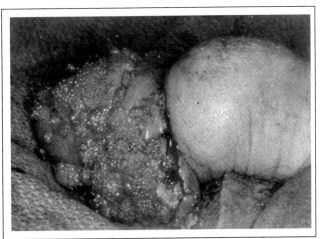

Figure 19-3 Condylomata acuminata. Multiple lesions devoid of surface keratinization obscure the foreskin and glans of the penis. (From Ferenczy A. Management strategies for genital HPV infection in men. Contemp Urology 1990;(Sep-Oct):10–22; and A. Ferenczy. Epidemiology and clinical pathophysiology of condylomata acuminate. Am J Obstet Gynecol 1995;1331–1339.)

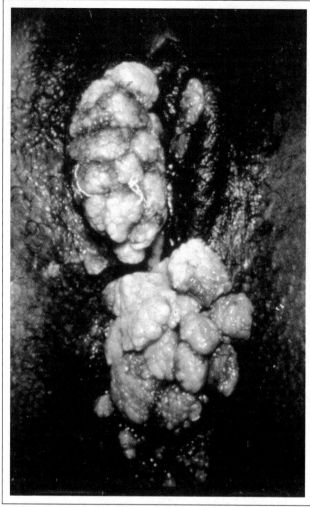

Figure 19-4 Condylomata acuminata. Hyperkeratotic, cauliflower-like lesions on the hairy skin of the vulva and perianal skin.

Table 19-1 Genital Condylomata Mimics

Epidermal inclusion cysts (mainly scrotum)

Giant condyloma of Buschke-Lowenstein

Herpes simplex virus

Human papillomavirus–related, basalo-verrucous VIN

Hypertrophy of sebaceous glands

Intradermal nevi, seborrheic keratosis, skin tag (achrochordon)

Micropapillomatosis labialis

Molluscum contagiosum

Pearly penile papules

Syphilis, chancre

Vulvar intraepithelial neoplasia

it may be appropriate to examine the cervix and vagina in individuals with EGWs. However, if unavailable, a cytologic sample taken from a clinically normal-appearing cervix is sufficient. In the author's experience, about 10% of women and 80% of homosexual men with perianal condylomata who had engaged in anoreceptive intercourse have intra-anal involvement of condyloma. Therefore in practices where colposcopy is readily available, it may be appropriate to examine these patients with high-resolution anoscopy, the anal equivalent of vaginal colposcopy. Lesional involvement is usually located at or below the anorectal junction (i.e., about 3 cm from the anal orifice). Meatal involvement by HPV infection manifests as acuminate- or papular-type condylomata, and the lesions are located in the fossa navicularis in more than 90% of cases. Urethrocystoscopy is only indicated if the condylomatous lesions are beyond colposcopic view.

Histologic evaluation of typical condylomata acuminata is optional. However, lesions should be histologically verified whenever the patient is treated with surgical techniques (e.g., electrosurgery, laser) or has atypical lesions where intraepithelial neoplasia or cancer is suspected (see Figure 19-7) or has lesions unrelated to HPV infections (e.g., molluscum contagiosum, nevi, skin tag, seborrheic keratosis) or invasive disease (Figure 19-10). In the surgically treated group, histologic evidence of disease serves as proof that the treatment was indicated or serves to identify noncondylomatous lesions that are treated differently from typical warts. In two large randomized, controlled trials determining the efficacy of the prophylactic HPV 6/11/16/18 vaccine (Gardasil), the agreement between a central laboratory and a panel of experts in gynecologic pathology was 80%, with a higher prevalence of HPV 6/11 in condylomatous lesions diagnosed by the panel (90%) compared with that of the central laboratory ($p < 0.001$).[18]

Colposcopy of the external anogenital skin is indicated in two situations: (1) to localize small papular or acuminate lesions that may be hidden in the hairy genital skin, allowing all lesional tissue to be included in the treatment field (see Figure 19-1, *A*, and 19-2); and (2) to explain the origin of a positive cytologic smear in patients whose cervix and vagina are devoid of lesional tissue by colposcopy, histology, and endocervical curettage. In such cases of a verified cytologic diagnosis, the epithelium of the introitus, labia minora, or both often contain HPV-related subclinical macules (see Figure 19-5). In such cases, the exfoliated cells are carried presumably by antiperistalsis cephalad in the vagina and recovered at the cervix level.

THE MALE PARTNER

Because external genital HPV infections are sexually transmitted, some recommend evaluating their male sexual partners.[19,20] However, in the author's opinion the compulsive tracing of contacts is not cost-effective for the current relationship because her partner already has subclinical HPV infection that has already spontaneously regressed or will

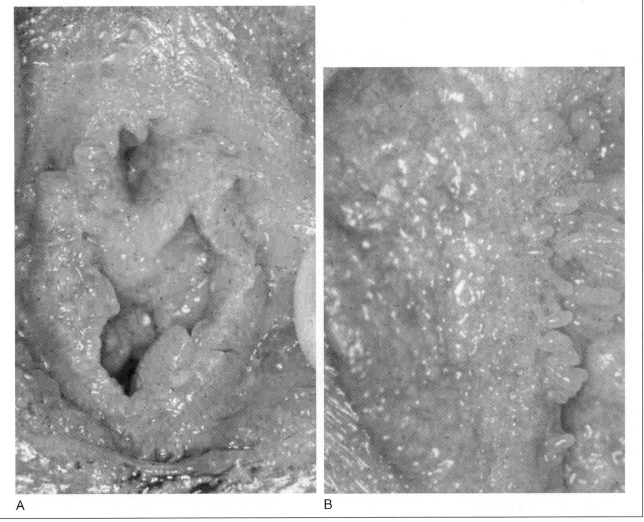

Figure 19-5 Condyloma mimic. **A,** The entire hymenal ring and labia minora contain confluent, micropapillary epithelium. This is an example of MPL. The patient complained of cyclic vulvitis, and vaginal culture showed *Candida glabrata*. **B,** Detailed view of MPL with each fingerlike projection having its own base compared with acuminate condylomata. (**A,** From Ferenczy A. Epidemiology and clinical parhophysiology of condylomata acuminate. Am J Obstet Gynecol 1995; 172:1331–1339, **B,** from Richart RM, Beutner K, Ferenczy A. Current management of genital warts. Contemp Obstet Gynecol 1997;(Nov):74–103.)

regress within a relatively short period of time, or the male partner carries latent HPV without lesional epithelium and is simply not the source of EGWs in his current partner.[21] This philosophy is in agreement with the latest recommendations of the Centers for Disease Control and Prevention in which examination of sex partners is not recommended.[22] Exceptions to this practice are the following:

1. Men with suspected condylomata acuminata
2. Symptomatic patients with pruritus and/or burning of the penis
3. Examination specifically requested by the patient

In the first two instances, evaluation of the external anogenital skin is often followed by therapy. In the third instance (in the absence of finding visible lesions), information on the natural history of HPV infection may be helpful in relieving anxiety, guilt, or both and may result in the modification of sexual practices, including consistently using condoms or engaging in long-term, mutual monogamy. Indeed, most

agree with the concept that a woman's cervical cancer risk depends not as much on her own sexual behavior but rather on that of her male sexual partners. Although the use of condoms has not been shown to prevent all HPV infections, they can substantially reduce (but not eliminate) the risk of HPV transmission.[19,20] The evidence on treatment results of women with vulvar warts suggests that in long-term, mutual monogamous sexual relationships, the untreated male partner does not represent a reservoir of reinfection.[11] In one study, only 23% of couples had the same HPV type in their genital specimens[21]; another study found that only 37% of partners were infected by the same HPV type.[20] One retrospective study comparing treated to untreated male patients failed to demonstrate a decrease in the post-treatment recurrence/failure rate for EGWs in the female partners.[23]

Table 19-2 contains the author's experience with 108 steady male sexual partners (6 months and longer) with penile HPV infections whose female partners had been treated for EGWs. The men were randomized to either surgery

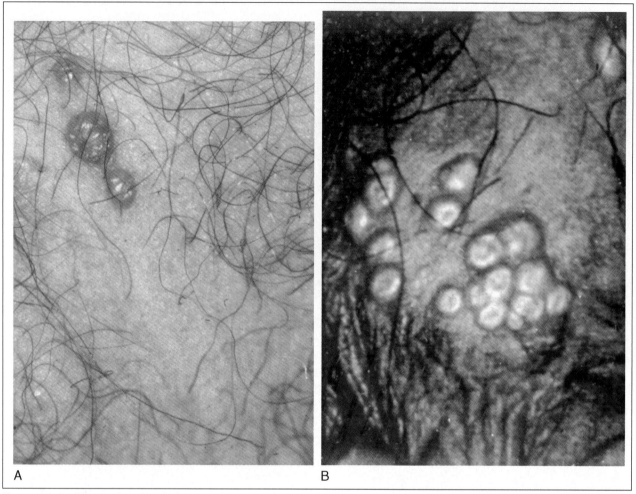

Figure 19-6 Condyloma mimic. **A,** Multiple papules with smooth surface and umbilicated center, typical of molluscum contagiosum. **B,** Detailed view of molluscum contagiosum. (**B,** From Ferenczy A, Kohn T, Shore M. Evaluating male partners of condyloma patients. Contemp Ob Gyn 1983;22:183–196.)

(CO$_2$ laser vaporization) or loop electrosurgical excision procedure (LEEP) and condom use (55 patients) or no therapy and no condom use (53 patients), and the entire cohort was followed for a minimum of 6 weeks to a maximum of 24 weeks (mean 12 weeks). The results clearly show that recurrence rates for women whose male partners were treated versus those whose partners were not treated are similar. The results are consistent with the concept that partners in stable sexual unions do not reinfect each other; rather, post-therapy recurrence is a reflection of later activation of latent HPV DNA that is present in the normal epithelium adjacent to previously treated fields in a large proportion of cases (Figure 19-11).

The author also questions the clinical benefit of removing subclinical lesions that coexist with clinically overt condylomata. Earlier reports suggested improved cure rates for EGWs (87%) and decreased number of repeat ablative procedures when both the subclinical macules and condylomata are treated using the so-called extended CO$_2$ laser vaporization technique. However, subsequent experience with extended laser vaporization for EGWs yielded only 40% cure rates, certainly not better than those reported

without extended laser therapy.[23] Also, extended laser therapy is often associated with more pain and delayed healing. Finally, a recent cross-sectional study of heterosexual couples found that the majority of flat, subclinical, penile lesions regressed simply with the use of condoms.[20]

THERAPY

General Considerations

There have been no new significant breakthroughs in the treatment of EGWs in the last 10 years. Treatment regimens continue to be numerous and are testimony of our failure to guarantee cure, at least with a single treatment session. Indeed, *there is no evidence to suggest that any treatment modality is significantly superior to another, nor is there evidence indicating that the currently available treatments eradicate or affect the natural history of HPV infection.* The removal of warts may or may not decrease infectivity. If left untreated, visible genital warts may resolve on their own in 20% to 30% of cases, remain unchanged, or increase in size or number.

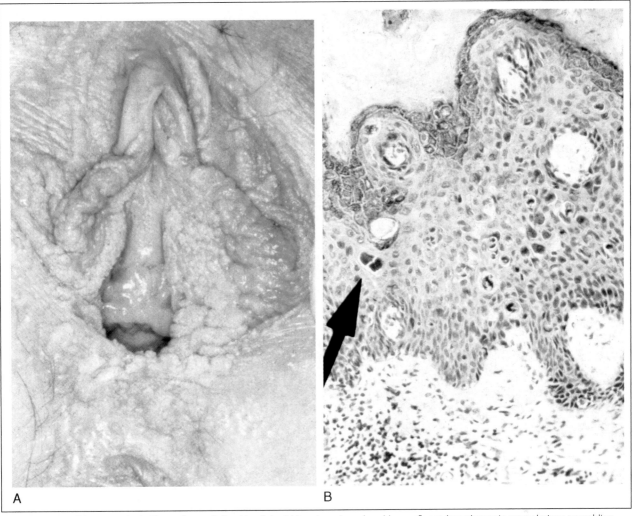

Figure 19-7 Condyloma mimic. **A,** The entire nonhairy skin of the labia minora is replaced by confluent, hyperkeratotic, warty lesions resembling condylomata acuminata. **B,** Histology of "warty" vulvar intraepithelial neoplasia. Papillary, hyperkeratotic surface and pleomorphic, poorly differentiated, neoplastic squamous cells. *Arrow* points to a "corps ronds," and there are several abnormal mitotic figures *(lower middle)*. (**A** and **B,** From Ferenczy A. Intraepithelial neoplasia of the vulva. In: Coppleson M (ed). Gynecologic Oncology, vol 1, ed 2. London: Churchill-Livingstone, 1992, pp 447–452; and Ferenczy A. Epidemiology and clinical pathophysiology of condylomata acuminata. Am J Obstet Gynecol 1995;172:1331–1339. **A,** Also from Ferenczy A. Using lasers to treat condylomas and VIN. Contemp Obstet Gynecol 1982;(20):57–75.)

The treatment of visible warts does not decrease the risk of developing cervical cancer.[22] *It is important to inform the patient that treatment often requires multiple (the average number is 5 sessions) rather than a single session of therapy, and recurrences are frequent (30% or more).* Fortunately, the majority of patients experience sustained disease-free periods within 3 months and recurrences are relatively infrequent 6 months after the last successful treatment.[24] In general, favorable response to therapy is much more likely in patients aged 20 years or younger regardless of extent of lesions; other good response predictors are lesions less than 10 cm^2 in total volume, lesions less than 4 months in duration and those in immunocompetent women.

Most patients in private practice have less than 10 genital warts, with a total wart area of 5.0 cm^2 or less that are responsive to most treatment modalities (Table 19-3). In contrast, in referral centers, many patients have EGWs between 20 and 50 cm^2 in total wart area. These patients often require longer treatment sessions and surgical rather than medical-type therapies. In general, factors that might influence selection of treatment in addition to patient preference include wart size, wart number, anatomic site of warts, wart morphology, the cost of treatment, convenience, adverse effects, and provider experience. Having a treatment plan is important because most patients are likely to require multiple therapeutic sessions. *EGWs with little or no keratinization located on moist surfaces and/or in intertriginous areas generally respond better to topical treatment (e.g., trichloroacetic acid [TCA], podophyllin, 0.5% podofilox, 5% imiquimod) than do their keratinized counterparts on drier surfaces* (Figure 19-12). The differential in therapeutic success rates is likely due to enhanced product absorption into HPV-infected keratinocytes.

A given treatment modality may be changed after four to six weekly provider-administered treatments or if warts have not completely cleared after eight weekly treatments. The

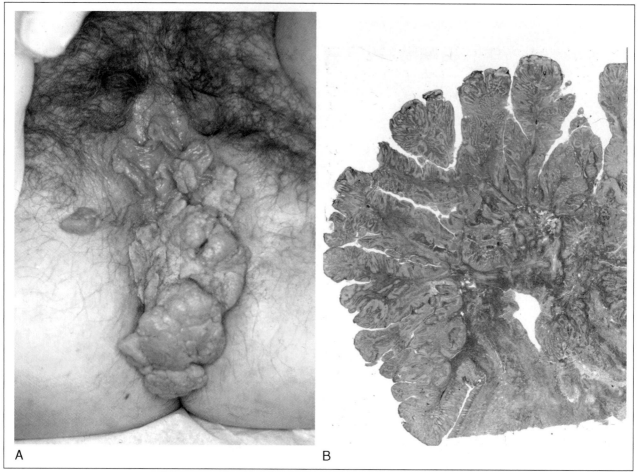

A   B

Figure 19-8 Condyloma mimic. **A,** Voluminous, confluent, exophytic lesions obscuring the anogenital skin. **B,** Histologically, confluent, club-shaped rete pegs extend superficially into the dermis, consistent with verrucous squamous cell carcinoma of vulva.

exception to this rule is the use of the immune system modulator, 5% imiquimod cream (Aldara), and the recently Food and Drug Administration (FDA)-approved pro-apoptotic polyphenon-E 15% ointment, both of which can be used for as much as 16 weeks of therapy. Using these treatment modalities, a substantial number of patients (about an additional 20%) may experience complete clearance between the eighth and sixteenth weeks of therapy.[24,25] In intractable, standard treatment-resistant cases, therapies that combine topical cytotoxins or immunomodulators with ablative/excisional methods may be indicated. Topical, off-label 1% cidofovir gel—a broad-spectrum antiviral agent—has also been shown to be successful in about 40% of recurrent EGWs in a small group of immune-suppressed, human immunodeficiency virus (HIV)-positive patients.[26]

When treatments for warts are employed properly, complications are rare. *Patients should be warned that scarring in the form of persistent hypopigmentation or hyperpigmentation is common with ablative treatment modalities.* Depressed or hypertrophic scars are rare but can occur, especially if the patient has had insufficient time to heal between treatments. Rarely, treatment can result in disabling chronic pain syndromes (e.g., vulvodynia, hyperesthesia of the treatment site).

In couples who are not in long-term, mutually monogamous sexual unions, treatment results are enhanced and recurrences prevented by the consistent and correct use of condoms prior to and during intercourse, as well as the practice of genital hygiene. Ultimately, the universal use of the prophylactic HPV vaccine containing HPV types 6 and 11 (Gardasil) is likely to provide the most successful preventive measure against most cases of EGWs.

Table 19-3 presents the summary data on provider-administered and patient-applied treatment results. *It is impossible to compare one method with another because of numerous variables, all of which can influence therapeutic results.* The most common confounding factors are age of patient (i.e., younger patients respond better than their older counterparts), number and size of EGWs, gender, treatment regimen, diagnostic ascertainment (histology versus clinical inspection), duration of EGWs (longer outbreaks are associated with a less-favorable response than shorter outbreaks), length of follow-up, and method of assessment of recurrences. It should be realized that treatment results obtained under perfect experimental conditions (per-protocol cohort) tend to be superior to intent-to-treat protocols that reflect *real-life* practices. Furthermore, in most reports recurrences are reported separately and not included in failure rates,

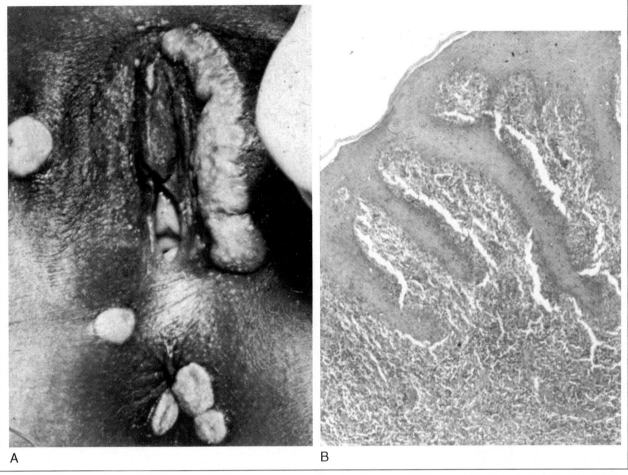

Figure 19-9 Condyloma lata. **A**, Multiple, raised, sharply demarcated, smooth-surfaced lesions mimicking condylomata. Both serology and histology were consistent with secondary syphilis in this sexually abused 7-year-old girl. **B**, Histology of acanthotic rete pegs and marked, chronic inflammatory exudate in subepithelial, papillary dermis.

whereas in *real life* the reason that the patient still has warts (recurrence or treatment failure) is not relevant. As a result, *to assess the true overall cure rate, one should only consider complete responders as cured and include recurrences in the group of those who failed to respond.*

Provider-Applied Therapies

Provider-applied therapies include the following:

1. **Podophyllin:** This is one of the oldest cytotoxic agents (podophyllotoxin). It is applied topically at concentrations ranging from 8% to 25% in compound tincture of benzoin. It interferes with mitosis of infected cells by "paralyzing" the mitotic spindle.

   Application: Once a week for as long as 6 weeks over total wart area of less than 10 cm^2 per application. It should be washed off with soap within 4 to 6 hours.

   Treatment results: *Complete clearance is obtained in about 50%; however, recurrences are in the order of 40%.*[27] It is ineffective on large, hyperkeratotic, dry lesions of the hairy skin of the lower genital tract (i.e., scrotum, labia majora, base of penis). Overall, the use of podophyllin has *limited* therapeutic value.

   Adverse effects: Pruritus, burning pain, erythema and edema. Podophyllin has the potential for massive systemic absorption that may result in bone marrow depression or coma. *It should not be used in pregnant women because it contains mutagenic substances.*[22,27]

2. **Trichloroacetic (TCA) or bichloroacetic acid (BCA):** These are keratolytic and keratinocytic chemo-coagulating agents. TCA and BCA are the most commonly used topical agents by North American gynecologists.

   Application: Once a week for as long as 8 weeks at a 50% to 90% concentration in 70% ethanol solution. Once TCA/BCA dries, a white frost develops on the surface of EGWs (Figure 19-13). This should not be washed off for at least 4 four hours. Burning discomfort may be reduced by topical perilesional application of 5% EMLA anesthetic cream or 25% benzocaine gel or by neutralizing TCA with sodium bicarbonate (baking soda).

   Treatment results: *Better than podophyllin, particularly for EGWs on moist genital epithelium.* No data are available as to whether TCA is superior to BCA or vice versa. Recurrences are as high as 36%.[27]

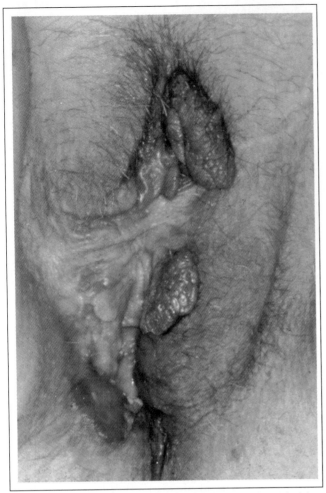

Figure 19-10 Invasive squamous cell carcinoma of vulva. This mid-adult organ transplantee has been treated for recurrent condylomata acuminata for a number of years. At the margin of previously treated area, a sharply demarcated, ulcerative lesion developed, which on excision was found to be invasive cancer. (From Ferenczy A. External genital human papillomavirus infections. Curr Obstet Gynaecol 1995;5:98–106.)

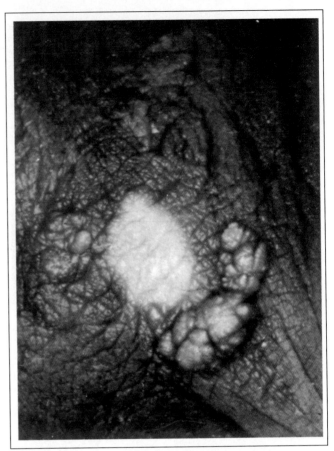

Figure 19-11 Koebner phenomenon. In this patient, multiple acuminate lesions developed peripherally to previous treatment sites (vitiligoid epithelium). They are believed to represent complications due to activation of latent HPV.

Adverse effects: Same type of skin reactions as for podophyllin; however, overapplication may produce *excessive pain, ulcerations, and scarring*. TCA/BCA are not absorbed into the systemic circulation and can be *safely used during pregnancy*.

3. **5-Fluorouracil (5-FU) cream (Efudex):** This is an antimetabolite interfering with nuclear DNA and ribonucleic acid (RNA) synthesis; it is a sort of DNA "splitter." In current practice, its use is *limited to meatal warts. The therapeutic response is difficult to evaluate.* It should not be used in pregnancy and generally has limited application.

4. **Cryotherapy:** This is the most commonly used means to treat EGWs by North American dermatologists and genitourinary medicine clinics in the United Kingdom.[28] Liquid nitrogen is the most common refrigerant used by dermatologists, and nitrous oxide is the most common refrigerant used by gynecologists. Regardless of cryogen

Table 19-2 Role of the Male Sexual Partner in Treatment Results of Vulvar/Anal Condylomata

Male Partners**	Recurrence of Vulvar Warts*	
	Number of Patients	**Percent (%)**
CO$_2$ laser/LEEP + condom (n = 55)	92	58
No therapy/no condom (n = 53)	98	62
Total: 108	160	100

LEEP, Loop electrosurgical excision procedure.
*After single CO$_2$ laser therapy or LEEP.
**With clinical/subclinical lesions.

Table 19-3 External Genital Warts: Summary Data of Treatment Results by Therapeutic Methods

Therapy	Complete Clearance (%)	Recurrence Rates (%)
Provider Applied		
Podophyllin	22–80	21–65
BCA/TCA	64–80	36
Cryotherapy, Electrosurgery, CO$_2$ laser	70–96	25–39
Excision	72–94	25–51
Interferons:	72–97	6–49
Systemic	89–93	19-22
Intralesional	7–82	23
Topical	36–52	21–25
	33	N/A
Patient Applied		
Podofilox (Condyline)	68–88	16–34
Imiquimod (Aldara)	50	13–19
Polyphenon-E (Veregen)	59	10.5

Adapted from K. Beutner and A. Ferenczy, Am J Med 1997;102:29, and A. Ferenczy, J SOGC Dec 1999:1307.
BCA, Bichloracetic acid; *TCA*, trichloracetic acid; *N/A*, data not available.

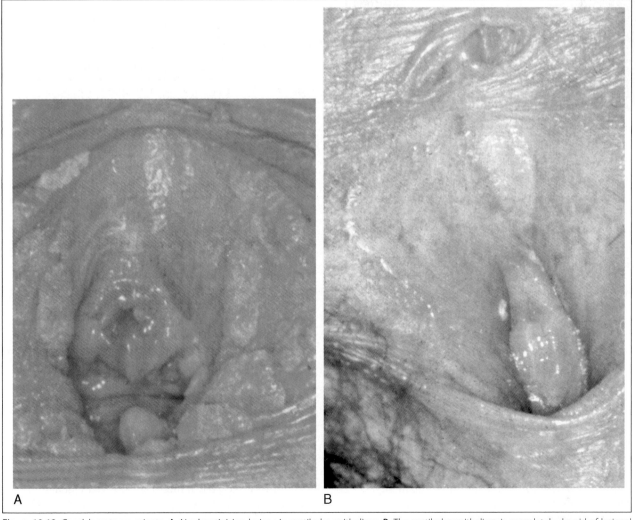

A   B

Figure 19-12 Condylomata acuminata. **A,** Nonkeratinizing lesions in vestibular epithelium. **B,** The vestibular epithelium is completely devoid of lesional epithelium 8 weeks after home therapy with imiquimod 5% cream.

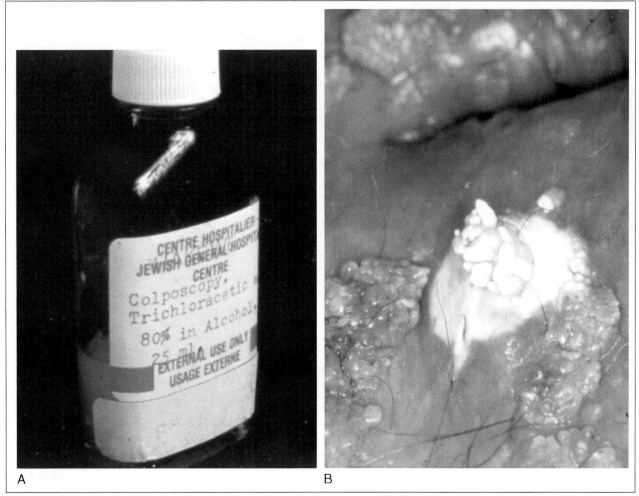

A   B

Figure 19-13 Topical trichloroacetic acid therapy. **A,** 80% TCA solution must be shaken to obtain a turbid fluid prior to application. **B,** Soon after application, the salt oxidizes, producing chemocoagulation of condylomata and 2 mm of the adjacent epithelium.

used, *the cryo-coagulative effect is particularly noticeable on small and keratinized lesions.*

Application: Therapy is delivered once a week for as long as 8 weeks using a modified cotton-tipped applicator or spray by dermatologists or cryoprobe by gynecologists. To optomize treatment results, it is important to *double- or triple-freeze with appropriate thaw periods (30 seconds) and extend the ice ball 2 to 5 mm beyond the margin of the lesion being treated* (Figure 19-14).

Treatment results: *Clearance rates as high as 80% are obtained; however, recurrences may be as high as 21%.*[27,28]

Adverse effects: The most frequent complaint is *pain during therapy;* however, the pain is generally only mild to moderate in severity and of short duration. In the case of severe discomfort, local anesthesia—either topical 5% EMLA cream or subepithelial injection of 2% lidocaine solution—may be used at treatment sites. Cryotherapy can safely be used during pregnancy.

5. **CO_2 laser therapy:** Heat generated by CO_2 laser light is selectively absorbed by intra- and intercellular water, resulting in instant vaporization of genital warts. Under magnification, the laser light is delivered with precision,

preventing excessive removal of normal tissues adjacent to lesional tissues. *With appropriate depth control, healing occurs without scarring.*

Application: The laser beam is best delivered either using a micromanipulator or handheld device at magnification (using colposcopy) (Figure 19-15). The procedure requires either local or general anesthesia depending on the extent and anatomic location of disease. *CO_2 laser therapy is indicated for extensive disease and that which has failed to respond to other forms of therapy.* Its major pitfall is the high cost of the equipment and its maintenance. The technique requires hands-on training and a relatively high volume of cases to acquire and maintain expertise.

Treatment results: *Success rates are 50% including recurrences after a single session and 70% to 80% after multiple treatments.*[27] Due to the coagulative property of the CO_2 laser beam, vaporization has been used for *treating heavily vascularized EGWs during pregnancy.* The lowest recurrence rates are observed when treatment is given during the last trimester (i.e., 32–34 weeks).[29]

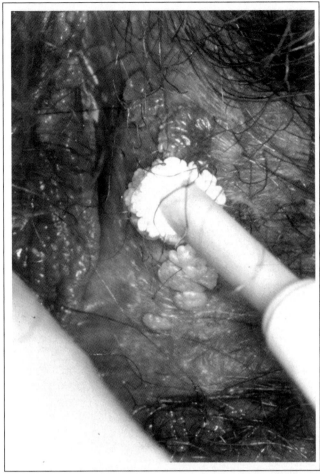

Figure 19-14 Cryotherapy. Cryogen in the form of nitrous oxide gas is delivered onto warts by a cryoprobe.

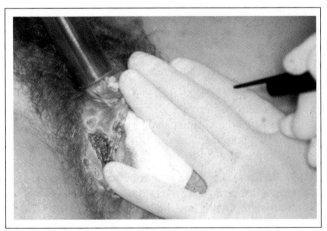

Figure 19-15 CO_2 laser vaporization. Laser light is delivered a handheld device, and a suction hose *(upper left)* is kept within 1 inch of the operative field to adequately remove the plume of smoke.

Adverse effects: *Using appropriate technique, the cosmetic results are excellent* (Figure 19-16). Poor depth control may lead to delayed healing, pain, scarring, perforations, and hyper- or depigmentation (vitiligo). The laser beam may ignite rectal gases in inappropriately

prepared patients to whom laser therapy is delivered for intra-anal warts. Adequate evacuation of the plume of smoke is critical to prevent inhaling allergens, carcinogens, and HPV DNA.

6. **Electrosurgery:** This technique uses high- (radio) frequency alternating current to electroexcise, desiccate, or fulgurate EGWs. Electrosurgery generates less smoke than the CO_2 laser surgery.

    Application: Electrosurgery is performed under local or general anesthesia. Loop-shaped and ball-type electrodes are used for excision and fulguration, respectively. The thermocoagulated eschar is removed by a wet cotton-tipped applicator or a curette (Figure 19-17).

    Treatment results: *After considering recurrences, complete clearance rates are similar to those obtained by CO_2 laser photovaporization, in the order of 50%.*[23] *Cure rates can be improved with repeated laser sessions.* The advantages of electrosurgery over laser therapy are the lower cost of the equipment and maintenance and easier depth control when electrofulguration is used.

    Adverse effects: Electroexcision with either loop or needle-shaped electrodes may cause *deep cuts into dermis that may lead to intraoperative bleeding and require suturing.* Electrofulguration or desiccation that extends to the deep dermis or subcutaneous fat may result in *hypertrophic scarring.*

7. **Surgical excision:** This is probably the *best and least costly option for a limited number (<10) of warts and may also be used for recurrent and large or extensive acuminate warts.*

    Application: Local or general anesthesia is required. Excisions are performed using either *scissors or cold or hot knife* (Figure 19-18). Another advantage of surgical excision is that it *provides specimens for histologic evaluation.* Bleeding sites from extensive excisions are sutured, whereas those from smaller sites are treated with topical Monsel's paste or electrofulguration.

    Treatment results: *After considering recurrences, complete clearance rates are in the order of 70% to 80% after one session and 90% after repeat excisions.*[27]

    Adverse effects: In unskilled hands, intraoperative bleeding due to poor depth control, postoperative pain, and delayed healing with or without scarring may occur.

8. **Interferons (IFNs):** Both natural and recombinant IFNs have antiproliferative, immunomodulating, and antiviral effects although they have not been shown to clear HPV DNA.[22,27] Prospective, randomized, placebo-controlled studies have shown that when IFNs are administered systemically (subcutaneous or intramuscular) at a site distant to the EGWs, they are ineffective.[30] Currently, *only IFN-α produced by virus-infected lymphocytes/lymphoblasts is approved by the FDA for intralesional use in the treatment of EGWs in the United States.*

    Application: The treatment protocol consists of sublesional (not intralesional) injections of recombinant

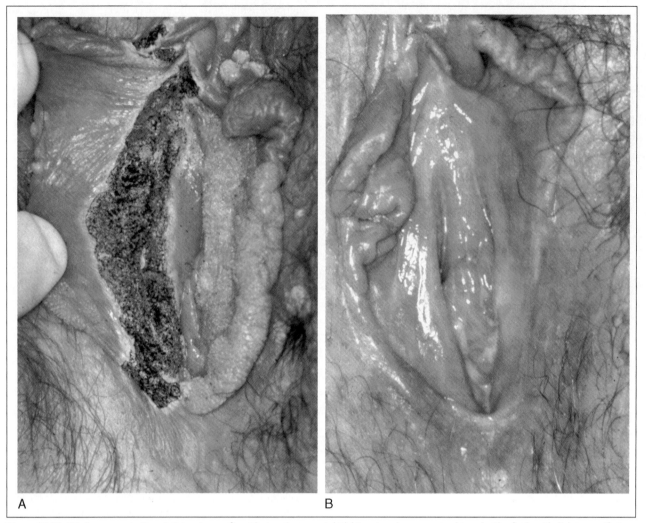

A   B

Figure 19-16 CO_2 laser vaporization. **A,** Extensive confluent lesions (seen on right labia minora) are vaporized to a depth of subepithelial stroma (first surgical plane). **B,** Complete re-epithelialization without scarring of treatment fields occurs by the eighth week after laser vaporization. (From Ferenczy A, Behelak Y, Wright TC, et al. Treating vaginal and external anogenital condylomas with electrosurgery vs CO_2 laser ablation. J Gynecol Surg 1995;11:42–43.)

IFN-α2b three times a week for 3 weeks; for natural IFN-α, injections are given twice a week for 8 weeks. Results following topically applied IFNs (in the form of cream) are not better than placebo. Another therapeutic approach uses IFN as an adjunct to conventional therapy.

Treatment results: *Intralesional IFNs produce two to four times better clearance rates than the placebo; however, the overall efficacy and recurrence rates are comparable to other forms of therapy*[31] (see Table 19-1).

Adverse effects: Patients frequently complain of *flulike symptoms, fever, and pain at injection sites and require frequent office visits.* For example, with IFN-α2b, only five EGWs can be treated in one sitting, whereas with natural IFNs, treatment is total dose limited. Additionally, IFN therapy is *expensive* (U.S. $900–1200 per month) and long-term therapy may result in leukopenia. Because of the shortcomings of IFN therapy, it is *rarely used as a treatment of EGWs and then only as a last resort.*

Patient-Applied Therapies

Patient-applied therapies have been developed primarily to improve patient compliance with therapy and reduce costs related to provider-administered therapies. They are available in liquid solution and solid (gel, cream, or ointment) formulations and include the following:

1. **Podophyllotoxin:** This is the main cytotoxic lignin of podophyllin resin, also referred to as *podophyllotoxin.* Unlike podophyllin, in which the concentration of podophyllotoxin is high and nonstandardized (8–25%), in podofilox the concentration is low and standardized to 0.5%. This results in a lower concentration of systemic podofilox, and it is therefore safer to use than podophyllin. Podofilox has been homologated worldwide and is available under the names of Condylox, Condyline, and Wartec.

Application: Podofilox is available as a 0.5% solution (3.5 ml), a 5% gel (3.5 g), and a 0.15% cream. Regardless of presentations, they are *applied topically twice a day, three*

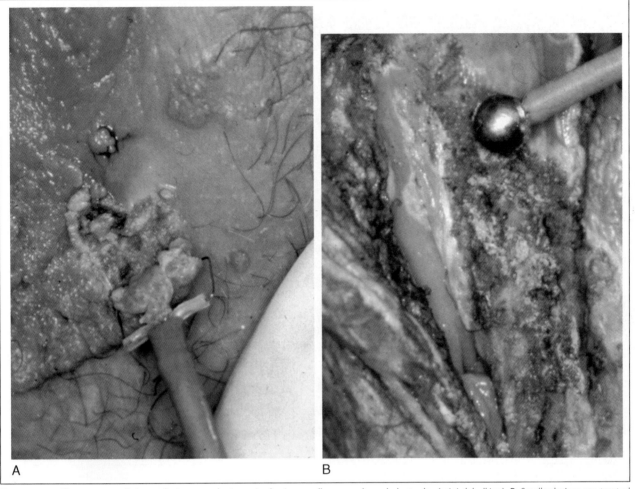

Figure 19-17 Electrosurgery. **A,** Larger lesions are electroexcised using small, square-shaped electrodes (mini-debulking). **B,** Smaller lesions are treated by electrofulguration with a ball-shaped electrode using coagulating power output. (From Ferenczy A, Behelak Y, Wright TC, et al. Treating vaginal and external anogenital condylomas with electrosurgery vs CO$_2$ laser ablation. J Gynecol Surg 1995;11:42–43.)

days per week for as long as 3 weeks. If a partial response is obtained by 3 weeks, treatment may be continued as off-label use for as long as 8 weeks. The solution is applied with cotton-tipped applicators, and the gel/cream formulations are applied with a finger. Total wart area treated should not exceed 10 cm². It is important to demonstrate the appropriate application technique to the patient in the office and indicate the location of EGWs to be treated.

Treatment results: Several comparative clinical trials showed better and faster therapeutic response with podofilox than podophyllin or placebo.[32] *Therapeutic response to solution is similar to gel formulation (30–70%); unfortunately, 35% to 90% of patients with wart clearance experience recurrences.*

Adverse effects: Moderate to severe reactions occur usually within the first 2 weeks of treatment and include burning pain (59%), erythema (40%), and erosions (30%) at treatment sites.[32] Although the concentration of podophyllotoxin is low, *podofilox should not be prescribed to pregnant women, as it has teratogenic and embryotoxic effects (FDA pregnancy category C).*

2. **Imiquimod 5% cream (Aldara):** Imiquimod *destroys HPV-infected keratinocytes by stimulating the cell-mediated immune system.* Imiquimod is a potent pro-inflammatory cytokine inducer in both animal models and humans. The main cytokines are IFN-α; interleukin-1, -6, and -8; and tumour necrosis factor. Induction of cytokines is rapid (8 hours after cream application) and sustained for 1 to 3 days.[33] Importantly, virus-presenting Langerhans cells (decreased CD-1), T cells (increased CD-4 and 8+), and T-cell activation (increased CD-29) are all stimulated by imiquimod at wart sites. Paralleling the increase in intralesional IFNs, HPV DNA L$_1$ and E$_7$ genes decreased dramatically from baseline value. The results indicate that imiquimod has powerful but nonspecific antiviral activity.

Application: Imiquimod is available in packets (sachets), each containing 0.25 g of 5% imiquimod vanishing cream. The cream is rubbed into the warts with a finger followed by handwashing. It is *applied in thin layers at bedtime three times a week for as long as 16 weeks.* The treatment sites are washed the next morning. Imiquimod is dispensed for a period of 4 weeks at a

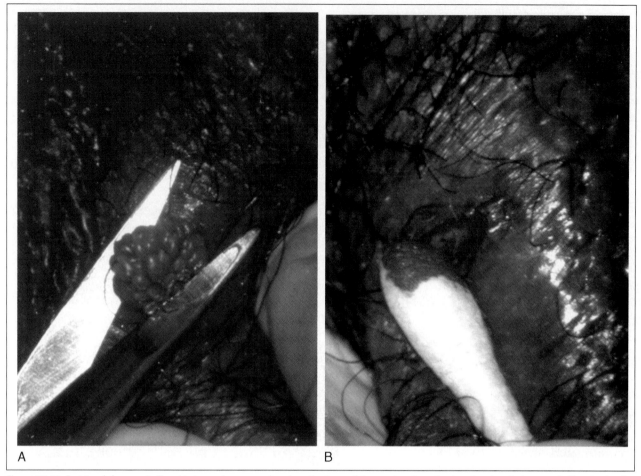

Figure 19-18 Excisional therapy. **A,** Fine, iris-type scissors are placed on the base of the wart and gently closed and pulled to cut. **B,** The depth of excision is shallow. Hemostasis is provided by Monsel's paste, which is then removed to prevent scarring of treatment sites.

time, and the patient is examined at the end of each month of therapy.

Treatment results: In a prospective, multicenter, randomized vehicle-controlled, double-blind study of 209 patients, *50% experienced total clearance of their EGWs compared with 11% for the placebo group* (intent-to-treat analysis).[24] More women (72%) than men (33%) responded favorably to imiquimod, presumably because of differences in bioavailability of the active agent, shorter outbreak, and younger age of female than male patients. Indeed, men had more keratinizing warts and longer outbreak (>6.5 months) and were older (>29 years) than their female counterparts. In addition to the total clearance rates, the *majority of patients experienced a 50% or greater reduction (partial response) of the total wart area.* Partial therapeutic response was observed in most patients by the fourth week of treatment, and close to 50% of patients were cleared of EGWs by the eighth week of therapy. *The most attractive feature of imiquimod was its association with a low recurrence rate (13%), similar to that experienced by the placebo group (10%).*

Adverse reactions: These are mainly limited to *application site reactions* such as burning (22%), pruritus (13%), pain (6%), erythema (61%), erosion (30%), and excoriation (32%). Most local skin reactions are mild to moderate and resolve spontaneously.[24] Patients, particularly those with fair skin complexions, may be hypersensitive to imiquimod and should be warned to apply imiquimod only once or twice a week. More frequent applications may be associated with severe local skin reactions including burning pain, severe erythema, and erosions.

Systemic IFN-like side effects are rare with imiquimod. It has not been clinically tested in pregnancy, although no complications (abortion or premature delivery) were observed in five pregnant patients treated with imiquimod (personal observation). Experimentally, imiquimod is not mutagenic, cytotoxic, teratogenic, or carcinogenic. Although it is classified as FDA pregnancy category B (no known fetotoxic effects), *whether it may be used in pregnancy remains to be determined.* Imiquimod *should not be used on open wounds, erosions due to infections or inflammatory* reactions, or as postsurgical therapy for EGWs or genital ulcers.

3. **Polyphenon-E ointment 15% (Veregen)** has recently received FDA approval for home therapy for EGWs (*www.bradpharm.com*). The active ingredient in polyphenon-E is a mixture of catechins extracted from green tea. Catechins are antioxidants and have possible anticarcinogenic, anti-inflammatory, antimicrobial, and antiviral activities.[34]

   Application: Three times a day (up to 250 μg) until clearance or 12 weeks maximum.

   Treatment results: In a prospective phase II/III, pivotal, randomized, controlled trial with placebo on 125 male and 117 female patients with EGWs, *complete clearance of pre-existent and post-baseline (new) warts was 59% versus 37.3% in the placebo group.*[25] Partial clearance (>50% total wart area) occurred in 54.5% of the active treatment group versus 51.8% for placebo. Recurrence rates were 10.6% and 10.3% in the active and placebo-treated groups, respectively. The median time to clearance was 16 weeks both in the active and placebo treatment groups.

   Adverse effects: These occurred in 8% of the subjects; most were related to *local application site reactions* and occurred more frequently in the 15% ointment group versus placebo. Local reactions occurred after 2 weeks of treatment and decreased gradually over the remaining study period. Only three patients discontinued participation in the study because of allergic dermatitis. Systemic adverse events were not encountered. *No information is available as to its safety in pregnant patients.*

Therapies for Intractable Disease

The management of EGWs, particularly in immunosuppressed patients including HIV-infected individuals, is frustrating because failure and recurrence rates are very high. Theoretically, imiquimod could be an attractive choice of therapy for this population because it boosts cell-mediated immunity. Unfortunately, in one randomized, controlled trial of 100 patients, complete response rates were only 11% versus 6% in the placebo group, whereas the partial response rate was 38% versus 14%.[35] Similarly, response rates have been lower (31%) in 75 highly active antiretroviral therapy (HAART)-treated HIV-positive subjects compared with 50 HIV-negative control subjects (62%). Nevertheless, overall *55% of the HIV-positive patients had either complete or partial response with 20% recurrence rates, findings that are highly acceptable considering the difficulties in treating this subset of the population.*[36]

Cidofovir 1% gel has been tried in desperate cases. It is given once a day at bedtime for five consecutive days for a maximum of 6 cycles, with 1 week off between treatment cycles. Cidofovir is a nucleotide analogue with a broad-spectrum antiviral (DNA) activity. *Cidofovir therapy causes necrosis of EGWs. It should only be used on external lesions, as its absorption through nonkeratinized, internal mucous membranes may lead to nephrotoxicity.* In one study of 10 patients, 40% complete response occurred within 2 weeks of treatment and 30% of patients had 50% or greater total wart reduction.[26]

Several off-label treatment combinations may be considered for intractable EGWs either simultaneously or concomitantly. These include simultaneous application of 80% to 90% TCA and podophyllin solutions; surgical ablation followed by topical application of either 85% TCA solution/1% cidofovir daily, or imiquimod 5% on newly recurrent lesions. Topical therapy may be replaced by systemic IFN therapy.[37–39] The author often uses 85% TCA solution to remove surface keratin layer on keratinized warts. This is then followed by home therapy with 5% imiquimod cream or polyphenon-E ointment. In open-labeled, noncontrolled clinical trials in HIV-positive men, electrofulguration or laser vaporization followed by application of intra-anal imiquimod suppositories reduced recurrences of intra-anal condylomata and viral load by 50%.[40] Laser vaporization followed by intramuscular injection of IFN has been standard therapy for juvenile onset of recurrent respiratory papillomatosis (JORRP) with relatively good results in reducing recurrent disease.[8] More recently, IFN therapy has been replaced by the phytochemical indole-3-carbinole (I-3-C). I-3-C is extracted from vegetables such as cabbage and broccoli and has a potent, direct antiproliferative effect in both estrogen-dependent and independent tumor cell lines by inducing a G1 cell cycle arrest and increasing p53-independent apoptotic response.[41] I-3-C is administered orally, has little side effects compared with IFN therapy, and reduces recurrences to the same magnitude as IFN therapy. Adjuvant IFN-α2b therapy has also been assayed after cryosurgery and CO_2 laser vaporization delivered for refractory EGWs. The results have been mixed; one controlled trial found no increased efficacy of cryotherapy combined with subcutaneous injection of IFN,[42,43] whereas others reported increased efficacy with systemic IFN-α prior to cryotherapy[44] as well as IFN-α prior to CO_2 laser vaporization.[40] In one study, better complete response rates (67%) were reported with intralesional IFN combined with podophyllin versus 42% with podophyllin alone. However, recurrence rates were the same: 67% and 65%, respectively.[38] Lower recurrences have been obtained when intralesional IFN was used as an adjunct to either CO_2 laser or 5-FU therapy (27%) compared with those without IFN therapy (24%).[39]

PROSPECT FOR HUMAN PAPILLOMAVIRUS VACCINES

Because EGWs are HPV induced, prevention by using prophylactic HPV vaccination in HPV 6/11-naïve individuals is the best approach. The recently FDA-approved *quadrivalent HPV 6/11/16/18 L_1-VLP (Gardasil) has been shown in multiple, large, randomized control trials (RCTs) to have a 95% to 99% efficacy of preventing HPV 6 or 11–positive EGWs.*[44] However, the impact of universal mass vaccination programs to reduce substantially EGWs will take several years, and parallel to prophylactic vaccination, it may be appropriate to develop therapeutic HPV vaccines to treat existing disease. *Unfortunately, clinical trials published to date fail to show cure rates any better, and sometimes even less favorable, than those existing with conventional medical or surgical treatment modalities.*[45]

Whereas prophylactic vaccination depends on the secretion of neutralizing antibodies against HPV (humoral immunity), induction of cell-mediated immunity including cytotoxic cells that are needed to regress anogenital warts is much more difficult.[46] In general, the target molecules of interest have been the HPV E_6 and E_7 gene products. So far, several phase I and II RCTs have been conducted using a variety of therapeutic vaccine designs including recombinant viruses, synthetic peptides, and dimeric virus-like particles. Despite induction of an adequate immune response, therapeutic vaccination that uses fusion protein of L_2 and E_7 from HPV type 6 (HPV L_2/E_7) and ASO_2A adjuvant fail to increase the efficacy of conventional therapies for EGWs.[45] In another uncontrolled study on 14 patients using HPV-16 E_7 protein fused to heat-shock protein 65 (Hsp65) from mycobacterium bovis, 3 of 14 (28%) patients completely cleared their EGWs.[46] However, this clearance rate is not greater than that reported in patients receiving placebo and might be due to a nonspecific effect of Hsp65.[24]

The failure of therapeutic vaccines may be due to (1) using a weak antigen such as L_2 as opposed to a more potent inducer of both neutralizing antibodies and cell-mediated immunity such as L; (2) E_7 may be expressed too late in the viral cycle as opposed to E_2 or E_4; and (3) E_7 protein may be "masked" from immunocytes by L_2, which is the predominant part in the L_2E_7-HPV-6 vaccine.

Many more and larger RCTs are needed to refine HPV research aimed at the development of effective therapeutic vaccines.

CONCLUSIONS

Genital warts are mostly caused by the low-risk HPV types 6 and 11. They represent a major burden of disease with a 10% lifetime risk of developing lesions and high medical, financial, and psychological costs. *Both external and internal genital warts need treatment because persistent lesions are a source of infection to sexual partners and rarely to newborn infants.* Treatment strategies should be discussed with the patient and be instituted after obtaining a mutual (patient–healthcare provider) agreement on the choice(s) of therapy (Figures 19-19 and 19-20).

Provider-administered and patient-applied therapies are appropriate either as first-line or second-line treatments. Their

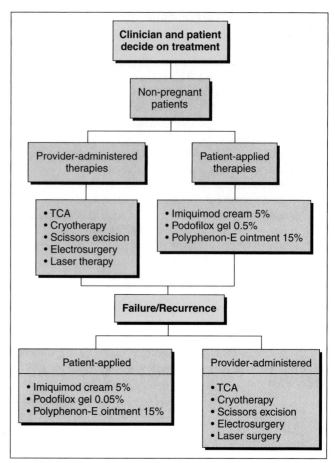

Figure 19-19 Treatment protocols for external genital warts. Flow chart to illustrate various therapeutic alternatives used for treating EGWs in nonpregnant patients. (Adapted from Ferenczy A. External anogenital warts: old and new therapies. J SOGC 1999;(Dec):1305–1313.)

choice depends on volume, distribution, and type of lesion as well as the patient's preference and financial resources.

A given treatment(s) should be discontinued if no response is obtained by 4 weeks or only partial response is observed at 8 weeks of therapy. Alternate therapies are to be instituted. Exception to the rule is 5% imiquimod cream and 15% polyphenon-E ointment, both of which are associated with a substantial rate of complete clearance if used for as long as 16 weeks.

Most single use of therapeutic agents or interventions result in an approximately 50% wart clearance, and recurrence rates range from close to 10% and 90% with an average of 30%. Patients have to be informed about the need for multiple applications of single or combined therapies and possible adverse effects associated with wart treatments. Overall, approximately 80% of patients will experience clearance of their warts within 1 year after multiple therapeutic attempts; the remaining 20% will need further therapies on a relatively long-term basis or follow-up without therapy. Short of efficacious HPV vaccines, the best preventive action is to practice long-term, mutual monogamy or the consistent and correct use of condoms. The ultimate solution will likely be provided by universal, mass, prophylactic vaccination with HPV 6/11-containing vaccines.

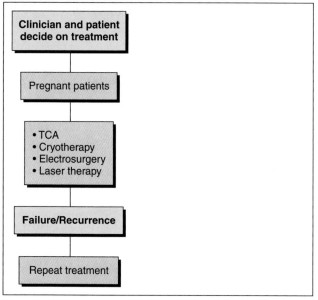

Figure 19-20 Treatment protocols for external genital warts. Flow chart to illustrate therapeutic alternatives, all of which are considered safe for both the pregnant patient and the fetus. In cases of recurrence, focus on vaginal and introital lesions that are potentially infectious to the baby during delivery, rather than attempting to remove all anogenital lesional tissue. (Adapted from Ferenczy A. External anogenital warts: old and new therapies. J SOGC 1999;(Dec):1305–1313.)

REFERENCES

1. Koutsky LA, Galloway DA,Holmes KK. Epidemiology of genital human papillomavirus infection. Epidemiol Rev 1988;10: 122–163.

2. Kjaer SK, Munk C, Tran TN, et al. The burden of genital warts: a study of nearly 70,000 women from four Nordic countries. Abstract SS21-1 presented at the 6th EUROGIN Congress, Paris, France, April 23–26, 2006.

3. Arduino JM, Roberts C, Skeldestad FE, et al. Cumulative incidence of genital warts by baseline HPV infection status in young, sexually active, Norwegian women. Abstract SS21-6 presented at the 6th EUROGIN Congress, Paris, France, April 23–26,2006.

4. Winer RL, Lee SK, Hughes JP, et al. Genital human papillomavirus infection: incidence and risk factors in a cohort of female university students [published erratum appears in Am J Epidemiol 200357:858]. Am J Epidemiol 2003;157:218–226.

5. Oriel JD. Natural history of genital warts. Br J Vener Dis 1971; 47:1–13.

6. Obalek S, Jablonska S, Favre M, et al. Condylomata acuminata in children: frequent association with human papillomaviruses responsible for cutaneous warts. J Am Acad Dermatol 1990; 23:205–213.

7. Sonnex C, Scholefield JH, Kocjan G, et al. Anal human papillomavirus infection in heterosexuals with genital warts: prevalence and relation with sexual behaviour. Br Med J 1991; 303:1243.

8. Sinclair KA, Woods CR, Kirse DJ, et al. Anogenital and respiratory tract human papillomavirus infections among children: age, gender and potential transmission through sexual abuse. Pediatrics 2005;116:815–825.

9. Sattler C. Personal communication.

10. Palefsky JM. Anal squamous intraepithelial lesions in human immunodeficiency virus-positive men and women. Semin Oncol 2000;27:471–479.

11. Ferenczy A, Coutlée F, Franco EL, et al. Human papillomavirus and HIV coinfection and the risk of neoplasias of the lower genital tract: a review of recent developments. CMAJ 2003;169:431–434.

12. Rosenberg PS, Greene MH, Alter BP. Cancer incidence in persons with Fanconi anemia. Blood 2003;101:822–826.

13. Spence AR, Franco EL, Ferenczy A. The role of human papillomavirus in cancer: evidence to date. Am J Cancer 2005;4: 49–64.

14. Bergeron C, Ferenczy A, Richart RM, et al. Micropapillomatosis labialis appears unrelated to human papillomavirus. Obstet Gynecol 1990;76:281–286.

15. Moyal-Baracco M, Leibowitch M, Orth G. Vestibular papillae of the vulva. Arch Dermatol 1990;126:1594–1598.

16. Ferenczy A, Richart RM, Wright TC. Pearly penile papules: absence of human papillomavirus DNA by the polymerase chain reaction. Obstet Gynecol 1991;78:118–122.

17. Li J, Rousseau M-C, Franco EL, et al. Is colposcopy warranted in women with external anogenital warts? J Lower Genital Tract Dis 2003;7:22–28.

18. Liaw K-L, Kurman RJ, Ronnett B, et al. Diagnosis of condylomata acuminata and vulvar and vaginal squamous intraepithelial lesions correlated with HPV 6/11 detection: comparison between a commercial central laboratory and an expert pathology panel. Abstract SS21-5 presented at EUROGIN 2006, Paris, France, April 23–26, 2006.

19. Dunne EF, Nielson CM, Stone KM, et al. Prevalence of HPV infection among men: a systematic review of the literature. J Infect Dis 2006;194:1044–1057.

20. Bleeker MCG, Snijders FJ, Voorhorst FJ, et al. Flat penile lesions: the infectious "invisible" link in the transmission of human papillomavirus. Int J Ca 2006;119;2505–2512.

21. Hippelainen MI, Yliskoski M, Syrjanen S, et al. Low concordance of genital human papillomavirus (HPV) lesions and viral types in HPV-infected women and their male sexual partners. Sex Transm Dis 1994;21:76–82.

22. CDC 2006 Guidelines for treatment of sexually transmitted diseases. Morbid Mortal Wkly Rep 2006;55(Aug 4 RR-11).

23. Ferenczy A, Behelak Y, Haber G, et al. Treating vaginal and external anogenital condylomas with electrosurgery vs CO_2 laser ablation. J Gynecol Surg 1995;11:41–50.

24. Edwards L, Ferenczy A, Eron L, et al. Self-administered topical 5% imiquimod cream for external anogenital warts. Arch Dermatol 1998;134:25-30.

25. Gross G, Meyer K-G, Pres H, et al. A randomized, double-blind, four-arm parallel-group, placebo-controlled Phase II/III study to investigate the clinical efficacy of two galenic formulations of polyphenon-E in the treatment of external genital warts. J Eur Acad Dermatol Venereol 2007;21:1404–1412.

26. Orlando G, Fasolo MM, Beretta R, et al. Intralesional or topical cidofovir (HPMPC, Vistide) for the treatment of recurrent genital warts in HIV-1-infected patients. AIDS 1999;13:1978–1980.

27. Beutner KR, Ferenczy A. Therapeutic approaches to genital warts. Am J Med 1997;102:28–37.

28. McClean H, Shann S. A cross-sectional survey of treatment choices for anogenital warts. Int J STD AIDS 2005;16:212–216.

29. Ferenczy A. Treating genital condyloma during pregnancy with the carbon dioxide laser. Am J Obstet Gynecol 1984; 148:9–12.

30. Condyloma International Collaborative Study Group. Randomized placebo-controlled double-blind combined therapy with laser surgery and systemic interferon-alpha 2a in the treatment of anogenital condylomata acuminata. J Infect Dis 1993; 167:824–829.

31. Douglas JM, Eron LJ, Judson FN, et al. A randomized trial of combined therapy with intralesional interferon alpha-2b and podophyllin versus podophyllin alone for the therapy of anogenital warts. J Infect Dis 1990;162:52–59.

32. Tyring SK, Edwards L, Cherry LK, et al. Safety and efficacy of 0.5% podofilox gel on the treatment of anogenital warts. Arch Dermatol 1998;134:33–38.

33. Tyring SK, Arany I, Stanley MA, et al. A randomized, controlled, molecular study of condylomata acuminata clearance during treatment with imiquimod. J Infect Dis 1998;178: 551–555.

34. Song J-M, Lee KH, Seong B-L. Antiviral effects of catechins in green tea on influenza virus. Antiviral Res 2005;68:66–74.

35. Gilson RJ, Shupack JL, Friedman-Kien AE, et al. A randomized, controlled, safety study using imiquimod for the topical treatment of anogenital warts in HIV-infected patients. AIDS 1999; 13:2397–2404.

36. Cusini M, Salmaso F, Zerboni R, et al. 5% imiquimod cream for external anogenital warts in HIV-infected patients under HAART therapy. Int J STD AIDS 2004;15:17–19.

37. Petersen CS, Bjerring P, Larsen J, et al. Systemic interferon alpha-2b increases the cure rate in laser treated patients with multiple persistent genital warts: a placebo-controlled study. Genitourin Med 1991;67:99–102.

38. Gross G, Roussaki A, Bauer S, et al. Systematically administered interferon alpha-2a prevents recurrence of condylomata acuminate following CO_2 laser ablation. The influence of the cyclic low-dose therapy regimen. Results of a multicentre, double-blind, placebo-controlled trial (letter). Genitourin Med 1996;72:71.

39. Klutke JJ, Bergman A. Interferon as an adjuvant treatment for genital condyloma acuminatum. Int J Gynecol Obstet 1995;49: 171–174.

40. Kaspari M, Gutzmer R, Kaspari T, et al. Application of imiquimod by suppositories (anal tampons) efficiently prevents recurrences after ablation of anal canal condyloma. Br J Dermatol 2002;147:757–759.

41. Wiatrek BJ, Wiatrak DW, Broker TR, et al. Recurrent respiratory papillomatosis: a longitudinal study comparing severity associated with human papilloma viral types 6 and 11 and other risk factors in a large pediatric population. Laryngoscope 2004;114:1–23.

42. Mayeux EJ, Harper MB, Barksdale W, et al. Noncervical human papillomavirus genital infections. Am Fam Physician 1995;52: 1137–1146.

43. Kirby PK, Kiviat N, Beckman A, et al. Tolerance and efficacy of recombinant human interferon gamma in the treatment of refractory genital warts. Am J Med 1988;85:183–188.

44. Ferenczy A, Franco EL. Prophylactic human papillomavirus vaccines: potential for sea change. Expert Rev Vaccines 2007;6:511–525.

45. Vandepapelière P, Barrasso R, Meijer CJ, et al. Randomized controlled trial of an adjuvanted human papillomavirus (HPV) type 6 L2E7 vaccine: infection of external anogenital warts with multiple HPV types and failure of therapeutic vaccination. J Infect Dis 2005;192:2099–2107.

46. Coleman N, Birley HD, Renton AM, et al. Immunologic events in regressing genital warts. Am J Clin Pathol 1994;102:768–774.

Lower Genital Tract Changes Associated with In Utero Exposure to Diethylstilbestrol

Raymond H. Kaufman

KEY POINTS

- In some parts of the United States, diethylstilbestrol (DES) continued to be prescribed widely through November 1971, when the association was reported between in utero exposure to DES and development of clear cell adenocarcinoma of the vagina and cervix.
- Gross vaginal findings observed in DES-exposed daughters include columnar epithelium, gland openings, nabothian cysts, acetowhite epithelium, mosaic, punctation, and areas that remain nonstaining after the application of Lugol's solution.
- The most frequent location of the vaginal epithelial changes is in the upper third of the vagina.
- The degree of vaginal epithelial changes is related to the dose and duration of DES exposure and to an early gestational age at first exposure.
- Careful palpation of the upper vagina may uncover small clear cell adenocarcinomas that are not readily identified on the basis of colposcopic examination.
- The colposcopic examination of the DES-exposed woman should include a careful examination of the cervix and the entire vagina.
- In a DES-exposed daughter, acetowhite epithelium, punctation, and a fine mosaic are most often associated with metaplasia. Despite this, such areas should be biopsied.
- On colposcopy, adenosis is visible as red, granular-appearing epithelium involving focal or extensive areas of the upper vagina, similar to columnar epithelium on the exocervix.
- The most common structural changes noted in the cervix include cervical collar, coxcomb, pseudopolyp, and hypoplastic cervix.
- Over time, many of these changes disappear, most often in women who have experienced a pregnancy.
- Any mode of surgical treatment may be associated with cervical stenosis in a substantial percentage of DES-exposed women.
- The risk of women exposed in utero to DES developing clear cell adenocarcinoma is less than 1 in 1000.
- Women exposed to DES in utero have demonstrated an increased risk of preterm delivery, ectopic pregnancy, spontaneous abortion, and infertility—primarily due to uterine and tubal problems.

Diethylstilbestrol (DES), a nonsteroidal estrogen, was used from 1941 through 1971 in the United States and through 1978 in Europe in the hope of improving pregnancy outcomes, especially in women with prior pregnancy loss and women with diabetes. DES was marketed by many companies under more than 70 different trade names. The peak years of its use were the 1940s and early 1950s, after which its popularity declined. Despite a report by Dieckman[1] in 1953, the medication continued to be used extensively. *In some parts of the United States, DES was prescribed widely through November 1971.* An estimated 2 to 4 million Americans received DES during pregnancy (DES mothers) or were exposed to the drug in utero (DES daughters and sons). *In 1971, a report by Herbst et al[2] demonstrated an association between in utero exposure to DES and development of clear cell adenocarcinoma of the vagina and cervix.* Seven of eight women with clear cell adenocarcinoma were delivered of mothers who had received estrogen during their relevant pregnancies. None of 32 normal control women was exposed to DES. After its use was associated with clear cell adenocarcinoma of the vagina and cervix, the drug was banned from use during pregnancy. Since that time, numerous studies have noted the relationship between in utero DES exposure and the presence of other changes in the offspring, including vaginal epithelial changes and structural changes of the cervix and upper genital tract. This review will be limited primarily to those changes noted in the cervix and vagina.

The preponderance of data relating to in utero DES exposure has been obtained from the studies carried out by the *National Cooperative Diethylstilbestrol Adenosis (DESAD) project.*[3] This multicenter study included Massachusetts General Hospital, the Mayo Clinic, the University of Southern California, and the Baylor College of Medicine. More than 4500 women were followed prospectively for a period of 10 years with annual examination and, since 1984, by questionnaire. The women studied were identified from several sources and included women determined to have been exposed to DES through review of their mothers' pregnancy records and a comparison group of women who had no prenatal exposure to DES, identified in a similar manner. Physicians referred additional women to the study clinics, and some women were self-referred for gynecologic examination and follow-up based on documented in utero DES exposure. The least biased of the women entered into the study (40%) were those identified through prenatal record review. Since 1992, several cohorts of DES-exposed daughters have been followed, including those patients originally identified in the DESAD project, the Dieckmann cohort in Chicago, and the Horne cohort in Boston. A fourth cohort was identified through the Women's Health Study, originally studied during the 1970s and 1980s.[4] In 1992, DES-exposed mothers and a comparison group of unexposed mothers were asked for permission to contact their offspring, who were then recruited into the current National Cancer Institute (NCI) follow-up study. A total of 7439 women from the various cohorts were identified as eligible for follow-up. Eighty-four of the DES-exposed offspring were already deceased, and 804 refused further contact. In 1994, 6551 women were mailed questionnaires with a response rate of 87%. Response rates since that time have varied between 90% and 93%. Information gleaned from the questionnaires mailed to the patients on a periodic basis will be discussed later in this chapter.

There has been considerable speculation as to the mechanism by which DES may be responsible for the changes identified in the exposed offspring. Walker and Kurth[5] have suggested that DES has a multigenerational effect that is transmitted through the blastocyst, and in fact the authors believed this to be consistent with a fetal germ cell mutation resulting from exposure to DES during pregnancy. It has also been suggested that in utero exposure to DES altered the manner in which the müllerian-derived epithelium was replaced by squamous epithelium advancing up from the urogenital sinus. Hajek et al,[6] using fluorescence in situ hybridization with centromeric probes for chromosomes 1, 7, 11, and 17, noted that the frequency of trisomy in the DES-exposed woman was greater than 5%. The frequency of trisomy in the control patients was less than

1.5% for all the probes used. More recently, evidence has suggested that mutagenicity is not the only or even most important mechanism for the effects of DES. Crews and McLachlan[7] have suggested that the *early exposure to DES may cause persistent epigenetic changes in some genes.* They felt that these changes may actually persist through generations of cells in a single organism and could even affect the next generation. They cited the work of Newbold,[8] who demonstrated that cancers in female DES-exposed mice were seen in the next generation of mice.

VAGINAL EPITHELIAL CHANGES

Vaginal epithelial changes include those changes observed in the vagina on the basis of colposcopic examination or iodine staining and microscopic changes in the vagina, including squamous metaplasis and epithelium of müllerian origin (endocervical, endometrial, tubal). *The gross findings observed included columnar epithelium, gland openings, nabothian cysts, acetowhite epithelium, mosaic, punctuation, and areas that remain nonstaining after the application of Lugol's solution. The microscopic changes included adenosis (columnar cells or their secretory products in the vagina) and squamous metaplasia.*

Studies differed in their estimation of the number of DES-exposed women with adenosis, with estimates ranging from 35% to 90%. Table 20-1 demonstrates the frequency of vaginal epithelial changes in the three study groups exposed in utero to DES.[9] Vaginal epithelial changes were found in 34% of the record review patients, 59% of the documented walk-in patients, and 65% of the documented referred patients. This certainly suggests some degree of selection bias in the latter two groups of women. *The most common location of the vaginal epithelial changes was in the upper third of the vagina, and only a small percentage of women were found to have changes in the lower third of the vagina.*

Patients with vaginal epithelial changes were found to have been exposed in utero to a higher total dose of DES over a prolonged period of time. Adenosis was observed in 73% of

Table 20-1 Greatest Extent of Colposcopically Observed Epithelial Change

Most Distal Extent of Change	Participant Classification			
	Record Reviews	Documented Walk-Ins	Documented Referrals	Changes, No Documentation
Vagina	435 (34%)	480 (59%)	473 (65%)	334 (84%)
Upper third	295 (23%)	319 (39%)	305 (42%)	213 (54%)
Middle third	117 (9%)	143 (18%)	134 (18%)	104 (26%)
Lower third	23 (2%)	18 (5%)	34 (5%)	17 (4%)
Total	1275 (100%)	815 (100%)	726 (100%)	396 (100%)

Data from O'Brien PC, Noller KL, Robboy SJ, et al. Vaginal epithelial changes in young women enrolled in the National Cooperative Diethylstilbestrol Adenosis (DESAD) project. Obstet Gynecol 1979;53:300–308.

subjects initially exposed during the first 2 months of pregnancy but in only 7% of those initially exposed in the 17th week of pregnancy or later.[10] *The frequency of these changes diminished with age, occurring less often among women older than 26 years.* Noller et al.[11] suggested that this finding represented a decrease in the frequency of vaginal epithelial changes over time. There was a decrease in the extent of these changes in 29.3% of women followed for a period of 3 years. Review of biopsy specimens taken at the initial examination of 3339 DES-exposed women revealed that only 45% of the women with vaginal epithelial changes had adenosis. Of significance is the fact that several reports noted a relationship between clear cell adenocarcinoma and adenosis, primarily the tuboendometrial type.

In evaluating the DES-exposed woman, careful colposcopic and cytologic examinations should be performed. *Careful palpation of the upper vagina is extremely important because small clear cell adenocarcinomas may be covered by a normal-appearing squamous epithelium and are not readily identified on the basis of colposcopic examination. Thus palpation alone may identify submucosal nodules, which require biopsy. In evaluating these women, it is important that a cytologic smear be obtained from the vaginal fornices in addition to one taken from the cervix. Unfortunately, even in the presence of a small clear cell adenocarcinoma, the cytology may be reported as negative.*

Colposcopic examination of the DES-exposed woman should include a careful examination of the cervix and the entire vagina. *Special attention should be paid to the anterior and posterior vaginal walls, which are frequently covered by the blades of the vaginal speculum; these changes may be missed.* White epithelium (Figure 20-1) after the application of 4% to 5% acetic acid most often represents the presence of squamous metaplasia. *The presence of punctation and a fine mosaic can occasionally be misleading because they are most often associated with metaplasia rather than with intraepithelial neoplasia. Despite this, such areas should be biopsied.* The colposcopic identification of adenosis is usually made on the basis of identification of *red, granular-appearing epithelium involving focal or extensive areas of the upper vagina and occasionally the mid- and lower vagina* (Figures 20-2 to 20-4). These foci have an appearance similar to columnar epithelium on the exocervix. Not uncommonly, small submucosal nabothian cysts (Figure 20-5) will be observed, and gland openings may extend onto the surface epithelium. Iodine staining of the vagina often reveals large areas of nonstaining epithelium. These areas frequently have a characteristic appearance (Figure 20-6).

STRUCTURAL CHANGES OF THE CERVIX AND VAGINA

A number of structural changes of the cervix and vagina have been observed in DES-exposed women. Some of these changes are so characteristic that their presence strongly suggests that the patient has been exposed to DES even though she does not present with a history of this exposure. The structural defects seen have been reported by Jefferies et al.

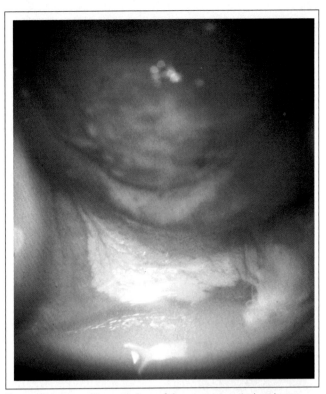

Figure 20-1 Acetowhite epithelium of the posterior vaginal vault area, representing the presence of squamous metaplasia.

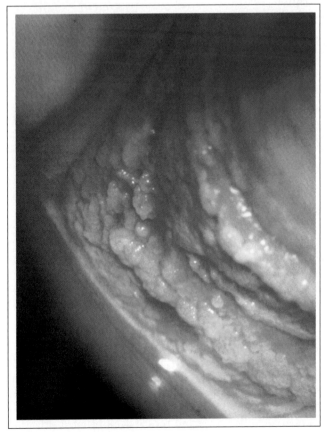

Figure 20-2 Adenosis of the cervicovaginal reflection.

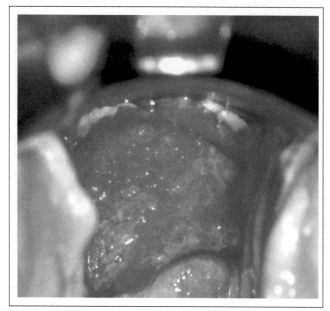

Figure 20-3 Anterior vaginal wall adenosis.

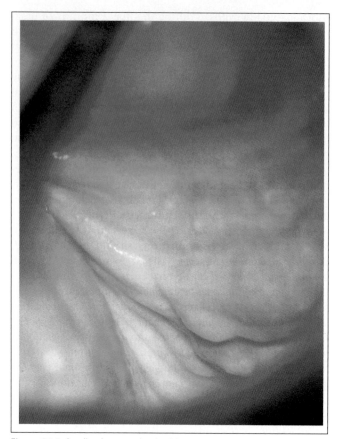

Figure 20-5 Small submucosal nabothian cyst.

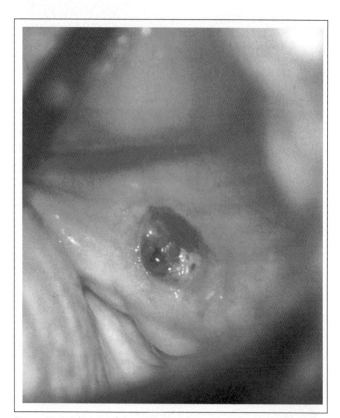

Figure 20-4 Adenosis of the posterior cul-de-sac.

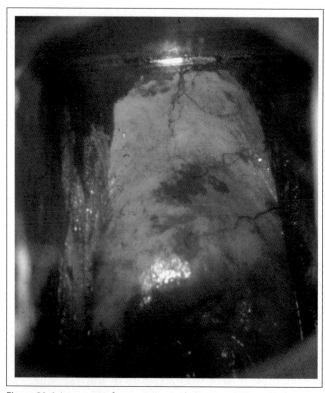

Figure 20-6 Large area of nonstaining epithelium in a DES-exposed woman.

and are listed in Table 20-2. The types and frequency of changes on the entry examination into the DESAD study are presented in Table 20-3.[12] Twenty-five percent of the women identified by record review demonstrated structural changes of the lower genital tract. Similar findings were

Table 20-2 Structural Defects

Abnormalities of Cervix and Vaginal Fornix

Coxcomb
Description	Raised ridge, usually on anterior cervix
Synonym	Hood, transverse ridge of cervix

Collar
Description	Flat rim involving part to all of circumference of cervix
Synonym	Rim, hood, transverse ridge of cervix

Pseudopolyp
Description	Polypoid appearance of cervix resulting from circumferential constricting groove, thickening of stroma of anterior or posterior endocervical canal
Synonym	Endocervical stromal hyperplasia

Hypoplastic cervix
Description	Cervix smaller than 1.5 cm in diameter
Synonym	Immature cervix

Altered fornix of vagina	Absence—complete or partial—of pars vaginalis; abnormality of fornices Fusion of cervix to vagina; partial or complete forniceal obliteration

Abnormalities of Vagina Exclusive of Fornix

Transverse septum, incomplete
Longitudinal septum, incomplete

Data from Jefferies JA, Robboy SJ, O'Brien PC, et al. Structural anomalies of the cervix and vagina in women enrolled in the diethylstilbestrol adenosis (DESAD) project. Am J Obstet Gynecol 1984;148:59–66.

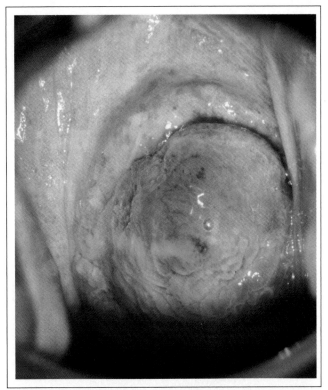

Figure 20-7 Cervical collar.

found in only 2% of nonexposed women. A total of 43% of the walk-in patients were found to have structural changes, and 49% of the referral patients had similar changes. *The most common structural changes noted in the cervix included cervical collar* (Figure 20-7), *coxcomb* (Figure 20-8), *pseudopolyp* (Figure 20-9), *and hypoplastic cervix* (Figure 20-10). Abnormalities of the vaginal fornix were also observed in the record review patients. These latter changes included a shortened fornix or vaginal strictures. As follow-up of the exposed women continues, it has been observed that *many of these changes disappear over time.* Regression of the cervical structural changes was noted in 41% of 361 women. An interesting observation was that *regression of these changes occurred most often among women who have experienced a pregnancy.*

Table 20-3 Types and Frequencies of Structural Changes Found on Entry Examination

Participant Classification	Structural Changes of Cervix and Vaginal Fornix (%)						
	Any Structural Changes	Any Type	Coxcomb	Collar	Pseudopolyp	Abnormal Fornix	Hypoplastic Cervix
Record review (n = 1655)	25.3	24.8	9.1	13.4	3.4	3.1	3.2
Control (n = 963)	2.3[†]	2.1[†]	0.9[†]	0.8[†]	0.1[†]	0.3[†]	0[†]
Walk-in (n = 800)	42.6	42.1	14	24.5	1.9	7	9.1
Referral (n = 1089)	48.6	47.8	16.1	30.9	4.5	5.7	6

Data from Jefferies JA, Robboy SJ, O'Brien PC, et al. Structural anomalies of the cervix and vagina in women enrolled in the diethylstilbestrol adenosis (DESAD) project. Am J Obstet Gynecol 1984;148:59–66.
*Values are percentages of persons in each classification who had the indicated abnormalities. Some participants had more than one abnormality.
[†]Significantly (p < 0.01) less than the record review group (chi-square test); two-sided P value = 0.059.

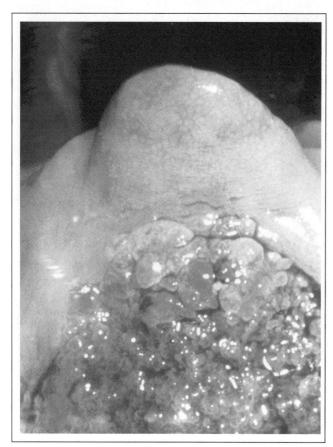

Figure 20-8 Coxcomb anterior lip.

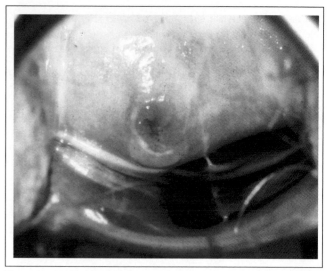

Figure 20-10 Hypoplastic cervix.

INTRAEPITHELIAL NEOPLASIA AND CLEAR CELL ADENOCARCINOMA OF THE VAGINA AND CERVIX

In 1984, Robboy et al.[13] reported that the incidence of intraepithelial neoplasia of the vagina and cervix was significantly higher in women exposed in utero to DES than in an unexposed matched cohort group (15.7 versus 7.9 cases per 1000 person-years of follow-up). In 2001, Hatch et al.[14] reviewed the records of 2899 DES-exposed and 1074 unexposed daughters who had been followed for 13 years (1982 to 1995). They obtained data on pathology and confirmed diagnoses of high-grade squamous intraepithelial neoplasia of the lower genital tract. They found that the relative risk among DES-exposed versus unexposed women, based on 111 cases of high-grade disease, was 2.1 (95% confidence interval [CI] 1.2–3.8). Relative risk was higher with earlier intrauterine exposure. When exposure occurred within 7 weeks of the last menstrual period it was 2.8 (95% CI 1.4 - 5.5). Their findings supported an association between in utero DES exposure and high-grade squamous intraepithelial neoplasia. They did suggest that more intensive screening among DES-exposed women could have been responsible for this observed excess of cases in the DES-exposed women. The last possibility, suggested by Camp et al.,[15] is that the immature metaplasia seen in the DES-exposed individual is often erroneously diagnosed as intraepithelial neoplasia (Figure 20-11). For this reason, *it is advisable to have all such diagnoses reviewed by a pathologist experienced in the interpretation of specimens obtained from the DES-exposed woman.*

Despite the potential increased risk for intraepithelial neoplasia, caution is advised when deciding on a mode of treatment. *Any mode of surgical treatment* (e.g., conization, cautery, cryosurgery) *may be associated with cervical stenosis in a substantial percentage of DES-exposed women,* and nearly 30% of DES daughters who underwent cervical cauterization or cryosurgery

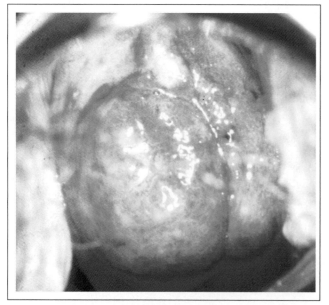

Figure 20-9 Complete cervical collar with pseudopolyp appearance.

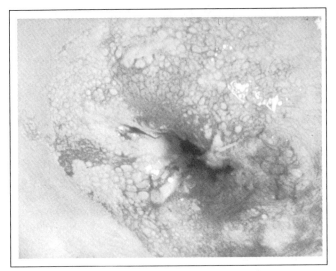

Figure 20-11 Immature metaplasia seen in a DES-exposed woman.

experienced at least one subsequent pregnancy loss.[16] *Treatment of a cervical ectropion for mucorrhea should be discouraged.* Treatment with laser vaporization may be less often associated with stenosis, but the risk is still present. There are no significant data available as to whether or not loop electrical excision of the transformation zone in the treatment of DES-exposed women with high-grade lesions will lead to cervical stenosis.

CLEAR CELL ADENOCARCINOMA OF THE VAGINA AND CERVIX

The report of Herbst et al. in 1971 brought to our attention the association of in utero exposure to DES and the development of clear cell adenocarcinoma of the vagina and cervix. Further studies have corroborated their findings. However, *the risk of women exposed in utero to DES developing clear cell adenocarcinoma is less than 1 in 1000.* The registry for research on hormonal transplacental carcinogenesis at the University of Chicago under the direction of Herbst has reviewed more than 700 cases of adenocarcinoma of the vagina and cervix. Approximately 60% of these women were exposed to DES. *The mean age of diagnosis of clear cell adenocarcinoma was 19 years, with the peak incidence occurring in 1975.* The frequency of diagnosis has decreased progressively since that time; *however, clear cell carcinoma has been diagnosed in DES-exposed women in their early 40s.* Whether there will be a secondary increase in incidence of this carcinoma in the DES-exposed women as they enter the years when this type of carcinoma is most often seen (the sixth decade of life and above) is unknown. Thus *continued careful surveillance of these women is necessary.*

Herbst et al.[17] evaluated the factors related to development of clear cell adenocarcinoma of the vagina and cervix in the DES-exposed woman. Their studies suggested that *the relative risk of clear cell adenocarcinoma was greater in those women whose mothers began DES before the twelfth week of pregnancy and in those women who were conceived during the winter.* A maternal history of at least one spontaneous

abortion appeared to increase the risk for the development of carcinoma. More recent data obtained from the follow-up of the DESAD cohort suggest that time of birth may not be related to the development of this carcinoma.

Waggoner et al.[18] detected p53 protein in tumors in 14 of 21 cases of clear cell adenocarcinoma. They were unable, however, to identify p53 mutations in any of the cases, which suggests that the tumors contained only wild-type p53. They hypothesized that p53 overexpression in clear cell adenocarcinoma was a response to generalized DNA damage, rather than a result of p53 protein half-life prolongation resulting from mutational inactivation. Waggoner et al. suggested that this overexpression of wild-type p53 protein in the clear cell adenocarcinomas might connote a more favorable prognosis compared with that of other gynecologic tumors containing mutated p53 protein. Waggoner et al.[19] further noted that the prognosis and metastatic behavior of clear cell adenocarcinoma of the vagina appeared to be influenced by DES exposure. *The DES-negative women had a worse prognosis and higher rate of metastasis than DES-exposed women.* They noted that these differences did not appear to be related to clinical prognostic factors such as tumor stage or diameter but rather suggested differences in tumor behavior.

Clear cell carcinoma may present as a firm granular lesion (Figure 20-12) *that is easily identified; however, it will occasionally present as a small, hemorrhagic nodule or as firm, submucosal nodules* (Figure 20-13). *Obviously, biopsy of such areas should be performed.*

RECENT FINDINGS IN DIETHYLSTILBESTROL-EXPOSED AND THEIR OFFSPRING

Since the institution of the questionnaire follow-up study in 1992, a wealth of data has been accumulated regarding various findings and health aspects of both the DES-exposed women and their offspring. These data will be summarized briefly.

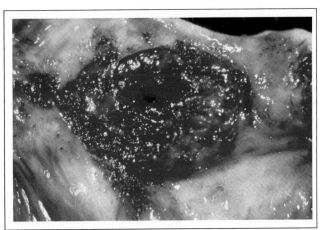

Figure 20-12 Clear cell carcinoma presenting as a firm, granular lesion.

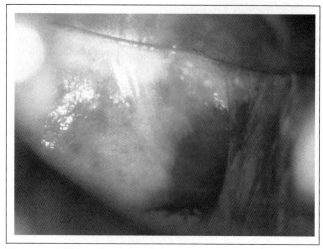

Figure 20-13 Clear cell carcinoma presenting as a small, firm, submucosal nodule.

Breast Cancer in Diethylstilbestrol-Exposed Women

In 2001, Palmer et al.[20] reported on the risk of breast cancer in the women exposed to DES in utero. The data were gleaned from the 1997 questionnaire, in which responses were obtained from 3916 exposed women and 1746 unexposed individuals. A total of 78 cases of breast cancer were reported, and the pathology reports and death certificates were obtained for 72 of them. The diagnosis was confirmed in all but 1 instance, and that case was excluded. The women had been followed for an average of 19 years. Overall, *the incidence of invasive breast cancer in exposed women was not significantly higher than in the unexposed population of women.* However, although DES exposure was not associated with an increased risk of breast cancer in women younger than age 40, in women aged 40 and older the rate ratio was 2.5 (95% CI, 1.0–6.3). A follow-up study was published in 2006[21] in which 3812 DES-exposed women and 1637 unexposed women responded to the 2001 questionnaire. At this time the median number of years followed was 24 years for the exposed women and 22 years for the unexposed women. A total of 102 cases of incident invasive breast cancer were identified. The overall age-adjusted incidence rate ratio (IRR) was 1.40 (95% CI, 0.89–2.22). For breast cancer occurring at or after age 40, the IRR was 1.91 (95% CI, 1.09–3.33), and in women age 50 or older the IRR was 3.00 (95% CI, 1.01–8.98). These findings strongly suggest that *women with prenatal exposure to DES have an increased risk of breast cancer after the age of 40 years* and support a hypothesis that prenatal hormone levels influence breast cancer risk.

Overall Cancer Risk

Titus-Ernstoff et al.[22] evaluated the long-term cancer risk in women given DES during pregnancy. They based their information on data obtained from a completed 1994 questionnaire or from death certificates. They reconfirmed a prior finding relative to a slight increased risk of breast cancer (IRR, 1.27; 95% CI, 1.07–1.52) in the mothers taking DES. However, there was no evidence that DES was associated with the risk of ovarian, endometrial, or other cancers in these women. In 2006, they published a follow-up to this study[23] and found that *DES exposure was associated with a small elevation of all-case mortality.* There was no increase in the number of cerebrocardiovascular deaths. Their findings again noted a slight increased risk of breast cancer death in the exposed women. *The data did not show an evaluated risk of mortality from cancer overall or gynecologic cancers.*

Hatch et al.[24] found, after 16 years of average follow-up, that *DES-exposed daughters did not demonstrate any increased cancer risk except for clear cell adenocarcinoma of the cervix, vagina, or both.* The DES-exposed daughters were only 38 years old at last follow-up, and thus the study does not provide information on longer-term risk of carcinoma in this population of women.

Reproductive Effects

Current studies have demonstrated an increased risk of preterm delivery, ectopic pregnancy, and spontaneous abortion in women exposed in utero to DES. In 2000, Kaufman et al.,[25] on the basis of the returned 1994 questionnaire, evaluated pregnancy outcomes in DES-exposed women. Questionnaires from 3373 exposed daughters and 1036 unexposed women were evaluated. Full-term infants were delivered in the first pregnancies of 84.5% of unexposed women compared with only 64.1% of exposed women identified by record review. *There was a significant increase in preterm delivery, ectopic pregnancy, and spontaneous abortion in the DES-exposed women as compared with the unexposed women.* This data further confirmed their prior findings.

The question of fertility in the DES-exposed woman had not been resolved until the review by Palmer et al. in 2001[26] on the basis of data obtained on 1753 exposed and 1051 unexposed women. The authors concluded that *DES exposure was significantly associated with infertility—primarily due to uterine and tubal problems,* with relative risks of 7.7 (95% CI, 2.3–25) and 2.4 (95% CI, 1.2–4.6), respectively. Hatch et al.[27] evaluated the age at natural menopause in women exposed to DES in utero. They estimated the occurrence of natural menopause in 4210 DES-exposed versus 1829 unexposed women based on responses to questionnaires mailed in 1994, 1997, and 2001. They reported that the DES-exposed women were 50% more likely to experience natural menopause at any given age. There appeared to be a dose-response effect with a greater than twofold risk for those exposed to greater than 10,000 mg DES. It was postulated that possibly a smaller follicle pool, more rapid follicle depletion, or changes in hormone synthesis and metabolism may be factors in the DES-exposed daughters.

Findings in Third-Generation Daughters

Because it has already been suggested that in utero DES exposure resulted in epigenetic alterations, it has been postulated that abnormalities might well be anticipated in the third generation offspring (daughters of mothers exposed in utero to DES). Kaufman and Adam[28] reported their results following examination of 28 third-generation daughters. Three of the daughters had been delivered from 1 mother. Review of the mothers' records demonstrated that 61.5% of the mothers exposed to DES during their pregnancies demonstrated structural changes of the cervix, upper vagina, or vaginal epithelial changes. None of the daughters were found to have changes usually associated with DES exposure. The authors believed that the absence of abnormalities in the lower genital tract in the third-generation women compared with the high frequency of these abnormalities in their mothers suggested that *a third-generation carryover related to structural affects was highly unlikely.* The number of women studied, however, was too small to generalize.

Titus-Ernstoff et al.[29] reviewed the menstrual and reproductive outcomes by mail questionnaire in 793 women whose mothers had documented information regarding in utero DES exposure. A total of 463 women were delivered of mothers exposed in utero to DES, and 330 were delivered of mothers who were not exposed to DES. *The mean age of menarche was the same in both groups (12.6 years); however, the daughters of the exposed women obtained menstrual regularization later (mean age of 16.2 years versus 15.8 years) (p = 0.05) and were more likely to report irregular menstrual periods than the unexposed daughters.* They found limited evidence that the daughters of the exposed women had more adverse reproductive outcomes; the daughters of exposed women had fewer live births (1.6 versus 1.9 in unexposed daughters) (p = 0.005). Thus it appears that there may be some carryover effect in the third-generation offspring, but additional long-term studies will be required to fully evaluate this prospect.

REFERENCES

1. Dieckman WJ, Davis ME, Ryukiewiez LM, et al. Does the administration of diethylstilbestrol during pregnancy have therapeutic value? Am J Gynecol 1953;66:1062–1081.
2. Herbst AL, Ulfelder H, Poskancer DC. Adenocarcinoma of the vagina: association of maternal stilbestrol therapy with tumor appearance in young women. N Engl Med 1971:284: 878–881.
3. Labarthe D, Adam E, Noller KL, et al. Design and preliminary observation of the National Cooperative Diethylstilbestrol Adenosis (DESAD) project. Obstet Gynecol 1978;51:453–458.
4. Colton T, Greenberg ER, Noller K. Breast cancer in mothers prescribed diethylstilbestrol in pregnancy. J Am Med Assoc 1993; 269:2096–2100.
5. Walker BE, Kurth LA. Multi-generational carcinogenesis from diethylstilbestrol investigated by blastocyst transfers in mice. Int J Cancer 1995;61:249–252.
6. Hajek RA, King DW, Hernández-Valero MA, Kaufman RH, Liang JC, Chilton JA, Edwards CL, Wharton JT, Jones LA. Detection of chromosomal aberrations by fluorescence in situ hybridization in cervicovaginal biopsies from women exposed to diethylstilbestrol in utero. Int J Gynecol Cancer. 2006 Jan-Feb; 16(1):318–324.
7. Crews D, McLachlan JA. Epigenitics, evolution, endocrine disruption, health and disease. Endocrinology 2006;147:S4–S10.
8. Newbold RR, Hanson RB, Jefferson WN, et al. Increased tumors but uncompromised fertility in the female descendents of mice exposed developmentally to diethylstilbestrol. Carcinogenesis 1998;19:1655–1663.
9. O'Brien PC, Noller KL, Robboy SJ, et al. Vaginal epithelial changes in young women enrolled in the National Cooperative Diethylstilbestrol Adenosis (DESAD) project. Obstet Gynecol 1979;53:300–308.
10. Herbst AL, Poskanzer DC, Robboy SJ, et al. Prenatal exposure to stilbestrol. N Engl J Med 1975;292:334–339.
11. Noller KL, Towsend DE, Kaufman RH, et al. Maturation of vaginal and cervical epithelium in women exposed in utero to Diethylstilbestrol (DESAD project). Am J Obstet Gynecol 1983;146:279–285.
12. Jefferies JA, Robboy SJ, O'Brien PC, et al. Structural anomalies of the cervix and vagina in women enrolled in the diethylstilbestrol Adenosis (DESAD) project. Am J Obster Gynecol 1984;148:59–66.
13. Robboy SJ, Noller KL, O'Brien PC, et al. Increased incidence of cervical and vaginal dysplasia in 3980 diethylstilbestrol-exposed young women. Experience of the National Collaborative Diethylstilbestrol Adenosis project. JAMA 1984;252: 2979–2983.
14. Hatch EE, Herbst AL, Hoover RN, et al. Incidence of squamous neoplasia of the cervix and vagina in women exposed prenatally to diethylstilbestrol (United States). Cancer Causes Control 2001;12:837–845.
15. Camp EA, Coker AL, Troisi R, et al. Who observed that the DES-exposed women exceeded the recommended frequency of pap smear screenings compared to the unexposed women. J Lower Genital Tract Dis (In press).
16. Herbst AL, Senekjian EK, Frey KW. Abortion and pregnancy loss among diethylstilbestrol-exposed women. Semin Endocrinol 1989:7:124–129.
17. Herbst AL, Anderson S, Hubby MM, et al. Risk factors for the development of diethylstilbestrol-associated clear cell adenocarcinoma: a case controlled study. Am J Obstet Gynecol 1986; 154:814–822.
18. Waggoner SE, Anderson SM, Luce MC, et al. P53 protein expression and gene analysis and clear cell adenocarcinoma of the vagina and cervix. Gynecol Oncol 1996;6:339–344.
19. Waggoner SE, Mittendorf FR, Biney N, et al. Influence of in utero diethylstilbestrol exposure on the prognosis and biologic behavior of vaginal clear-cell adenocarcinoma. Gynecol Oncol 1994;55:238–244.
20. Palmer JR, Hatch EE, Rosenberg CL, et al. Risk of breast cancer in women exposed to diethylstilbestrol in utero: preliminary results (United States). Cancer Causes Control 2002;13: 753–758.
21. Palmer JR, Wise LA, Hatch EE, et al. Prenatal diethylstilbestrol exposure and risk of breast cancer. Cancer Epidemiol Biomarkers Prev 2006;15:1509–1514.
22. Titus-Ernstoff L, Hatch EE, Hoover RN, et al. Long term cancer risk in women given diethylstilbestrol (DES) during pregnancy. Br J Cancer 2001;84:126–133.
23. Titus-Ernstoff L, Troisi R, Hatch EE, et al. Mortality in women given diethylstilbestrol during pregnancy. Br J Cancer 2006; 95:107–111.
24. Hatch E, Palmer JR, Titus-Ernstoff L, et al. Cancer risk in women exposed to diethylstilbestrol in utero. J Am Med Assoc 1998;280:631–634.

25. Kaufman RH, Adam E, Hatch E, et al. Continued follow-up of pregnancy outcome in diethylstilbestrol-exposed offspring. Obstet Gynecol 2000;96:483–489.

26. Palmer JR, Hatch EE, Rao RF, et al. Infertility among women exposed prenatally to diethylstilbestrol. Am J Epidemiol 2001;154:316–321.

27. Hatch EE, Troisi R, Wise LA, et al. Age at natural menopause in women exposed to diethylstilbestrol in utero. Am J Epidemiol 2006;164:682–688.

28. Kaufman RH, Adam E. Finding in female offspring of women exposed in utero to diethylstilbestrol. Obstet Gynecol 2002; 99:197–200.

29. Titus-Ernstoff L, Troisi R, Hatch EE, et al. Menstrual and reproductive characteristics of women whose mothers were exposed in utero to diethylstilbestrol (DES). Int J Epidemiol 2006; 35:862–868.

CHAPTER 21

Colposcopy in Pregnancy

David G. Weismiller

KEY POINTS

- The Papanicolaou (Pap) test is a reliable screening test in pregnancy. Approximately 5% to 8% of cytology results in pregnancy are abnormal; invasive cancer is rare (1 in 3000 pregnancies).
- The goal of colposcopy in pregnancy is to exclude the presence of invasive cancer and to provide support for conservative management of intraepithelial lesions.
- Colposcopy is preferred for pregnant, nonadolescent women with HPV-positive ASC-US and low-grade squamous intraepithelial lesion, but deferring the initial colposcopy until at least 6 weeks postpartum is acceptable. If no high grade disease is found, post parturm follow up is recommended. There are no specific guidelines for pregnant women with ASC-H.
- Colposcopy is recommended for all pregnant women including adolescents with high-grade squamous intraepithelial lesion (HSIL). Biopsy of lesions suspicious for CIN 2,3 or cancer is preferred. Diagnostic excision is unacceptable unless invasion is suspected based on colposcopic findings, cytology or histology.
- The initial evaluation for pregnant women with atypical glandular cells (AGC) is identical to the nonpregnant women except that endocervical curettage and endometrial biopsy are unacceptable.
- Because of the physiologic alterations of the cervix during pregnancy, colposcopy can be challenging and should be performed by experienced colposcopists.
- The transformation zone is usually fully visualized during pregnancy because the endocervical columnar epithelium becomes everted by about the 20th week of gestation (satisfactory colposcopic examination).
- Colposcopically directed ectocervical biopsies should be performed in pregnancy if the results will assist the practitioner in making management decisions about invasive disease.
- Neither precancerous nor cancerous lesions progress more rapidly during pregnancy.
- Despite significant morbidity that can occur as a result of conization during pregnancy, pregnant women with suspected microinvasion should undergo cervical conization.
- Progression of early-stage cervical cancer in pregnancy is rare. Based on limited data, postponing therapy until fetal lung maturity has been achieved does not seem to reduce survival in women receiving standard therapy.

Cervical cancer during pregnancy constitutes a threat to mother and baby. As most women at risk for cervical intraepithelial neoplasia (CIN) or cervical cancer are of childbearing age, pregnancy presents an opportune moment to screen women who otherwise would not avail themselves of routine health maintenance but who do seek prenatal care.[1,2] Cytology screening has dramatically reduced cancer rates among young women, but cancers are still identified during pregnancy. The accepted standard of care is to screen all women for cervical cancer at the first prenatal visit.[3] When results are abnormal, clinicians must balance the threat of cancer against the potential harm to the pregnancy resulting from diagnostic and therapeutic interventions.

Cervical cancer screening and colposcopy during pregnancy have two functions. For those women with mildly abnormal cytology, colposcopy can be used to identify those with occult high-grade disease. For women presenting with highly abnormal cytology, colposcopy can help direct management by distinguishing preinvasive from invasive disease. *Because of the physiologic, cytologic, histologic, and colposcopic changes of the cervix that normally occur in during pregnancy, a significant degree of expertise is required of the colposcopist.* Invasive cervical cancer can present as a small, localized, occult lesion, and its appearance may be influenced by the dramatic physiologic changes on the cervix during pregnancy.

CIN does not occur more commonly during pregnancy. The incidence of abnormal Papanicolaou (Pap) tests has been reported to be 5% to 8% in pregnancy,[2,4–8] which is identical to nongravid women.[9] It is estimated that 1.2% of these women with abnormal Pap tests (*only 1 in 3000 pregnancies*) has cervical cancer.[7] The percentage of squamous carcinomas (greater than 80%) and adenocarcinomas (up to 20%) during pregnancy is similar to the nonpregnant population.[10–12]

Although rare, cervical cancer is the most common reproductive tract malignancy associated with pregnancy. Approximately 30% of women diagnosed with cervical cancer are in their reproductive years, and 3% of cervical cancers are diagnosed during pregnancy.[4] This increased incidence of cervical cancer during pregnancy is likely due to improved surveillance during prenatal care with improved access to healthcare during pregnancy.[13] This improved surveillance accounts for the fact that cervical cancer is three times more likely to be identified at stage I in pregnant women than in their nonpregnant matched controls.[14] Overall, *cervical cancer is encountered in its earlier stages during pregnancy compared with the general population* and is two to three times more likely to be diagnosed in an operable stage of disease.[15] In two series of pregnant women with cervical cancer,[10,15] 69% to 83% were in International Federation of Gynecology and Obstetrics (FIGO) stage I, 11% to 23% were in stage II, 3% to 8% were in stage III, and 0% to 3% were in stage IV; whereas these numbers were 42%, 35%, 21%, and 2%, respectively, in a control group.[15] This observation might be explained by the frequent pelvic examinations performed during prenatal care and the fact that advanced stages will prevent conception. *When they are matched by age, stage, and year of diagnosis, there appears to be no difference in survival between pregnant and nonpregnant women with cervical cancer.* The difficulty in managing cervical cancer during pregnancy relates primarily to the clinical decision of whether to delay therapy to achieve optimal fetal outcome.

The diagnosis of invasive carcinoma during pregnancy poses a complicated therapeutic dilemma and underscores the importance of optimal cytologic screening, detection, and follow-up of CIN in pregnancy and the postpartum period. *The risk that CIN will progress during pregnancy to invasive cancer is very low, whereas the rate of regression from low-grade lesions during pregnancy to normal after has been found to be as high as 65%.* The rate of regression from high-grade lesions to normal during pregnancy in women who were evaluated sequentially by colposcopy and not by biopsy ranged from 30% to 54%. Recent literature supports a trend of conservative management of cytologic abnormalities during pregnancy.

PHYSIOLOGY OF THE CERVIX DURING PREGNANCY

Pregnancy produces dramatic alterations in the gross and colposcopic appearance of the cervix as well as in the cytology and histology of cervical pathology specimens (Table 21-1).

During pregnancy, the cervix undergoes glandular and stromal changes similar to those occurring in the endometrium.[16] Most of these changes are the result of the high estrogen state. Cervical epithelium is highly sensitive to alterations in estrogen levels. The cervical stroma undergoes extensive destruction of its collagen by collagenases and accumulation of gel-like mucopolysaccharides, as well as increased fluid content. This results in softened and edematous cervical lips that roll out onto the vagina and evert a considerable portion of the endocervix beyond the external os. The dimensions of the cervix increase appreciably with associated remodeling of surface contours.

The endocervical glands become hyperplastic, resulting in a polypoid protrusion, microglandular hyperplasia, or both. They also become hypersecretory, a state known as *endocervical gland hyperplasia*, contributing to a thick mucous plug that seals off the endometrial cavity from the vagina. Increased vascularity and abundant mucus production are clearly evident (Figure 21-1).

The increased vascularity of the cervical epithelium and stroma produces a bluish hue (Chadwick's sign)

Table 21-1 Alterations in the Cervix in Pregnancy*

Ectocervix
Alterations are mostly the result of the high estrogen status in pregnancy.
Increased vascularity produces a bluish hue.
Dilute acetic acid reaction of the metaplastic epithelium in pregnancy is exaggerated.
There is an increase in cervical volume through hypertrophy of the fibromuscular stroma.

Endocervix
Endocervical canal is everted, particularly in the primiparous woman.
There is gaping of the endocervical canal, particularly in the multiparous woman.
Everted epithelium, exposed to the acidity of the vaginal environment, usually results in significant squamous metaplasia.

*Pregnancy produces dramatic alterations in the colposcopic appearance of the cervix. The appearance is determined largely by gestational age.

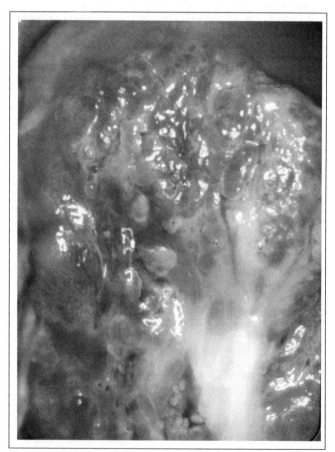

Figure 21-1 Microglandular hyperplasia resulting in a polypoid surface to the cervix along with extensive squamous metaplasia and abundant mucus production.

(Figure 21-2). The gross appearance of the cervix is determined largely by the gestational age, especially in the primigravida.[2,17] Increased estrogen content in early pregnancy

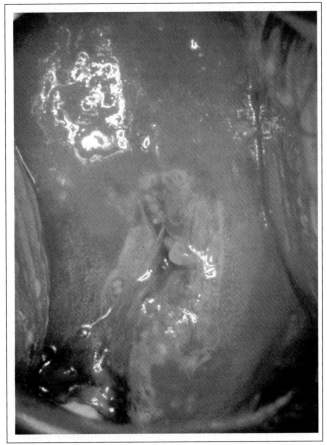

Figure 21-2 Cervix in the second trimester with vascular engorgement leading to the bluish hue called Chadwick's sign. There are also several fine, milia-like white spots that represent decidualization hypertrophy of the stromal cells.

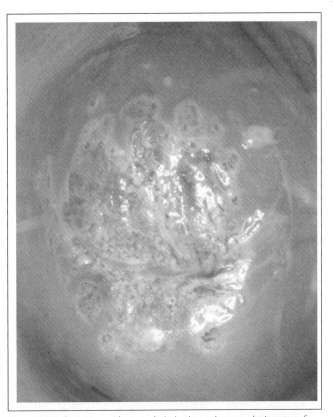

Figure 21-3 Ectropion with metaplasia in the early second trimester of pregnancy.

produces a significant expansion in cervical volume through hypertrophy of the fibromuscular stroma. Consequently, the endocervical canal is everted onto the ectocervix (Figure 21-3). The extent of eversion varies among individuals and with parity, being most common and most marked in the primiparous gestation. The eversion process begins during the early weeks of pregnancy and is usually clearly apparent in the early second trimester. A substantial amount of immature squamous metaplasia will subsequently occur. The stroma can also undergo focal or massive decidualization and may cause vaginal spotting in pregnancy[18] (Figure 21-4). In subsequent pregnancies, the extent of eversion of the endocervical canal is less significant, but gaping of the endocervical canal may result in a similar exposure of endocervical columnar epithelium to the acidic vaginal environment (Figure 21-5).

CYTOLOGY

The Pap test in the pregnant woman reflects the physiologic changes of pregnancy. Cellular components are altered in this high-estrogen environment, resulting in squamous metaplasia and cells with hypervacuolated cytoplasm and atypical nuclei reflecting endocervical gland

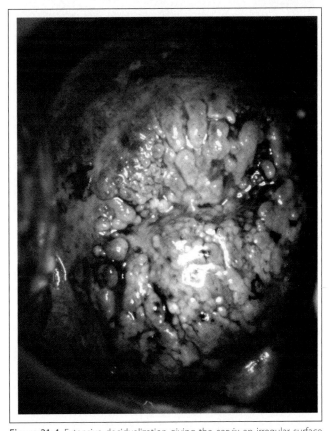

Figure 21-4 Extensive decidualization giving the cervix an irregular surface contour.

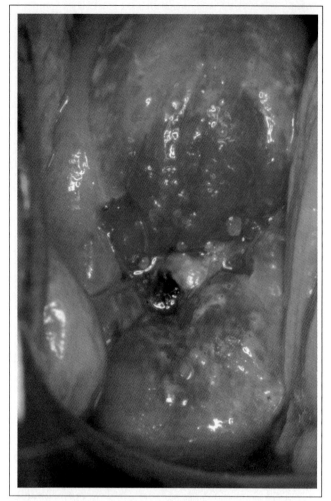

Figure 21-5 Normal cervix of a multiparous woman in the late second trimester.

hyperplasia. *As a result of the physiologic structural changes in the cervix, evaluation and interpretation of cytologic tests is more difficult during pregnancy* (Table 21-2).

Numerous reports have been published with emphasis on various aspects of pregnancy-related cellular changes and their diagnostic pitfalls[19–25]: basal cell hyperplasia, immature metaplasia, decidualization of the cervical stroma, nuclear clearing of glandular cells (endocervical gland hyperplasia), and the Arias-Stella reaction.

Cervical decidualization is not an uncommon event in pregnancy. Schneider and Barnes[26] examined 191 resected

Table 21-2 Cytologic Assessment in Pregnancy

Papanicolaou smear interpretation is more difficult.
Immature metaplasia
Basal cell hyperplasia
Decidualization
Arias-Stella reaction
Squamous intraepithelial lesion is the same as in the nonpregnant state.

gravida uteri, looking for the frequency and pattern of ectopic decidual reaction in the cervix. They found decidua in 38% of cases, of which 12 (34%) had decidual cells on Pap tests. The decidua was found in loose stroma directly beneath the overlying squamous epithelium that was commonly eroded or ulcerated. *This decidualization with erosion can result in vaginal bleeding and can be grossly and histologically mistaken for cancer.* Degenerated decidua can also mimic high-grade squamous intraepithelial lesion (HSIL). Although the cervix is the source of most decidual cells on a Pap test, some will exfoliate from the uterus. It is postulated that they slough from the free surface of the uterus by the friction of the chorion against the endometrium.[27]

Endocervical gland hyperplasia is not an uncommon event in pregnancy.[18] If recognized, it should not pose diagnostic difficulty. However, in cases of microglandular hyperplasia, the glandular atypia can be striking and may be misdiagnosed as HSIL or adenocarcinoma.[28]

The Arias-Stella reaction is a lesion that can closely mimic clear cell carcinoma.[29,30] It is a physiologic response to the presence of viable trophoblasts and increased hormonal levels. The cells are characterized by abundant, vacuolated cytoplasm; enlarged nuclei with prominent nucleoli; or smudged chromatin that can be easily mistaken for viral cytopathic effect or endocervical carcinoma.[31,32]

The presence of pregnancy-induced cytologic changes, immature metaplasia, and inflammatory infiltrate may lead to cytologic misdiagnosis. Navicular cells, low karyopyknotic and eosinophilic indexes, and marked cytolysis owing to the abundance of lactobacilli that thrive in the glycogen-rich environment[33,34] may all lead to diagnostic errors, particularly when inflammatory changes or human papillomavirus (HPV) infection are present (Figure 21-6). Conversely, actual dysplastic changes could be incorrectly attributed to pregnancy changes, leading to false-negative cytology.

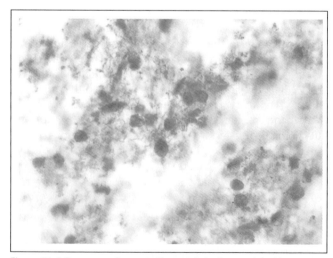

Figure 21-6 Pap smear demonstrating cytolysis. Bare nuclei without cytoplasm are seen with some nuclear irregularities. In the background, relatively large bacterial rods are identified, which are typical of lactobacilli. These are the features of cytolysis (Doderlein cytolysis).

All these changes may hinder Pap test interpretation. For the cytopathologist, these factors add to the complexity of the cytologic interpretation. Despite this, cytometric studies have shown that *CIN is morphologically identical in pregnant and nonpregnant patients.*

COLPOSCOPY IN PREGNANCY

The literature supports the role of colposcopy and directed biopsy in pregnancy as accurate and reliable.[35] *Compared with examination of the cervix in the nonpregnant patient, examination of colposcopic changes of the cervix during pregnancy demands more experienced pattern-recognition skills by the colposcopist* (Table 21-3). During pregnancy, some benign changes may cause suspicious colposcopic patterns that mimic severe lesions.[2] Examples include cervical ectropion with a coarse, grapelike appearance; large villi separated by deep longitudinal folds; coarse surface contour; and increased vascularity with confusing angioarchitecture that may result in a suspicious vascular pattern (Figure 21-7).

Transient atypical findings associated with active squamous metaplasia may be present on the transformation zone (TZ) during pregnancy. The new squamous epithelium produced during this active metaplastic transformation, or the extensive immature metaplastic epithelium itself, may exaggerate the acetowhite appearance (Figure 21-8). A fine punctation and mosaic pattern may be seen within acetowhite areas of physiologic metaplasia (Figure 21-9) and may be misinterpreted as disease. The surface contour changes associated with mucus-filled glands and decidual reaction are also confusing. Eversion of the endocervical columnar epithelium takes place after the first trimester of pregnancy and tends to be observed more commonly in primigravidas.[36,37] When prominent vascular changes accompany decidual reaction, the appearance may mimic an invasive cancer. *A small focal area of invasive cancer is sometimes difficult to detect because of the intensity of the acetowhite effect and the marked increase in vascular abnormalities.*

The squamocolumnar junction (SCJ) everts and is completely visible by 20 weeks of gestation in most pregnant women.[38] Serial colpomicrographs of the cervix throughout pregnancy confirm progressive eversion of the

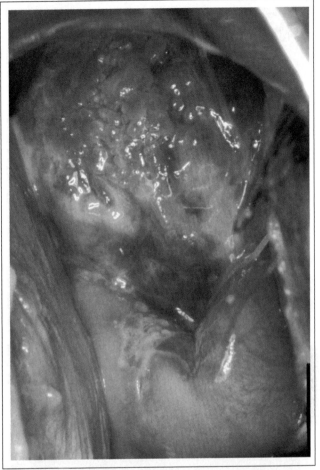

Figure 21-7 An asymmetric ectropion with increased vascularity, large crevices from hypertrophy of the epithelium, and acetowhite epithelium from metaplasia.

epithelium from the lower endocervical canal to an ectocervical position (Figure 21-10). *Thus, if colposcopy is considered unsatisfactory early in pregnancy, it may be repeated later in pregnancy when the colposcopic examination will often become satisfactory.*

Increased cervical perfusion may cause acetowhite epithelial changes to appear less prominent. This change may make high-grade lesions appear more like low-grade lesions in the nongravid state. Additionally, as physiologic eversion expands during pregnancy, new areas of acetowhite squamous metaplasia may appear. Everted columnar epithelium exposed to the acidity of the vaginal environment, particularly in the first pregnancy, enters a strikingly dynamic phase of squamous metaplasia that progresses throughout the pregnancy (Figure 21-11). Toward the end of the first trimester, eversion and the resulting metaplasia produce areas of fusion of columnar villi, with islands of immature metaplastic epithelium (Figure 21-12). This process rapidly progresses through the second trimester, producing a layer of smooth, opaque squamous metaplasia that appears acetowhite after application of 3% to 5% acetic acid (Figure 21-13). The acetowhite appearance of squamous metaplasia may be difficult to distinguish from dysplastic

Table 21-3 Colposcopic Changes of the Cervix in Pregnancy

Increased prominence of vascular patterns
Decreased prominence of acetowhite epithelium due to increased cervical perfusion.
Immature metaplasia difficult to distinguish from low-grade squamous intraepithelial lesion
Decidualization
Fine punctation and mosaic pattern within metaplasia.

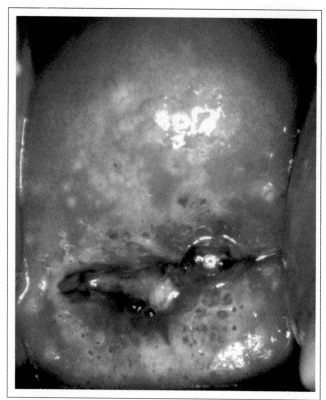

Figure 21-8 Immature metaplasia in a pregnant woman with a normal Pap smear. Several islands of columnar epithelium are present in the field of acetowhite metaplastic epithelium on the posterior lip of the cervix.

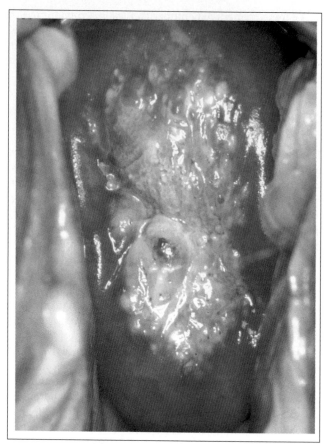

Figure 21-10 Eversion of columnar epithelium in the second trimester of pregnancy. Several small nabothian cysts are present, outlining the peripheral limits of the TZ. Acetowhite epithelium is present on the posterior lip of the cervix. Biopsy revealed decidual changes only.

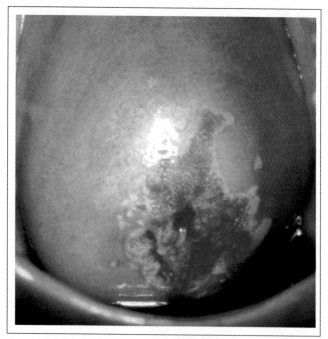

Figure 21-9 Example of a fine mosaic pattern on the anterior lip of the cervix in a pregnant patient with an ectropion and active metaplasia.

lesions except that it is typically paler, with less distinct borders than true dysplastic lesions; however, *the prominence of squamous metaplasia may still make colposcopy more difficult than in the nonpregnant state.* The vast expanse of immature metaplasia also may be difficult to distinguish from precancerous lesions.

In the third trimester, eversion of the endocervix and progressive metaplasia continues until about 36 weeks of gestation and then essentially stops. The area of metaplasia persists during the prenatal period and returns to its endocervical position in the puerperium. The metaplasia may also mature to squamous epithelium. In subsequent pregnancies, the preexisting area of metaplasia may again be everted, but not usually as dramatically as in the first pregnancy.

Similar epithelial changes occur in later pregnancies but to a limited degree. Gaping of the endocervical canal is more prominent than eversion and progresses throughout pregnancy, particularly during the third trimester (Figure 21-14). Squamous metaplasia tends to occur predominantly later in pregnancy. *The dynamic phase of squamous metaplasia associated with the first pregnancy is considered critical, representing the stage at greatest risk for initiation of cervical carcinogenesis.*

The vascularity of the cervix also tends to be more prominent during pregnancy, making it more important to distinguish benign vascular patterns from atypical vascular patterns associated with high-grade and invasive disease.[39] Lastly, *tenacious*

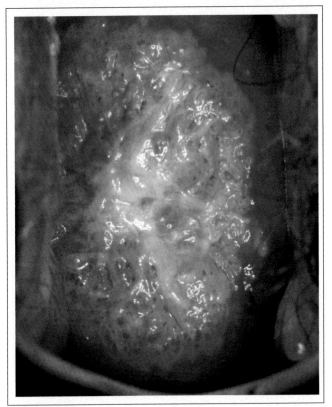

Figure 21-11 Example of a large eversion of columnar epithelium onto the portio of the cervix. Extensive metaplasia and copious thick mucus are present.

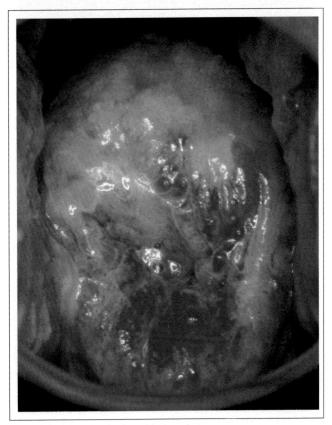

Figure 21-13 Large ectropion with metaplasia.

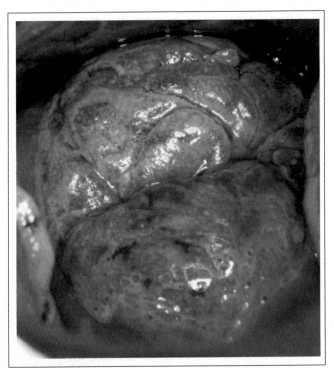

Figure 21-12 Pregnancy-related metaplasia with fusion of villi. The individual grapelike clusters of the columnar epithelium are no longer evident.

endocervical mucus develops during pregnancy and can hinder colposcopic assessment (Figure 21-15).

HISTOLOGY

During pregnancy, the cervix is characterized histologically by stromal edema, decidualization, increased vascularity, and enlargement of glandular structures associated with an acute inflammatory response[40] (Figure 21-16). The enlarged stromal glands are frequently mucus-filled and distort the architecture (Figure 21-17). Stromal decidualization occurs in the second and third trimesters in approximately 30% of pregnant women. The endocervical columnar epithelium responds to the estrogen surge by proliferating and folding into polypoid projections (Figure 21-18).

TECHNIQUE OF COLPOSCOPY IN PREGNANCY

Colposcopy is safe and should be performed in pregnancy when warranted.[38] The patient may feel anxious about the outcome and worry about possible adverse effects of the examination. Although colposcopic assessment will not impair the pregnancy or harm the fetus, the patient needs reassurance of this fact. *The goal of the colposcopic examination in the pregnant patient with abnormal cervical cytology is to exclude the presence of invasive cancer, avoiding the need for*

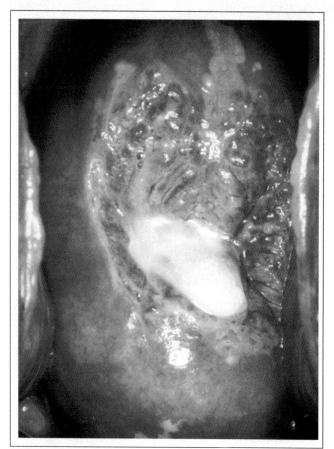

Figure 21-14 Gaping os with eversion of the SCJ onto the portio of the cervix. There is a small area of low-grade CIN on the anterior lip with a fine mosaic pattern.

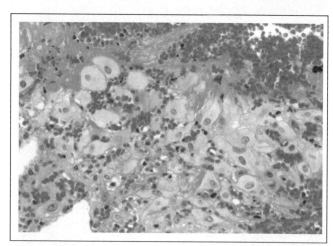

Figure 21-16 Decidual cells in stroma. These cells are large and have poorly defined cell borders. The nuclei are quite uniform with small nucleoli and a fine vesicular chromatin (×400).

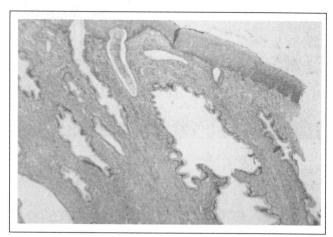

Figure 21-17 Example of glands in a cervical biopsy. The epithelium demonstrates CIN 2.

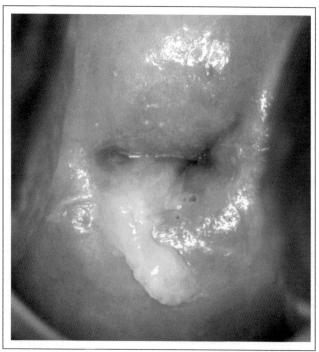

Figure 21-15 Example of thick mucus and dilated gland openings.

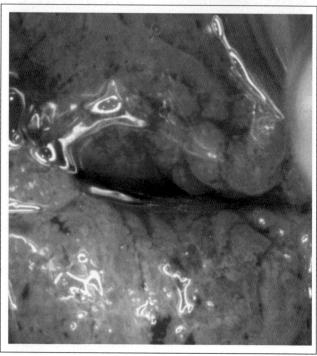

Figure 21-18 Polypoid appearance of hypertrophied endocervical tissue related to pregnancy.

418

cervical conization and allowing treatment to be deferred until the postpartum period.

In addition to the colposcopic interpretive challenges discussed previously, physical changes in the lower genital tract make the procedure of colposcopy technically more difficult in the pregnant patient. The colposcopist is challenged with the increased laxity of the vaginal walls, which prolapse through the speculum blades, interfering with proper visualization of the cervix. *A large vaginal speculum will usually be necessary—the largest speculum that the patient can comfortably tolerate should be used.* For small degrees of vaginal redundancy, gentle traction with a wooden tongue blade may facilitate visualization. A condom, latex glove finger, or endovaginal ultrasound probe sheath with the tip removed may be rolled onto the speculum for better visualization. Vaginal sidewall retractors can be inserted after the speculum is in place. Tenacious endocervical mucus encountered in pregnancy can be a significant obstacle to adequate visualization (Figure 21-19). The application of 5% acetic acid to the cervix provides a mucolytic effect and will aid in mucus removal. Mucus that cannot be satisfactorily removed may be gently manipulated using cotton-tipped applicators or an endocervical brush. If the overall size of the

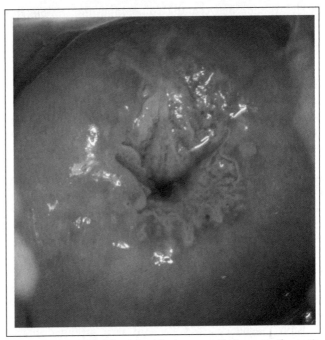

Figure 21-20 Example of eversion of columnar epithelium onto the portio of the cervix yielding an adequate examination. Acetowhite epithelium is present at 12 o'clock, representing CIN 2 and peripherally milder acetowhite epithelium that was CIN 1.

cervix precludes visualizing the entire TZ in a single colposcopic field, the cervix can be analyzed in four separate quadrants.

The examination should be gentle because tissue fragility is more common in pregnancy. If the highly vascular cervical epithelium is traumatized and bleeds, the view can be further compromised. The TZ is fully visualized in the majority of women by the 20th week of gestation[41] (Figure 21-20). For this reason, an unsatisfactory colposcopy occurs less frequently in pregnant women than in nonpregnant women.[35] Despite the eversion of the endocervical columnar epithelium in most women, further instrumentation is sometimes needed to adequately evaluate the endocervical canal and to visualize the entire SCJ. An endocervical speculum is often too narrow, especially later in pregnancy. A ring forceps or two cotton-tipped applicators can be used to gently evert the epithelium. If the clinician cannot complete an adequate examination, the patient needs to be referred to a more experienced colposcopist.

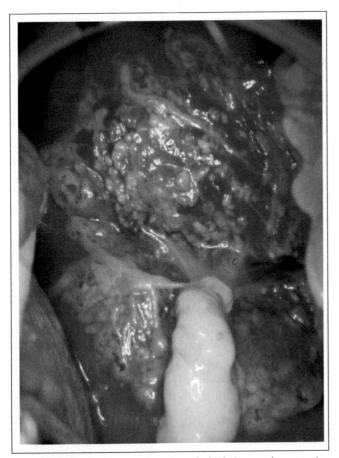

Figure 21-19 Large, normal cervix in the early third trimester demonstrating very active metaplasia, decidualization changes, and thick mucus. The bumpy white areas, noted especially on the anterior lip of the cervix, are hypertrophied stromal cells (decidualization reaction).

COLPOSCOPIC-DIRECTED BIOPSY AND ENDOCERVICAL CURETTAGE IN PREGNANCY

It is rare that cervical cancer will be undiagnosed during the prenatal period if colposcopy and directed biopsy are used to evaluate abnormal cervical cytology.[35,42] If uncertainty or discrepancy between the colposcopic impression and the index test exists, the use of the directed biopsy is strongly recommended and presents minimal risk to the patient.[43,44]

Controversy surrounds the question of whether biopsies should be performed during pregnancy in the absence of a colposcopic suspicion of invasive cervical cancer. It is natural to be reluctant in taking biopsies from the pregnant cervix with the theoretical risk of morbidity for the patient. Some centers recommend biopsy only when cancer is suspected colposcopically.[42,45] However, other data suggest that when biopsy is limited in this way, some cancers may be missed,[46] and still other centers recommend biopsy for lesions with a high-grade colposcopic appearance[46] or of the most abnormal-appearing area.[5,46,47] However, *a large number of reports support the use of directed biopsy in pregnancy with little morbidity.*[5,9,35] The risks of hemorrhage and infection are low, and the risk of premature birth is not increased after directed biopsy.[48] The preponderance of evidence suggests that cervical biopsy during pregnancy should not be deferred if it will assist in making a necessary triage decision. Pregnancy losses have not been attributed to colposcopic biopsy, and biopsy of any lesion may maximize diagnostic accuracy.[38]

A sharp biopsy forceps should always be used. Marked edema and vascularity of the cervix may contribute to significant bleeding after punch biopsy; however, hemostasis is usually attained without considerable difficulty. *Because of the increased risk of bleeding during pregnancy, the number of biopsies should be minimized.* If possible, one biopsy of the most severe area should be done to establish the histologic diagnosis.

Cotton-tipped applicators soaked in thickened Monsel's solution should be kept immediately at hand. *As soon as the specimen is taken with one hand, the Monsel's solution–soaked applicators are pressed firmly onto the bleeding site with the other hand. The applicators should be held in place for about* 30 *seconds.* The women should avoid vigorous activity for approximately 48 hours after the procedure. Occasionally, some spotting and discharge may continue for several days. Counseling the patient of these possibilities in advance can help relieve her anxiety. The ability of skilled colposcopists to establish the presence of CIN by colposcopically directed biopsy, both before[42] and after childbirth, has been consistently demonstrated.

Endocervical curettage is unacceptable during pregnancy because of the potential risk of premature rupture of membranes, premature onset of labor, and uncontrolled bleeding.[17] No trials have or will be performed to quantify the risks of intracervical instrumentation during pregnancy. Given that benefits of endocervical curettage remain the subject of debate, risks seem to exceed possible benefits.[49] More recently, the use of an endocervical brush sampler has been shown to improve the yield of endocervical cells obtained from the endocervical canal, and it can be used as a substitute for diagnostic endocervical curettage, if needed.[50] *Careful use of the endocervical brush has been demonstrated to be safe in pregnancy.*[51,52] Because unsatisfactory colposcopy may become satisfactory as the pregnancy progresses, a repeat colposcopy in 6 to 12 weeks for women with unsatisfactory colposcopic findings is recommended.[49] Fortunately, eversion of the SCJ during pregnancy improves access to the endocervix and decreases the necessary volume of tissue to be removed.

MANAGEMENT OF ABNORMAL CYTOLOGY IN PREGNANCY

Pregnant women are unique in that treatment is unnecessary unless cancer cannot be excluded. Management of the pregnant patient with abnormal cervical cytology (Table 21-4, Figure 21-21) focuses on documenting the presence of intraepithelial neoplasia while excluding the

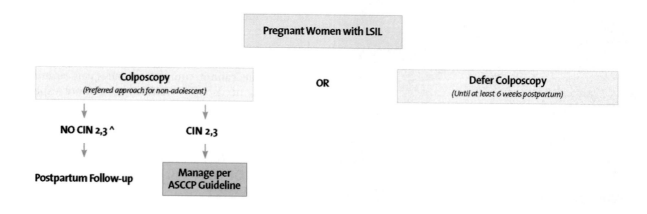

Management of Pregnant Women with Low-grade Squamous Intraepithelial Lesion (LSIL)

Pregnant Women with LSIL

Colposcopy
(Preferred approach for non-adolescent)

OR

Defer Colposcopy
(Until at least 6 weeks postpartum)

NO CIN 2,3 ^   CIN 2,3

Postpartum Follow-up   Manage per ASCCP Guideline

^ In women with no cytological, histological, or colposcopically suspected CIN 2,3 or cancer

Figure 21-21 Reprinted from *The Journal of Lower Genital Tract Disease* Vol. 11 Issue 4, with the permission of ASCCP © American Society for Colposcopy and Cervical Pathology 2007. No copies of the algorithms may be made without the prior consent of ASCCP.

Table 21-4 Management of Abnormal Cytology in Pregnancy

Atypical Squamous Cells of Undetermined Significance (ASC-US)
Management options for pregnant women over the age of 20 years with ASC-US are identical to those described for nonpregnant women, with the exception that it is acceptable to defer colposcopy until at least 6 weeks postpartum. **(CIII)** Endocervical curettage is unacceptable in pregnant women. **(EIII)**

Atypical Squamous Cells: Cannot Exclude High-Grade SIL (ASC-H)
There are no special guidelines for ASC-H in pregnant women.

Low-Grade Squamous Intraepithelial Lesion (LSIL)
Colposcopy is preferred for pregnant, nonadolescent women with LSIL cytology. **(BII)** Endocervical curettage is unacceptable in pregnant women. **(EIII)** Deferring the initial colposcopy until at least 6 weeks postpartum is acceptable. **(BIII)** In pregnant women who have no cytologic, histologic, or colposcopically suspected CIN 2,3 or cancer at the initial colposcopy, postpartum follow-up is recommended. **(BIII)** Additional colposcopic and cytologic examinations during pregnancy are unacceptable for these women. **(DIII)**

High-Grade Squamous Intraepithelial Lesion (HSIL)
Colposcopy is recommended for pregnant women with HSIL. **(AII)** It is preferred that the colposcopic evaluation of pregnant women with HSIL be conducted by clinicians who are experienced in the evaluation of colposcopic changes induced by pregnancy. **(BIII)** Biopsy of lesions suspicious for CIN 2,3 or cancer is preferred; biopsy of other lesions is acceptable. **(BIII)** Endocervical curettage is unacceptable in pregnant women. **(EIII)** Diagnostic excision is unacceptable unless invasive cancer is suspected based on the referral cytology, colposcopic appearance, or cervical biopsy. **(EII)** Reevaluation with cytology and colposcopy is recommended no sooner than 6 weeks postpartum for pregnant women with HSIL in whom CIN 2,3 is not diagnosed. **(CIII)**

Atypical Glandular Cells (AGC)
The initial evaluation in pregnant women should be identical to that of nonpregnant women except that endocervical curettage and endometrial biopsy are unacceptable (BII)

From Ref. 59.

presence of invasive cancer. The trend of managing abnormal Pap tests during pregnancy has changed over the decades from an aggressive approach with more liberal use of conization to a more conservative approach of observation with cytologic and colposcopic surveillance during the antenatal period or even deferring colposcopy until the postpartum period.

The risk that CIN 2,3 will progress to invasive cancer during pregnancy is low. Trials have not been performed to compare various strategies for antepartum and postpartum observation, so the yield and cost-effectiveness of antepartum observation of preinvasive lesions is unknown. Although repeated antepartum colposcopy and cytology may be useful, ideal intervals for reevaluation have not been defined.[49] Most women with preinvasive cervical lesions are able to continue routine obstetric care, and a vaginal delivery can be anticipated. However, because cervical cancer is a relative contraindication to vaginal delivery, identification of invasive disease may be important to avoid bleeding from a lacerated cancer or from implants in vaginal lacerations.[49]

A significant number of dysplastic lesions regress from the antenatal to postnatal period. The regression rate of CIN has been recognized for many years, but the reported rates appear widely different.[5,8,53] *Some studies report spontaneous regression rates of HSIL range from 6% to 31% in nonpregnant women and 30% to 54% in pregnancy.*[54–56] One study of 153 pregnant women with CIN 2,3 who were followed during pregnancy reported a 69% rate of spontaneous regression and identified no invasive cancers postpartum.[44,57] Ahdoot et al. found an overall postpartum regression rate

for women with HSIL of 48%.[58] The regression was most significant for women who delivered vaginally as compared with cesarean section. In contrast, Kaneshiro et al.[59] and Yost et al.[44] found that mode of delivery did not influence the natural history of dysplastic lesions. Gravid and nongravid women had similar regression rates. When available, Kaneshiro et al. included colposcopy and biopsy results, the current gold-standard diagnostic technique, whereas Ahdoot et al. analyzed cytologic data alone. Additionally, Kaneshiro et al. analyzed women who reached active labor but subsequently underwent cesarean section in the vaginal delivery group (intention to treat). This stratified women into groups who experienced similar levels of cervical trauma, a factor hypothesized to be important in cervical dysplasia regression.[60] They found no correlation between route of delivery and persistence of disease.

The most commonly cited theories for high regression rates of HSIL include the following[44,61,62]:

- Cervical trauma with labor and delivery. Trauma may lead to the desquamation of dysplastic cells, followed by subsequent postpartum cervical epithelial repair.
- The cervix undergoes extensive metaplastic change during pregnancy and postpartum.
- Postpartum resolution of immunosuppression is believed to occur during pregnancy.
- Resolution of the enhanced expression of the HPV genome appears to occur during the third trimester.
- Removal of the lesion or a portion of the lesion by biopsy and the accompanying inflammatory process may enhance the resolution of CIN.

Most of the recommendations for managing abnormal cytology and CIN during pregnancy are based on expert opinion and retrospective studies. Table 21-4 outlines the current recommendations for management of abnormal cytology in pregnancy. These recommendations are based on currently published guidelines by the American Society of Colposcopy and Cervical Pathology (ASCCP).[63,64]

TREATMENT OF CERVICAL INTRAEPITHELIAL NEOPLASIA AND CERVICAL NEOPLASIA IN PREGNANCY

Definitive diagnostic workup and treatment of CIN (Table 21-5) are reserved for the puerperium unless invasive disease is discovered or suspected during the prenatal period. *Should a histologic diagnosis of CIN be made in pregnancy, there is good rationale for keeping the lesion under observation but not intervening in the form of treatment with a diagnostic excisional procedure. Intraepithelial disease poses no immediate risk to the mother or fetus, and gynecologic oncologists are increasingly moving toward conservative management of invasive cancer during pregnancy.* Although cancer cannot be completely excluded in women with CIN and unsatisfactory colposcopy, the likelihood of occult carcinoma is low, especially when biopsy shows only CIN 1.[65,66] Follow-up, rather than a diagnostic excisional procedure, is recommended for all pregnant women with CIN 1 regardless of whether their colposcopy is satisfactory.

For women with invasive disease, delay in therapy must be balanced against benefit of improved fetal outcome. Unfortunately, published studies are primarily retrospective,

and their conclusions are conflicting. *Progression of early-stage cervical cancer during pregnancy has rarely been reported,[68] and postponing therapy until fetal maturity is achieved does not seem to reduce survival in women receiving standard treatment.[69]* Treatment risks include pregnancy loss and hemorrhage requiring transfusion. Although comparative trials of delayed versus immediate treatment have not been performed, these risks seem unjustifiable in the absence of benefit. Invasive cancer is rare but can occur in association with only minor cytologic atypia. *If any suspicion of invasion exists on cytology, discussion between the colposcopist and the pathologist should ensue before triage decisions are made.* A large biopsy specimen is mandatory if colposcopy indicates possible early invasion. If there is genuine suspicion of cancer, wedge biopsy or conization is mandatory to exclude invasive disease and to determine depth of invasion.

Many factors must be considered in counseling pregnant women with invasive cervical carcinoma. These include the following[70]:

- Patient's desire for continuation of the pregnancy
- Stage of the disease
- Number of weeks remaining to achieve fetal viability or lung maturity
- Effect of treatment on subsequent fertility or ability to maintain a normal pregnancy

Older reports of the use of conization suggest unacceptable risk, but the advent of loop electrosurgical excision was viewed by some as a form of safe conization in pregnancy.[71] However, *loop excision of the cervix during pregnancy does not consistently produce diagnostic specimens and is associated with a significant rate of residual disease. Residual CIN has been reported in 43% to 53% of women who underwent electrosurgical biopsy during pregnancy.[72–74]*

Loop excisional procedures performed during pregnancy are associated with complications that include significant bleeding and preterm births.[1,74] Heavy cervical bleeding has been reported in 5% to 15% of patients, with spontaneous abortion in as many as 25%.[65,72] One series demonstrated that all women with significant morbidity had loop excision performed between 27 and 34 weeks (third trimester). This would suggest that complications may be less frequent if loop excision is limited to the second trimester.[72] Until refinements in technique occur, loop excision during pregnancy should be reserved for women with evidence or suspicion of carcinoma by biopsy or colposcopy[74] with no defined risk of preterm labor or delivery.[75]

Cold-knife conization is reserved for suspicion of microinvasion or persistent cytologic evidence of invasive carcinoma in the absence of colposcopic confirmation. Conization is typically avoided in the first trimester due to the high rate of associated miscarriage and in the third trimester due to the risk of hemorrhage.[76] Conization during pregnancy is associated with a 12% bleeding complication rate, a 5% perinatal mortality rate from preterm delivery and maternal chorioamnionitis, and an increase in the rate of preterm labor from 4% to 30%.[72] In addition, as many as 50% of pregnant

---

Table 21-5 Management of Cervical Intraepithelial Neoplasia (CIN) in Pregnancy

CIN 1

The recommended management of pregnant women with a histologic diagnosis of CIN 1 is follow-up without treatment. **(BII)** Treatment of pregnant women for CIN 1 is unacceptable. **(EII)**

CIN 2,3

In the absence of invasive disease or advanced pregnancy, additional colposcopic and cytologic examinations are acceptable in pregnant women with a histologic diagnosis of CIN 2,3 at intervals no more frequent than every 12 weeks. **(BII)** Repeat biopsy is recommended only if the appearance of the lesion worsens or if cytology suggests invasive cancer. **(BII)** Deferring reevaluation until at least 6 weeks postpartum is acceptable. **(BII)** A diagnostic excisional procedure is recommended only if invasion is suspected. **(BII)** Unless invasive cancer is identified, treatment is unacceptable. **(EII)** Reevaluation with cytology and colposcopy is recommended no sooner than 6 weeks postpartum. **(CIII)**

From Ref. 67.

women have residual CIN after conization. *The second trimester seems to be the optimal period for conization to minimize fetal and maternal complications.*[5,42,77]

POSTPARTUM ISSUES

All women with CIN diagnosed during pregnancy should undergo postpartum colposcopy with cytologic or histologic evaluation before proceeding with therapy. This is especially important among women with antepartum HSIL. Reevaluation with cytology and colposcopy is recommended no sooner than 6 weeks postpartum. Definitive diagnostic evaluation of women with known HSIL during pregnancy may occur 8 to 12 weeks postpartum or no sooner than 6 weeks, which is the amount of time it takes the cervix to completely return to a normal physiologic state.[58] Premature colposcopy with biopsy risks bleeding and misdiagnosis.[49] Even if the postpartum Pap test is negative, the patient with an antepartum Pap test or colposcopic impression or histology with HSIL should have a complete colposcopic evaluation, including directed biopsies if indicated.

About 11.1% of prenatal women with histologic CIN have normal postpartum cytology.[38] The postpartum diagnosis rarely exceeds the diagnosis during pregnancy. *Because of the high regression rate of cervical dysplasia in the postpartum period, many colposcopic examinations result in findings of no dysplasia. If the postpartum colposcopy is adequate and normal, cytology and/or colposcopy should be repeated according to the ASCCP consensus guidelines.* It is estimated that as many as one third of women who have abnormal cytology during pregnancy and normal colposcopy postpartum will be found to have CIN within 1 year[78].

CONCLUSION

The current ASCCP guidelines recommend a conservative approach to the pregnant patient.[63,64] The risks of malignancy in pregnancy are small, and there is a strong likelihood that CIN will regress during the antenatal period.[79] Colposcopy should be undertaken as dictated by the clinical circumstances and, if uncertainty exists, directed biopsy poses minimal risk to the mother or her baby. Unless invasive disease is detected, treatment should be deferred until after delivery. The consensus recommendation is an initial colposcopy at the point of referral because of an abnormal index test and, if invasion is excluded (by colposcopic assessment and/or the use of directed biopsy in selected cases where appropriate), no further colposcopy until after pregnancy. Optimally, colposcopic evaluation should be performed 8 to 12 weeks postpartum when most of the local inflammatory reactions and reparatory processes have resolved. If assessment at this time is suggestive of persistence or progression of preinvasive disease, then appropriate treatment can be undertaken. Noncorrelation among cytology, colposcopic assessment, and histologic findings should alert the clinician to the possible need for follow-up in the antenatal period.

MANAGEMENT SCENARIOS

Scenario 1

Sentinel Pap: Atypical squamous cell of undetermined significance (ASC-US) or low-grade squamous intraepithelial lesion (LSIL)
Trimester of pregnancy: Any
Colposcopic findings or histologic cell type if a biopsy was done: No squamous intraepithelial lesion (SIL) found, or only CIN 1 is suspected and no biopsy is done
HPV testing for high-risk (oncogenic) HPV types: Positive (This test is relevant only in women with ASC-US and should only be done in that group. In women with LSIL, it is cost-inefficient.)
Satisfactory colposcopy: Yes
Fertility desires: Not applicable (N/A) (The patient is pregnant.)

The management options for pregnant adult women with ASC-US or LSIL are identical to those described for nonpregnant women, with the exception that is acceptable to defer colposcopy until at least 6 weeks postpartum.[62] In the first trimester, the relatively mild degree of cervical changes and the length of time until the postpartum evaluation (if delayed until then) favor colposcopy during pregnancy. As pregnancy progress, the balance gradually shifts in favor of delaying the colposcopy until the postpartum period. In the third trimester, colposcopy for ASC-US or LSIL can almost always be postponed.

Another change in the management of these women relates to the management of pregnant women whose colposcopy is unsatisfactory. In the past, the recommendation was to repeat the colposcopy at about 20 weeks' gestation when the cervix was more everted and the colposcopy was more likely to be satisfactory. No solution is generally offered if the colposcopy remains unsatisfactory at this point because colposcopy done even later in pregnancy becomes technically difficult. However, with the new ASC-US and LSIL guidelines, no distinction is made between satisfactory and unsatisfactory colposcopy with respect to subsequent management, so no further colposcopy is needed if the TZ is not fully visualized. Additional colposcopic and cytologic examinations during pregnancy are unacceptable for these women. The patient should be reevaluated postpartum with colposcopy regardless of the results of her postpartum cytology. Finally, when only CIN 1 is suspected, no biopsy is indicated.

Scenario 2

Sentinel Pap: HSIL
Trimester of pregnancy: First
Colposcopic findings or histologic cell type if a biopsy was done: CIN 3 is suspected at the ectocervical os, but cancer is not suspected. Biopsy confirms CIN 3.
HPV testing for high-risk (oncogenic) HPV types: Positive (This test is not relevant in women with HSIL and should not be done. It is cost-inefficient, and the management would be the same even if the result were negative.)

Satisfactory colposcopy: No
Fertility desires: N/A (The patient is pregnant.)

All pregnant women with HSIL should undergo colposcopy. Generally in the first trimester, colposcopy mirrors what is seen in the nonpregnant state and thus is more likely to be unsatisfactory than later in pregnancy. In a nonpregnant patient, an unsatisfactory colposcopy with disease at the os would be an indication for an endocervical curettage, but endocervical curettage is unacceptable in pregnant women. In a nonpregnant patient, an unsatisfactory colposcopy with disease in the os would be an indication for a diagnostic excision, but diagnostic excision is unacceptable in pregnancy unless invasive cancer is suspected based on the referral cytology, colposcopic appearance, or cervical biopsy. No invasive disease is suspected in this patient. This leaves two options. One option is to repeat the colposcopy in the mid-second trimester, when the endocervix everts more and the TZ is more likely to be completely visible. The colposcopy can be repeated again in the third trimester if the colposcopist is still not sufficiently reassured that no invasion is present. The other option is to refer the patient to a clinician who is experienced in the evaluation of colposcopic changes induced by pregnancy. Experienced clinicians are more likely to have the skills necessary to manipulate the cervix and obtain a satisfactory colposcopy without causing bleeding that will alarm the patient and interfere with the colposcopy.

Scenario 3

Sentinel Pap: Any result
Trimester of pregnancy: First or second
Colposcopic findings or histologic cell type if a biopsy was done:
  Microinvasive cancer is suspected. Biopsy shows invasion
  of less than 3 mm
HPV testing for high-risk (oncogenic) HPV types: N/A
Satisfactory colposcopy: Yes or No
Fertility desires: N/A (The patient is pregnant.)

This patient may have microinvasion. Although the biopsy shows invasion of less than 3 mm, in the absence of a conization specimen, one cannot be sure that deeper invasion is not present elsewhere in the cervix. The management of pregnant women in whom cancer is suspected or diagnosed should be conducted by clinicians who are experienced in the management of cervical cancer in conjunction with specialists in maternal-fetal medicine and neonatologists who can cooperatively balance delay in diagnosis and therapy against the benefit of improved fetal outcome.

Loop excisional procedures and cone biopsies are contraindicated during pregnancy in the absence of suspected cancer because of the morbidity involved to the fetus and the pregnancy including significant bleeding, chorioamnionitis, premature rupture of membranes, and preterm birth. Furthermore, in an attempt to minimize these complications, many specimens are too small, creating nondiagnostic and nontherapeutic confusion. Depending on the extent of disease, the cancer specialist may choose to do a wedge resection of the cervix, knowing that it is nontherapeutic and

not fully diagnostic but will minimize complications. Women in whom fully invasive cancer is not diagnosed would then undergo a diagnostic/therapeutic cold-knife conization postpartum. Assuming that there is no clinical evidence of stage IB disease, progression of microinvasive cancer during pregnancy is rare, and postponing therapy until fetal maturity is achieved does not seem to reduce neonatal survival.

COUNSELING

Abnormal Pap smears and minor and major grades of CIN are encountered in pregnancy. However, invasive cancer is an extremely rare event. Furthermore, progression of lower grades of CIN and CIN 3 to cancer are even rarer. Because of this, the 2006 ASCCP guidelines emphasize that colposcopy for LSIL or ASC-US is only needed once during the pregnancy and can even be deferred until the postpartum period diagnostic excision for CIN 3 is contraindicated during pregnancy unless cancer is suspected. The message is very clear: Cervical disease is rarely a problem that requires intervention in pregnancy. Nevertheless, women who are told that their Pap smear is abnormal during pregnancy and that they need to undergo a diagnostic test (colposcopy) are very scared and concerned. They want the pregnancy preserved and their baby to be normal. Any hint of lack of normalcy threatens one of the most important events in their life and is very emotionally traumatic. After the call from their healthcare provider's office, they may feel that their life and health are threatened, as is the survival of their unborn child. Any bleeding that results from the colposcopy is immediately attributed to the pregnancy, and women are concerned that it portends a miscarriage or preterm labor. Furthermore, the slightest concern expressed by the healthcare provider or his or her office staff is instantly magnified in the mind of the patient as an imminent threat to her pregnancy. The healthcare provider needs to understand appropriate triage so that the patient can be confidently reassured that the abnormal Pap test, although it needs follow-up postpartum, is not an imminent threat to the patient, the pregnancy, or the unborn child. It must be explained in advance that colposcopy may cause bleeding due to slight trauma to fragile tissue but that it does not threaten the pregnancy. A clinician who is overly cautious because of inexperience in managing colposcopy in pregnant women is not doing the patient a favor. If the clinician is inexperienced, these patients are better referred to others who are experienced in the evaluation of colposcopic changes and the management of abnormal cytology and histology during pregnancy.

REFERENCES

1. Connor JP. Noninvasive cervical cancer complicating pregnancy. Obstet Gynecol Clin North Am 1998;25:331–342.
2. Campion MJ, Sedlacek TV. Colposcopy in pregnancy. Obstet Gynecol Clin North Am 1993;20:153–163.

3. Gilstrap LC, Oh W (eds). Guidelines for Perinatal Care, ed 5. Washington, D.C.: American Academy of Pediatrics and the American College of Obstetricians and Gynecologists, 2002.

4. Nguyen C, Montz FJ, Bristow RE. Management of stage 1 cervical cancer in pregnancy. Obstet Gynecol Surv 2000;55:633–643.

5. Economos K, Perez-Veridiano N, Delke I, et al. Abnormal cervical cytology in pregnancy: a 17-year experience. Obstet Gynecol 1993;81:915–918.

6. Palle C, Bangsbøll S, Andreasson B. Cervical intraepithelial neoplasia in pregnancy. Acta Obstet Gynecol Scand 2000;79: 306–310.

7. Kaminski PF, Lyon DS, Sorosky JI, et al. Significance of a typical cervical cytology in pregnancy. Am J Perinatol 1992;9: 340–343.

8. Vlahos G, Rodolakis A, Diakomanolis E, et al. Conservative management of cervical intraepithelial neoplasia (CIN(2–3)) in pregnant women. Obstet Gynecol Invest 2002;54: 78–81.

9. Coppola A, Sorosky J, Casper R, et al. The clinical course of cervical carcinoma in situ diagnosed during pregnancy. Gynecol Oncol 1997;67:162–165.

10. Jones WB, Shingleton HM, Russell A, et al. Cervical carcinoma and pregnancy. A national patterns of care study of the American College of Surgeons. Cancer 1996;77:1479–1488.

11. Lishner M. Cancer in pregnancy. Ann Oncol 2003;14(suppl 3): iii31–iii36.

12. Sood AK, Sorosky JI, Mayr N, et al. Radiotherapeutic management of cervical carcinoma that complicates pregnancy. Cancer 1997;80:1073–1078.

13. Wright TC Jr, Cox JT, Massad LS, et al. Consensus guidelines for the management of women with cervical cytological abnormalities. J Am Med Assoc 2002;287:2120–2129.

14. Solomon D, Davey D, Kurman R, et al; Forum Group Members; Bethesda 2001 Workshop. The 2001 Bethesda System: terminology for reporting results of cervical cytology. J Am Med Assoc 2002;287:2114–2119.

15. Zemlickis D, Lishner M, Degendorfer P, et al. Maternal and fetal outcome after invasive cervical cancer in pregnancy. J Clin Oncol 1991;9:1956–1961.

16. Hendrickson MR, Kempson L. Uterus and fallopian tubes. In: Sternberg SS (ed). Histology of Pathologists. New York: Raven Press, 1992, p 809.

17. Ostergard DR. The effect of pregnancy on the cervical squamocolumnar junction in patients with abnormal cervical cytology. Am J Obstet Gynecol 1979;134:759–760.

18. Michael CW, Esfahani FM. Pregnancy-related changes: a retrospective review of 278 cervical smears. Diagn Cytopathol 1997; 17:99–107.

19. VanNiekerk WA. Cervical cytological abnormalities caused by folic acid deficiency. Acta Cytol 1966;10:67–73.

20. Danos ML. Postpartum cytology: observations over a four year period. Acta Cytol 1968;12:309–312.

21. Soloway HB. Vaginal and cervical cytology of the early puerperium. Acta Cytol 1969;13:136–138.

22. Klaus H. Quantitative criteria of folate deficiency in cervicovaginal cytograms, with report of a new parameter. Acta Cytol 1971;15:50–53.

23. Fiorella RM, Cheng J, Kragel PJ. Papanicolaou smears in pregnancy; positivity of exfoliated cells for human chorionic gonadotropin and human placental lactogen. Acta Cytol 1993;37:451–456.

24. Kobayashi TK, Yuasa M, Fujimoto T, et al. Cytologic findings in postpartum smears. Acta Cytol 1980;24:328–334.

25. Murad TM, Terhart K, Flint A. Atypical cells in pregnancy and postpartum smears. Acta Cytol 1981;25:623–630.

26. Schneider V, Barnes LA. Ectopic decidual reaction of uterine cervix; frequency and cytologic presentation. Acta Cytol 1981;25:616–622.

27. Danos M, Holmquist ND. Cytologic evaluation of decidual cells: a report of two cases with false abnormal cytology. Acta Cytol 1967;11:325–330.

28. Valente PT, Schantz HD, Schultz M. Cytologic atypia associated with microglandular hyperplasia. Diag Cytopathol 1994;10: 326–331.

29. Arias-Stella J. Atypical endometrial changes associated with the presence of chorionic tissue. Arch Pathol 1954;58:112–128.

30. Arias-Stella J. A topographic study of uterine epithelial atypia associated with chorionic tissue: demonstration of alteration in the endocervix. Cancer 1959;12:782–790.

31. Shrago SS. The Arias-Stella reaction. A case report of a cytologic presentation. 1977;21:310–313.

32. Mulvany NJ, Khan A, Ostor A. Arias-Stella reaction associated with cervical pregnancy; report of a case with cytologic presentation. Acta Cytol 1994;38:218–222.

33. Dupre-Froment J. Cytologie Gynecologique. Paris: Flamarion Medicine Science, 1974.

34. Meisels A, Morin C. Cytopathology of the Uterine Cervix. Chicago: ASCP Press, 1991.

35. Baldauf JJ, Dreyfus M, Ritter J, et al. Colposcopy and directed biopsy reliability during pregnancy: a cohort study. Eur J Obstet Gynecol Reprod Biol 1995;62:31–36.

36. Coppleson M, Reid B. A colposcopic study of the cervix during the pregnancy and the puerperium. J Obstet Gynaecol 1966; 73:575–585.

37. Singer A. The uterine cervix from adolescence to the menopause. Br J Obstet Gynaecol. 1975;82:81–99.

38. LaPolla JP, O'Neill C, Wetrich D. Colposcopic management of abnormal cervical cytology in pregnancy. J Reprod Med Obstet Gynecol 1988;33:301–306.

39. Brown D, Berran P, Kaplan K, et al. Special situations: abnormal cervical cytology during pregnancy. Clin Obstet Gynecol 2005;48:178–185.

40. Bertini-Oliveira AM, Keppler MM, Luisi A, et al. Comparative evaluation of abnormal cytology, colposcopy and histopathology in preclinical cervical malignancy during pregnancy. Acta Cytol 1982;26:636–644.

41. Behnam K, Mariano E. The value of colposcopy in evaluating cervical intraepithelial neoplasia during pregnancy. Diagn Gynecol Obstet 1982;4:133–135.

42. Benedet JL, Selke PA, Nickerson KG. Colposcopic evaluation of abnormal Pap smears in pregnancy. Am J Obstet Gynecol 1987;157:932–937.

43. Jain AG, Higgins RV, Boyle MJ. Management of low-grade squamous intraepithelial lesions during pregnancy. Am J Obstet Gynecol 1997;177:298–302.

44. Yost NP, Santoso JT, McIntire DD, et al. Postpartum regression rates of antepartum cervical intraepithelial neoplasia II and III lesions. Obstet Gynecol 1999;93:359–362.

45. DePetrillo AD, Townsend DE, Morrow CP, et al. Colposcopic evaluation of the abnormal Papanicolaou test in pregnancy. Am J Obstet Gynecol 1975;121:441–445.

46. Cristoforoni PM, Gerbaldo DL, Philipson J, et al. Management of the abnormal Pap smear during pregnancy: lessons for quality improvement. J Lower Genital Tract Dis 1999;3: 225–230.

47. Lurain JR, Gallup DG. Management of abnormal Pap smears in pregnancy. Obstet Gynecol 1979;53:484–488.

48. Baldauf JJ, Dreyfus M, Ritter J. Benefits and risks of directed biopsy in pregnancy. J Lower Genital Tract Dis 1997;1:214–220.

49. Massad SL, Wright TC, Cox TJ, et al. Managing abnormal cytology results in pregnancy. J Lower Genital Tract Dis 2005;9:146–148.

50. Anderson W, Frierson H, Barber S, et al. Sensitivity and specificity of endocervical curettage and the endocervical brush for the evaluation of the endocervical canal. Am J Obstet Gynecol 1988;159:702–707.

51. Orr JW Jr, Barrett JM, Orr PF, et al. The efficacy and safety of the cytobrush during pregnancy. Gyncol Oncol 1992;44:260–262.

52. Lieberman RW, Henry MR, Laskin WB, et al. Colposcopy in pregnancy: directed brush cytology compared with cervical biopsy. Obstet Gynecol 1999;94:198–203.

53. Siddiqui G, Kurzel RB, Lampley EC, et al. Cervical dysplasia in pregnancy: progression versus regression postpartum. Int J Fertil Womens Med 2001;46:278–280.

54. Kiguchi K, Bibbo M, Hasegawa T, et al. Dysplasia during pregnancy: a cytologic follow-up study. J Reprod Med 1981;26:66–72.

55. Yoonessi M, Wieckowska W, Mariniello D, et al. Cervical intraepithelial neoplasia during pregnancy. Int J Gynaecol Obstet 1982;20:111–118.

56. Kaplan AL, Kaufman RH. Diagnosis and management of dysplasia and carcinoma in situ of the cervix in pregnancy. Clin Obstet Gynecol 1967;10:871–878.

57. Paraskevaidis E, Koliopoulos G, Kalantaridou S, et al. Management and evolution of cervical intraepithelial neoplasia during pregnancy and postpartum. Eur J Obstet Gynecol Reprod Biol 2002;104:67–69.

58. Ahdoot D, Van Nostrand KM, Nguyen NJ, et al. The effect of route of delivery on regression of abnormal cervical cytologic findings in the postpartum period. Am J Obstet Gynecol 1998;178:1116–1120.

59. Wright TC Jr, Massad LS, Dunton CJ, Spitzer M, Wilkinson EJ, Solomon D; for the 2006 ASCCP-Sponsored Consensus Conference. 2006 Consensus guidelines for the management of women with abnormal cervical screening tests. J Low Genit Tract Dis. 2007 Oct;11(4):201–222.

60. Kaneshiro BE, Acoba JD, Holzman J, et al. Effect of delivery route on natural history of cervical dysplasia. Am J Obstet Gynecol 2005;192:1452–1454.

61. Brinton LA, Reeves WC, Brenes MM, et al. Parity as a risk factor for cervical cancer. Am J Epidemiol 1989;130:486–496.

62. Rock JD, Thompson JA. Te Linde's Operative Gynecology, ed 8. Philadelphia: Lippincott-Raven, 1997, p 1403.

63. Wright TC, Massad LS, Dunton CJ, et al, for the 2006 ASCCP-sponsored Consensus Conference. 2006 consensus guidelines for the management of women with abnormal cervical cancer screening tests. Am J Obstet Gynecol, in press.

64. Wright TC, Massad LS, Dunton CJ, et al, for the 2006 ASCCP-sponsored Consensus Conference. 2006 consensus guidelines for the management of women with cervical intraepithelial neoplasia or adenocarcinoma in-situ. Am J Obstet Gynecol, in press.

65. Averette HE, Nasser N, Yankow SL, et al. Cervical conization in pregnancy: analysis of 180 operations. Am J Obstet Gynecol 1970;106:543–549.

66. Patsner B. Management of low-grade cervical dysplasia during pregnancy. South Med J 1990;83:1405–1406.

67. Wright TC, Massad LS, Dunton CJ, et al. 2006 Consensus Guidelines for the Management of Women with Cervical Intraepithelial Neoplasia or Adenocarcinoma In Situ. J Lower Genital Tract Dis 2007;11:223–239.

68. Dudan RC, Yon JL, Ford JH, et al Carcinoma of the cervix and pregnancy. Gynecol Oncol 1973;1:283–289.

69. Sorosky JI, Squatrito R, Ndubisi BU, et al. Stage I squamous cell carcinoma in pregnancy: Planned delay in therapy awaiting fetal maturity. Gynecol Oncol 1995;59:207–210.

70. Apgar BS, Zoschnick LB. Triage of the abnormal Papanicolaou smear in pregnancy. Prim Care Clin North Am 1998;24:483–503.

71. Dunn TS, Ginsburg V, Wolf D. Loop-cone cerclage in pregnancy: a 5-year review. Gynecol Oncol 2003;90:577–580.

72. Hannigan EV, Whitehouse HH 3rd, Atkinson WD, et al. Cone biopsy during pregnancy. Obstet Gynecol 1982;60:450–455.

73. Hacker NF, Berek JS, Lagasse LD, et al. Carcinoma of the cervix associated with pregnancy. Obstet Gynecol 1982;59:735–746.

74. Robinson WR, Webb S, Tirpack J, et al. Management of cervical intraepithelial neoplasia during pregnancy with LOOP excision. Gynecol Oncol 1997;64:153–155.

75. Althuisius SM, Schornagel U, Dekker GA, et al. Loop electrosurgical excision procedure of the cervix and time of delivery in subsequent pregnancy. Int J Gynecol Obstet 2001;72:31–34.

76. Ward RM, Bristow RE. Cancer and pregnancy: recent developments. Curr Opin Obstet Gynecol 2002;14:613–617.

77. Larsson G, Grundsdell H, Gullberg B, et al. Outcome of pregnancy after conization. Acta Obstet Gynecol Scand 1982;61:461–466.

78. Hellberg D, Axelsson O, Gad A, et al. Conservative management of the abnormal smear during pregnancy. A long-term follow-up. Acta Obstet Gynecol Scand 1987;66:195–199.

79. Siddiq TS, Twigg JP, Hammond RH. Assessing the accuracy of colposcopy at predicting the outcome of abnormal cytology in pregnancy. Euro J Obstet Gynecol Reprod Bio 2006;124:93–97.

CASE STUDY 1 QUESTIONS

HISTORY

This 30-year-old gravida 2, para 1, at 20 weeks' gestation, presents with a Pap test showing a low-grade squamous intraepithelial lesion (LSIL). She has never had an abnormal Pap smear prior to this one. She is sexually active and has had seven partners in the past, although she has been with her current partner for 6 years.

- Is the transformation zone fully visualized?
- Describe what you see.
- What is the differential diagnosis for this lesion?
- Is a biopsy necessary?
- Should you perform an endocervical curettage (ECC)?
- What is your pathologic diagnosis?
- What is the next step in this patient's evaluation?

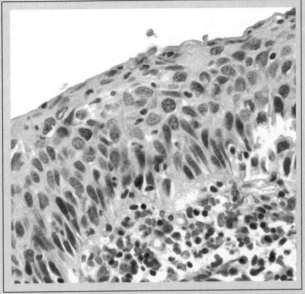

Figure 21-23 is a biopsy of the worst colposcopic lesion.

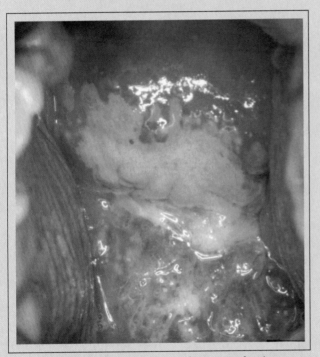

Figure 21-22 This is a colpophotograph of her cervix after the application of 5% acetic acid.

CASE STUDY 1 ANSWERS

FIGURE 21-22

The cervix is somewhat cyanotic as a result of pregnancy. In this colpophotograph, the TZ is not fully visualized. Although the SCJ can be seen on the posterior lip of the cervix, thick mucus in the endocervical canal blocks its view on the anterior lip. It is often possible to manipulate this mucus to visualize the SCJ. On the anterior lip of the cervix there is a flat, acetowhite lesion with a geographic border and no vascular markings. The color is somewhat grayish in nature, but the cyanosis of the cervix can cause the color of the lesion to be undergraded. This is consistent with a low-grade lesion (CIN1/condyloma); however, a somewhat higher-grade lesion could not be definitely excluded. A biopsy is not mandatory, and the decision to take one should be based on the comfort level of the colposcopist that he or she has definitely excluded cancer or any other diagnosis that would adversely affect the patient or the pregnancy should its diagnosis be delayed. An ECC is unacceptable in

Continued

CASE STUDY 1 ANSWERS—Cont'd

pregnancy, as there is a theoretical risk that it will result in rupture of the fetal membranes or in hemorrhage.

FIGURE 21-23

The biopsy shows CIN 3 with crowding and irregularity of the cells along the basal layer, with lack of maturation involving the lower two thirds of the epithelium.

In a nonpregnant woman, an unsatisfactory colposcopy in association with a high-grade lesion would necessitate a diagnostic excision procedure. However, the risk of complications such as hemorrhage and preterm labor makes this procedure particularly undesirable in a pregnant patient. Also, the endocervical canal will continue to evert as the pregnancy progresses, raising the possibility that the colposcopy that was unsatisfactory earlier in pregnancy will become satisfactory later. As long as the colposcopist can be confident that the patient does not currently have an invasive cancer, she can be followed through the pregnancy and reevaluated postpartum. If the colposcopist lacks confidence in his or her evaluation, the patient should be referred to a more experienced colleague before resorting to conization.

KEY POINT OF CASE 1

As long as the colposcopist can be confident that the patient does not currently have an invasive cancer, even a high-grade lesion can be followed through the pregnancy and reevaluated postpartum.

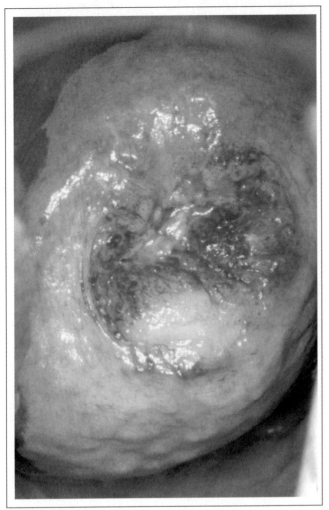

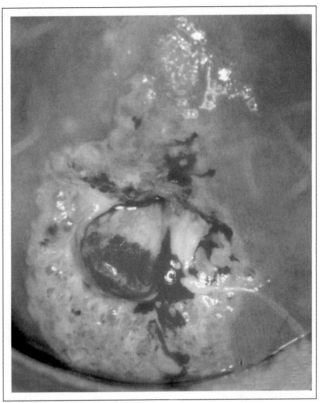

Plate 21-1 Large area of CIN 1 covering most of the cervix, along with a focal area of dense acetowhite epithelium at 6 o'clock. The exam is adequate, and there is hypertrophy of the endocervical tissue. A biopsy at 6 o'clock revealed CIN 3.

Plate 21-2 Second-trimester cervix with a large decicidual polyp noted centrally and surrounding metaplasia and thick mucus at the os.

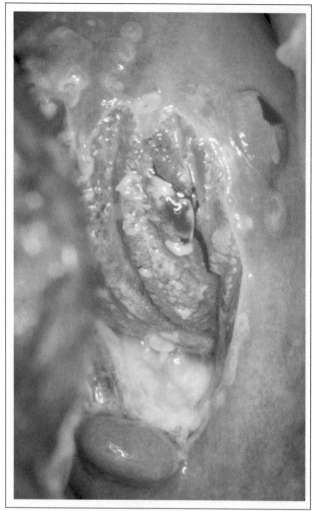

Plate 21-3 This patient has a normal cervix with some distortion of the surface contour from a prior LEEP. Thick mucus is present in the os, and metaplasia is occurring in the area of ectropion on the anterior lip of the cervix.

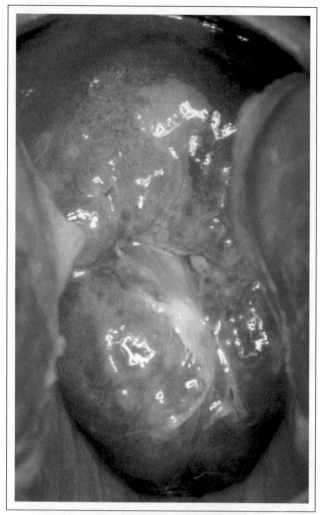

Plate 21-4 Area of CIN 1 on the anterior lip of a cervix in a woman who is 28 weeks pregnant. The remaining cervix is normal with thick mucus and increased vascular congestion, giving the cervix a blue-purple appearance.

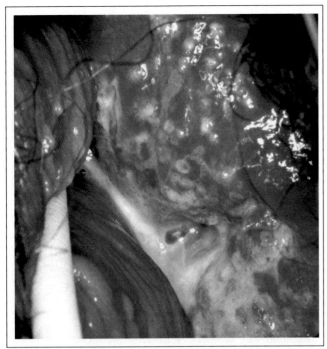

Plate 21-5 Example of normal cervix in the third trimester with purple appearance due to vascular engorgement and redundant vaginal walls partially obstructing the view of the cervix.

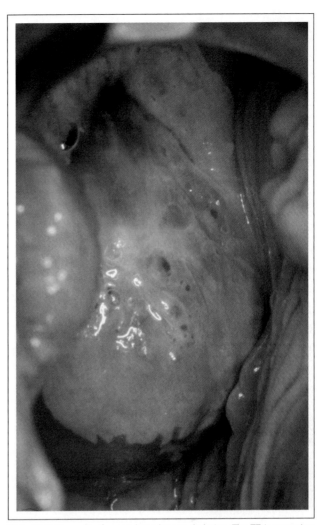

Plate 21-7 Example of a very large low-grade lesion. The TZ is extensive and cannot be seen entirely in this view.

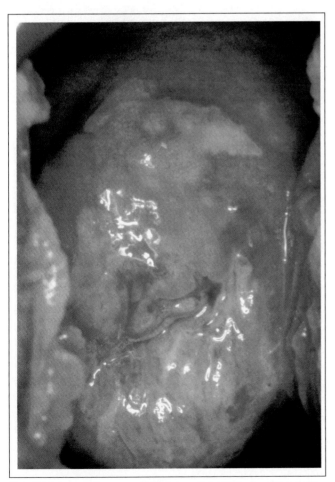

Plate 21-6 Low-grade geographic lesion on the anterior lip of the cervix.

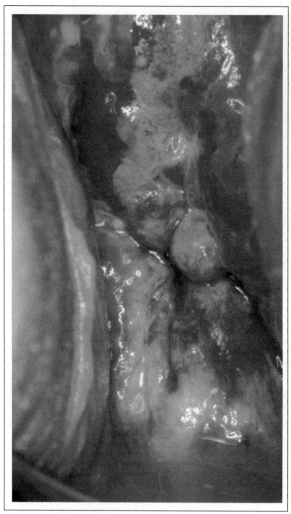

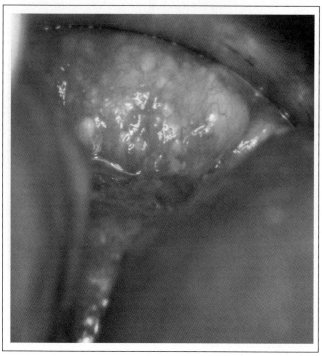

Plate 21-9 Large TZ with multiple nabothian cysts and redundant vaginal walls. Only a portion of the posterior lip can be visualized.

Plate 12-8 Large TZ with a fine mosaic pattern at 12 o'clock, contact bleeding, and acetowhite epithelium. The SCJ cannot be seen in this view. Biopsies were negative.

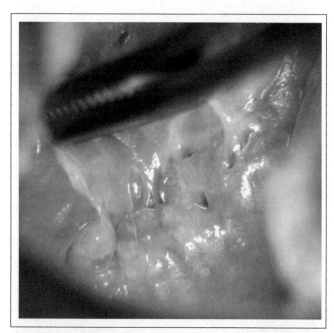

Plate 21-10 Example of dilated gland openings, associated copious mucus production, and nabothian cysts.

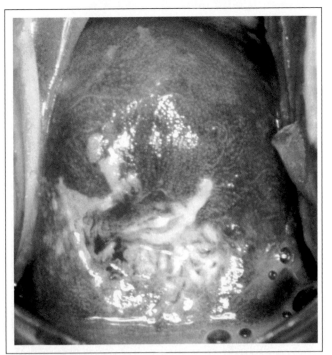

Plate 21-11 Diffuse decidual changes with fine, milia-like white areas present. In addition, dense acetowhite epithelium is present at the 9- to 12-o'clock position. Biopsy revealed CIN 2.

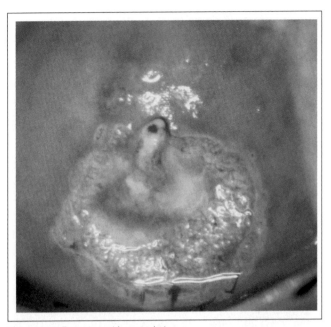

Plate 21-13 Ectropion with metaplasia.

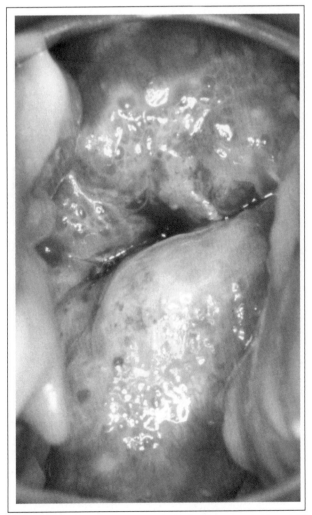

Plate 21-12 High-grade CIN on a early third-trimester cervix. Normal TZ components are seen on the anterior lip of the cervix.

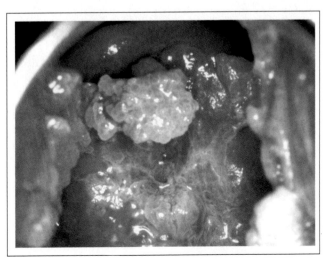

Plate 21-14 Large exophytic condyloma of the anterior cervix at 20 weeks' gestation.

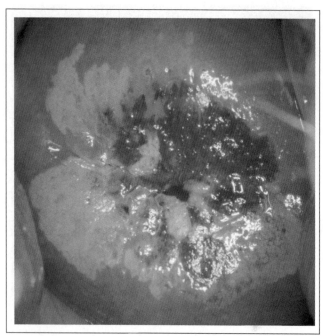

Plate 21-15 Ectropion along with dense acetowhite epithelium at 9 o'clock, with some peeling of the margins and subsequent bleeding.

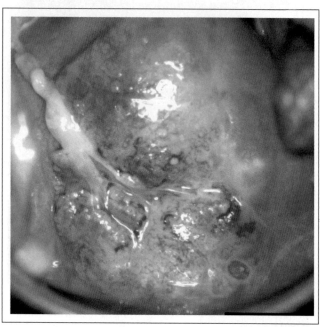

Plate 21-17 Coarse mosaic and atypical blood vessels in a pregnant woman with HSIL. Biopsies revealed microinvasive cancer. A cone biopsy is necessary to rule out invasive cancer.

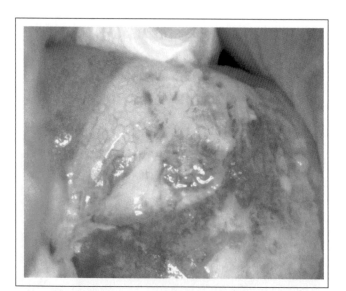

Plate 21-16 High-grade CIN with coarse mosaic and dense acetowhite epithelium.

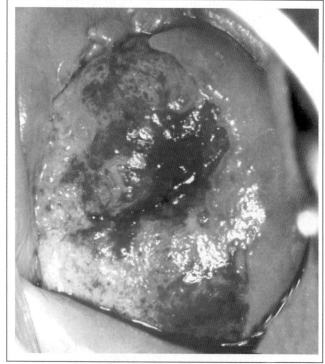

Plate 21-18 This 20-week-pregnant woman had a Pap smear suggestive of cancer, her cervix felt firm to palpation, and the image reveals dense acetowhite epithelium with atypical vessels involving half of her cervix. Biopsy confirmed invasive cancer.

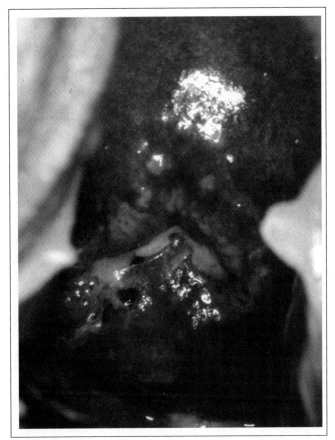

Plate 21-19 Deep purple appearance of cervix in late pregnancy, called *Chadwick's sign*. There is also accentuation of normal vascular markings along with metaplasia and mucus near the os.

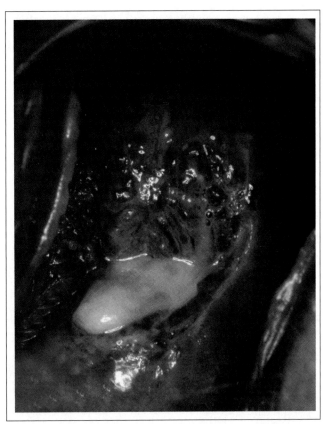

Plate 21-20 Low-grade lesion on the anterior lip with faint acetowhite epithelium and a fine mosaic pattern. The cervix has a cyanotic appearance, and thick mucus is present at the os.

CHAPTER 22

Human Papillomavirus Infections in Adolescents

Anna-Barbara Moscicki

KEY POINTS

- The physiologic changes of the cervix that occur in adolescents make them vulnerable to human papillomavirus (HPV) infections.
- Most HPV and HPV-associated changes are transient, resulting in fairly rapid clearance of HPV.
- Guidelines for triage of adolescents with abnormal cytology should primarily be conservative; invasive procedures should be avoided.

Recent attention regarding human papillomavirus (HPV) has focused on adolescent populations. This is somewhat surprising because anogenital cancers are rarely diagnosed in this age group. On the other hand, HPV infections and abnormal cytology occur most frequently in this age group, raising the question, "Why do we care about HPV in adolescents?" *Adolescents show high rates of acquisition with equally high rates of clearance. This is paralleled with high rates of abnormal cytology. In contrast, cervical cancer is extremely rare in this group.* However, there is a long gap between first infection (usually before 21 years of age) and development of invasive cancer in women several decades later. The strong relationship between HPV and cervical cancer attests that not all HPV acquired during adolescence has a "benign" outcome. Adolescence is a time of dynamic biological and psychological development, and both the biological and psychological changes may contribute to the high rates of HPV prevalence and incidence. On the other hand, it is most likely that the biological development during adolescence contributes to the vulnerability of the adolescent to eventual cancer development. This chapter will discuss rates of and risks for HPV acquisition, low-grade squamous intraepithelial lesion (LSIL) and high-grade squamous intraepithelial lesion (HSIL) development in sexually active adolescents, biological changes unique to adolescents, screening strategies, management of adolescents with abnormal cytology, and preferred treatment recommendations for abnormal histology.

RISKS FACTORS AND EPIDEMIOLOGY

Prevalence and Incidence of Human Papillomavirus in Adolescents

HPV is predominantly an infection of younger women, with six- to eightfold higher rates of HPV infection in adolescents than in adult women. Rates have ranged from 12% to 56% in women younger than 21 years compared with 2% to 7% in women older than 35 years.[1-4] This difference is fairly consistent among countries.[5] De Sanjose in a recent meta-analysis showed a peak HPV prevalence of 23% for women younger than age 20, with a rapid decline with increased age, resulting in a prevalence of 10% by 30 years of age. The analysis initially showed a slight increase in older women (>65 years), but after controlling for study design, sampling collection device, and HPV assay, the prevalence was flat in the older women. However, in some countries the rates do not show such dramatic differences.[4] For example, in Hanoi, Vietnam, a sampling study showed prevalence rates less than 5% in all age groups including women younger than 20 years. Sampling in Nigeria also showed no age-specific rates but did show high prevalence rates, ranging from 32% in women younger than 20 years to 25% in women aged 45 years and older. The reasons for these differences are not clear and may have resulted from testing biases.

Because no treatment for HPV exists, the dramatic decrease in HPV prevalence after the age of 25 years seen in most countries suggests that clearance of the virus is common and rapid. Because age is often inversely related to number of current sexual exposures, this observed age-related decrease in the prevalence of HPV infection has been thought to be due to sexual behavior. However, incidence studies show the same age-related differences, which suggests that young women are biologically more vulnerable. Munoz et al.[6] reported incidence rates of HPV in women who were normal cytologically and HPV negative at entry. The incidence of HPV was highest in adolescents aged 15 to 19 years of age, with a cumulative incidence of 17% at 1 year and 35.7% at 3 years. The incidence rates gradually decreased through age groups, with a 3-year incidence of 24.1% in the 20- to 24-year-old group and 8.1% in women aged 45 years and older. This risk of age remained independently significant in the final models that controlled for number of recent sexual partners. One possible explanation not related to biology is that the male sexual partner of the older women was also less likely to carry HPV, decreasing the chance of infection. Another possible explanation is that older women may have already been exposed to a variety of HPV types and developed immunity to them, so the likelihood that they will be exposed to a new HPV type to which they are not already immune decreases with each subsequent exposure.

In comparison, higher rates of acquisition have been observed for U.S. adolescents. In one study, approximately 55% of adolescents and young women who were HPV negative at entry acquired a cervical HPV infection within 36 months after joining the study[7] and more than 20% had prevalent infections.[1] *This means that 75% of young women in this study had cervical HPV infection within 5 to 7 months after initiating intercourse.* In another study of 60 adolescents, Brown et al.[8] intensely tested adolescents with weekly vaginal samples and cervical samples every 3 months. Thirty-six percent had a cervical infection detected within 2 years of follow-up, and 77% had a positive sample from either the vaginal swab or cervical swab. This is not surprising, as many more samples from the vagina were obtained in this study than from the cervix. On the other hand, this finding also suggests that many of the vaginal infections do not cause cervical infections and will not lead to cervical cancer. Similarly high rates of infection have been reported in slightly older women as well. In their study of college students, Winer et al.[9] included some women who were virgins at the time of entry. Interestingly, those virgin women who became sexually active had similar rates of acquisition as the already sexually experienced group, with approximately 50% acquiring HPV by 36 months.

Prevalence of Squamous Intraepithelial Lesion

Similar to HPV, rates of low-grade squamous intraepithelial lesion (LSIL) are highest among younger women. LSIL rates have been reported to range from 2% to 14%[10-13] in adolescents, whereas in older women (>30 years) the rates range from 0.6% to 1%. Even within the small timeframe of adolescence, there is a striking increase with age: rates of squamous intraepithelial lesion (SIL) are reported in fewer than 1% of girls screened who were younger than 16 years but in 7% to 14% in girls younger than 19 years.[14,15] Although high-grade squamous intraepithelial lesion (HSIL) is not as common as LSIL in adolescents, the rate of HSIL in adolescents is similar to that in older women. In a review of cytology findings, Mount et al.[13] found that 0.7% of 15- to 19-year-olds had HSIL compared with 0.8% of women aged 20 to 29 years and 0.7% of

women aged 30 to 39 years. What is unknown is what proportion of the HSIL is cervical intraepithelial neoplasia (CIN) 2 versus CIN 3. Countries with CIN 3 registries report that the peak age for CIN 3 is 27 to 29 years, which suggests that the majority of HSIL in adolescents is CIN 2, not CIN 3. (See Natural History for further discussion.)

SEXUAL RISK FACTORS AND HUMAN PAPILLOMAVIRUS

The most significant risk factor for HPV infection among adolescents is multiple partners and frequent intercourse. Hence, in countries where the number of partners does not vary with age, little change in HPV infection may be observed with changing age.[3] This of course would have to include men, because in countries where men have large number of partners but women have few, high rates of HPV are still detected. Not surprisingly, a new sexual partner appears more important than the number of lifetime partners.[6,7,9] Among adolescents, Moscicki et al.[7] showed that *the risk was more than tenfold for each new partner reported per month since the last visit 4 months earlier.* Winer et al.[9] reported a two- to threefold risk for cervical infection when reporting a new partner compared with no new partners. However, in contrast to Moscicki et al.,[7] Winer's group found that the risk due to the new partner was higher if the new partner was reported 5 to 8 months prior to testing rather than within 4 months. This difference is not easily explained, as it has been thought that HPV infection is established within 1 to 3 months after exposure.

The question remains: "Are adolescents particularly biologically vulnerable to HPV, or is the risk all linked to sexual behavior?" Although adolescents on the whole report more recent sexual partners than adult women, the differences are not dramatic. National survey data in the United States report that by 19 years of age, 75% to 77% report having had sexual intercourse and 50% report having had 4 or more partners with a median of 4 partners.[16,17] However, national survey data also show that adolescents do not necessarily have regular sex. According to data collected from the Centers for Disease Control and Prevention (CDC), 43% of adolescent females reported no sexual partners in the past 12 months compared with only 13% of 20- to 24-year-old females and 7.4% of 25- to 44-year-old females.[17] But when the number of partners was reported, 22% of the 15- to 19-year-old females reported two or more partners in the past 12 months, compared with 12% of the 25- to 44-year-old women.[17] The group of 20- to 24-year-old females had the highest rates, with 26% reporting two or more partners in the past 12 months. Interestingly, 15- to 19-year-old males reported similar rates, with 23% reporting two or more partners compared with 15% of 25- to 44-year-old males.

Biological Risk Factors and Human Papillomavirus

The ease of sexual transmission of HPV in adolescents does not seem to be explained by sexual behavior alone, as seen in the study by Munoz et al.[6] In addition to acquiring HPV at higher rates, young age at first intercourse also places women at a greater future risk for the development of cancer in later life. *There appears to be a three- to fourfold increased risk of developing invasive cancer if a women initiates intercourse before age 18 compared with age 20 or older.*[18,19] Certainly, the adolescent cervix in general is biologically different than the adult cervix.[20] During embryologic development, the cervix is initially lined by Müllerian columnar epithelium and later replaced by urogenital squamous epithelium from the vagina toward the endocervical os. The replacement is incomplete with an abrupt squamocolumnar junction (SCJ) occurring on the ectocervix in the majority of neonates. This SCJ remains relatively unchanged until puberty. The adolescent enters puberty with relatively large areas of columnar epithelium (Figure 22-1) and as the adolescent ages, the cervix undergoes relatively dramatic changes. *The initial changes are thought to be due to the increased estrogenic activity of puberty resulting in glycogenation of the vaginal epithelium, which leads to an increase in vaginal lactobacilli that in turn produce more lactic acid and subsequently acidify the vagina. This acidity induces uncommitted generative cells of the columnar epithelium to begin a process referred to as* squamous metaplasia; *that is the columnar epithelium transforms itself into squamous epithelium.* The changes of squamous metaplasia are described in more detail in Chapter 7. Eventually a new SCJ exists that advances toward the cervical os with advancing age (Figure 22-2). Biologically, the predominant cell type in adults is the mature squamous cell (Figure 22-3), whereas in an adolescent both columnar

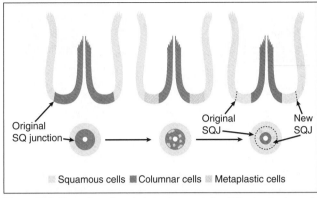

Figure 22-2 Illustration of cervical development; the SCJ migrates toward the os as the patient ages.

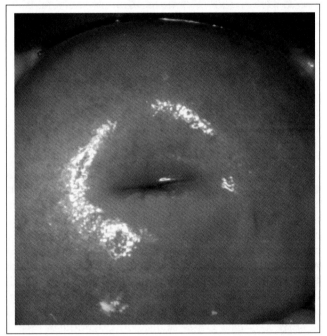

Figure 22-3 Typical example of a mature cervix with little to no columnar epithelium visible. The entire cervix is covered by mature squamous epithelium.

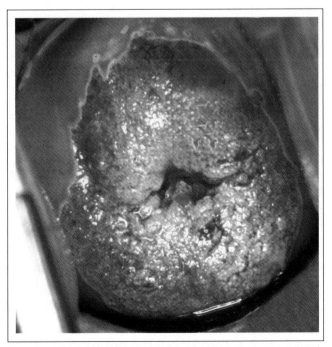

Figure 22-1 Typical immature cervix of an adolescent. The cervix is primarily covered by columnar epithelium, giving a red hue to the epithelium. There are also pockets of squamous metaplasia (11 to 2 o'clock), which are seen as white epithelium after the application of 3% acetic acid.

and metaplastic squamous cells predominate (Figure 22-4). One of the vulnerabilities of adolescents to HPV may be the thinness of columnar epithelium (one cell layer thick) compared with the thicker squamous epithelium (60 to 80 cell layers thick). Easy access to basal epithelial cells is thought to be important for the establishment of HPV infections.

Possibly more important than the presence of columnar epithelium is the presence of metaplastic epithelium. The importance of the TZ is known, as all squamous cell cancers of the cervix appear to arise within this area. HPV requires host cell replication and differentiation for its survival (see Chapter 2). Both replication and differentiation are hallmarks of squamous metaplasia; hence, the process of

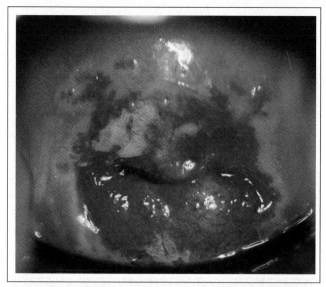

Figure 22-4 Picture of an adolescent cervix with a mixture of columnar, metaplasia, and squamous epithelium. The process of metaplasia can be somewhat random and often occurs in patches. As seen in this cervix, there is a patch of metaplasia at 10 o'clock surrounded by columnar epithelium.

metaplasia is fertile ground for acquiring and establishing HPV infections. Aside from puberty, sexual activity is also a trigger for squamous metaplasia. *Adolescents with exposure to multiple sexual partners have cervixes that appear more adult-like, with little to no ectopy.*[21,22] It may be that women with multiple partners are more likely to be exposed to sexually transmitted infections (STIs), which induce inflammation, repair, and metaplasia, or that semen itself may induce metaplasia.[23] *The high rates of LSIL in adolescents may be explained by these high rates of metaplasia.* That is, squamous metaplastic tissue inherently supports HPV replication. HPV expression of the proteins E6 and E7 initially result in mild basal cell proliferation and nuclear enlargement, and E4 expression results in cytologic changes referred to as *koilocytic halos*. These changes are diagnostic of LSIL.[24] A study of adolescent women showed that those with evidence of ongoing metaplasia visible on colpophotographs were more likely to develop LSIL if infected with HPV than adolescents with relatively quiescent cervices, which underscores the importance of metaplasia in supporting HPV replication.[25]

Few studies have attempted to examine the biological vulnerability of epithelial types to specific HPV type infections. Castle et al.[26] detected more alpha nine HPV types (16, 31, 33, 35, 52, 58, and 67) in women with large areas of ectopy, whereas these types were not common in women with mature cervixes. The prevalence of other HPV types (61, 71, 72, 81, 83, 84, 89), which are nononcogenic, increased with increasing maturity. Many of these observed differences, however, may not be due to epithelial type; rather they are due to immune factors related to age. *Because the incidence of HPV appears to decrease over time, some immunity against repeated HPV infection may develop with age, which may or may not be associated with epithelial cell change.*

Although the lifetime risk of HPV is high, it has been shown that most infections occur shortly after the onset of sexual activity.[7,9] *If some protection is offered after a single infection is cleared, it would help explain the lowering rates of HPV seen by each of the age groups.* In unpublished data, Moscicki observed a population of young women and found that 66% of adolescents and young women with incident HPV had a second incident HPV infection with a new type; of those with two infections, 47% had a third detected infection; and of those with 3 infections, half had a fourth infection. This suggests that some protection may develop over time.

In summary, *the protective barrier reflected by the mature squamous epithelium may be an important factor why adult women have lower rates of infection and the high rate of metaplastic epithelium not only may be fertile ground for LSIL development but also may be fertile grounds for the establishment of HPV persistence.* It is important to emphasize that HPV detection in adolescents is most commonly associated with normal cytology; approximately three fourths of HPV-infected adolescents have normal cytology.[7] The role of HPV persistence in these women without evidence of microscopic abnormalities remains to be elucidated.

NATURAL HISTORY OF HUMAN PAPILLOMAVIRUS

The natural history of prevalent HPV infection differs between adolescents and adults because *detection of HPV most likely reflects a persistent infection in older women and an incident infection in adolescents.* On the other hand, incident infections are not likely to differ. *Numerous studies have documented the transient nature of incident HPV infections in adolescents and young women; approximately 50% of women will clear infection within 6 months, and 90% will clear within 24 months.*[27-29] This has been true for 15- to 19-year-old women as well as 25- to 29-year-old women. Few studies have examined the natural history of incident infection in older women because most detected infections in older women are prevalent. In addition, detection of HPV may reflect recurrence of a latent infection in older women, blurring true regression rates in this age group.

Some evidence suggests that infection with multiple HPV types slows clearance of HPV in adolescents.[30,31] This may reflect a global defect in the immune response in adolescents or possibly a synergist effect of HPV. These studies are also difficult to interpret, as the reproducibility for the detection of multiple types is low. Sexually transmitted diseases are another factor that may influence clearance. *Chlamydia trachomatis*, a common infection in adolescents, has been shown in one study to enhance HPV persistence.[32,33] The mechanism of this association is not clear.

The natural history of LSIL also appears to differ for adolescents. A study of adolescents and young women showed that *92% of LSIL regressed within 36 months of observation,*[31] *whereas only 3% of the adolescent women went on to develop HSIL.* These rates significantly differ from older women.

Differences are likely due to two reasons. The first is *misclassification*. It has been well described that the majority of CIN 3 is diagnosed in women referred for LSIL. *Because the rates of CIN 3 are higher in older than younger women, it is more likely that an older woman with LSIL will be misclassified by chance alone.* Second, the LSIL detected in an older woman may already reflect a persistent infection and consequently be less likely to regress.

Human Papillomavirus Persistence and Squamous Intraepithelial Lesion

The important role of HPV persistence in the development of invasive cervical cancer has been established. However, the length of persistence required for the development of LSIL, HSIL, or cancer remains controversial. *LSIL in adolescents has been shown to develop within 3 months to 3 years after infection.* Moscicki et al.[7] found that 25% of adolescents developed detectable LSIL within 3 years, with the risk of developing LSIL cytology diminishing after 3 years. In a college population who only recently became sexually active, Winer et al.[34] found similar findings.

Time to HSIL appears to have a similar timeframe as LSIL. If CIN 2 and 3 are separated, the time to CIN 3 appears to be somewhat longer than CIN 2. Several countries that have collected rates for CIN 3 show that *rates of CIN 3 appear to peak in women aged 27 to 30 years, or 7 to 10 years after peak rate for HPV infections.*[35] In comparison, the risk of developing HSIL/CIN 2 may be more rapid. Woodman et al.[36] noted that 7% of adolescents developed HSIL within 19 months of acquiring HPV. HSIL in this case was a combination of CIN 2,3. Because CIN 2 is more common than CIN 3 in adolescents, these HSIL most likely reflect CIN 2 lesions. The similar timeframe for the development of LSIL and HSIL most likely reflects the difficulty in the ability of pathologists to reproducibly distinguish CIN 1 from CIN 2.[37]

Given these limitations, it can be summarized that *CIN 1 and 2 develop shortly after infection in some women, with detection in other women taking as long as 1 to 3 years. This may be a factor of size of lesion and not latency. Most women appear not to develop CIN 3 shortly after infection, although individual cases have been reported.*[34]

NATURAL HISTORY OF SQUAMOUS INTRAEPITHELIAL LESION

Progression of SIL also differs for adolescents. In general, *LSIL in adolescents is most likely to clear, with only a few cases progressing.* In a longitudinal study of LSIL, only 3% of adolescents went on to develop HSIL within 3 years, whereas 92% regressed.[31] In contrast, a retrospective chart review of adolescents <19 years of age with cytologic LSIL reported that 31% progressed to HSIL by 36 months.[38] Because this study involved chart reviews, it is not clear whether the HSIL reflected new lesions or actual progression of LSIL, and two thirds of the original cohort were lost

to follow-up. None of the studies found invasive cancer. Cox et al.[39] showed that 12.8% of older women (>30 years) will progress from LSIL or atypical squamous cells of undetermined significance (ASC-US)/HPV positive to HSIL within 2 years. One of the limitations of all these studies of cytology or histology is the poor sensitivity of cytology at any single event to detect true disease. HPV persistence by DNA detection is much more likely to predict HSIL development,[40] underscoring the importance of HPV persistence in the development of disease.

There are very few studies of HSIL in adolescents because of the ethical concerns in monitoring these lesions without treatment. As mentioned previously, CIN 2 is not a very reproducible diagnosis by pathologists, and there is considerable debate as to whether CIN 2 behaves more like CIN 1 or more like CIN 3.[41] Although there are no published CIN 2 follow-up studies of adolescents, most data suggest that the majority of HSIL in adolescents is CIN 2, rather than CIN 3,[10,13] and most importantly, rates of invasive cancer are extremely low in this age group. According to the most recent U.S. Surveillance, Epidemiology, and End Results (SEER) statistics (1995–1999), the incidence of invasive cancer in women younger than 20 years is 0 to 3 per million.[42] *This suggests that even in those with CIN 2 or 3, progression in this age group is uncommon. On the other hand, as women age past 25 years of age, the incidence of invasive cancer begins to rise. Interestingly, despite the decreasing age of sexual debut and sexual risk behavior, cancer rates in U.S. adolescents have not changed during the last 2 decades.*

SCREENING GUIDELINES

Cervical Cancer Screening

Translation of the recent natural history studies have resulted in new changes in the guidelines for cervical cancer screening in adolescents. Older guidelines in the United States recommended that all adolescents begin screening once sexually active.[43,44] These guidelines resulted in an overwhelming number of unnecessary referrals to colposcopy, even though spontaneous regression of SIL would have most likely been the natural history. Recently, guidelines were constructed based on risk behaviors (i.e., initiating sexual activity) with an allowable timeframe for regression to occur.[45] *Modeling has shown the cost-effectiveness of initiating screening 3 years after the onset of sexual activity or by 21 years of age, whichever comes first.* These guidelines were also believed to encompass screening in high-risk groups (i.e., those initiating sexual activity at early ages).

Although the upper age limit for initiating screening is much higher in many other countries, the upper age limit used by the American Cancer Society was considered a realistic age for compliance and access to patients, particularly considering that the United States has no mandatory organized screening program. A cap was believed necessary for women who are unwilling or unable to report sexual activity. In countries with organized screening, such as the

United Kingdom, new recommendations are to begin screening at 25 years of age.[46] In contrast, Australia has new guidelines recommending that screening begin at the age of 18 years, or 1 to 2 years after first sexual intercourse, whichever is later.[47]

COLPOSCOPIC FINDINGS

Colposcopic Findings in Adolescents

Dysplasia and cancer look no different in adolescents compared with adult women except that many dysplastic lesions are small because they are more likely early in the natural history than those seen in adult women. More importantly, atypical metaplasia, which is common in adolescents, has a strong resemblance to dysplasia. The colposcopic appearance of metaplasia includes numerous changes that often coexist. Some have divided the squamous metaplastic process colposcopically into five stages.[48] Stage 1 shows a pallor within the grapelike villi composed of columnar epithelium. In stage 2 the new squamous epithelium begins to grow down the sides of the villi and the colposcopic appearance results in attachment of adjacent villi. In stage 3 the fusion is completed; the new epithelium appears smooth and pink. In stage 4 maturation continues but capillary networks remain near the surface, giving the appearance of punctation and mosaic that may be associated with dysplasia. Finally, in stage 5 the capillary structures are compressed, forming a network under the epithelium that results in tissue indistinguishable from original squamous epithelia. This process is not uniform; topographically, the presence of any one of these stages is quite variable. It is not uncommon that several stages are present on the cervix simultaneously with islands of villi adjacent to smooth epithelium (Figure 22-5). This is especially true in an adolescent cervix. Stages 3 and 4 share common features with dysplastic lesions and are often referred to as *atypical squamous metaplasia*. These include coarse punctation, mosaic, and dense acetowhite epithelium (Figure 22-6) that can be difficult to distinguish from CIN 2,3.

HISTOLOGY

Histology of Squamous Metaplasia

CIN is no more reproducible in adolescents than in adult women. This is likely the main reason why the natural histories often differ. CIN 2 lesions in adolescents behave more like CIN 1. On review, these CIN 2 lesions are often recategorized to CIN 1 lesions. Because CIN 1 is extremely common in adolescents, chance alone contributes to increased chance of misclassification.[13] Furthermore, unlike in adults, in whom CIN 3 is highly reproducible, CIN 3 is poorly reproducible in adolescents.[49]

Squamous metaplasia has also been misclassified as CIN by inexperienced pathologists specifically when there are adjacent components of columnar and metaplastic

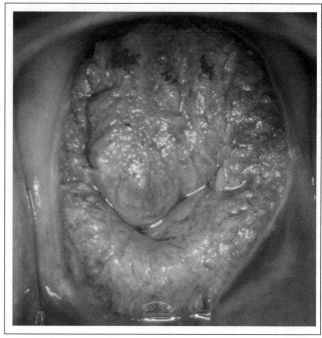

Figure 22-5 Adolescent cervix with several types of epithelium present. After the application of 3% acetic acid, mature squamous epithelium *(smooth pink areas)*, mature metaplastic epithelium *(thicker white areas)*, early metaplasia *(more translucent white areas)*, and columnar epithelium *(red areas)* can be visualized.

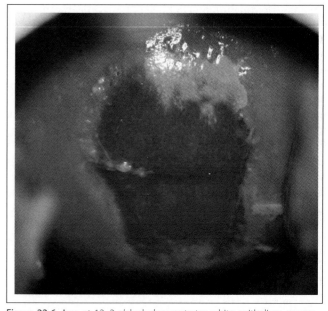

Figure 22-6 Area at 12–2 o'clock demonstrates white epithelium, coarse punctation, and mosaicism after the application of 3% acetic acid. This area is often referred to as *atypical squamous metaplasia*. This is often confused with CIN.

epithelium. Early features of squamous metaplasia found in stage 1 and 2 are multilayered undifferentiated sheets of cells toward the top of the villus and degeneration of the original basement membrane underlying the columnar epithelium with a formation of a new one.[48] Within the newly formed squamous epithelium, there are often residual columnar-lined surfaces with columnar cells. As the epithelium matures, it is common to see patches of smooth-surfaced epithelium with occasional stromal papillae projecting into the epithelium, representing the original stromal cores of the fused villi. Sometimes columnar epithelium can be seen underlying the new metaplastic epithelium and metaplastic epithelium within clefts of columnar epithelium. All these changes can be confusing, and the pathologist must be careful to differentiate these from squamous neoplasia and adenocarcinoma.

MANAGEMENT

Rationale

The rationale for management of abnormal cytology in adolescents was based primarily on the (1) observed high rates of HPV infections, (2) high rates of HPV and LSIL regression, and (3) low rates of CIN 3 and cervical cancer. Natural history studies show the low rates of CIN 3 and cervical cancer and the high rates of HPV and LSIL regression are likely related. Cost-effective strategies are based on the identification of women with HPV persistence, not incident infection. In adolescents, in whom incident infections are common, persistence is not common, and the risk of CIN 2,3 lesions (if present) progressing is rare, "time" is the best management strategy for distinguishing between incident and prevalent infection. *Because time is important, it is critical to give adequate time for regression.* Moscicki et al.[31] found that 60% of lesions regressed during the first year, but 92% regressed by 3 years, underscoring the importance of allowing adequate time for regression. *Another rationale for observation without treatment is the risk of the procedure versus the perceived benefit.* A recent meta-analysis of cervical excisional procedures showed increased risk of preterm delivery, low birth weight, and premature rupture of membranes.[50] With treatment comes the high risk of repeat treatment, as young women carry a high risk of repeated HPV infection and repeat lesions. Consequently, observation becomes important in the management of adolescents with HPV infection.

Furthermore, *because of the high rates of multiple incident HPV infection in adolescents, follow-up with HPV testing for any reason (ASC0US, LSIL follow-up) is of questionable value.* Boardman et al.[51] found that as many as 77% of adolescents with ASC-US will be positive for high-risk HPV types, calling into question its value in ASC-US triage in adolescents (defined as younger than 21 years).[52] No cost-effectiveness analysis for HPV testing in this age group has been performed, but most experts agree that HPV triage for ASC-US and HPV testing follow-up in LSIL is not cost-effective.

Management of Abnormal Cytology for Adolescents (<21 Years Old)

Human Papillomavirus Testing in Adolescents

Although HPV testing is being used more often for adult women in triage strategies, the evidence for its use in adolescents remains weak. *Repeat cytology is now favored over HPV triage in all the triage algorithms.*[52] Also, because adolescents experience multiple sequential HPV infections, a repetitively positive HPV test in this age group may represent repeated transient infections rather than a persistent infection.

Atypical Squamous Cells of Undetermined Significance and Low-Grade Squamous Intraepithelial Lesion Triage for Adolescents

Conservative observation of ASC-US and LSIL by cytology is recommended with repeat cytology rather than immediate referral to colposcopy.[52,53] HPV testing for ASC-US in adolescents is discouraged, and any results obtained are not helpful. *It is recommended that ASC-US/LSIL can be followed with repeat cytology at 12-month intervals for 2 years.*[52] During the 2 years of follow-up, a threshold of HSIL or greater is recommended before referral to colposcopy. After 2 years, a threshold of ASC or greater is recommended before referral to colposcopy. HPV testing for follow-up is not recommended. See Table 22-1 and Figure 22-7.

Atypical Squamous Cells of Undetermined Significance/Suggestive of High-Grade Squamous Intraepithelial Lesion

Triage recommendations are similar to that for adults (see Chapter 11).

High-Grade Squamous Intraepithelial Lesion

The majority of cases of CIN 2,3 especially in adolescents and young adults, spontaneously regress.[54,55] Moreover, recent studies have highlighted the potential negative impact of loop electrosurgical excision procedure (LEEP) on subsequent pregnancies. LEEP appears to approximately double the risk that a woman will subsequently have preterm delivery, a low-birth weight infant, or premature rupture of membranes.[50] See Table 22-2 and Figure 22-8.

Table 22-1 2006 American Society for Colposcopy and Cervical Pathology Atypical Squamous Cells of Undetermined Significance and Low-Grade Squamous Intraepithelial Lesion Guidelines in Adolescent Women

In adolescents with ASC-US and LSIL, follow-up with annual cytologic testing is recommended. **(BII)** At the 12-month follow-up, only adolescents with HSIL or greater on the repeat cytology should be referred to colposcopy. At the 24-month follow-up, those with an ASC-US or greater result should be referred to colposcopy. **(AII)** HPV DNA testing and colposcopy are unacceptable for adolescents with ASC-US and LSIL. **(EII)** If HPV testing is inadvertently performed, the results should not influence management.

ASC-US, atypical squamous cells of undetermined significance; *LSIL,* low-grade squamous intraepithelial lesion; *HSIL,* high-grade squamous intraepithelial lesion; *HPV,* human papillomavirus; *DNA,* deoxyribonucleic acid.
From Wright TC Jr, Massad LS, Dunton CJ, Spitzer M, Wilkinson EJ, Solomon D; for the 2006 ASCCP-Sponsored Consensus Conference. 2006 consensus guidelines for the management of women with abnormal cervical screening tests. J Low Genit Tract Dis. 2007 Oct;11(4):201–22.

Management of Adolescent Women with Either Atypical Squamous Cells of Undetermined Significance (ASC-US) or Low-grade Squamous Intraepithelial Lesion (LSIL)

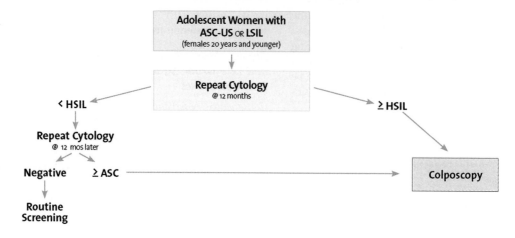

Figure 22-7 Reprinted from *The Journal of Lower Genital Tract Disease* Vol. 11 Issue 4, with the permission of ASCCP © American Society for Colposcopy and Cervical Pathology 2007. No copies of the algorithms may be made without the prior consent of ASCCP.

Table 22-2 2006 American Society for Colposcopy and Cervical Pathology High-Grade Squamous Intraepithelial Lesion Guidelines in Adolescent Women

In adolescents with HSIL, colposcopy is recommended. Immediate LEEP (i.e., see and treat approach) is unacceptable in adolescent women. **(AII)** When CIN 2,3 is not identified histologically, observation for up to 24 months using both colposcopy and cytology at 6-month intervals is preferred, provided the colposcopic examination is satisfactory and endocervical sampling is negative. **(BIII)** In exceptional circumstances, a diagnostic excisional procedure is acceptable. **(BIII)** If during follow-up a high-grade colposcopic lesion is identified or HSIL cytology persists for 1 year, biopsy is recommended. **(BIII)** If CIN 2,3 is identified histologically, management should follow the 2006 Consensus Guideline for the Management of Women with Cervical Intraepithelial Neoplasia. **(BIII)** If HSIL persists for 24 months without identification of CIN 2,3, a diagnostic excisional procedure is recommended. **(BIII)** After two consecutive "negative for intraepithelial lesion or malignancy" results, adolescents and young women without a high-grade colposcopic abnormality can return to routine cytologic screening. **(BIII)** A diagnostic excisional procedure is recommended for adolescents and young women with HSIL when colposcopy is unsatisfactory or CIN of any grade is identified on endocervical assessment. **(BII)**

LEEP, loop electrosurgical excision procedure;
HSIL, high-grade squamous intraepithelial lesion; *CIN*, cervical intraepithelial lesion. From Wright TC Jr, Massad LS, Dunton CJ, Spitzer M, Wilkinson EJ, Solomon D; for the 2006 ASCCP-Sponsored Consensus Conference. 2006 consensus guidelines for the management of women with abnormal cervical screening tests. J Low Genit Tract Dis. 2007 Oct;11(4):201–22.

TREATMENT DECISIONS

Treatment of Cervical Intraepithelial Neoplasia, Grade 1

In general, treatment of CIN 1 in adolescents is considered unwarranted.[52,53,56] Follow-up of histologically proven CIN 1 is recommended, similar to ASC-US/LSIL, with cytology at 12-month intervals. HSIL on cytology at 2 years warrants re-referral. As long as CIN 1 remains the histologic diagnosis, observation is warranted. See Table 22-3 and Figure 22-9.

Treatment of Cervical Intraepithelial Neoplasia, Grades 2,3

Although the recommendations for adult women with HSIL include immediate treatment, this approach should be avoided in adolescents. Excising the TZ by LEEP without biopsy confirmation is not recommended. Nearly 90% of such referred adolescents have no HSIL found on the specimen undergoing an LEEP, and the risk of side effects exceeds the potential benefit for patients without dysplasia.[57] In addition, recurrent lesions are not uncommon. Hence, cumulative effects of multiple treatments must be considered.[50] Hillard et al.[58] reported that 9% of adolescents undergoing LEEP developed pelvic inflammatory disease (PID) within 1 month of treatment. This underscores the importance of screening for STIs prior to treatment in adolescents. Some have recommended that cryotherapy be used over LEEP for suitable cases (small accessible lesions) in adolescents because of the lower rate of

Management of Adolescent Women (20 Years and Younger) with High-grade Squamous Intraepithelial Lesion (HSIL)

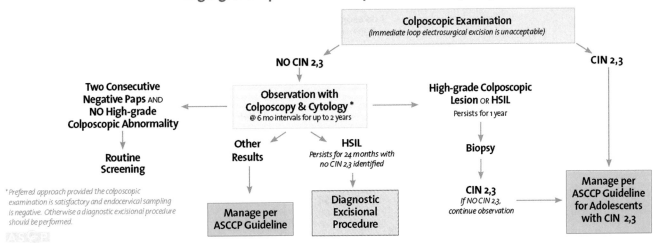

Figure 22-8 Reprinted from *The Journal of Lower Genital Tract Disease* Vol. 11 Issue 4, with the permission of ASCCP © American Society for Colposcopy and Cervical Pathology 2007. No copies of the algorithms may be made without the prior consent of ASCCP.

Table 22-3 2006 American Society for Colposcopy and Cervical Pathology Cervical Intraepithelial Neoplasia 1 Guidelines in Adolescent Women[56]

Follow-up with annual cytologic assessment is recommended for adolescents with CIN 1. **(AII)** At the 12-month follow-up, only adolescents with HSIL or greater on the repeat cytology should be referred to colposcopy. At the 24-month follow-up, those with an ASC-US or greater result should be referred to colposcopy. **(AII)** Follow-up with HPV DNA testing is unacceptable. **(EII)** Treatment of adolescents for CIN 1 is unacceptable. **(EII)**

CIN, cervical intraepithelial neoplasia; *HSIL*, high-grade squamous intraepithelial neoplasia; *ASC-US*, atypical squamous cells of undetermined significance; *HPV*, human papillomavirus; *DNA*, deoxyribonucleic acid.
From Wright TC Jr, Massad LS, Dunton CJ, Spitzer M, Wilkinson EJ, Solomon D; 2006 Amercian Society for Colposcopy and Cervical Pathology-sponsored Consensus Conference. 2006 consensus guidelines for the management of women with cervical intraepithelial neoplasia or adenocarcinoma *in situ*. J Low Genit Tract Dis. 2007 Oct;11(4):223–39.

complication associated with cryotherapy, but no recent studies have confirmed this.

Once CIN 2 is diagnosed, adolescents who are considered reliable candidates for follow-up can be observed. Observation is recommended at 6-month intervals with colposcopy and cytology.[52] If the lesion progresses to CIN 3 or greater or remains persistent at 2 years, treatment is recommended. If CIN 3 is diagnosed, treatment is recommended as in adult women. *Unfortunately, histologic diagnosis of CIN 2 and 3 are often not distinguished. Because CIN 2 lesions are more common than CIN 3 in adolescent girls, it is recommended that the CIN 2,3 be treated similar to CIN 2. If compliance is doubtful, treatment is the better option. If CIN 2,3 is treated, recommendations for follow-up in adolescents are similar to those in adults.* See Table 22-4 and Figure 22-10.

MANAGEMENT SCENARIOS

Scenario 1

Age: 15 years (any age < 21 years)
Sentinel Pap: Atypical squamous cells of undetermined significance (ASC-US)
Colposcopic findings or biopsy result (if a biopsy was done): Not performed
HPV testing for high-risk (oncogenic) HPV types: High-risk HPV types *(HPV testing should not have been done and any results from such a test should be ignored [see discussion].)*
Satisfactory colposcopy: Not applicable (N/A)
Fertility desires: Yes

This 15-year-old female began sexual activity 2 years ago and has had three partners and a history of *C. trachomatis. The Pap smear in this case should not have been obtained.* The new guidelines suggest that cervical cancer screening should begin 3 years after the onset of sexual activity regardless of number of sexual partners and history of STI. Most likely this ASC-US is benign with little clinical relevance. The recommendation in this case is to *ignore the HPV testing* and treat similarly to LSIL. At this point, the clinician is now obligated to *follow* the patient. Recommendations are to repeat the Pap test in 1 year. If the results are less than HSIL, the Pap test should be repeated in another 12 months. If the repeat is HSIL, then the patient should be referred for colposcopy.

Scenario 2

Age: 19 years (any age < 21 years)
Sentinel Pap: persistent LSIL for 2 years
Colposcopic findings or biopsy result (if a biopsy was done): Patient is found to have CIN 3 on histology; a single quadrant is involved

Management of Adolescent Women (20 Years and Younger) with a Histological Diagnosis of Cervical Intraepithelial Neoplasia - Grade 1 (CIN 1)

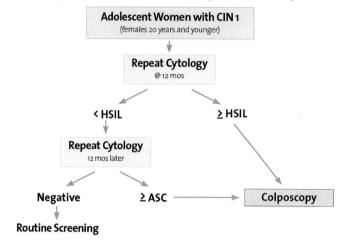

Figure 22-9 Reprinted from *The Journal of Lower Genital Tract Disease* Vol. 11 Issue 4, with the permission of ASCCP © American Society for Colposcopy and Cervical Pathology 2007. No copies of the algorithms may be made without the prior consent of ASCCP.

Table 22-4 2006 American Society for Colposcopy and Cervical Pathology Cervical Intraepithelial Neoplasia 2,3 Guidelines in Adolescent Women

For adolescents and young women with biopsy confirmed CIN 2,3, not otherwise specified, either treatment or observation for up to 24 months using both colposcopy and cytology at 6-month intervals is acceptable, provided colposcopy is satisfactory. **(BIII)** When a histological diagnosis of CIN 2 is specified in these women, observation is preferred; treatment is acceptable. When a histological diagnosis of CIN 3 is specified or when colposcopy is unsatisfactory, treatment is recommended. **(BIII)** If the colposcopic appearance of the lesion worsens or if HSIL cytology or a high-grade colposcopic lesion persists for 1 year, repeat biopsy is recommended (BIII). After 2 consecutive "negative for intraepithelial lesion or malignancy" results, adolescents and young women with normal colposcopy can return to routine cytological screeing (BII). Treatment is recommended if CIN 3 is subsequently identified or if CIN 2,3 persists for 24 months (BII).

CIN, cervical intraepithelial neoplasia; *HSIL,* high-grade squamous intraepithelial neoplasia.
From Wright TC Jr, Massad LS, Dunton CJ, Spitzer M, Wilkinson EJ, Solomon D; 2006 American Society for Colposcopy and Cervical Pathology-sponsored Consensus Conference. 2006 consensus guidelines for the management of women with cervical intraepithelial neoplasia or adenocarcinoma *in situ.* J Low Genit Tract Dis. 2007 Oct;11(4):223–39.

HPV testing for high-risk (oncogenic) HPV types: N/A
Satisfactory colposcopy: Yes
Fertility desires: Yes

This young woman is an example of the importance of following LSIL. Persistent LSIL, like persistent HPV, is a risk for the development of CIN 3. The recommendation for the management of adolescents with CIN 3 is identical to the management of CIN 3 in adult women. CIN 3 lesions should be treated. The two best options are those best to preserve her fertility. Either cryotherapy, as the lesion is located in a single quadrant, or a small LEEP targeting the lesion is warranted. Because the immature TZ may be much larger in adolescents, one must take care not to *excise large portions of the cervix* to *a great depth* in the zealous attempt to cure the patient. The area closest to the lesion and the SCJ should be excised to an appropriate depth while the remaining portion of the TZ should be ablated or excised to a shallower depth.

Scenario 3

Age: 16 years (any age < 21 years)
Sentinel Pap: HSIL
Colposcopic findings or biopsy result (if a biopsy was done):
    Biopsy showed atypical squamous metaplasia and LSIL.
    Endocervical curettage was normal
HPV testing for high-risk (oncogenic) HPV types: N/A
Satisfactory colposcopy: Yes
Fertility desires: Yes

Common to young women, the colposcopic and histologic examination revealed no CIN 2,3 lesion despite the HSIL cytology. In young women, regression of HSIL is common. In this case, the lesion most likely regressed by the time the patient was referred to colposcopy, or the HSIL was an overcall. *This emphasizes the importance of not performing LEEPs on adolescents without histologic confirmation of CIN 3.* This young woman would best be followed by repeat cytology in 6 to 12 months. Repeat colposcopy is probably unnecessary unless HSIL is present.

Management of Adolescent and Young Women
with a Histological Diagnosis of Cervical Intraepithelial Neoplasia - Grade 2,3 (CIN 2,3)

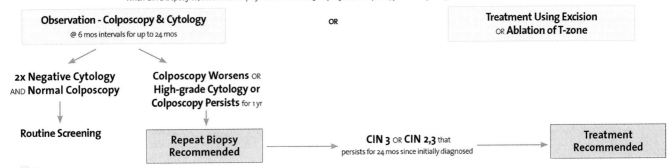

Figure 22-10 Reprinted from *The Journal of Lower Genital Tract Disease* Vol. 11 Issue 4, with the permission of ASCCP © American Society for Colposcopy and Cervical Pathology 2007. No copies of the algorithms may be made without the prior consent of ASCCP.

Scenario 4

Age: 14 years (any age < 21 years)
Sentinel Pap: LSIL
Colposcopic findings or biopsy result (if a biopsy was done):
   Colposcopy not performed
HPV testing for high-risk (oncogenic) HPV types: N/A
Satisfactory colposcopy: Not applicable
Fertility desires: Yes

This 14-year-old female began sexual intercourse at the age of 11 years. Her first Pap smear revealed LSIL. LSIL is quite common in young women, as is HPV detection. Although she has been sexually active for 3 years, it is best to follow the LSIL cytology rather than evaluating it with colposcopy. A repeat cytology should be performed in 12 months. As in an adult, HPV testing is not helpful in triage of the initial Pap, but *in adolescents it is also not helpful in follow-up because an HPV test that remains positive may indicate a serially positive result (a positive test that resolved followed by a new infection) rather than a persistently positive test.* If the repeat Pap remains LSIL or lower, observation can be continued for another year with follow-up cytology in 12 months. If the repeat cytology reveals HSIL, referral to colposcopy should be made.

Scenario 5

Age: 15 years (any age < 21 years)
Sentinel Pap: LSIL
Colposcopic findings or biopsy result (if a biopsy was done):
   Colposcopy shows a moderate- to high-grade lesion; CIN 2,3 is confirmed by histology
HPV testing for high-risk (oncogenic) HPV types: N/A
Satisfactory colposcopy: Yes
Fertility desires: Yes

As in adults, most CIN 2,3 among adolescents is diagnosed after a referral cytology of LSIL or less. However, as in adolescents with LSIL/CIN 1, much of CIN 2 also regresses in adolescents. *When histologic diagnoses are combined, CIN 2 is the most statistically likely diagnosis in adolescents. Hence, the patient should be managed based on a diagnosis of CIN 2, and follow-up is the management of choice.* This young woman can be followed with colposcopy and cytology at 6-month intervals for as long as 2 years. If the lesion persists for 2 years, treatment is recommended. In adolescents in whom the histology or colposcopy is suggestive of true CIN 3 *(not just a high-grade CIN)* or if compliance is questioned at any visit, treatment is preferred.

SUMMARY

Although HPV is extremely common in adolescents, spontaneous clearance occurs in the majority. These high rates of infection are due either to sexual behavior, biological vulnerability, or a combination of both. The association between age of first intercourse and invasive cancer cannot be ignored. Consequently, initiating screening at appropriate times in this vulnerable group is essential. Because infections frequently come and go in this age group, studies show that observation for most HPV-associated lesions is preferred. Even with the increase in risky sexual behavior among adolescents, the risk of progression to cancer in the adolescent years appears miniscule. Because of the frequent comings and goings of HPV, HPV testing is not cost-effective in any screening or triage strategy. With the HPV vaccine, it will be essential to vaccinate children prior to the onset of sexual activity—prior to acquisition of HPV. Accordingly, adolescents who initiate sexual activity may not have yet developed an HPV infection and should receive vaccination as well. All adolescents vaccinated must be counseled about the important of continued cancer screening.

REFERENCES

1. Moscicki AB, Palefsky J, Gonzales J, et al. Human papillomavirus infection in sexually active adolescent females: prevalence and risk factors. Pediatr Res 1990;28:507–513.

2. Moscicki AB, Ellenberg JH, Vermund SH, et al. Prevalence of and risks for cervical human papillomavirus infection and squamous intraepithelial lesions in adolescent girls: impact of infection with human immunodeficiency virus. Arch Ped Adolesc Med 2000;154:127–134.

3. Burchell A, Winer R, de Sanjose S, et al. Epidemiolgoy and transmission dynamics of genital human papillomavirus infection. Vaccine Monographs 2006;24:52–62.

4. Franceschi S, Herrero R, Clifford GM, et al. Variations in the age-specific curves of human papillomavirus prevalence in women worldwide. Int J Cancer 2006;119:2677–2684.

5. De Sanjose S. La investigacion sobre la infeccion por virus del papiloma human y el cancer de cuello uterino en Espana. In: de Sanjose S, Garcia A (eds). El Virus del Papiloma Human y Cancer: Epidemiologia y Prevencion. Madrid: EMISA, 2006.

6. Munoz N, Mendez F, Posso H, et al. Incidence, duration, and determinants of cervical human papillomavirus infection in a cohort of Colombian women with normal cytological results. J Infect Dis 2004;190:2077–2087.

7. Moscicki AB, Hills N, Shiboski S, et al. Risks for incident human papillomavirus infection and low-grade squamous intraepithelial lesion development in young females. J Am Med Assoc 2001;285:2995–3002.

8. Brown DR, Shew ML, Qadadri B, et al. A longitudinal study of genital human papillomavirus infection in a cohort of closely followed adolescent women. J Infect Dis 2005;191:182–192.

9. Winer RL, Lee SK, Hughes JP, et al. Genital human papillomavirus infection: incidence and risk factors in a cohort of female university students. Am J Epidemiol 2003;157:218–226.

10. Sadeghi SB, Hsieh EW, Gunn SW. Prevalence of cervical intraepithelial neoplasia in sexually active teenagers and young adults. Am J Obstet Gynecol 1984;148:726–729.

11. Bjorge T, Gunbjorud AB, Langmark F, et al. Cervical mass screening in Norway—510,000 smears a year. Cancer Detect Prevent 1994;18:463–470.

12. Schydlower LTM, Greenberg MH, Patterson CPH. Adolescents with abnormal cervical cytology. Clin Pediatrics 1981;20:723–726.

13. Mount SL, Papillo JL. A study of 10,296 pediatric and adolescent Papanicolaou smear diagnoses in northern New England. Pediatrics 1999;103:539–546.

14. Moscicki AB. Genital HPV infections in children and adolescents. Obstet Gynecol Clin North Am 1996;23:675–679.

15. Monteiro DL, Trajano AJ, da Silva KS, et al. Pre-invasive cervical disease and uterine cervical cancer in Brazilian adolescents: prevalence and related factors. Cad Saude Publica 2006;22:2539–2548.

16. Santelli JS, Brener ND, Lowry R, et al. Multiple sexual partners among U.S. adolescents and young adults. Fam Plann Perspect 1998;30:271–275.

17. Mosher WD, Chandra A, Jones J. Sexual behavior and selected health measures: men and women 15–44 years of age, United States, 2002. Adv Data 2005;362:1–55.

18. Green J, Berrington de Gonzalez A, Sweetland S, et al. Risk factors for adenocarcinoma and squamous cell carcinoma of the cervix in women aged 20-44 years: the UK National Case-Control Study of Cervical Cancer. Br J Cancer 2003;89:2078–2086.

19. Sierra-Torres CH, Tyring SK, Au WW. Risk contribution of sexual behavior and cigarette smoking to cervical neoplasia. Int J Gynecol Cancer 2003;13:617–625.

20. Moscicki AB, Singer A. The cervical epithelium during puberty and adolescence. In: Jordan JA, Singer A (eds). The Cervix, ed 2. Malden, MA: Blackwell, 2006, pp 81–101.

21. Singer A. The uterine cervix from adolescence to the menopause. Br J Obstet Gynaecol 1975;82:81–99.

22. Moscicki AB, Ma Y, Holland C, Vermund SH. Cervical ectopy in adolescent girls with and without human immunodeficiency virus infection. J Infect Dis 2001;183:865–870.

23. Schachter J, Hill EC, King EB, et al. Chlamydial infection in women with cervical dysplasia. Am J Obstet Gynecol 1975;123:753–757.

24. Solomon D, Davey D, Kurman R, et al. The 2001 Bethesda System: terminology for reporting results of cervical cytology. J Am Med Assoc 2002;287:2114–2119.

25. Moscicki AB, Grubbs-Burt V, Kanowitz S, et al. The significance of squamous metaplasia in the development of low grade squamous intra-epithelial lesions in young women. Cancer 1999;85:1139–1144.

26. Castle PE, Jeronimo J, Schiffman M, et al. Age-related changes of the cervix influence human papillomavirus type distribution. Cancer Res 2006;66:1218–1224.

27. Moscicki AB, Shiboski S, Broering J, et al. The natural history of human papillomavirus infection as measured by repeated DNA testing in adolescent and young women. J Pediatr 1998;132:277–284.

28. Ho GY, Bierman R, Beardsley L, et al. Natural history of cervicovaginal papillomavirus infection in young women. N Engl J Med 1998;338:423–428.

29. Evander M, Edlund K, Gustaffson A, et al. Human papillomavirus infection is transient in young women: a population-based cohort study. J Infect Dis 1995;171:1026–1030.

30. Moscicki AB, Ellenberg JH, Fahrat S, et al. HPV persistence in HIV infected and uninfected adolescent girls: risk factors and differences by phylogenetic types. J Infect Dis 2004;190: 37–45.

31. Moscicki AB, Shiboski S, Hills NK, et al. Regression of low-grade squamous intra-epithelial lesions in young women. Lancet 2004;364:1678–1683.

32. Silins I, Ryd W, Strand A, et al. *Chlamydia trachomatis* infection and persistence of human papillomavirus. Int J Cancer 2005;116:110–115.

33. Samoff E, Koumans EH, Markowitz LE, et al. Association of *Chlamydia trachomatis* with persistence of high-risk types of human papillomavirus in a cohort of female adolescents. Am J Epidemiol 2005;162:668–675.

34. Winer RL, Kiviat NB, Hughes JP, et al. Development and duration of human papillomavirus lesions, after initial infection. J Infect Dis 2005;191:731–738.

35. Bosch FX, de Sanjose S. Chapter 1: Human papillomavirus and cervical cancer—burden and assessment of causality. J Natl Cancer Inst Monogr 2003;31:3–13.

36. Woodman CB, Collins S, Winter H, et al. Natural history of cervical human papillomavirus infection in young women: a longitudinal cohort study. Lancet 2001;357:1831–1836.

37. Heatley MK. How should we grade CIN? Histopathology 2002;40:377–390.

38. Wright JD, Davila RM, Pinto KR, et al. Cervical dysplasia in adolescents. Obstet Gynecol 2005;106:115–120.

39. Cox JT, Schiffman M, Solomon D, ASCUS-LSIL Triage Study (ALTS) Group. Prospective follow-up suggests similar risk of subsequent cervical intraepithelial neoplasia grade 2 or 3 among women with cervical intraepithelial neoplasia grade 1 or negative colposcopy and directed biopsy. Am J Obstet Gynecol 2003;188:1406–1412.

40. Kjaer SK, van den Brule AJ, Paull G, et al. Type specific persistence of high risk human papillomavirus (HPV) as indicator of high grade cervical squamous intraepithelial lesions in young women: population based prospective follow up study. Br Med J 2002;325:572–578.

41. Syrjanen K, Kataja V, Yliskoski M, et al. Natural history of cervical human papillomavirus lesions does not substantiate the biologic relevance of the Bethesda System. Obstet Gynecol 1992;79:675–682.

42. Chan PG, Sung HY, Sawaya GF. Changes in cervical cancer incidence after three decades of screening US women less than 30 years old. Obstet Gynecol 2003;102:765–773.

43. American College of Obstetricians and Gynecologists. Recommendations on frequency of Pap test screening.1995;152.

44. American Medical Association. Guidelines for adolescent preventive services. Chicago, IL: American Medical Association, 1992.

45. Saslow D, Runowicz CD, Solomon D, et al. American Cancer Society guideline for the early detection of cervical neoplasia and cancer. CA Cancer J Clin 2002;52:342–362.

46. NHS Cancer Screening Programmes. NHS Cervical Screening Programme: NHS Cervical Screening Programme, *www.cancerscreening.nhs.uk/cervical/index.html#invited*. Accessed 2006.

47. National Health and Medical Research Council. *www.nhmrc.gov.au/publications*. Vol. 2006, 2005. Accessed August 2007.

48. Singer A, Jordan JA. The functional anatomy of the cerivx, the cerivcal epithelium and the stroma. In: Jordan JA, Singer A, eds. The Cervix, ed 2. Malden, MA: Blackwell, 2006, pp 13–37.

49. Moscicki AB, Powers A, Ma Y, et al. Years sexually active and oral contraceptives are a risk for CIN 3 in adolescents and young women. Presented at the 23rd International Papillomavirus Conference 2006, Prague, September 2006.

50. Kyrgiou M, Koliopoulos G, Martin-Hirsch P, et al. Obstetric outcomes after conservative treatment for intraepithelial or early invasive cervical lesions: systematic review and meta-analysis. Lancet 2006;367:489–498.

51. Boardman LA, Stanko C, Weitzen S, et al. Atypical squamous cells of undetermined significance: human papillomavirus testing in adolescents. Obstet Gynecol 2005;105:741–746.

52. Wright TC Jr, Massad LS, Dunton CJ, Spitzer M, Wilkinson EJ, Solomon D; for the 2006 ASCCP-Sponsored Consensus Conference. 2006 consensus guidelines for the management of women with abnormal cervical screening tests. J Low Genit Tract Dis. 2007 Oct;11(4):201–22.

53. American College of Obstetricians and Gynecologists. ACOG Guidelines for Women's Health Care. Washington, DC: ACOG, 1996.

54. Melnikow J, Nuovo J, Willan AR, et al. Natural history of cervical squamous intraepithelial lesions: a meta- analysis. Obstet Gynecol 1998;92:727–735.

55. Peto J, Gilham C, Deacon J, et al. Cervical HPV infection and neoplasia in a large population-based prospective study: the Manchester cohort. Br J Cancer 2004;91:942–953.

56. Wright TC Jr, Massad LS, Dunton CJ, Spitzer M, Wilkinson EJ, Solomon D; 2006 American Society for Colposcopy and Cervical Pathology-sponsored Consensus Conference. 2006 consensus guidelines for the management of women with cervical intraepithelial neoplasia or adenocarcinoma in situ. J Low Genit Tract Dis. 2007 Oct;11(4):223–39.

57. Sadler L, Saftlas A, Wang W, et al. Treatment for cervical intraepithelial neoplasia and risk of preterm delivery. J Am Med Assoc 2004;291:2100–2106.

58. Hillard PA, Biro FM, Wildey L. Complications of cervical cryotherapy in adolescents. J Reprod Med 1991;36:711–716.

CHAPTER 23

Anal Disease

Teresa M. Darragh • J. Michael Berry •
Naomi Jay • Joel M. Palefsky

KEY POINTS

- Anal cancer is increasing in incidence in both men and women in the general population.
- The primary risk factor that anal and cervical cancer share is the human papillomavirus (HPV), mostly HPV type 16.
- Groups at increased risk of AIN and anal cancer include human immunodeficiency virus (HIV)-positive men and women, HIV-negative men who have sex with men (MSM), HIV-negative women at high risk of HIV infection, and recipients of organ transplants with iatrogenic immunosuppression to prevent graft rejection.
- The incidence of anal cancer among HIV-positive MSM is estimated to be double that of HIV-negative MSM. The incidence of anal cancer has increased since the introduction of highly active antiretroviral therapy (HAART).
- Anal intercourse is not an absolute requirement to acquire anal HPV infection.
- The prevalence of anal HPV does not decline with age, as does cervical infection.
- The incidence of high-grade AIN is high in HIV-positive MSM. HAART appears to have little beneficial effect on AIN.
- There is support for screening for anal cancer in all men and women with HIV disease and in all MSM. An anoscope is unnecessary for specimen collection. The goal of anal cytology is to sample the entire anal canal from the distal rectal vault to the anal verge.
- The sensitivity and specificity of anal cytology are similar to conventional cervical cytology. Liquid-based cytology improves the quality of an anal specimen.
- Anal cytology is reported like gynecologic cytology using the same Bethesda terminology as the cervix.
- The epithelial abnormalities on anal cytology mirror the cervix and include low-grade squamous intraepithelial lesion (LSIL), high-grade squamous intraepithelial lesion (HSIL), and atypical squamous cells of undetermined significance (ASC-US).
- The anal TZ is the area undergoing dynamic squamous metaplastic change. Most high-grade AIN is located in or near the TZ.
- The goal of high-resolution anoscopy (HRA) is to systematically visualize the entire anal canal and perianal skin to determine the presence or absence of HPV-associated disease and to select appropriate areas for biopsy.
- HIV-negative MSM with no prior history of anal squamous intraepithelial lesion (SIL) can be screened cytologically every 2 to 3 years. HIV-positive persons should be screened annually. Persons with LSIL on anal cytology, normal digital rectal exam (DRE), and no high-grade AIN on HRA can be followed every 6 months. Those with HSIL, a normal DRE, and no lesions on HRA should be followed at 4-month intervals. Persons with high-grade AIN should be treated regardless of immune status. Persons diagnosed with invasive anal cancers should be referred to anal disease specialists.

EPIDEMIOLOGY AND NATURAL HISTORY OF ANAL HUMAN PAPILLOMAVIRUS INFECTION AND ANAL HUMAN PAPILLOMAVIRUS-RELATED NEOPLASIA

The incidence of anal cancer is growing in the general population and particularly among certain high-risk groups such as those with immunosuppression and/or a history of receptive anal intercourse. Anal cancer and its putative precursor, anal intraepithelial neoplasia (AIN), share extensive biological similarity with cervical cancer and cervical intraepithelial neoplasia (CIN), including anatomic similarities and an etiologic relationship with human papillomavirus (HPV). *The approach to the understanding of the biology and natural history of anal cancer and AIN has therefore borrowed heavily from approaches used to study cervical disease, including HPV detection techniques, cytology, anoscopy using a colposcope, and biopsy.* Although the results of these studies indicate many similarities between CIN and AIN, there are several key differences in the epidemiology and natural history of these two diseases, which will be discussed in this chapter.

Epidemiology of Anal Cancer

The relationship between cervical HPV infection, CIN, and cervical cancer has been appreciated for several decades. *Compared with CIN and cervical cancer, AIN and anal cancer are poorly understood, largely because attention was focused on anal disease only recently, and much of this interest was stimulated by the advent of the human immunodeficiency virus (HIV) epidemic that began in the United States in the 1980s.* Prior to this time, there was relatively little interest in anal cancer because of its rarity in the general population.

Historically, anal cancer was a disease of individuals over the age of 60 years, with a female:male ratio of about 1.6 to 1.[1] However, several landmark papers published in the 1980s demonstrated an increased risk among specific subgroups, particularly those with a history of receptive anal intercourse, especially men who have sex with men (MSM).[2–4] The incidence of anal cancer among MSM prior to the HIV epidemic was estimated to be as high as 37/100,000,[3] indicating that the incidence of anal cancer was roughly equivalent to that of cervical cancer in the general population in the United States prior to the introduction of cervical Papanicolaou (Pap) smear screening. *Risk factors for anal cancer included a history of receptive anal intercourse, external genital warts, number of sexual partners, and smoking.* Other investigators have also demonstrated a relationship between cervical and anal cancer.[5,6] Women with a history of CIN or cervical cancer are more likely to develop anal cancer than colon cancer (odds ratio [OR] 5.2, 95% confidence interval [CI] 3.3–8.3). The primary etiologic factor that these two diseases share is HPV. *Several studies have demonstrated a high prevalence of HPV directly in anal cancer tissues, mostly HPV 16.[7–10] After cervical cancer, anal cancer has the highest proportion of HPV positivity among anogenital cancers.*

Although less common than cervical cancer, anal cancer is increasing in incidence in both women and men in the general population, doubling from about 10 cases per million to 20 cases per million from 1973 to 2000.[11] In 2006, there were 4660 cases of anal cancer and 660 deaths in the United States. Some of this increase may be attributable to an increase in incidence among HIV-positive MSM. Data from matches of cancer and acquired immune deficiency syndrome (AIDS) registries show that the relative risk of invasive anal cancer was 37 in HIV-positive MSM compared with the general population.[12] *The incidence of anal cancer among HIV-positive MSM is estimated to be double that of HIV-negative MSM and at the time of an AIDS diagnosis is 80 times higher than in the general population.[13] HIV-positive women have a nearly sevenfold higher risk of anal cancer than the general population of women.[12]*

With longer survival associated with the introduction of highly active antiretroviral therapy (HAART), the incidence of anal cancer continues to increase.[1,14–17] Although HAART has increased survival, it has not reduced the incidence of anal cancer. Likewise, the female:male ratio of anal cancer has been steadily decreasing, reflecting the increase of anal cancers among MSM.[1] In a study from a match between the San Francisco AIDS Surveillance Registry and California Cancer Registry, *the incidence of anal cancer has increased since the introduction of HAART in San Francisco (relative hazard 2.7) after adjustment for age at time of AIDS diagnosis, race, risk group, calendar year, and HAART use.[18]* Finally, an increased risk of anal cancer is not limited to immunosuppression related to HIV infection; recipients of organ transplants with iatrogenic immunosuppression to prevent graft rejection are at a tenfold increased risk of anal cancer compared with the general population.[19,20] *These data indicate that immunosuppression is a key risk factor for anal cancer although an additional direct role for HIV infection cannot be excluded.*

In summary, although anal cancer remains a comparatively rare disease, its incidence is increasing. The incidence of anal cancer is particularly high in specific risk groups, including those with a history of receptive anal intercourse and immunosuppression. The incidence of anal cancer has seen a steady rise among MSM with the onset of the HIV epidemic and, more recently, with the longer survival

associated with HAART. This has been accompanied by a change in the female:male ratio of the disease in the United States, as well as a reduction in the mean age at time of diagnosis. However, the relationship between anal cancer and immunosuppression is complex, at least among those with HIV infection. Earlier studies had suggested that progression to invasive cancer was not as clearly related to immunosuppression as progression to AIN 2,3, the putative anal cancer precursor.[12,21] Instead, progression from AIN 2,3 to invasive cancer may be related more to the accumulation over time of genetic changes associated with HPV-induced chromosomal instability (Table 23-1).[22] If true, this may partly explain the lack of benefit of HAART-associated immune reconstitution in reducing the incidence of anal cancer, similar to its lack of effect on cervical cancer.

Epidemiology and Natural History of Anal Human Papillomavirus Infection

The spectrum of HPV types found in the anal canal is similar to that seen in the cervix. Studies of anal HPV infection in at-risk groups consistently show a high prevalence of anal HPV infection. *In a study of sexually active HIV-negative MSM from four cities in the United States, the prevalence of anal HPV infection was high, between 50% and 60%, and remained so for each of the age groups studied, from younger than 25 years to older than 55 years.[23]* This is in contrast to studies of cervical HPV infection in women, some of which show a marked decline in the prevalence of HPV after the age of 30 years.[24] Although the reason for this difference is not clear, it is speculated that this reflects *a higher number of new sex partners and exposures among the population of MSM after age 30 as compared with women.*

Anal HPV infection is even more common in HIV-positive MSM than in HIV-negative MSM.[21,25] *Anal HPV infection was found in almost all HIV-positive MSM, usually with multiple HPV types, including one or more oncogenic HPV types. The primary risk factor in these men is having a lower CD4+ level.*

Anal HPV infection is also common in other HIV-positive populations. This includes HIV-positive men without a history of receptive anal intercourse[26] and HIV-positive women. In a study of HIV-positive and HIV-negative women in San Francisco for whom concurrent anal and cervical HPV data were available, anal HPV was more common than cervical HPV in both HIV-positive (79% anal versus 53% cervical) and HIV-negative women (43% anal versus 24% cervical).[27] This finding is consistent with results of another study of HIV-positive women living in Denmark.[28] About one half of the women had at least one HPV type in their cervical and anal samples, and the others did not, despite having had multiple HPV types at each site. *Because the overall distribution of HPV types appears to be similar in the anal canal and cervix, this finding implies that many of these infections were the results of separate exposures, rather than spread from one anatomic site to another.* However, with at least one HPV type in common between the cervix and the anus in about half of the women, the results are also consistent with a role for the anal canal being a potential

Table 23-1 Effect of Highly Active Antiretroviral Therapy on Anal Intraepithelial Neoplasia

Reference	Study Area	HPV Infection and Related Disease	Study Design	Impact of HAART on Disease
42	USA	HR HPV AIN	Comparison of the natural history of ASIL in HIV-positive men before and after initiation of HAART	Limited positive effect
36	France	HR HPV AIN	Prevalence of ASIL and HPV infection in HAART treated patients	No effect
34	USA	HG AIN	Prevalence of HG AIN among HIV-positive MSM in the post-HAART era	No effect
68	USA	HPV DNA AIN	Association of HAART with HPV and ASIL in HIV-positive	Positive

HPV, Human papillomavirus; *HAART*, highly active antiretroviral therapy; *HR HPV*, high-risk HPV; *AIN*, anal intraepithelial neoplasia; *ASIL*, anal squamous intraepithelial lesions; *HIV*, human immunodeficiency virus; *HG*, high grade; *MSM*, men who have sex with men; *DNA*, deoxyribonucleic acid.

reservoir for cervical HPV infection in women, or vice versa. Overall, HPV infection in HIV-positive women and, to a lesser extent, in HIV-negative women, should be considered a "field" infection of the anogenital region, rather than a site-specific infection.

In the San Francisco study, the HIV-negative women were at high risk for HIV infection and most had a history of working in the commercial sex trade or of intravenous drug use.[27] Hernandez et al. studied healthy women (presumably at low risk of HIV infection) in Hawaii and found that 27% had anal HPV infection, 29% had cervical HPV infection, and 13% had concurrent infection at both sites.[29] *Having cervical HPV infection was associated with increased risk of anal HPV infection, and genotype concordance was high in this study.* Interestingly, the prevalence of anal HPV infection did not decline with age as did cervical infection, consistent with the study of HIV-negative MSM described earlier.[23]

Patients with immunosuppression due to causes other than HIV are also at risk of anal HPV infection. Patel et al. showed that 23% of patients with a new renal transplant had anal HPV infection.[20] Patients who had had a renal transplant for a longer period of time had a 47% prevalence of anal HPV infection, implying that reactivation of prior HPV infection may be playing a role, in addition to new exposures.

The relationship between anal HPV infection and receptive anal intercourse is not entirely clear. Determining the role of anal intercourse in MSM is technically difficult given the high proportion of study MSM who engaged in this activity. Anal intercourse was not a clear risk factor for anal HPV infection in HIV-positive women[27] but was a significant risk factor in the Hawaiian study among women who had anal HPV infection in the absence of cervical infection.[29] *Clearly, anal intercourse is not an absolute requirement to acquire anal HPV infection, especially given the high prevalence of anal HPV infection among HIV-positive men without a history of anal intercourse.*[26] However, the data in the Hawaiian study, the high prevalence of anal HPV infection in MSM, and the fact that anal intercourse is a risk factor for anal cancer for both men and women indicate that anal intercourse is likely to increase the risk of anal HPV infection. Other methods of introduction of HPV to the anal canal may include spread from other genital sites or insertion of fingers, toys, or other objects into the anal canal.

Clearly, anal HPV infection is clinically important for its role in development of anal cancer. However, given the unexpected ubiquity of anal HPV infection in the population and comparative rarity of anal cancer, the data suggest that on a per-infection basis, *the anal canal is not as susceptible to malignant transformation as the cervix.* However, given the relationship to cervical HPV infection and concordance between anal and cervical HPV types in some studies, the anus may constitute an important reservoir of HPV infection. Movement of fluids from the anus to the anterior genital region is not uncommon, as shown by the frequency of urinary tract infections in women caused by fecal organisms. It is possible, although as yet unproven, that in addition to its role in causation of anal cancer, anal HPV infection may also be important in modulating the biology of cervical HPV infection if it persists in the anus and is intermittently shed to the cervix over time. Prospective studies over a number of years will be needed to address this issue.

Epidemiology and Natural History of Anal Intraepithelial Neoplasia

Given the biological similarity between cervical cancer and anal cancer, and between CIN and AIN, it is assumed that if cervical cancer is preceded by CIN, then anal cancer might be preceded by AIN. As in the cervix, it is assumed that low-grade intraepithelial neoplasia does not progress directly to cancer, whereas high-grade intraepithelial neoplasia may do so in a small percentage of cases and over a period of many years. In the anus, the former would be classified as AIN 1 and the latter as AIN 2 or AIN 3. Using techniques adapted from those for evaluation of the cervix, including anal cytology and colposcopy-based high-resolution anoscopy (HRA), several investigators have described the prevalence and natural history of AIN. *Data on the prevalence and natural history of AIN in the general population are still relatively scarce.*

Among HIV-negative MSM, the prevalence of AIN based on anal cytology was between 18% and 23% across the age spectrum, from younger than 25 years to older than 55 years.[30] Like the prevalence of anal HPV infection in this population, the overall prevalence of AIN varied little with age. The prevalence of AIN 2,3 increased after the age of 40 although this increase was not statistically significant. Risk factors for prevalent AIN 1 included having more than five male receptive anal sex partners, use of poppers (alkyl nitrites) in the previous 6 months or use of injection drugs two or more times per month during the previous 6 months, older age at first receptive anal intercourse, and infection with a higher number of HPV types. *Risk factors for prevalent AIN 2,3 included having any anal HPV infection and infection with a higher number of HPV types.* Because anal cytology has limited sensitivity, this study likely underestimated the true prevalence of AIN. In a study of HIV-negative MSM in San Francisco, abnormal anal cytology was associated with anal HPV positivity and with the number of anal HPV types detected.[31] High-risk HIV-negative women are also at risk for AIN, with 8% having abnormal anal cytology.[32]

The prevalence of AIN among HIV-positive men and women is substantially higher than among their HIV-negative counterparts.[32,33] Consistent with the high prevalence of anal HPV infection in HIV-positive MSM, the prevalence of AIN was also very high in this population (36%).[34] In a more recent study, *AIN was found in 81% of HIV-positive MSM.*[35] Risk factors for AIN 2,3 included having anal HPV infection and being on HAART. Among HIV-positive women, the prevalence of abnormal anal cytology was 26%, with risk factors including anal HPV infection, lower CD4+ level, and higher HIV plasma viral load. After adjustment for anal HPV infection and CD4+ level, risk factors included history of anal intercourse and diarrhea for more than 1 month.[32] AIN is also common in HIV-positive men with no history of receptive anal intercourse,[26,36] and it is common among immunosuppressed individuals with renal transplant, with 20% having AIN in one study.[20]

The incidence of high-grade AIN is high in HIV-positive MSM,[27,33,37] with 49% developing high-grade AIN over a 4-year period in one study.[33] In *HIV-positive MSM, anal HPV infection and lower CD4+ cell count were the main risk factors associated with incident AIN.*[27,37]

Because a lower CD4+ level was shown to be an important risk factor for prevalent and incident AIN, it was hoped that HAART might exert a beneficial effect on AIN natural history. However, as described earlier, *HAART has not led to a reduction in the incidence of anal cancer or cervical cancer.*[17,18,38–40] Most of the data on the effect of HAART

on cancer precursors to date have been generated from studies of CIN in women. The impact of HAART on the natural history and treatment of CIN has been somewhat variable among the different studies. Overall, however, some studies have shown no effect, and the positive benefits of HAART shown in other studies have been only modest.[41] HAART has never been shown to result in clearance of cervical HPV infection, and to date there has not been a HAART-associated reduction in the incidence of cervical cancer.

Likewise, and consistent with the lack of reduction in the incidence of anal cancer associated with HAART, most data in men suggest that HAART has little beneficial effect on AIN (see Table 23-1).[36,42] Among HIV-positive MSM, a high prevalence of AIN 2,3 has been observed among men on HAART.[35] No studies have yet reported on the effect of HAART on the natural history of AIN in women.

In summary, *risk groups that have been shown to be at particularly high risk of AIN and anal cancer include HIV-negative MSM, HIV-positive MSM and women, HIV-negative women at high risk of HIV infection, and men and women iatrogenically immunosuppressed due to organ transplant.*

Given the relatively recent history of the study of AIN and anal cancer, several key questions remain to be answered. These include the following:

1. What are the molecular factors that drive progression of AIN 2,3 to invasive anal cancer?
2. Does treatment of AIN 2,3 prevent anal cancer?
3. What is the optimal treatment for AIN 2,3?
4. Does anal HPV infection modulate the biology of cervical HPV infection, CIN, and cervical cancer?
5. What is the natural history of AIN and anal cancer among healthy young women and men?
6. Will vaccination against HPV prevent anal HPV infection and, ultimately, AIN 2,3 and anal cancer?

ANAL CANCER SCREENING

Anal cancer and cervical cancer can be considered to be the same disease affecting different organs. The number of new anal cancer cases has been increasing for many years in the United States. The American Cancer Society estimates that in 2007 about 4650 new cases of anal cancer will be diagnosed and about 690 people will die of the disease (*www.cancer.org*). *The pathology of HPV-related disease of the anal canal mimics that seen in the cervix, both cytologically and histologically.* Because the Pap test has been such a successful tool in cervical cancer screening, it was logical to attempt to use anal cytology for anal cancer screening. Indeed, in populations at risk for anal cancer and its precursor lesions, including MSM and those with HIV disease, anal cytology is beginning to be used as a screening test in a manner analogous to the Pap test. Accumulating research supports screening for anal cancer in all men and women with HIV disease and in all MSM.[21,26,32–34]

Other populations potentially at risk for anal cancer that may benefit from anal cancer screening (Table 23-2)

Table 23-2 Candidates for Anal Cancer Screening

High-Risk Groups
Men and women with HIV
All MSM

Possible High-Risk Groups
Organ transplant patients
Patients on chronic steroid therapy
Patients with other causes of immunosuppression
Women with lower genital tract HPV-related disease, especially high-grade VIN
Men and women with perianal condyloma

HIV, Human immunodeficiency virus; *MSM,* men who have sex with men; *HPV,* human papillomavirus; *VIN,* vulvar intraepithelial neoplasia.

include those immunosuppressed on the basis of drug therapy for organ transplantation[19,20] or connective tissue diseases or cancer chemotherapy, any patient with perianal condyloma (regardless of sex or sexual orientation), and women with high-grade dysplasia of the lower genital tract,[43–45] especially high-grade vulvar disease.

Anal cytology has shown similar strengths and weaknesses as the Pap test—the most successful cancer screening test we currently have available. *The sensitivity and specificity of anal cytology are similar to conventional cervical cytology.*[46–48] Liquid-based cytology also improves sample quality of an anal specimen.[49,50] Interobserver variability among pathologists is similar in the interpretation and diagnosis of anal cytology and biopsy samples.[51] Anal cytology has been shown to be cost-effective as a screening test for anal cancer in the at-risk populations of both HIV-positive and HIV-negative MSM.[52,53]

ANAL CYTOLOGY

Sample Collection and Preparation

Collection of a cytologic sample from the anal canal is a relatively simple procedure. Patients should be instructed not to use an enema or insert anything per rectum 24 hours prior to collection of an anal cytology specimen. Ideally, they should avoid receptive anal intercourse during this time as well. Typically, the sample is collected with the patient in either the left lateral recumbent (knee-chest) or dorsal lithotomy position. *The specimen is collected without direct visualization of the anal canal; an anoscope is not needed. The sample itself is collected using a tap water–moistened, synthetic-fiber (e.g., Dacron) swab.* A cytobrush may be used, but many patients find it uncomfortable, and an adequate sample can be obtained using the Dacron swab. Lubrication should not be used, as the lubricant may interfere with the processing and interpretation of the sample. To collect a sample for anal cytology, first gently separate the buttocks. If in the lateral knee-chest position, the patient may retract the upper cheek to facilitate the view of the anal verge. From the external anal opening or anal verge, the swab should be inserted into the anal canal until it reaches the distal rectal vault. One feels slight resistance as the swab passes the anal sphincters, where the walls of the anal canal are opposed at rest. Care should be taken to insert the sampling device with gentle pressure but not force. If significant resistance or patient discomfort is encountered, remove the swab and reinsert it in a different angle or position. Reinsertion of the swab with a slight posterior orientation may be helpful. A slight decrease in resistance can be appreciated as the swab tip enters the rectal vault, then resistance is again felt as the swab gently abuts the distal rectal wall. Depending on how far the patient's buttocks are held apart (and the anal verge is exposed), the "distance" that the swab is inserted varies; it can be as much as 2 to 2.5 inches or 5 to 6 cm. Once the swab is past the sphincter, the patient should be asked to release the hold on the buttocks. The collecting swab is slowly rotated circumferentially, while firm pressure is applied against the lateral walls of the anal canal, as it is slowly withdrawn from the anal canal in a spiral motion (Figure 23-1 *A, B). The goal of anal cytology is to sample the entire anal canal from the distal rectal vault to the anal verge. At rest, the mucosa in this region is opposed.*

The cellular sample is then transferred from the collecting device to a vial that contains liquid preservative for liquid-based cytology (e.g., SurePath, ThinPrep) or smeared directly on a glass slide and fixed for conventional cytology. In general, *liquid-based preparation are preferred; liquid samples increase cell yield and reduce compromising factors such as obscuring fecal material, air-drying, and mechanical artifacts, all of which are relatively common on direct smears.*[49,50] Patients can also be trained to successfully collect their own samples for liquid-based cytology.[54,55]

Terminology in Anal Cytology: The Bethesda System

The Bethesda 2001 conference was instrumental in increasing awareness of anal cytology as a cancer screening test.[56] According to the Bethesda 2001 guidelines, anal cytology should be reported in a manner similar to gynecologic cytology although modified as needed for the anus. *The Bethesda guidelines recommend using the same terminology for anal cytology as is used for cervical cytology: atypical squamous cells of undetermined significance (ASC-US), atypical squamous cells: cannot exclude high-grade squamous intraepithelial lesion (ASC-H), low-grade squamous intraepithelial lesion (LSIL), high-grade squamous intraepithelial lesion (HSIL), and so on.* The presence or absence of anal transformation zone (TZ) components (squamous metaplastic cells, rectal columnar cells, or both) should be indicated on the report. Criteria are similar to those for cervical Pap.

Specimen Adequacy and Normal Components

According to the Bethesda guidelines,[56] a minimum of 2000 to 3000 nucleated squamous cells are needed for conventional smears. For liquid-based anal samples, this is equivalent to 1 to 2 nucleated squamous cells per high-power field (hpf) for ThinPrep (with a diameter of

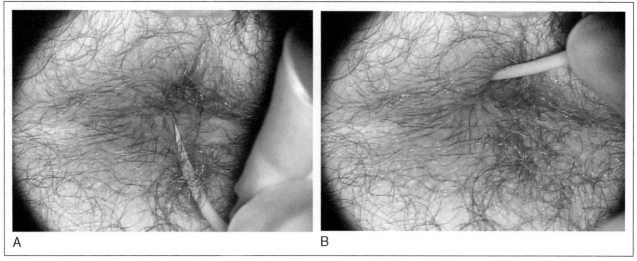

Figure 23-1 A, B, The Dacron swab should bend slightly to assure that adequate pressure is being used.

20 mm) and 3 to 6 nucleated squamous cells/hpf for Sure-Path (with a diameter of 13 mm). Others have suggested more stringent cellularity guidelines of at least 6 nucleated squamous cells/hpf for an adequate anal cytology sample.[47] Although specimen cellularity varies and is typically somewhat less than on a cervical cytology, the cellularity of a well-collected anal sample can equal that of cervical cytology.

The normal cellular components seen on anal cytology include rectal columnar cells from the distal rectum, squamous metaplastic cells from the anal TZ, nonkeratinized squamous cells (both intermediate and superficial types), and anucleated squames from the keratinized portion of the distal anal canal (Figures 23-2 to 23-4). Reactive and reparative changes are not seen as frequently on anal cytology as on cervical Pap tests; on anal cytology, these changes often accompany infectious agents such as herpes virus infection.

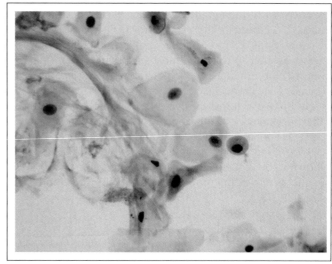

Figure 23-3 Normal components of an anal cytology: nucleated squamous cells and squamous metaplastic cells.

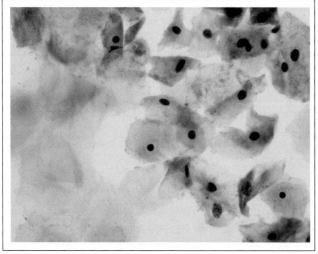

Figure 23-2 Normal components of an anal cytology: anucleated squames and nucleated squamous cells.

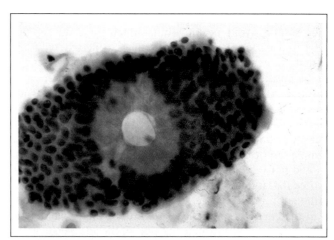

Figure 23-4 Rectal columnar cells on anal cytology.

Organisms

A number of different organisms can be seen on anal cytology. Some of these are similar to those encountered on gynecologic cytology (e.g., herpes simplex virus, *Candida* species) (Figures 23-5 and 23-6) and may cause local disease within the anal canal. Other organisms are unique to anal samples and may be localized to the anal canal (e.g., pinworm) or simply traveling through the anal canal from more proximal sites (e.g., ameba) (Figures 23-7 and 23-8). Clinical correlation and additional studies (e.g., stool for ova and parasites) may be needed to determine whether the organisms are pathogenic or nonpathogenic species.

Epithelial Cell Abnormalities

On anal cytology, the spectrum of HPV-related squamous abnormalities mirrors that seen on gynecologic cytology. Diagnostic criteria are similar. However, degenerative changes and low-grade and high-grade lesions with cytoplasmic keratinization are more commonly encountered on anal cytology.

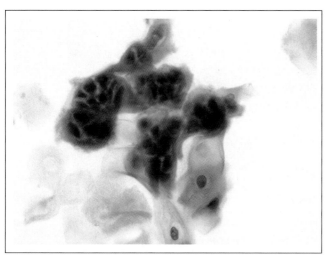

Figure 23-5 Herpes simplex virus infection, anal cytology.

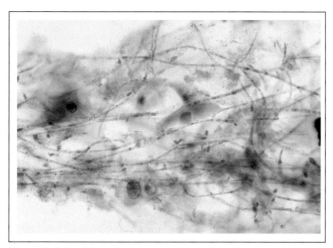

Figure 23-6 *Candida,* anal cytology.

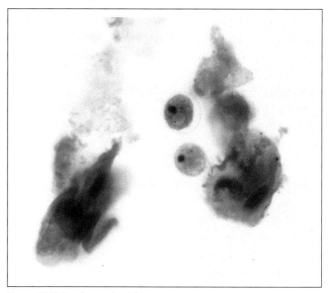

Figure 23-7 Ameba, anal cytology.

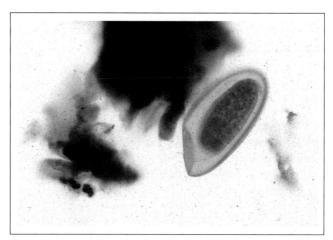

Figure 23-8 Pinworm eggs, anal cytology.

LSIL is characterized by abnormal nuclei in mature superficial or intermediate-type squamous cells. These cells have enlarged nuclei with hyperchromasia and nuclear contour or chromatin irregularities. The cytoplasm is abundant and may display HPV-related cytopathic effect or koilocytosis. When the cells have abundant cytoplasmic keratin, this perinuclear halo, characteristic of HPV infection, may not be distinct. Degenerative changes with nuclear karyorrhexis and empty cytoplasmic halos may be seen (Figures 23-9 to 23-11).

In HSIL the dysplastic cells are seen singly or in small cell clusters. The abnormal nuclei are seen in parabasal-type cells with scant cytoplasm. Often, dense metaplastic cytoplasm surrounds the dysplastic nuclei, signaling their origin from the immature squamous metaplasia at the leading edge of the anal TZ. *A pattern of relatively small dysplastic nuclei within a squamous metaplastic cell is common on anal cytology. Mixtures of both LSIL and HSIL in the same sample are commonly seen on anal cytology* (Figures 23-12 to 23-14).

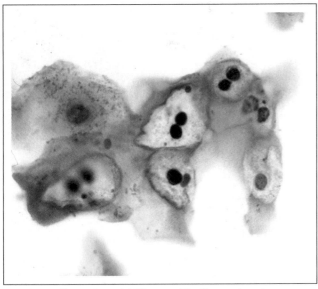

Figure 23-9 Classic LSIL with HPV cytopathic effect, anal cytology.

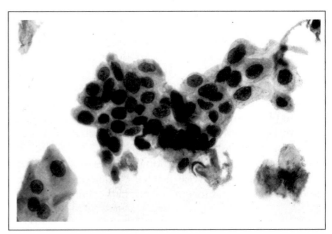

Figure 23-12 HSIL, anal cytology.

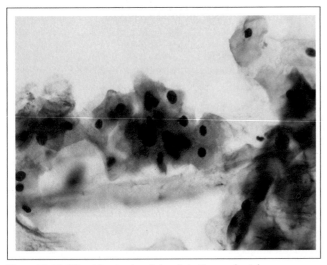

Figure 23-10 LSIL with cytoplasmic keratinization, anal cytology.

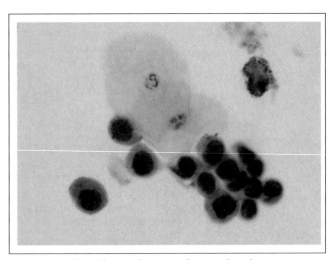

Figure 23-13 HSIL with metaplastic cytoplasm, anal cytology.

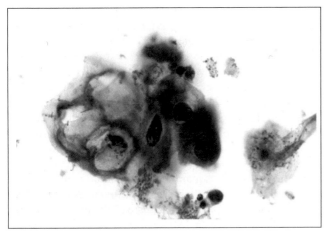

Figure 23-11 LSIL with degenerative changes, anal cytology.

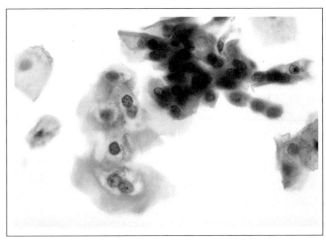

Figure 23-14 HSIL and LSIL seen together on anal cytology.

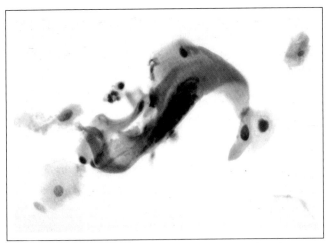

Figure 23-15 Keratinized squamous cell carcinoma on anal cytology.

Atypical squamous cells that lack (either quantitatively or qualitatively) sufficient changes to warrant an interpretation of SIL can be seen on anal cytology; this is similar to the cervical Pap test. In the spectrum of HPV-related disease, ASC-US is the cytologic interpretation when the atypical cells are suspicious but not diagnostic of LSIL; in ASC-H, the atypical cells are suspicious but not diagnostic of HSIL.

In general, *anal cytology tends to undercall the grade of lesion ultimately diagnosed on HRA with biopsy.*[47,57] Clinically significant *overcalls* are unusual.[58] An interpretation of ASC-US or above on anal cytology has a high predictive value for the detection of anal dysplasia on subsequent biopsies.[46,58] Cytologic *undercalls* may be secondary to incomplete sampling of the lesion(s) present. Because both low-grade and high-grade lesions are frequently present in the same patient, the low-grade lesion may be sampled or more readily recognized cytologically than its high-grade counterpart. Indeed, although squamous cell carcinoma of the anal canal is being seen with increasing frequency in the at-risk populations, the prospective diagnosis of squamous cell carcinoma on anal cytology is infrequent. When this interpretation is made, malignant squamous cells, similar to those seen on cervical cytology, can be seen (Figure 23-15). Cytologic clues for invasion such as tumor diathesis are not readily appreciated on samples from the anal canal.[59]

There is no known HPV-related glandular disease of the rectum, the counterpart of endocervical adenocarcinoma *in situ* (AIS) *and adenocarcinoma.* Colorectal polyps and adenocarcinomas can be seen in the populations at risk for squamous cell carcinoma of the anus; however, these lesions are rarely encountered on anal cytology.

HUMAN PAPILLOMAVIRUS TESTING

The populations that can potentially benefit from anal cancer screening are also those with a high baseline prevalence of anal HPV infection, especially high-risk HPV types.[31,48] Some researchers believe that this may limit the utility of *reflex* HPV DNA testing in these populations and advocate that all patients with ASC-US and higher on anal cytology

be triaged to HRA. Others, however, have found that *the high negative predictive value of HPV DNA testing may be useful in the triage of the patient with ASC-US on anal cytology.*[58,60]

HISTOPATHOLOGY OF HUMAN PAPILLOMAVIRUS–RELATED ANAL DISEASE

The histologic classification of anal dysplasia again mimics that used for cervical disease. Morphologically the lesions are essentially identical. Pathologists may use a variety of equivalent terms in the diagnosis of HPV-related lesions of the anogenital tract: the various grades of dysplasia (mild, moderate, severe dysplasia, and carcinoma *in situ*); *AIN 1, 2, and 3* (akin to CIN 1, 2, and 3); or low-grade and high-grade AIN or SIL.

Although the SIL classification system was originally proposed (in the Bethesda system) as a cytologic classification system for gynecologic cytology, many pathologists now use this terminology in the histologic diagnosis of all HPV-related anogenital disease. The context usually determines whether these terms are applied to the cytologic interpretation or a histologic diagnosis.

Anal Transformation Zone

Just as in the cervical TZ, there is a region of squamous metaplasia in the anal canal that comprises the anal transformation zone (AnTZ) (Figure 23-16). The columnar or cuboidal epithelium of the rectum extends distally into the upper portion of the surgical anal canal (whose proximal extent is the top of the internal anal sphincter—the mucosa of the entire surgical anal canal is opposed at rest). Here, above the level of the dentate or pectinate line, an irregular transition from glandular to squamous mucosa begins. Metaplastic squamous epithelium can be seen overlying rectal columnar glands. It often appears as a squamocuboidal type of epithelium and is sometimes referred to as the *transitional epithelium of the anal mucosa.* This blends into the stratified squamous epithelium that covers the rectal columns and sinuses above the dentate line. Below the dentate line, the stratified squamous mucosa is nonkeratinized and lacks underlying mucous glands or skin appendages; it is firmly attached to the underlying muscular and fibrous tissue of the external anal sphincter (the anatomic anal canal). At about the level of the anal verge, the surface of the epithelium becomes keratinized. Skin appendages, such as hair follicles and sebaceous glands, appear in the perianal skin.[61]

The histologic appearance of low-grade and high-grade AIN is identical to cervical disease. Specific diagnostic criteria will not be reviewed here; it is sufficient to state that the same morphologic criteria are used for grading HPV-related disease from any anogenital site. Low-grade AIN can be flat or have warty contour changes, such as micropapillary or condylomatous. It can be either nonkeratinized or keratinized; the warty lesions are frequently keratinized (Figures 23-17 to 23-19). The abnormal nuclei, characteristic of HPV-related dysplasia, are seen in *mature* squamous epithelium, with abundant cytoplasm. High-grade AIN of

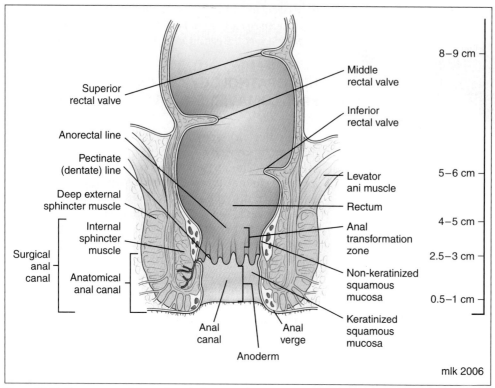

Figure 23-16 The anatomy of the anal canal. (Courtesy of Marya Krogstad.)

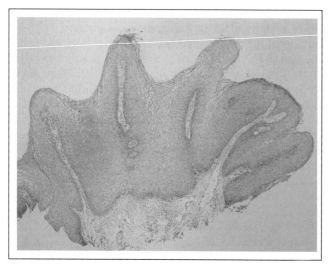

Figure 23-17 Low-grade AIN, warty.

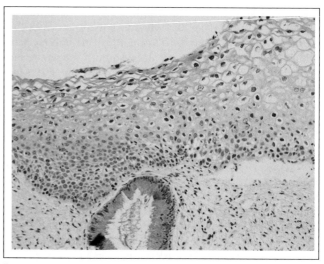

Figure 23-18 Low-grade AIN, flat.

the anal canal tends to be flat lesions and is frequently found in the region of squamous metaplasia; rectal-type glands are found underlying the dysplastic squamous epithelium (Figures 23-20 to 23-21). The dysplastic nuclei are seen in *immature* squamous cells with little or no cytoplasmic maturation (hence, high nucleus:cytoplasmic ratios) over the full thickness of the epithelium.

Invasion is present when the neoplastic squamous cells breach the basement membrane and invade the underlying fibroconnective stroma. *There is no counterpart in the anal canal to microinvasive squamous cell carcinoma of the cervix, with its well-defined clinical prognostic features; rather, early invasion is typically*

termed superficially invasive squamous cell carcinoma (Figure 23-22). Frankly invasive squamous cell carcinomas of the anal canal can have a variety of histologic patterns, particularly keratinized or nonkeratinized cancers (Figure 23-23).

HIGH-RESOLUTION ANOSCOPY

The goal of HRA is to systematically visualize the entire anal canal and perianal skin to determine the presence or absence of HPV-associated disease and, if indicated, to select areas for biopsy—the gold standard for diagnosis.

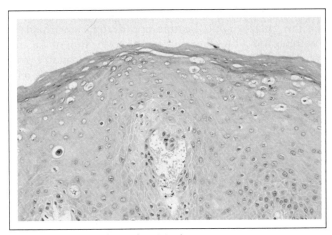

Figure 23-19 Low-grade AIN, keratinized.

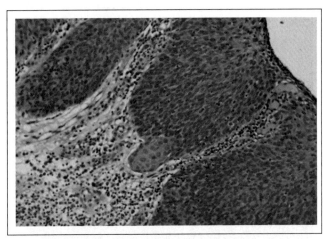

Figure 23-22 Superficially invasive squamous cell carcinoma of anus.

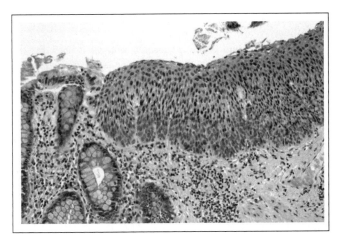

Figure 23-20 High-grade AIN at SCJ.

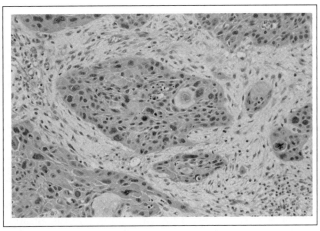

Figure 23-23 Invasive squamous cell carcinoma of anus.

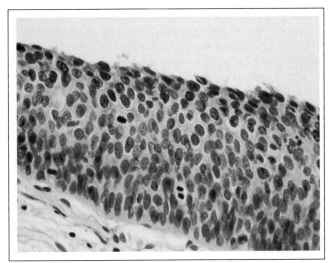

Figure 23-21 High-grade AIN, high power.

Much of the equipment for HRA is similar to that used for cervical colposcopy, with the following differences: metal or disposable plastic anoscopes, 3% acetic acid for the internal exam (although 5% can be used for the perianal exam), and small biopsy forceps. Anal biopsies are typically smaller than cervical biopsies to minimize bleeding, and so *the preferred forceps are baby Tischlers, flexible endoscopy, and nose or ear forceps* (Figure 23-24). The flexible endoscopy forceps affords the smallest biopsies and minimizes bleeding but requires an assistant to hold the anoscope while the clinician manipulates the forceps.

Clean technique is more difficult to maintain with HRA than with cervical colposcopy because the clinician must hold the anoscope during the entire exam. Wrapping parts of the colposcope that are touched during the exam (e.g., the colposcope's magnification dials, fine focus knobs, eyepieces) with plastic wrap will help keep the colposcope clean. An experienced clinician can complete a careful and complete HRA exam, including biopsies, in approximately 10 to 20 minutes. Exams requiring biopsies of both internal anal mucosa and the perianal areas typically take 30 to 40 minutes to complete. Additional time may be needed for patient counseling, especially for an initial visit.

HRA can be performed in several positions including left or right lateral, dorsal lithotomy, or prone positions. Most patients prefer the left lateral position; this includes women who may have just completed a cervical exam in the dorsal

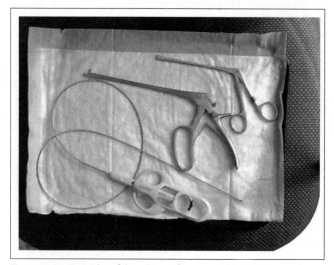

Figure 23-24 Examples of three biopsy forceps used for HRA. Pictured are a flexible endoscopy forceps, baby Tischler, and nasal forceps.

lithotomy position. *It is very important to be clear and consistent when describing the location of lesions and the position used. The* anal clock *is different than the* gynecologic clock (Figure 23-25). In the prone position, posterior is 12 o'clock, whereas in the dorsal lithotomy position, anterior is 12 o'clock. Because treatment referrals may be to colorectal surgeons, describing lesion locations both anatomically as well as with the *clock* for shorthand will minimize errors.

After the collection of the anal cytology and before the HRA, a thorough digital rectal exam (DRE) should be performed by inserting a finger liberally lubricated with a mixture of K-Y jelly and 2% to 5% lidocaine gel. Care should be taken to palpate for warts, masses, scar tissue, ulcerations, fissures, or areas of thickening or induration. Attention should be paid to focal areas of discomfort or pain. The visual exam can then be correlated with these areas. Areas that are hard, firm, indurated, or immobile may be suspicious for cancer, whereas a typical wart may be palpated but will usually be soft and mobile.

After the DRE, the anoscope is inserted using additional lubrication. The anoscope's obturator is removed, and a cotton-tipped applicator wrapped in gauze that has been soaked

in 3% acetic acid is inserted. The anoscope is removed, leaving the gauze-wrapped, cotton-tipped applicator in place. The vinegar is allowed to saturate the epithelium of the anal canal for 1 to 2 minutes. After soaking, the cotton-tipped applicator and gauze are removed and the anoscope is reinserted. The visualization aspect of the HRA can now begin.

The anal canal is observed through the colposcope while the anoscope is slowly removed. When fully inserted, the end of the anoscope will be partially into the distal rectum in most patients. The anoscope is then slowly withdrawn until the anal squamocolumnar junction (SCJ) and AnTZ comes into focus. To maintain focus, the colposcope has to be continually repositioned slightly while the anoscope is moved or withdrawn. The length of the anal canal differs widely (e.g., 1–5 cm). In some patients, the SCJ (indicating the proximal end of the anal canal) will immediately be viewed; in others (especially in women), the anal canal is quite short and the SCJ may not be seen until the anoscope is withdrawn nearly to the verge.

Once the SCJ and AnTZ are located, vinegar is reapplied frequently, using proctoswabs or cotton-tipped applicators, throughout the exam. To visualize all aspects of the AnTZ, it is necessary to manipulate the anoscope or use cotton-tipped applicators to view areas hidden by mucosal folds, normal anal papillae, hemorrhoids, or prolapsed mucosa. These structures can make an adequate HRA exam, in which the entire TZ has been visualized, challenging. However, with careful manipulation of the mucosa, it is rare for an anal HRA to be unsatisfactory.

After the AnTZ has been thoroughly examined, the anoscope is slowly withdrawn while the rest of the anal canal is observed. Although most high-grade AIN is found at the AnTZ, it is common to find skipped or off-transformation zone (OTZ) lesions especially in patients whose AnTZ may have been partially ablated or altered by prior treatments. Low-grade AIN, primarily condyloma acuminata, may be found anywhere in the anal canal. The anal margin will appear toward the end of the HRA and can also be viewed through the anoscope or by gently separating the buttocks. The anal margin begins at the verge and represents the transition from mucosal to epidermal epithelium and extends to the perianal skin. By consensus, the region designated *perianal skin* is considered to extend approximately 5 cm from the anal margin (Figure 23-26). *A complete HRA includes evaluation of the entire anal canal including the AnTZ and the perianal skin.*

Anal Biopsies

Biopsies are directed at the lesions thought to represent the highest-grade abnormality by colposcopic impression. Anal biopsies are usually smaller than those typically taken from the cervix, using forceps with bites no larger than 2 to 3 mm. Internal anal biopsies do not require anesthesia. External anal biopsies require local anesthesia, similar to vulvar biopsies (e.g., 1–2% lidocaine preceded by lidocaine gel or spray). Monsel's solution or silver nitrate may be used for homeostasis, although the pressure of the anal walls, which are opposed at rest, will usually stop all bleeding for internal anal biopsies. Patients

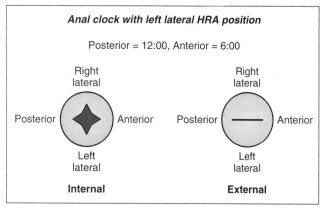

Figure 23-25 The anal HRA "clock" in the left lateral recumbent position.

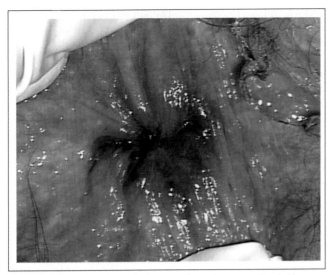

Figure 23-26 View of the anal margin and transition to perianal skin.

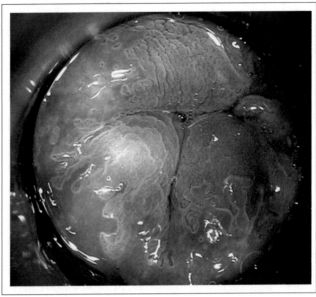

Figure 23-28 The AnTZ is seen here as an acetowhite, thin line at the current SCJ. Acetowhite ringed gland openings can be seen on the upper left.

are advised to expect slight bleeding with bowel movements for several days following an internal anal biopsy. Complications such as infection or problematic bleeding are extremely rare. Patients are also advised to avoid receptive anal intercourse for as long as 2 weeks following biopsy.

Recognition of the Anal Squamocolumnar Junction and Anal Transformation Zone

The anal SCJ may be more subtle and difficult to locate than on the cervix. It is rarely viewed in its entirety without manipulation of the anoscope, anal mucosa, or both. Repeated application of 3% acetic acid helps distinguish anal squamous epithelium from rectal columnar epithelium. The squamous epithelium will appear lighter or pinker in color, whereas columnar epithelium is darker and redder in color (Figure 23-27). The SCJ is the area

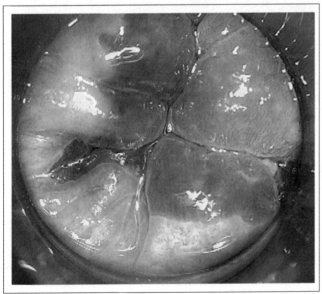

Figure 23-27 View of normal anal and rectal epithelium. The SCJ is where the white- or pink- appearing epithelium of the anus (squamous) joins the redder epithelium of the rectum (columnar).

where the fully mature anal squamous epithelium is adjacent to the columnar epithelium of the colon. Although more difficult to visualize compared with the cervix, an original anal SCJ and a current SCJ exist. The current SCJ is easier to appreciate and can be seen easily in Figure 23-27. The AnTZ represents the area that is undergoing dynamic squamous metaplastic changes (Figure 23-28).

Features of the Normal Anal Transformation Zone

Like the cervix, the AnTZ has distinguishing features such as squamous metaplasia and gland openings that help determine its location. Because dysplasia often occurs in areas undergoing squamous metaplasia, identification of features indicating metaplasia helps to locate potential abnormal epithelium. *Most high-grade AIN will be located in or near the TZ; recognition of the AnTZ enables the clinician to better locate these abnormalities.*

Anal squamous metaplasia is a normal process of change during which the stratified squamous epithelium covers the simple columnar epithelium of the distal rectum. The mechanism for metaplasia in the anus has not been identified although it is assumed that trauma to the anal epithelium plays a role. Metaplasia can be seen in different stages including early, mid, and late (Figure 23-29). In early metaplasia, the coalescing and clustering of columnar epithelium is just beginning. In mid metaplasia, the coalescing is more pronounced and may appear faintly acetowhite. The coalescing is nearly complete in late squamous metaplasia; these areas may mimic lesions in appearance. The grapelike clustering of the coalescing columnar epithelium of the cervical TZ is not as pronounced in the AnTZ.

Gland openings and islands of columnar epithelium within fully mature squamous epithelium are normal findings that occur during the metaplastic process in the AnTZ. These areas were skipped during the process of squamous

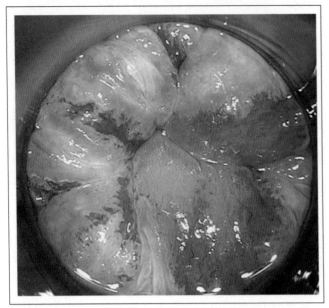

Figure 23-29 Active squamous metaplasia in all three stages.

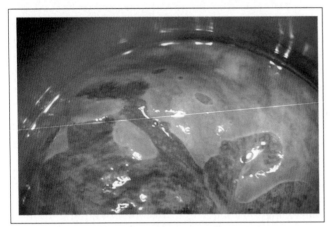

Figure 23-30 Acetowhite gland openings and islands of columnar epithelium surrounded by fully mature squamous epithelium indicating an area that has undergone metaplasia.

metaplasia; they help identify where the original SCJ was and where metaplasia has occurred (Figure 23-30).

Atypical Anal Transformation Zone

Similar to cervical colposcopy, common epithelial and vascular changes are found in the atypical or abnormal anal TZ. Most are only visible with the use of colposcopic magnification and illumination and with application of 3% acetic acid, Lugol's solution, or both. Unlike cervical colposcopy, little has been published describing specific colposcopic features of AIN, with the exception of the article by Jay.[62] Acetowhite epithelium is identified after the application of 3% acetic acid; acetowhitening is a transient change in the squamous epithelium that can be associated with areas of low or high-grade AIN, or normal squamous metaplasia. Repeated application of 3% acetic acid is needed to visualize some lesions. *When a patient is referred with an*

abnormal anal cytology, it is important to reapply the 3% acetic acid even after soaking for several minutes if a lesion does not appear immediately (Figures 23-31 to 23-34).

Lesion characteristics used to describe cervical lesions have been validated for anal disease.[62] The findings are similar to cervical colposcopy, but some differences have been noted and will be described below. *To maintain consistency between the disciplines, cervical colposcopic descriptors and terminology have been adapted for anal lesions. Lesions are evaluated for their acetowhitening, margins, vascular changes, surface contour, and Lugol's staining for the following characteristics:*

1. Acetowhitening: *Lesions may have distinct or very minor, barely visible coloring* (Figures 23-35 and 23-36).
   - Evaluate for color: snowy white, oyster white, or gray.
   - Evaluate for faint versus distinct color.
2. Borders/margins: *The border adjacent to the rectum is frequently indistinct, and the lesion's edge may be blurred and difficult to distinguish from the rectal mucosa.* Figures 23-37 and 23-38 illustrate different margin patterns.
   - Evaluate for distinct versus indistinct margins.
   - Evaluate for distinctly different lesions within lesions.

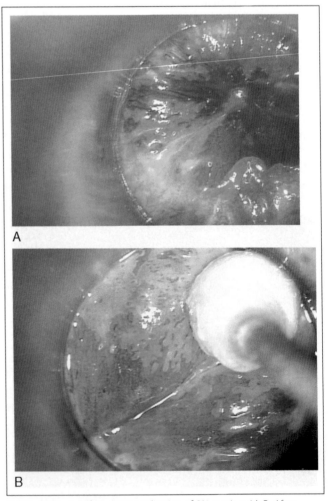

Figure 23-31 A, Before direct application of 3% acetic acid. B, After application of 3% acetic acid using a cotton-tipped swab to apply it directly to the anal epithelium.

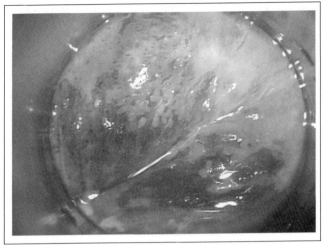

Figure 23-32 View of lesion depicted in Figure 23-31, *B*. Lesion is acetowhite with atypical-appearing squamous metaplasia. Histology revealed AIN 2,3.

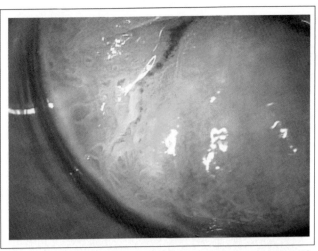

Figure 23-34 Magnified view of Figure 23-33, *B*. Lesion is acetowhite with epithelial honeycombing. Biopsy revealed AIN 3.

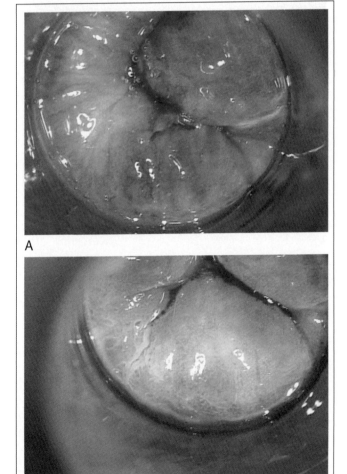

A

B

Figure 23-33 A, Before direct application of 3% acetic acid. **B**, After application of 3% acetic acid using a cotton-tipped swab to apply it directly to the anal epithelium.

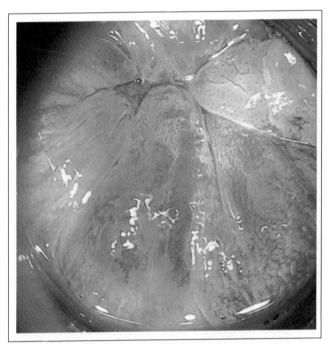

Figure 23-35 Indistinct acetowhitening seen in an example of high-grade AIN (AIN 3).

3. Vascular pattern: *Punctation and mosaic patterns are similar to the cervix but are usually coarse and rarely fine.* Striated vessels are elongated patterns of vessels that can be especially common in patients who have previously had fulgarative procedures. *Atypical vessels may be thickly dilated and nonbranching with bizarre shapes; they can be seen with both HSIL and anal cancer.* Warty vessels are looped and are often found in conjunction with warty papillae.

- Punctation (Figure 23-39)
- Mosaic pattern (Figure 23-40)
- Striated vessels (Figure 23-41)
- Atypical or abnormal vessels (Figure 23-42)
- Warty vessels (Figure 23-43)

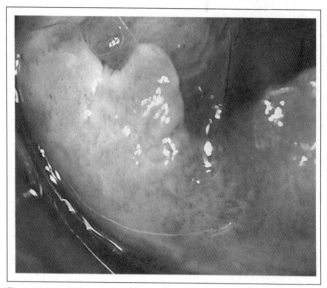

Figure 23-36 Distinct acetowhitening seen in an example of low-grade AIN.

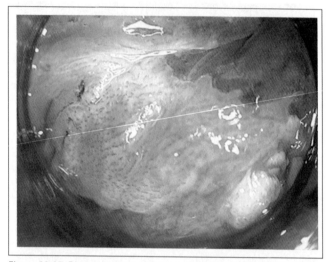

Figure 23-37 Distinct margins seen in an example of high-grade AIN (AIN 2).

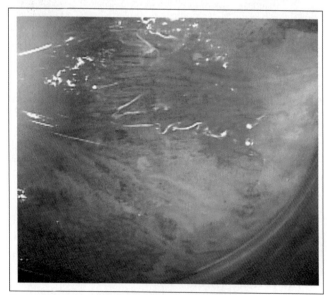

Figure 23-38 Indistinct margins seen in an example of high-grade AIN.

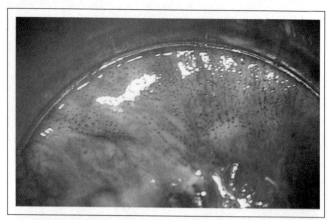

Figure 23-39 Vascular punctation.

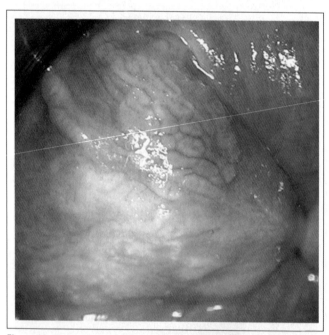

Figure 23-40 Mosaic pattern.

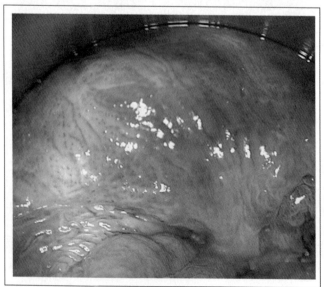

Figure 23-41 Striated vessel pattern.

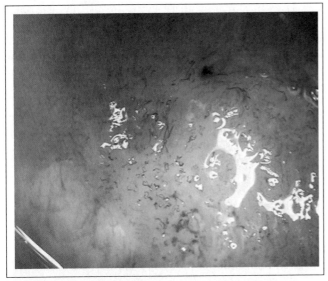

Figure 23-42 Atypical or abnormal vessels.

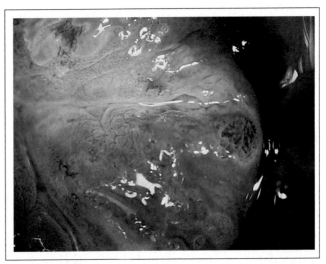

Figure 23-44 Lesion with flat contour.

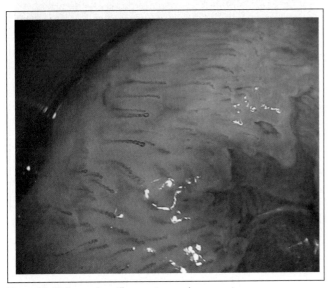

Figure 23-43 Looped capillary warty vessels.

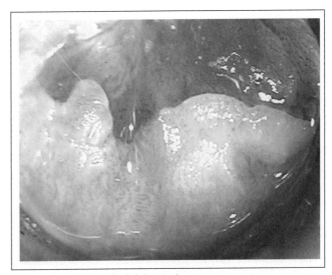

Figure 23-45 Lesion with slightly raised contour.

4. Contour: *Lesions can be flat, slightly raised (thickening of the epithelium) with associated granularity or micropapillae, or raised. Raised lesions are often associated with other warty features such as papillae and warty vessels.*
   - Flat (Figure 23-44)
   - Slightly raised (Figure 23-45)
   - Raised (verrucous) (Figure 23-46)
5. Lugol's staining: *Staining patterns are similar to the cervix. Normal epithelium will have a dark, mahogany color, as will many warts. Negative staining is not specific for high-grade AIN, but most high-grade AIN will be Lugol's negative. The utility of Lugol's staining has not been published for anal lesions, but it may help in certain situations. When HSIL is found on cytology and only warts are seen on HRA,*

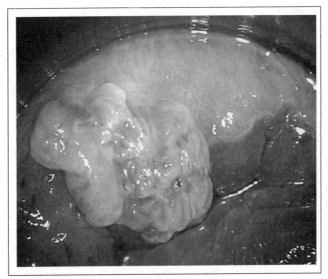

Figure 23-46 Lesion with raised contour.

Lugol's-negative areas within the warts may be high-grade AIN; this may help guide the choice of areas to biopsy. Lugol's staining also may help determine the margins of a lesion for treatment (Figures 23-47 and 23-48).

- Complete (mahogany, normal uptake)
- Partial (mixture of mahogany and non-stain)
- Negative (non-stain, yellow)

Typical Lesion Patterns

The classical features of low- and high-grade AIN and cancer on HRA are summarized in Table 23-3. Here, LSIL includes AIN 1 or mild dysplasia and condyloma. HSIL includes AIN 2 or moderate dysplasia, as well as AIN 3 encompassing severe dysplasia and carcinoma *in situ*.

Low-grade lesions can be flat or raised; smooth, micropapillary, granular, or papillary; and faintly acetowhite or distinct snowy white. Vascular changes, if present, are usually punctation, but occasionally mosaic patterns are seen. Warty vessels with *hairpin* capillary loops are usually associated with low-grade AIN. The Lugol's staining can be positive or complete (dark mahogany brown in color), partial (mottled or tortoiseshell), or negative (yellow). In other words, *several different presentations of low-grade lesions can be encountered on HRA.* A typical *warty* low-grade AIN may be acetowhite, raised, and papillary with warty vessels and may stain Lugol's partial or positive. A typical flat low-grade AIN may be acetowhite with punctation and may stain Lugol's negative or partial. Slightly raised, granular, low-grade AIN may also occur. An indistinct area with micropapillary changes and Lugol's partial staining is often low-grade AIN; it may also represent atypical changes or areas where older warts have resolved or been treated (Figures 23-49 to 23-53).

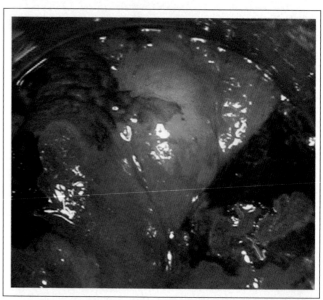

Figure 23-48 Same lesion as in Figure 23-47 with Lugol's solution applied. Note the more distinct and larger lesion margins as compared with that seen with vinegar on Figure 23-47.

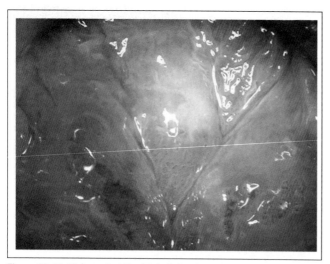

Figure 23-47 High-grade AIN with indistinct margins.

Table 23-3 Classical Features of Anal Intraepithelial Neoplasia and Cancer on High-Resolution Anoscopy

Classical Features of Low-Grade AIN				
DRE	**Surface Changes**	**Epithelial Changes**	**Vascular Changes**	**Lugol's Staining**
Granular, gritty, soft, warty nodularity	Flat or raised	Papillae or micropapillae	None, fine or coarse punctation, warty vessels	Negative, partial, or complete
Classical Features of High-Grade AIN				
Nonpalpable or subtle thickening	Flat or slightly raised	Smooth or honeycombing	Coarse punctation, mosaic	Negative
Classical Features of Cancer				
Firm mass, indurated or distinct thickening	Raised, ulcerated, occasionally flat	Peeling or denuding, heaping edges	Atypical, large, nonbranching vessels	Negative

AIN, Anal intraepithelial neoplasia; *DRE,* digital rectal examination.

High-grade lesions are usually acetowhite and flat with coarse punctation and mosaic patterns; they typically stain negative with Lugol's iodine solution (Figures 23-54 to 23-61). Areas of thickened acetowhitening are more often high-grade AIN than low-grade disease. Coarse punctation, mosaic patterns, or both are common with high-grade lesions. In AIN 3 lesions, there may be shallow ulcerations and friability of the epithelium. The Lugol's staining is usually negative. Negative Lugol's iodine staining indicates the absence of glycogen; the epithelium stains yellow. Normal rectal columnar epithelium does not contain glycogen and turns yellow when iodine is applied; it is important to directly observe where the iodine is applied and remember where the SCJ is located because lesions at both the SCJ and columnar epithelium will turn yellow with iodine (Figures 23-62 to 23-65). *Approximately 10% of lesions with a typical warty appearance will prove to be HSIL on biopsy.*[62,63] This underscores the importance of obtaining biopsies of lesions with different patterns,

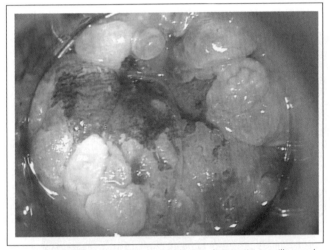

Figure 23-49 Diffuse acetowhitening with granularity, micropapillae, and warty vessels with flat and raised areas. Biopsy of a raised cerebriform area on the right revealed condyloma.

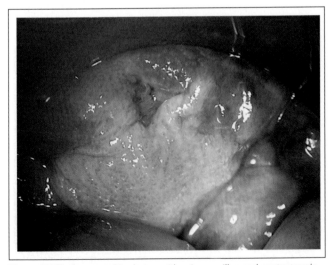

Figure 23-50 An acetowhite lesion with micropapillae and warty vessels. Biopsy of the ulcer revealed AIN 1.

especially when high-grade AIN is suspected due to a patient's cytologic findings or other history.

Signs of cancer on HRA include abnormal or atypical vessels, ulceration, and denuding or peeling of the epithelium. These areas should be biopsied to exclude invasion (Figures 23-66 to 23-70). Although the colposcopic or HRA impression is important, the diagnosis is established by biopsy of the most abnormal-appearing area or areas. In some cases, reactive squamous metaplasia or low-grade AIN may have colposcopic features suggestive of high-grade AIN (see Figures 23-64, 23-65, and 23-71). Probably more commonly than on the cervix, *atypical appearing squamous metaplasia seen at the SCJ is more likely to be a high-grade lesion; it is often AIN 3* (see Figures 23-58 to 23-59).

Other Findings on High-Resolution Anoscopy

Other findings, both normal and abnormal, can be recognized on HRA; they may be unrelated to HPV infection. Anal crypts are small glandular cavities. It is common to see acetowhite epithelium in crypts. These may contain AIN and should be biopsied to exclude disease; however, they often contain just squamous metaplastic tissue. *Anal tags* are normal redundant tissue secondary to resolved hemorrhoids or surgery. However, they can become irritated and inflamed with frequent bowel movements, and fissures may be seen at their base. *Anal warts* can sometimes be confused with these tags and may also develop in their tips. *Anal fissures* are small linear tears that can be recurrent, chronic, and very painful.

Hemorrhoids are common and must be differentiated from lesions. Most hemorrhoids will be soft, whereas a true lesion such as cancer may be hard, granular, or indurated. Hemorrhoids may also be painful. Figure 23-72 shows anal tags adjacent to a hemorrhoid. The acetowhite epithelium on the lesion highlights this as a lesion compared with the tag, but otherwise they can be similar in appearance. *Fistula tracts* may be caused by an abscess; the resulting cavity may be seen as a hole.

Anal ulcerations are sometimes associated with HPV infection, including the entire spectrum of HPV disease: low-grade AIN, high-grade AIN, and invasive carcinoma. Ulcerations should always be biopsied, especially nonhealing ulcers, which can be worrisome for cancer. Recurrent ulcerations and fissures may be herpetic or may simply represent areas that are difficult to heal following a surgical procedure and do not necessarily represent HPV-related disease. Patients may develop ulcerations following surgery for warts and high-grade AIN. *Biopsies of these areas will determine whether AIN has recurred.* Figure 23-73 shows a shallow ulceration in a high-grade AIN; Figure 23-74 is an ulcer associated with low-grade AIN.

Scar tissue related to prior treatments or surgery is another common finding; its appearance can be confusing. Scarred epithelium is typically less elastic than normal tissue. It may have vessels that mimic abnormal or atypical vessels, and it does not pick up Lugol's stain in an area that otherwise would have been expected to be Lugol's positive. *Because AIN can recur in scar tissue, biopsies of these areas may be indicated* (Figure 23-75).

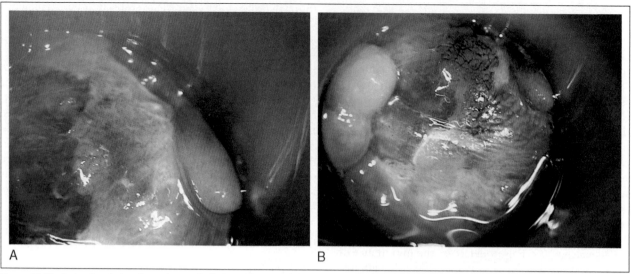

A   B

Figure 23-51 A, Another lesion that colposcopically is consistent with low-grade AIN. Partial Lugol's staining is seen. **B,** The bulbous structure on the right is a hypertrophied anal papilla that is not pathologic.

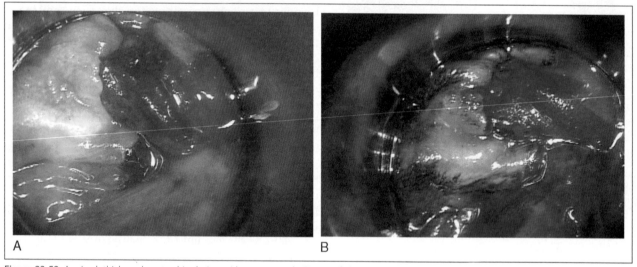

A   B

Figure 23-52 A raised, thickened acetowhite lesion with warty vessels. Biopsy of the Lugol's-negative staining area revealed AIN 1.

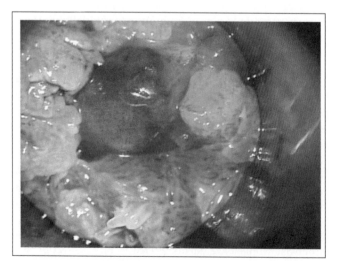

Figure 23-53 Circumferential condyloma with typical papillae and warty vessels. Histology of the warty lesion on the right was AIN 1.

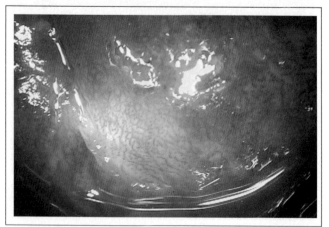

Figure 23-54 Coarse punctation and mosaic consistent with HSIL. Anal cytology was AIN 2,3.

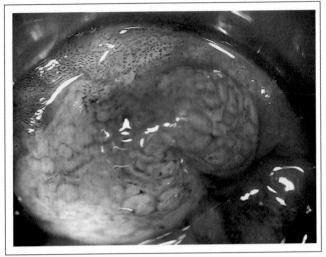

Figure 23-55 The central part of this lesion with very coarse punctation and mosaic was biopsied. Histology was high-grade AIN with features suggestive of invasion.

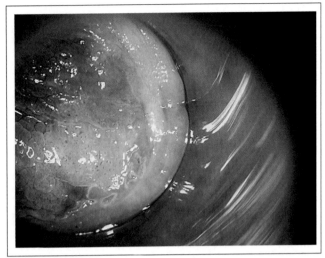

Figure 23-58 This acetowhite lesion that extends over the rectal mucosa has a predominance of ringed glands and is an example of atypical-appearing squamous metaplasia. Histology was AIN 3.

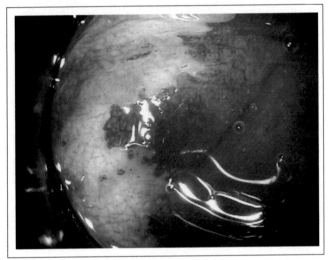

Figure 23-56 Acetowhite lesion with punctation and mosaic. Histology was AIN 3.

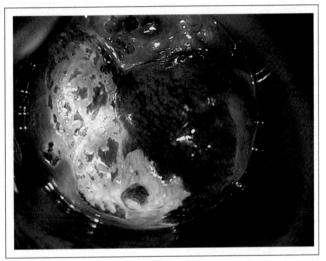

Figure 23-59 Atypical-appearing squamous metaplasia with ringed glands and mosaic extending from the SCJ over the rectal columnar epithelium. Histology was AIN 3.

MANAGEMENT OF ANAL INTRAEPITHELIAL NEOPLASIA AND CANCER

Once AIN is identified, a management strategy is individually tailored for each patient. All patients are assessed with a problem-focused history, looking for the presence of any anal symptoms such as itching, irritation, pain and bleeding, history of anal disease, sexual history and HIV status, and an assessment of overall health including comorbid illnesses or history of prolonged immunosuppression. *All patients are examined with anal cytology, DRE (specifically feeling for masses, ulceration, induration, or thickening), and HRA with biopsy of the most abnormal areas.* The goals are to determine whether any clinical suspicion of cancer is present. If so, can a diagnosis be made in the office, or does the patient need to be examined under anesthesia? Are there symptoms related to AIN that could be improved with

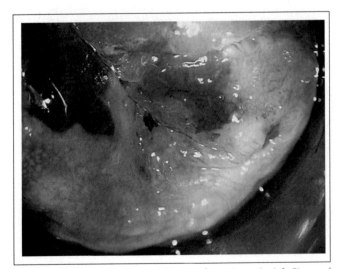

Figure 23-57 Acetowhite lesion with areas of mosaic on the left. Biopsy of the ulcer revealed AIN 3.

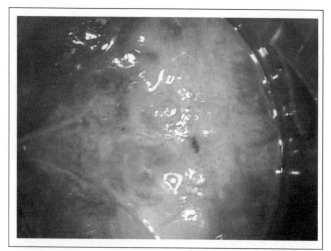

Figure 23-60 Acetowhite lesion with coarse punctation and mosaic. Histology was AIN 3.

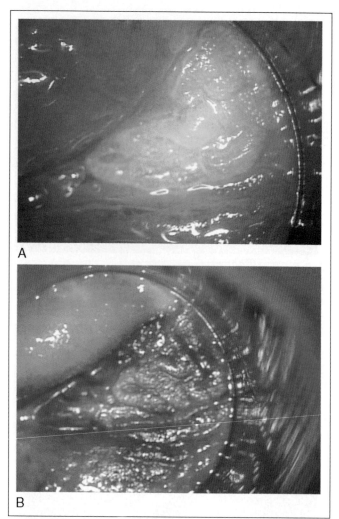

Figure 23-62 A, Granular, raised, acetowhite lesion that looks like low-grade AIN. **B,** Lugol's staining, however, was negative, and biopsy revealed AIN 2,3.

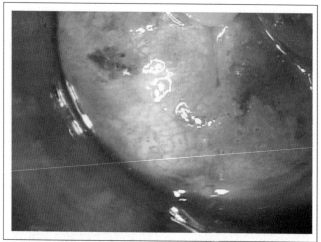

Figure 23-61 Acetowhite lesion with coarse punctation and mosaic. Histology was AIN 2,3.

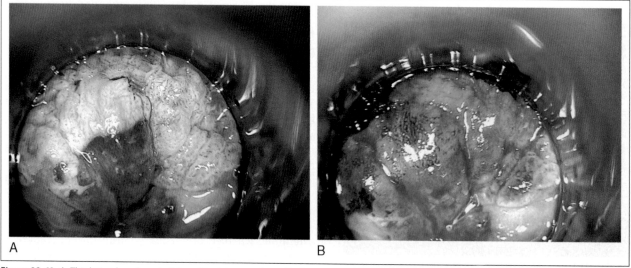

Figure 23-63 A, This lesion has characteristics of both low-grade and high-grade AIN. **B,** After Lugol's staining, biopsy of the most negative-staining area in the center of the lesion revealed AIN 3.

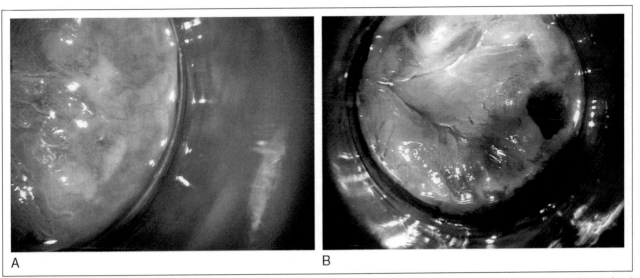

Figure 23-64 A, An acetowhite lesion is seen at the SCJ with high-grade vascular features **B,** After Lugol's, the negative-staining area was biopsied and revealed atypical squamous metaplasia, suggestive of high-grade AIN.

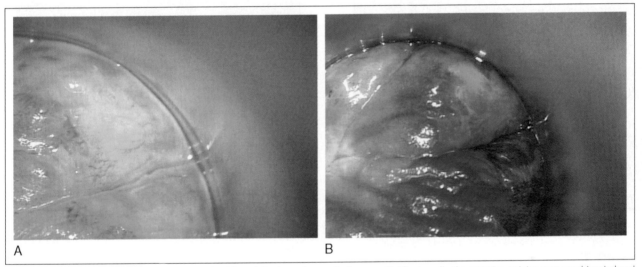

Figure 23-65 A, An acetowhite lesion is seen at the SCJ with high-grade vascular features. **B,** After Lugol's, the negative staining area was biopsied and revealed AIN 1.

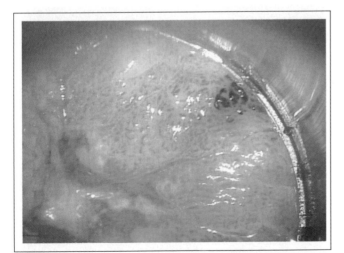

Figure 23-66 Atypical vessels and coarse punctation in a patient with perianal superficially invasive cancer. Biopsy of the dilated abnormal vessels at the upper right edge of the anoscope revealed AIN 3.

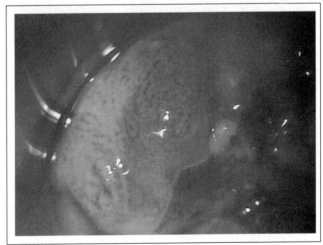

Figure 23-67 Lesion with atypical vessels was not palpable and was detected only by vascular changes detected during HRA. Excision of the lesion revealed superficially invasive squamous cell cancer.

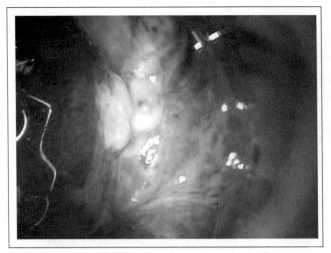

Figure 23-68 Epithelial thickening and atypical vessels. Histology was squamous cell carcinoma.

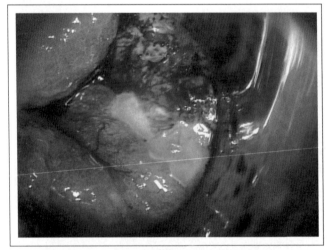

Figure 23-69 Atypical vessels with friable and peeling epithelium. Thickening felt on DRE. Initial clinic biopsy only suggested invasion. Operating room biopsy revealed squamous cell carcinoma.

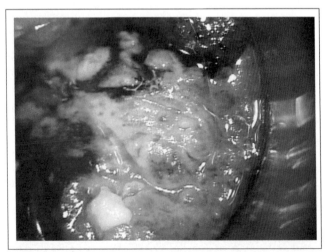

Figure 23-70 Atypical vessels with a friable, palpable mass. Initial biopsy in clinic did not confirm invasion, but clinical suspicion of cancer was very high. In the operating room, a deeper biopsy definitively established invasive squamous cell carcinoma.

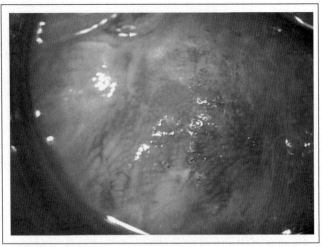

Figure 23-71 Acetowhite lesion with mosaic at the lower left edge at the anoscope was biopsied. Histology was reactive squamous metaplasia with chronic inflammation.

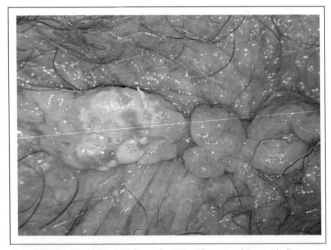

Figure 23-72 An external high-grade AIN with acetowhite epithelium adjacent to hemorrhoidal tags. Without the vinegar, the lesion can easily be mistaken for another hemorrhoid.

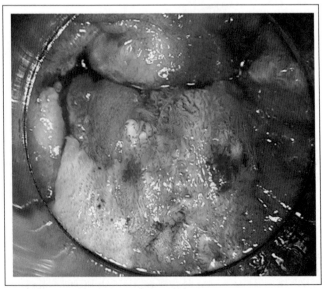

Figure 23-73 Denuded epithelium or shallow ulcerations in an AIN 3 lesion.

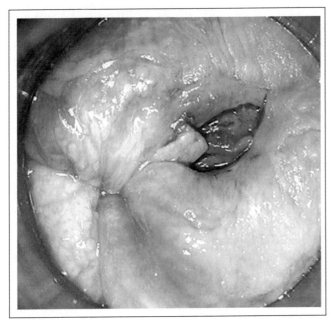

Figure 23-74 Biopsies in the center and edge of this ulcer revealed low-grade AIN.

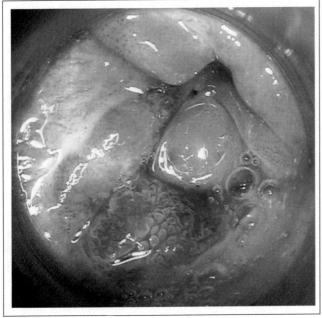

Figure 23-75 Scar tissue.

treatment? Is this patient at risk to progress to cancer because of high-grade AIN? The magnitude of that risk determines the ensuing management strategy. A general approach to patients is detailed here.

Patients who have a normal DRE, negative anal cytology, and no lesions seen on HRA are considered to have a normal exam with no evidence of anal neoplasia. Patients should continue screening based on their immune status and their anticipated risk of exposure to HPV. For HIV-negative MSM with no prior

history of anal SIL, anal cytology screening every 2 to 3 years should be adequate. HIV-positive persons should be seen at least annually.

Patients with *ASC-US* on anal cytology and a normal DRE with no significant lesions noted on HRA who are HIV-negative can be seen once a year. HIV-positive patients are seen every 6 months.

Patients with *ASC-H* on either cytology or biopsy of lesions that show atypical squamous cells suggestive of HSIL are followed more frequently, at 4- to 6-month intervals. The natural history of anal ASC-H is not well established although generally patients with atypia are followed rather than treated.

Patients with LSIL on anal cytology, normal DRE, and no evidence of high-grade AIN during HRA can be followed every 6 months. Because patients with LSIL are at increased risk for progression to high-grade AIN, they should continue to be followed regularly. Patients with large intra-anal warts or those who are symptomatic from their warts should be offered treatment. Following treatment, patients should continue to be followed at intervals determined by their response to treatment and their immune status.

Patients with HSIL on anal cytology, a normal DRE, and no lesions found on HRA should be followed more frequently, such as at 4-month intervals. In this situation, no high-grade disease was found on HRA, even though the anal cytology showed HSIL; close clinical follow-up is warranted. Because the high-grade disease cannot be treated unless it is located, it is reasonable to follow these patients in a fashion similar to patients with untreated, biopsy-proven, high-grade AIN.

Patients with high-grade AIN identified in biopsies should be treated, if at all possible, regardless of immune status. Currently, we consider this the best way to prevent anal cancer. Only a small number of people with high-grade AIN will progress to invasive anal cancer, but at the present time there is no certain way to determine who will and who will not progress.

Patients with high-grade AIN who cannot be treated should be followed closely and regularly. As previously stated, only a small number of people with high-grade AIN will progress to cancer, but when progression to cancer occurs, lesions may grow at a rapid pace. Based on our experience with several patients who had untreated high-grade AIN and developed detectable anal cancers over a 3- to 4-month period, we recommend that *patients should be seen at least at 4-month intervals.* We believe this interval will permit the early detection of a cancer, should it develop. Early anal cancers may be more easily treated and cured than larger, more advanced cancers.

Patients with exams that are suspicious for invasive anal cancer and who cannot be biopsied in clinic or for whom the exam is not adequate should be referred to an experienced surgeon for an examination under anesthesia.

Patients diagnosed with invasive anal cancers should be referred to providers experienced in managing this type of cancer. Patients with high-grade lesions are preferentially treated in the office whenever possible; this will be described in the next section, followed by a discussion of the role of surgery in managing patients with anal neoplasia.

OFFICE-BASED THERAPIES

Office-based therapies include chemical or physical ablation of lesions. It is appropriate to treat both low-grade and high-grade AIN, depending on the presentation. Patients with symptomatic low-grade lesions are usually offered treatment. Most patients receiving office procedures have a low volume of disease requiring simple treatments. However, even office-based therapy can be complex, lasting for 2 or more hours.

Chemical Ablation

Bichloracetic acid or trichloroacetic acid (BCA/TCA) 80% to 90% solution is a chemical ablative therapy that can be applied to AIN with a cotton-tipped applicator. It is best used for limited disease. Large, thick lesions are unlikely to respond to chemical ablation because the acid may not penetrate to the base of the lesion. Using TCA in conjunction with liquid nitrogen may improve its efficacy. There is minimal discomfort during or following the procedure. However, if the lesions are not successfully treated by the fourth application, an alternative method should be found. Podophyllin is an extract from the podophyllum plant. It is rarely used in current practice because, as a plant-based extract, the quality of the solution may vary. It has a potential for toxicity and may induce carcinogenic changes and thus is no longer recommended.[64] Condylox, a purified podophyllin derivative, can be effective for the treatment of external warts; it is approved by the Food and Drug Administration (FDA) only for external use.

Physical Ablation

Several techniques are available for physical ablation or destruction of anal lesions. These therapies include electrocautery, cryotherapy, infrared coagulation (IRC), and laser therapy. *Cryotherapy can only be used for external disease* and, similar to chemical ablation, often requires more than one treatment. IRC is a newer technique now validated for treatment of HSIL.[65] It has been used in the past for the treatment of external anal warts, hemorrhoids, and tattoo removals. In IRC, the heat from a light source is directed through a probe that is applied to the lesion. The heat is at a lower range compared with laser or cauterization. As such, it does not burn the lesions but rather coagulates the tissue so that it sloughs; the coagulated tissue is then removed by abrasion with a swab, curette, or the end of the anoscope (Figure 23-76, A to C). *A large volume of disease (involving 50–70% of the circumference of the anal canal) can be effectively treated with the IRC in the office with minimal discomfort both during and following the procedure.* For IRC, patients are anesthetized prior to treatment with 5% lidocaine gel followed by the injection of 1% lidocaine into the areas to be treated. The IRC procedure can last an hour or longer, but post-treatment recovery is brief (several days) and it has few of the risks associated with surgical intervention. Bleeding may last for 2 to 3 weeks and, with the exception of the first few days, is usually slight. Pain requiring medication is generally only a concern for 1 to 3 days and is usually restricted to bowel movements. Recurrences of disease can occur with any therapeutic modality, and patients should be counseled to expect this, although in most cases, treatment will be successful over time.

SURGICAL TREATMENT

Patients with AIN may need to be examined under anesthesia and/or treated in the operating room to reduce symptoms, to treat bulky or rapidly growing warts where high-grade AIN or superficially invasive cancer may be present, and to treat high-grade AIN to prevent invasive cancer. If invasive cancer is clinically suspected and a diagnosis cannot be made in the office, then patients should have an examination under anesthesia (EUA). **Clinical signs of invasive cancer include an abnormal DRE with thickening, induration, an anorectal mass, extensive perianal lesions with ulceration, the presence of an ulcerated lesion with abnormal vessels, and focally tender lesions.** If a biopsy reveals high-grade AIN with features suggestive of invasion, then patients should have these areas excised in the operating room to establish the diagnosis. Unlike the cervix, the entire anal SCJ cannot be removed circumferentially without significant morbidity. Because these are mucosal lesions, treatment should be superficial and treatment morbidity must be balanced with the low but uncertain potential for high-grade AIN to progress to cancer. Clinical trials demonstrating that treatment of high-grade AIN definitely prevents anal cancer have yet to be performed.

Other reasons for an EUA or surgical treatment include extensive or nearly circumferential lesions, significant perianal lesions, lesions present in the distal anal canal near the verge or opening to the anus, patients who have failed repeat treatments with IRC and have recurrent high-grade AIN, women who have coexistent VIN that requires laser treatment, patients with comorbidities such as low platelets or significant hemorrhoids, and those who are very anxious or needle phobic or who have poor tolerance of office-based HRA.

In the operating room, patients are usually treated in the prone-jackknife position with buttocks taped apart; patients can also be treated in the dorsal lithotomy position. Patients are treated with heavy sedation and placement of a perianal block; spinal or general anesthesia can also be used. The DRE is repeated to assess for suspicious areas of induration or anal masses. It is important to allow adequate time to apply sufficient amounts of vinegar to adequately visualize lesions, similar to office-based procedures. The entire SCJ is examined carefully with the operating microscope or colposcope to determine areas to biopsy. If extensive disease is present, it is important to decide whether the goal of surgery is therapeutic or diagnostic. If disease is circumferential, epithelial bridges to avoid stenosis are left in place to avoid stenosis of the anal canal. With electrocautery or laser ablation, burns should be superficial and débrided down to the submucosa. IRC can also be used in the operating room. It is advisable to avoid extensive

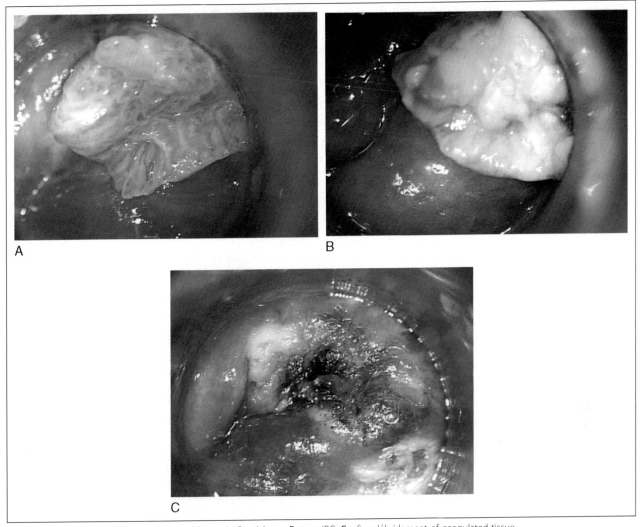

Figure 23-76 Typical IRC ablation of a condyloma. **A,** Condyloma; **B,** post-IRC; **C,** after débridement of coagulated tissue.

resections and use of skin flaps, and instead selectively excise areas suspicious for invasion and target destruction of remaining abnormal tissue. To avoid circumferential burns, some patients may require staged procedures. The decision to treat must be based on the patient's overall health, immune function, and risk of progression for invasive disease.

Postoperative care includes avoiding constipation and maintaining soft bowel movements and using 5% anorectal lidocaine cream (LMX5 or Lidosense) and Silvadene cream (used similar to patients with burns). Liberal and adequate analgesia, such as oxycodone, is prescribed in addition to nonsteroidal anti-inflammatory medication. *Soaking in hot water 6 to 8 times per day is probably the most important postoperative care instruction; it provides relief from anal spasms, particularly after bowel movement.* Patients are typically excused from work for 2 to 3 weeks, depending on the extent of treatment. They are cautioned to call if they develop fever, inability to urinate, excessive bleeding, or uncontrolled pain. Rarely, patients have developed urinary retention or required treatment for bleeding. Most patients recover well;

occasionally a few develop fissures, have prolonged healing times, or both. Infection is uncommon. Stenosis has been an uncommon complication with less than circumferential treatment of the anal canal, but it can occur with multiple procedures. Incontinence has not occurred.

There is a paucity of literature regarding treatment of high-grade AIN. Older articles describe the treatment of perianal Bowen's disease, mapping procedures, and wide local excisions with skin grafting. Recurrences were common, and patients were not followed very closely after treatment. The efficacy of surgical treatment of high-grade AIN at the University of California–San Francisco (UCSF) was reported in 29 HIV-positive and 8 HIV-negative MSM; it is the first study documenting the use of HRA to guide surgical treatment of high-grade AIN.[66] *No recurrence of high-grade AIN was seen in HIV-negative patients, but 79% (23 of 29) of HIV-positive patients had a recurrence of HSIL within 12 months. Sixteen of 29 patients reported uncontrolled pain that lasted a mean of 2.9 weeks.* No stenosis, incontinence, infection, or significant bleeding occurred postoperatively. Subsequently, the 10-year surgical experience at UCSF from 1996 to 2006 for treating high-grade AIN in 245 patients was reported[67] and is summarized here; the patients included 71% who were HIV positive, 8% who were immunocompromised due to other causes, and 21% who were HIV negative or whose immune status was not documented. On average at 14 months, recurrent or persistent high-grade AIN was found in 158 (64.5%), but only 47 (30%) required retreatment in the operating room. The remaining patients with recurrent disease were treated in the office with TCA, IRC, or both. Patients must be followed carefully and regularly because recurrent, persistent, and metachronous lesions are common. Patients who have been followed regularly after surgical treatment have not progressed to invasive cancer. Progression to cancer has occurred in at least 2 of our patients who did not return for follow-up.

REFERENCES

1. Chiao EY, Krown SE, Stier EA, et al. A population-based analysis of temporal trends in the incidence of squamous anal canal cancer in relation to the HIV epidemic. J Acquir Immune Defic Syndr 2005;40:451–455.

2. Daling JR, Weiss NS, Klopfenstein LL, et al. Correlates of homosexual behavior and the incidence of anal cancer. J Am Med Assoc 1982;247:1988–1990.

3. Daling JR, Weiss NS, Hislop TG, et al. Sexual practices, sexually transmitted diseases, and the incidence of anal cancer. N Engl J Med 1987;317:973–977.

4. Holly EA, Whittemore AS, Aston DA, et al. Anal cancer incidence: genital warts, anal fissure or fistula, hemorrhoids, and smoking. J Natl Cancer Inst 1989;81:1726–1731.

5. Scholefield JH, Sonnex C, Talbot IC, et al. Anal and cervical intraepithelial neoplasia: possible parallel [see comments]. Lancet 1989;2:765–769.

6. Melbye M, Sprogel P. Aetiological parallel between anal cancer and cervical cancer. Lancet 1991;338:657–659.

7. Palefsky JM, Holly EA, Gonzales J, et al. Detection of human papillomavirus DNA in anal intraepithelial neoplasia and anal cancer. Cancer Res 1991;51:1014–1019.

8. Zaki SR, Judd R, Coffield LM, et al. Human papillomavirus infection and anal carcinoma. Retrospective analysis by in situ hybridization and the polymerase chain reaction. Am J Pathol 1992;140:1345–1355.

9. Frisch M, Glimelius B, van den Brule AJ, et al. Sexually transmitted infection as a cause of anal cancer [see comments]. N Engl J Med 1997;337:1350–1358.

10. Parkin DM. The global health burden of infection-associated cancers in the year 2002. Int J Cancer 2006;118: 3030–3044.

11. Johnson LG, Madeleine MM, Newcomer LM, et al. Anal cancer incidence and survival: the surveillance, epidemiology, and end results experience, 1973-2000. Cancer 2004;101: 281–288.

12. Frisch M, Biggar RJ, Goedert JJ, et al. Human papillomavirus-associated cancers in patients with human immunodeficiency virus infection and acquired immunodeficiency syndrome. J Natl Cancer Inst 2000;92:1500–1510.

13. Melbye M, Cote TR, Kessler L, et al. High incidence of anal cancer among AIDS patients. The AIDS/Cancer Working Group. Lancet 1994;343:636–639.

14. Cress RD, Holly EA. Incidence of anal cancer in California: increased incidence among men in San Francisco, 1973-1999. Prev Med 2003;36:555–560.

15. Bower M, Powles T, Newsom-Davis T, et al. HIV-associated anal cancer: has highly active antiretroviral therapy reduced the incidence or improved the outcome?. J Acquir Immune Defic Syndr 2004;37:1563–1565.

16. Diamond C, Taylor TH, Aboumrad T, et al. Increased incidence of squamous cell anal cancer among men with AIDS in the era of highly active antiretroviral therapy. Sex Transm Dis 2005;32:314–320.

17. Bower M, Palmieri C, Dhillon T, et al. AIDS-related malignancies: changing epidemiology and the impact of highly active antiretroviral therapy. Curr Opin Infect Dis 2006;19: 14–19.

18. Hessol NA, Pipkin S, Schwarcz S, et al. The impact of highly active antiretroviral therapy on non-AIDS-defining cancers among adults with AIDS. Am J Epidemiol 2007;165(10): 1143–1153.

19. Adami J, Gabel H, Lindelof B, et al. Cancer risk following organ transplantation: a nationwide cohort study in Sweden. Br J Cancer 2003;89:1221–1227.

20. Patel HS, Silver AR, Northover JM, et al. Anal cancer in renal transplant patients. Int J Colorectal Dis 2005;22:1–5.

21. Palefsky JM, Holly EA, Hogeboom CJ, et al. Virologic, immunologic, and clinical parameters in the incidence and progression of anal squamous intraepithelial lesions in HIV-positive and HIV-negative homosexual men. J Acquir Immune Defic Syndr Hum Retrovirol 1998;17:314–319.

22. Gagne SE, Jensen R, Polvi A, et al. High-resolution analysis of genomic alterations and human papillomavirus integration in anal intraepithelial neoplasia. J Acquir Immune Defic Syndr 2005;40:182–189.

23. Chin-Hong PV, Vittinghoff E, Cranston RD, et al. Age-specific prevalence of anal human papillomavirus infection in HIV-negative sexually active men who have sex with men: the EXPLORE study. J Infect Dis 2004;190:2070–2076.

24. Schiffman MH. New epidemiology of human papillomavirus infection and cervical neoplasia [editorial; comment]. J Natl Cancer Inst 1995;87:1345–1347.

25. Kiviat N, Rompalo A, Bowden R, et al. Anal human papillomavirus infection among human immunodeficiency virus-seropositive and -seronegative men. J Infect Dis 1990;162: 358–361.

26. Piketty C, Darragh TM, Da Costa M, et al. High prevalence of anal human papillomavirus infection and anal cancer precursors among HIV-infected persons in the absence of anal intercourse. Ann Intern Med 2003;138:453–459.

27. Palefsky JM, Holly EA, Ralston ML, et al. Prevalence and risk factors for anal human papillomavirus infection in human immunodeficiency virus (HIV)-positive and high-risk HIV-negative women. J Infect Dis 2001;183:383–391.

28. Melbye M, Smith E, Wohlfahrt J, et al. Anal and cervical abnormality in women—prediction by human papillomavirus tests. Int J Cancer 1996;68:559–564.

29. Hernandez BY, McDuffie K, Zhu X, et al. Anal human papillomavirus infection in women and its relationship with cervical infection. Cancer Epidemiol Biomarkers Prev 2005;14: 2550–2556.

30. Chin-Hong PV, Vittinghoff E, Cranston RD, et al. Age-related prevalence of anal cancer precursors in homosexual men: the EXPLORE study. J Natl Cancer Inst 2005;97:896–905.

31. Palefsky JM, Holly EA, Ralston ML, et al. Prevalence and risk factors for human papillomavirus infection of the anal canal

in human immunodeficiency virus (HIV)-positive and HIV-negative homosexual men. J Infect Dis 1998;177: 361–367.

32. Holly EA, Ralston ML, Darragh TM, et al. Prevalence and risk factors for anal squamous intraepithelial lesions in women. J Natl Cancer Inst 2001;93:843–849.

33. Palefsky JM, Holly EA, Ralston ML, et al. Anal squamous intraepithelial lesions in HIV-positive and HIV-negative homosexual and bisexual men: prevalence and risk factors. J Acquir Immune Defic Syndr Hum Retrovirol 1998;17:320–326.

34. Palefsky JM, Holly EA, Ralston ML, et al. High incidence of anal high-grade squamous intraepithelial lesions among HIV-positive and HIV-negative homosexual/bisexual men. AIDS 1998;12:495–503.

35. Palefsky JM, Holly EA, Efirdc JT, et al. Anal intraepithelial neoplasia in the highly active antiretroviral therapy era among HIV-positive men who have sex with men. AIDS 2005;19: 1407–1414.

36. Piketty C, Darragh TM, Heard I, et al. High prevalence of anal squamous intraepithelial lesions in HIV-positive men despite the use of highly active antiretroviral therapy. Sex Transm Dis 2004;31:96–99.

37. Critchlow CW, Surawicz CM, Holmes KK, et al. Prospective study of high-grade anal squamous intraepithelial neoplasia in a cohort of homosexual men: influence of HIV infection, immunosuppression and human papillomavirus infection. AIDS 1995;9:1255–1262.

38. International Collaboration on HIV and Cancer. Highly active antiretroviral therapy and incidence of cancer in human immunodeficiency virus-infected adults. J Natl Cancer Inst 2000;92:1823–1830.

39. Dorrucci M, Suligoi B, Serraino D, et al. Incidence of invasive cervical cancer in a cohort of HIV-seropositive women before and after the introduction of highly active antiretroviral therapy. J Acquir Immune Defic Syndr 2001;26:377–380.

40. Clifford GM, Polesel J, Rickenbach M, et al. Cancer risk in the Swiss HIV Cohort Study: associations with immunodeficiency, smoking, and highly active antiretroviral therapy. J Natl Cancer Inst 2005;97:425–432.

41. Heard I, Palefsky JM, Kazatchkine MD, et al. The impact of HIV antiviral therapy on human papillomavirus (HPV) infections and HPV-related diseases. Antivir Ther 2004;9: 13–22.

42. Palefsky JM, Holly EA, Ralston ML, et al. Effect of highly active antiretroviral therapy on the natural history of anal squamous intraepithelial lesions and anal human papillomavirus infection. J Acquir Immune Defic Syndr 2001;28: 422–428.

43. Edgren G, Sparen P. Risk of anogenital cancer after diagnosis of cervical intraepithelial neoplasia: a prospective population-based study. Lancet Oncol 2007;8:311–316.

44. Stier EA, Krown SE, Chi DS, et al. Anal dysplasia in HIV-infected women with cervical and vulvar dysplasia. J Low Genit Tract Dis 2004;8:272–275.

45. Jamieson DJ, Paramsothy P, Cu-Uvin S, et al. Vulvar, vaginal, and perianal intraepithelial neoplasia in women with or at risk for human immunodeficiency virus. Obstet Gynecol 2006;107: 1023–1028.

46. Palefsky JM, Holly EA, Hogeboom CJ, et al. Anal cytology as a screening tool for anal squamous intraepithelial lesions. J Acquir Immune Defic Syndr Hum Retrovir 1997;14:415–422.

47. Arain S, Walts AE, Thomas P, et al. The anal Pap smear: cytomorphology of squamous intraepithelial lesions. CytoJournal 2005;2:4.

48. Fox PA, Seet JE, Stebbing J, et al. The value of anal cytology and human papillomavirus typing in the detection of anal intraepithelial neoplasia: a review of cases from an anoscopy clinic. Sex Transm Infect 2005;81:142–146.

49. Darragh TM, Jay N, Tupkelewicz BA, et al. Comparison of conventional cytologic smears and ThinPrep preparations of the anal canal. Acta Cytol 1997;41:1167–1170.

50. Sherman ME, Friedman HB, Busseniers AE, et al. Cytologic diagnosis of anal intraepithelial neoplasia using smears and Cytyc Thin-Preps. Mod Pathol 1995;8:270–274.

51. Lytwyn A, Salit IE, Raboud J, et al. Interobserver agreement in the interpretation of anal intraepithelial neoplasia. Cancer 2005;103:1447–1456.

52. Goldie SJ, Kuntz KM, Weinstein MC, et al. The clinical effectiveness and cost-effectiveness of screening for anal squamous intraepithelial lesions in homosexual and bisexual HIV-positive men. J Am Med Assoc 1999;281:1822–1829.

53. Goldie SJ, Kuntz KM, Weinstein MC, et al. Cost-effectiveness of screening for anal squamous intraepithelial lesions and anal cancer in human immunodeficiency virus-negative homosexual and bisexual men. Am J Med 2000;108:634–641.

54. Cranston RD, Darragh TM, Holly EA, et al. Self-collected versus clinician-collected anal cytology specimens to diagnose anal intraepithelial neoplasia in HIV-positive men. J Acquir Immmune Defic Syndr 2004;36:915–920.

55. Lampinen TM, Latulippe L, van Niekerk D, et al. Illustrated instructions for self-collection of anal-rectal swab specimens and their adequacy for cytological examination. Sex Transm 2006;33:386–388.

56. Darragh TM, Birdsong GG, Luff RD, et al. Anal-rectal cytology. In: Solomon D, Nayar R(eds): The Bethesda System for Reporting Cervical Cytology: Definitions, Criteria and Explanatory Notes, ed 2. New York: Springer, 2004, pp 169–176.

57. Panther LA, Wagner K, Proper J, et al. High resolutions anoscopy findings for men who have sex with men: Inaccuracy of anal cytology as a predictor of histologic high-grade intraepithelial neoplasia and the impact of HIV serostatus. Clin Infect Dis 2004;38:1490–1492.

58. Walts AE, Thomas P, Bose S. Anal cytology: is there a role for reflex HPV DNA testing?. Diagn Cytopathol 2005;33:152–156.

59. Friedlander, MA, Stier E, Lin O. Anal-rectal cytology as a screening tool of anal squamous lesions. Cancer (Cancer Cytopathol) 2004;102:19–26.

60. Walts AE, Thomas P, Bose S. Anal cytology: Is there a role for reflex HPV DNA testing? Diagn cytopatnol 2005; 33152–33156.

61. Netter FH. Lower digestive tract. In: Oppenheimer E (ed). The CIBA Collection of Medical Illustrations: Digestive System. New York: Ciba Pharmaceutical, 1975, pp 57–60.

62. Jay N, Berry JM, Hogeboom CJ, et al. Colposcopic appearance of anal squamous intraepithelial lesions: relationship to histopathology. Dis Colon Rectum 1997;4:919–928.

63. Scholefield JH, Ogunbiyi OA, Smith JH, et al. Anal colposcopy and the diagnosis anal intraepithelial neoplasia in high-risk gynecologic patients. Int J Gynecologic Cancer 1994;4:119–126.

64. Von Krogh G, Longstaff E. Podophyllin office therapy against condyloma should be abandoned. Sex Transm Infect 2001;77:409–412.

65. Goldstone SE, Kawalek AZ, Huyett JW, et al. Infrared coagulator: a useful tool for treating anal squamous intraepithelial lesions. Dis Colon Rectum 2005;48:1042–1054.

66. Chang GJ, Berry JM, Jay N, et al. Surgical treatment of high-grade anal squamous intraepithelial lesions: a prospective study. Dis Colon Rectum 2002;45:453–458.

67. Pineda C, Welton M, Berry J, et al. High resolution anoscopy targeted surgical destruction of anal high-grade squamous intraepithelial lesions: a ten year experience. Presented at the 2007 annual meeting of the American Society of Colon and Rectal Surgeons, June 2–6, 2007, St Louis.

68. Wilkin TJ, Palmer S, Brudney KF, Chiasson MA, Wright TC. Anal intraepithelial neoplasia in heterosexual and homosexual HIV-positive men with access to antiretroviral therapy. J infect Dis 2004;190(9):1685–1689.

CASE STUDY

The patient was a 50-year-old, HIV-positive MSM who presented with a 9-month history of anal soreness and discomfort with intercourse. He had a history of warts previously treated with podophyllin. Although HIV-positive, he was healthy and had been receiving antiretroviral therapy for the last year. His CD4+ lymphocyte count was 500 cells/mm^3 with a nadir of 200. His HIV viral load was undetectable. A local surgeon biopsied the area of irritation at the anal verge, which showed condyloma with focal high-grade AIN. Topical therapy was ineffective and he was referred to a dermatologist, who referred him to the UCSF Anal Neoplasia Clinic.

On initial examination, his DRE was unremarkable and anal cytology revealed HSIL. Figures 23-77 to 23-81 illustrate principles related to management of AIN. On HRA, the external lesion, seen in Figure 23-77, shows ulceration and coarse punctation; this is worrisome for invasive cancer. Intra-anally, the lesions seen in Figure 23-78, A, B were biopsied. Due to his symptoms and the need to rule out invasive cancer (because of the appearance of the external lesion), he was taken to the operating room (Figures 23-79 and 23-80). Fortunately,

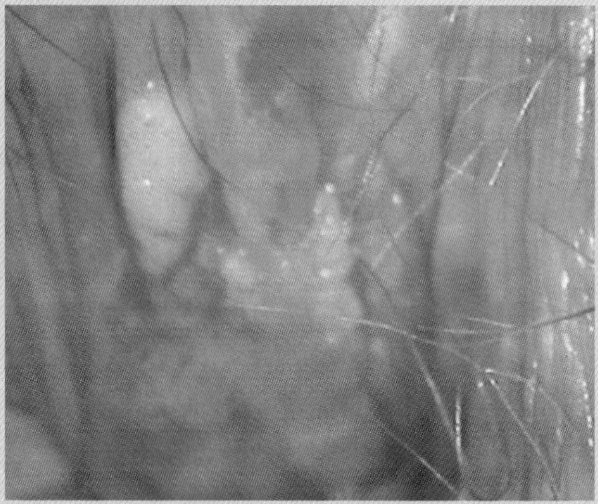

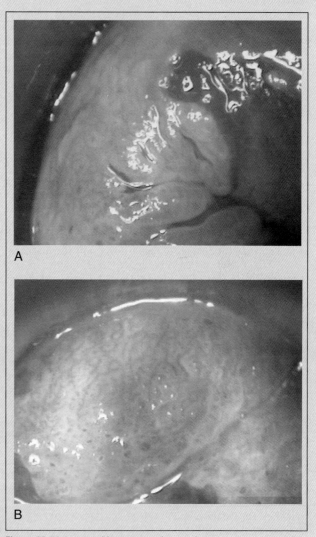

A

B

Figure 23-77 Case illustrating treatment principles. This HIV-positive MSM presented with an ulcerated lesion at the verge worrisome for invasive cancer.

Figure 23-78 Intra-anal lesions were biopsied prior to surgery, revealing AIN 2,3 in **A** and AIN 3 in **B**.

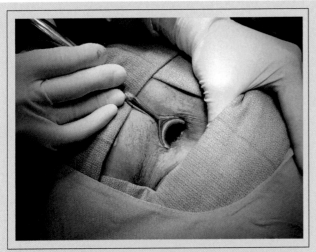

Figure 23-79 In the operating room the lesion was excised and fortunately was only AIN 3. The remaining lesions were destroyed using electrocautery.

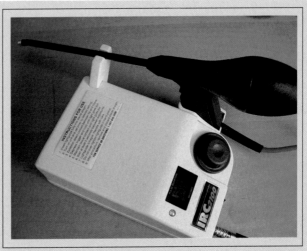

Figure 23-81 The IRC 2100 Infrared Coagulator (Redfield, Rochelle Park, N.J.).

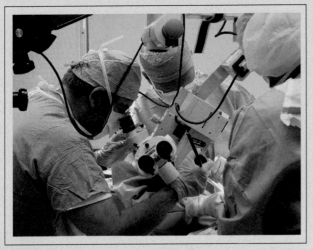

Figure 23-80 Surgery was guided by HRA. The most worrisome areas were excised, and remaining areas of dysplasia were ablated by targeted destruction using electrocautery.

this external lesion was AIN 3; no invasion was identified. Three months later, he had healed from surgery; anal cytology showed ASC-US. Seven months after surgery, he had two small recurrences of high-grade AIN, both easily treated with IRC, shown in Figure 23-81. Twelve months later he had a second high-grade recurrence detected that was treated with IRC but was completely healed and otherwise asymptomatic. He continues in follow-up and has had no evidence of high-grade AIN, now 18 months after the last procedure.

CHAPTER 24

Androscopy: Examination of the Male Partner

John L. Pfenninger

Human papillomavirus (HPV) infection in men has fewer health consequences than in women. It is not necessary to evaluate all male partners of women with condyloma or cervical intraepithelial neoplasia (CIN). However, the androscopy procedure (evaluation of the male genitalia and anorectal area with a colposcope) may assist in diagnosing and treating HPV-associated lesions in men.

RISK FACTORS AND EPIDEMIOLOGY

HPV infects both male and female genitalia.[1] Although penile HPV infection is very common and oncogenic HPV types are associated with penile cancer, the male is not at particularly high risk for developing cancer of the penis.[2,3] In the United States, HPV infection is associated with less than 1% of all malignancies in men.[4] The primary risk factors for penile carcinoma appear to be infection with HPV, sex outside of a monogamous relationship, smoking, and lack of genital hygiene.[5] The absolute number of sexual partners alone is not a high-risk indicator.[6,7] In cultures where a man may be *monogamous* with four or five wives, there is no increased risk of cancer of the cervix or penis.[8–10] Immunosuppression, such as occurs with human immunodeficiency virus (HIV) infection, increases the risk of development of more severe disease.[11]

Men who have sex with men and women who have anal-receptive intercourse are at markedly increased risk for anal and rectal carcinoma.[12–14] Cancer of the anal canal in these men and women is more likely to be associated with HPV.[15] The mechanism seems to involve HPV infection of the dentate or pectinate line in the rectum, which is analogous to the squamocolumnar junction (SCJ) of the cervix.[16,17] Some experts also advocate cytologic sampling of the anal canal to detect preinvasive and invasive lesions (see Chapter 23).

Sexual partners of women with genital warts or with preinvasive or invasive disease of the lower genital tract are invariably HPV infected themselves.[18–20] Women who have sex with men whose previous female partners had high-grade cervical lesions or cervical cancer have a much higher incidence of cervical dysplasia and cancer.[21]

The author wishes to thank Pat Wolfgram (Librarian, Mid-Michigan Medical Center) for research and assistance and Kay Pfenninger for secretarial support.

Although men have a much lower risk of developing HPV-related cancer than their female partners, men often act as unknowing vectors in the transmission of HPV infection. Furthermore, HPV is transmissible through nonpenetrative sexual contact in both the men and women.[22,23] Male partners should be informed of the risks of HPV transmission and the benefits of eliminating high-risk behaviors.[24]

HPV infection has several clinical manifestations in men. Condylomata may exist on the penis, scrotum, anus, or suprapubic area and in the urethral meatus (Figures 24-1 to 24-5).[25] The lesions may be acuminate and visible to the naked eye, or they may be flat and visible only after application of 5% acetic acid. The virus may also be latent, with no clinical signs.

Unlike cervical lesions, the histology of penile lesions is difficult to predict based on clinical appearance even when they are observed under colposcopic magnification. Some lesions with the appearance of classic condylomata are actually squamous intraepithelial lesions (SIL) or bowenoid carcinoma *in situ*. Others that appear dysplastic are simply genital warts. The lesions can be differentiated only by histology.[25]

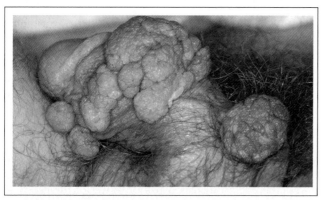

Figure 24-1 Several large condylomata acuminata of the penis. (Courtesy of the National Procedures Institute, 2007.)

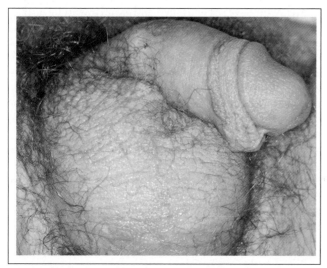

Figure 24-2 White scrotum syndrome: diffuse acetowhite epithelium from HPV. (Courtesy of the National Procedures Institute, 2007.)

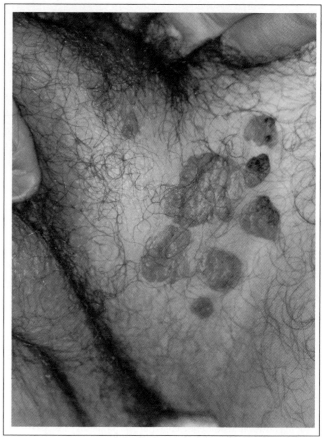

Figure 24-3 Pigmented condyloma. (Courtesy of the National Procedures Institute, 2007.)

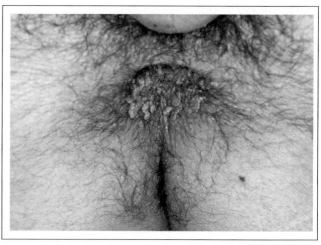

Figure 24-4 Perianal condyloma. (Courtesy of the National Procedures Institute, 2007.)

The differential diagnosis of penile lesions is outlined in Table 24-1. Because patients may be embarrassed about discussing genital lesions, their chief complaints may be misleading. It is only after clinical examination and possibly biopsy that a definitive diagnosis can be made.

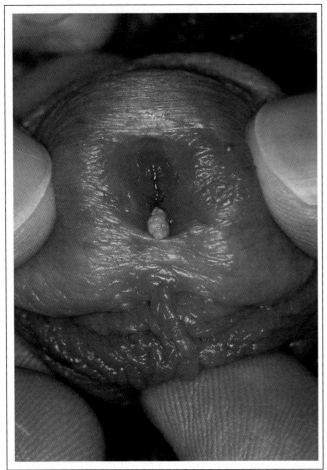

Figure 24-5 Condyloma of the penile meatus. (Courtesy of the National Procedures Institute, 2007.)

Table 24-1 Differential Diagnosis of Anogenital Lesions in Men

Infectious Lesions
Condylomata acuminata
Herpes simplex virus
Molluscum contagiosum
Chancre of Syphilis
Condylomata lata
Tinea pubis

Noninfectious Benign Lesions and Conditions (Including Normal Variants)
Anal polyp
Contact dermatitis
Cysts
Nevus
Normal variant, papular lesions of the frenulum
Normal variant, papular lesions of the corona (pearly penile papules)
Seborrheic keratosis
Sentinel "polyp" on a chronic fissure
Skin tags

Preneoplastic and Neoplastic Lesions
Penile intraepithelial neoplasia
Erythroplasia of Queyrat
Bowen's disease
Bowenoid papulosis
Cancer (squamous cell carcinoma of the penis and anus, prolapsing adenocarcinoma of the rectum)

ANDROSCOPY

Procedure

Early papers described *colposcopy of the penis* as a tool used to identify HPV lesions in men. Later, the terms *penoscopy* and *androscopy* were used.[26–30] The procedure involves applying 5% acetic acid to the penis, scrotum, perineum, and anal areas and then visualizing these areas under magnification with illumination. *Unlike colposcopy, the purpose of androscopy is not to identify the most severe lesions. Rather, it is to identify all lesions, especially small ones; to be sure all lesions have been removed in their entirety; to enhance directed biopsy and treatment of those lesions; to reassure the man regarding the extent of the infection (or lack thereof); and to provide an opportunity for patient education.*

Indications

The indications for androscopy are listed in Table 24-2.[26,30] *It is not essential that every man with condyloma undergo androscopy.* When a partner is found to have HPV-related disease, the role of androscopy is controversial. Some experts question the value of androscopy in men without grossly visible lesions,[31] whereas others suggest that men whose partners have HPV-related disease should be *screened*.[32] When male genitalia are examined without magnification, only 20% of lesions are identified.[23,28,33] However, there is no evidence that use of androscopy decreases the rate of genital cancers in men or recurrence in sexual partner.

Men often present requesting evaluation for the presence of infection after being exposed to HPV. Those exposed to HPV may have contracted the virus despite consistent condom use. The U.S. Food and Drug Administration (FDA) has been petitioned to require condom manufacturers to state on packages that *condoms do not offer full protection from infection with HPV*.[34] Nevertheless, in women who were followed closely from first intercourse and whose partners used condoms 100% of the time, no cervical SIL were detected in 32 patient-years at risk, whereas 14 incident lesions were detected during 97 patient-years at risk among women whose partners did not use condoms. Despite the fact that protection is far from complete, women whose partners always used condoms were 70% less likely to acquire any new infection. Condom use appeared to protect from both low- and high-risk HPV types.[37]

Table 24-2 Potential Indications for Androscopy

Identification of the presence or absence of anogenital skin lesions
Identification of lesions, allowing directed biopsy and removal of these lesions
Chronic pruritus/irritation of unknown cause

Table 24-3 Materials and Equipment for Androscopy

Examination table with stirrups (preferably a power table)
5% acetic acid (vinegar) in a spray bottle
2% lidocaine without epinephrine in a 5-mL syringe, 30-gauge needle
Colposcope with low power or a quality magnification lens or loupe
Quality tissue scissors (small, curved Metzenbaum)
#15 surgical blade (blade handle optional)
3- and 4-mm sharp, disposable dermatologic curettes
Toothed forceps
Formalin for tissue specimens
4 × 4 gauze pads
Ferric subsulfate (Monsel's solution) or aluminum chloride (Drysol)
85% trichlorocetic acid (for possible treatment)
Cotton-tipped applicators
Antibiotic ointment or petroleum jelly
Ive's slotted anoscope, if indicated

Treatment of HPV infection in men as a method to reduce recurrence of disease in their female partners has been a source of controversy.[38,39] Although some experts initially recommended that all male partners of infected females be examined and treated, this approach is of little value.[40] Additionally, studies do not support the suggestions that large or multiple lesions in the male may shed more virus.[41]

Patient History

The purpose of obtaining a history is to assess the patient's risk for HPV infection. Age at first intercourse helps define possible length of exposure to HPV. A history of sexual abuse should be ascertained. History of genital warts, how they were treated, recurrences, and any partners with HPV infection should be discussed. Patients should be queried about exposure to other sexually transmitted infections (STIs). The patient should be encouraged to be tested for HIV and should be offered screening for other STIs, including syphilis.

Equipment

Materials and equipment for performing androscopy are listed in Table 24-3.

It is important to have sharp, high-quality tissue scissors (i.e., small, curved Metzenbaum scissors). Low-quality or dull instruments may pinch or crush tissue rather than cut it sharply. Punch biopsy instruments such as Keyes' dermatologic punches are generally not indicated for biopsy of penile, scrotal, or anal lesions. Even perineal lesions can be biopsied with a scalpel blade using a shave technique or scissors excision. A sharp, 3- to 4-mm dermatologic disposable curette readily removes most small lesions. *Warts are superficial, so deep biopsies are unnecessary.* Topical astringents or light cautery will control any bleeding.

Rather than use a colposcope for magnification, some clinicians prefer to wear loupes or to use a handheld lens. The colposcopic technique of examination of the male genitalia, however, is easy to learn if the instrumentation is available.

Technique

In the examination room, *the patient is instructed to saturate the entire penis, scrotum, perineum, and anal area using a spray* bottle of warm 5% acetic acid (vinegar). The genitalia are soaked for least 5 minutes, and then the process is repeated, resulting in two thorough soakings.

During the 5-minute interval while the genitalia are being soaked, the clinician may use the opportunity to review the history and explain the procedure to the patient. No written informed consent is necessary unless a biopsy is performed. The patient should be advised regarding pain, bleeding, recurrence, and possible scarring from excision or other procedures. The patient is asked to assume the dorsal lithotomy position with his feet in stirrups such that the genitals are positioned at the end of the table, similar to the position for a pelvic examination. The entire genital area is moistened with 5% acetic acid once again and examined, first with the naked eye and then with the colposcope on low-power setting.[42]

The technique of androscopy is slightly different from that of colposcopy. When the cervix is visualized with a colposcope, the depth of field is quite shallow. Also, because the cervix is stationary, it is unnecessary to adjust the colposcope frequently to maintain the focus. *In the male,* the area examined (glans penis to suprapubic and anal area) is larger, and the distance from the colposcope to the genitalia varies considerably, so *the colposcope must be focused more frequently.* It may be easier to keep the colposcope stationary and to move the area to be examined into the plane of focus.

The genitals are kept saturated with 5% acetic acid during the entire examination. The penis, urethral meatus, scrotum, suprapubic area, perineum, and perianal tissues are examined. *Lesions in the hair-bearing areas are often difficult to detect. It is best to palpate these areas to ensure that no lesions are missed.*

Anoscopy is not indicated on a routine basis, and a digital examination is not performed unless genital warts are present or other indications exist. If external perianal lesions are identified, treating these lesions first may theoretically reduce the risk of tracking HPV infection intra-anally due to trauma from insertion of the anoscope. *If a digital examination is indicated, it should be performed at the time of anoscopic inspection.* Some lesions in the anus are not easily palpable because they are small or filamentous, whereas others may be concealed in mucosal folds. *Using both methods of examination will decrease the likelihood of missing any lesions.*

In the past, cystoscopy was recommended to rule out urethral or bladder lesions caused by HPV. Although some bladder cancers have been associated with HPV,[43] *routine cystoscopy is not currently recommended for men with genital warts* because evidence is lacking that it improves outcomes in men with genital HPV.

Although the entire procedure can take as little as 15 minutes, additional time will allow an opportunity to obtain a relevant history, to treat lesions, and to educate the patient. If more extensive lesions are present, another appointment may be required. If lesions were treated, a follow-up examination is usually scheduled in 4 to 6 weeks to determine the need for further treatment.

Clinical Findings

HPV lesions on male genitalia turn white after the application of 5% acetic acid. The lesions may be totally flat or raised (acuminate). Inflammation in the groin area may also turn white. At times, the entire scrotum will exhibit a faint acetowhite reaction (white scrotum syndrome).[33] Biopsies may confirm HPV infection. However, carcinoma of the scrotum is extremely rare.[44] Inflammation alone of the scrotum and groin area can produce an acetowhite reaction.

Krebs evaluated 155 men with androscopy and found lesions between 1 and 45 mm in diameter (median 3 mm).[24] Eighty-seven percent had lesions on the penile prepuce near the frenulum, 42% had involvement of the penile shaft, 20% had lesions on the glans, 11% had lesions on the corona, 6% had lesions on the urethral meatus, 6% had lesions on the urethra, 5% had lesions on the scrotum, 2% had lesions along the crural fold, 1% had lesions on the symphysis pubis, and 3% had lesions in the anus.

No lesion in the male genital area is analogous to leukoplakia in the female genital area. Occasionally, chronic perianal dermatitis in men can become lichenified and appear white before the application of 5% acetic acid. However, the process is more diffuse and generalized rather than focal, as leukoplakia is in women.

Pearly penile papules (PPPs), frequently observed around the glans corona, are 1- to 3-mm excrescences that may be misinterpreted as condylomata acuminata by patients and clinicians (Figure 24-6). *Unlike condylomata, PPPs are smooth and white before application of 5% acetic acid.* They have no clinical significance and are a normal variant. The frenulum may also exhibit papular lesions that appear wartlike. When in doubt, a biopsy should be performed.

Unlike colposcopy in the female, there are few reliable colposcopic signs to differentiate SIL from simple HPV lesions in men.[45] Leukoplakia and mosaic changes are virtually never observed. Classic punctation is also rarely seen, and on the male genitalia it more closely resembles the punctate vascularity seen with verrucae of the hands and feet. SILs of the male genitalia, are likely to be slightly hyperpigmented or inflamed. *The only reliable way to define the nature of penile lesions is by biopsy.* Bowen's disease (squamous cell carcinoma *in situ* or penile intraepithelial neoplasia [PIN]) is generally indistinguishable from a classic wart (Figure 24-7). Bowenoid papulosis lesions are multiple and erythematous

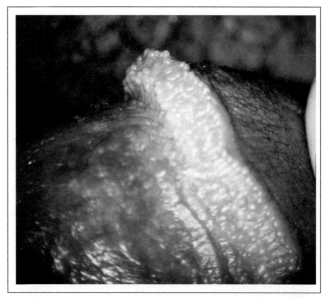

Figure 24-6 Penile pearly papules along the corona of the penis. (Courtesy of the National Procedures Institute, 2007.)

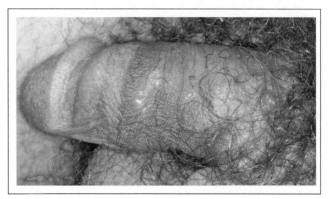

Figure 24-7 PIN 3. (Courtesy of the National Procedures Institute, 2007.)

and occur on a thin, scaly base. *In patients younger than 40 years, this disease is usually considered benign and self-limited. In patients older than 40 years, bowenoid papulosis is considered a cancer precursor. The diagnosis can be made only by biopsy.*[46]

Erythroplasia of Queyrat is another name for carcinoma *in situ* or PIN 3 that generally occurs under the foreskin (Figures 24-8 and 24-9). Although the lesions may have been present for years and may be similar in appearance to benign condylomata acuminata, the presence of friability and ulceration should raise the suspicion of penile carcinoma that can resemble a condyloma.

BIOPSY

Biopsy of a lesion on the male genitalia is obtained using sharp tissue scissors (small, curved Metzenbaum scissors), a scalpel blade, a dermal curette, or a radiofrequency loop electrode (Figure 24-10). It is not necessary to biopsy a typical condyloma before treatment, but *lesions that do not resolve after two treatment sessions should be biopsied to differentiate them from verrucous carcinoma or condylomata lata of syphilis.*

Most biopsies of the penis, scrotum, perineum, and perianal areas are readily obtained. First, the involved skin is

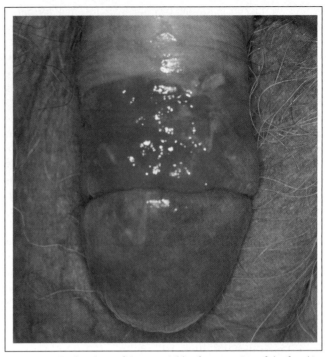

Figure 24-9 Erythroplasia of Queyrat visible after retraction of the foreskin. (Courtesy of the National Procedures Institute, 2007.)

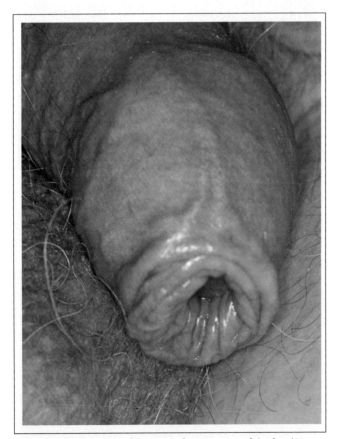

Figure 24-8 Erythroplasia of Queyrat before retraction of the foreskin. (Courtesy of the National Procedures Institute, 2007.)

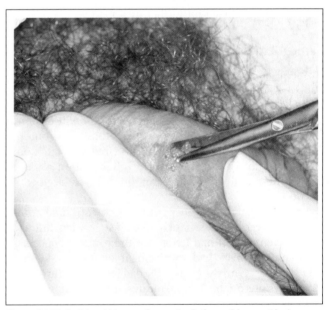

Figure 24-10 Excisional biopsy of a penile shaft condyloma with sharp tissue scissors. (Courtesy of the National Procedures Institute, 2007.)

pinched between the thumb and the index finger to tent the tissue and the lesion. Next, 0.1 to 0.2 mL of 2% lidocaine without epinephrine is injected with a 30-g needle. The lesion is then simply snipped off with scissors, curetted away, or shaved off with a scalpel blade. A 3-mm tissue sample is sufficient for histologic diagnosis. With large lesions, radiofrequency excision may be used. Bleeding is generally minimal and may be controlled with either direct pressure or application of Monsel's solution or aluminum chloride. At times, Monsel's solution or silver nitrate can leave a stain on the skin, of which the patient should be advised.

A biopsy obtained with a dermatologic punch biopsy instrument or a cervical biopsy forceps may excise too deep a sample on the male genitalia. Intra-anal lesions, on the other hand, are most readily biopsied or excised using a small cervical biopsy forceps. The flexible sigmoidoscopy biopsy forceps also makes an excellent biopsy tool when inserted through the anoscope. Urethral meatal lesions are generally not biopsied unless they fail to respond to treatment.

TREATMENT

In placebo-controlled studies, genital warts clear spontaneously in 20% to 30% of patients within 3 months.[41]

There is little benefit to attempting to eradicate all mildly acetowhite findings on the male genitalia. Asymptomatic, flat, faintly acetowhite changes on the male genitalia do not require treatment and rarely need biopsy for diagnostic confirmation. The goal of treatment in men should be to eliminate visible or symptomatic lesions, to educate the patient about the disease process, and to discuss methods to prevent recurrence and spread. Examination with magnification allows recognition of small lesions, making them easier to treat. It also ensures removal of entire lesions. However, studies have shown that even after the most aggressive treatments, residual HPV DNA can be detected.[47] Therefore the eradication of all evidence of HPV should not be a goal of treatment.[48]

Methods of treatment in men are similar to those in women (Table 24-4), although no head-to-head comparisons have been studied.[49-51] If only a few small lesions are present, it is quicker to remove them by a method similar to that described for biopsy.

Topical Therapies (Patient Applied)

Imiquimod and podofilox cost about $200 to $250 per month to treat average-sized lesions. A second month's use is frequently required. Patients can apply these preparations, thus reducing the number of office visits. Imiquimod is an immune enhancer and works through a different mechanism than that of podofilox, which is a caustic agent and is the purified active ingredient of podophyllin.[41,52,53]

Use of 5-fluorouracil cream has been described in three situations: for lesions of the urethral meatus, for perianal lesions, and prophylactic use to reduce recurrence following treatment with other modalities. No comparative studies are available, and use is limited because of potential ulceration. Imiquimod may prove to be a better agent for this indication, with fewer side effects.

Topical Therapies (Clinician Applied)

Another effective treatment for condylomata is 85% TCA. The preparation is inexpensive but must be applied by the clinician every 1 to 3 weeks. For small lesions, the wooden end of a cotton-tipped applicator is dipped in TCA solution and then applied to the lesions. For larger areas, the cotton-tipped end of the applicator is used. On application, the tissue immediately turns a snow-white color (Figure 24-11). The application site may burn intensely for 5 minutes. Applying TCA quickly to all lesions may minimize the length of time of discomfort. *Use of topical anesthesia before treatment with TCA or vaseline to "protect the normal tissue" should be discouraged because it may actually protect the warts from the effects of therapy.* TCA does not need to be neutralized or removed after treatment, and the area may be washed after the patient arrives home without decreasing

Table 24-4 Treatment of Condyloma in the Male: Methods and Reported Efficacy

Medical	Efficacy
Trichloroacetic acid, 85%	81%
Podofilox, 0.5% liquid/gel	45–50%
Imiquimod cream	52%
Interferon injection	19–62%
Surgical	Efficacy
Cryotherapy	63–88%
Electrodesiccation	94%
Surgical removal (radiofrequency, curettage, shave)	93%
Laser	31–94%
Infrared coagulation	50–76%

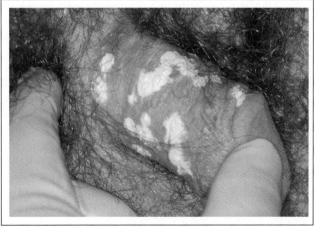

Figure 24-11 Appearance of penis after application of 85% TCA. (Courtesy of the National Procedures Institute, 2007.)

efficacy. The destruction of viable tissue occurs almost immediately, and sloughing occurs in a few days.

Interferon is rarely used except when all other modalities have failed. Drawbacks include its cost and frequent side effects.[41]

Most lesions may be treated with cryotherapy using a close-tipped nitrous oxide unit or liquid nitrogen. The close-tipped cryotherapy provides more control, but the liquid nitrogen is quicker. The latter can be applied with a small nozzle and a spray gun (Brymill or Wallach) or by dipping a cotton-tipped applicator into the liquid nitrogen and then applying it to the wart. For the treatment to be effective, an ice ball must form at least 3 mm beyond the lesion. After the treated area thaws, immediate re-treatment will enhance effectiveness. Depending on the amount of tissue to be treated, topical or injectable local anesthesia can be used. Scarring is rare, and the patient's potential to have and maintain an erection is not compromised. Some hypopigmentation may result. After treatment the area may become edematous, and bullae may form. The bullae may later slough, producing an open lesion. The bullae may be left intact or removed. The efficacy of treatment varies among reported studies.

Surgical Treatment

Condylomata may be removed using any of a number of surgical techniques. Before the application of any of these modalities, the skin must be anesthetized. Two percent lidocaine without epinephrine is injected superficially with a 30-g needle just beneath each lesion. For extensive penile lesions, a dorsal penile block or ring block may be used. Additional anesthesia is used at the frenulum because this area is particularly difficult to anesthetize.

For smaller lesions, the methods described previously for biopsy work best: sharp tissue scissors or a sharp dermal curette (disposable). When larger lesions exist, more aggressive intervention is needed.

Laser ablation of external lesions is highly effective when properly used and has excellent cosmetic results. Drawbacks include the high cost of equipment and the need for greater operator expertise. HPV and HIV have been documented in laser smoke plumes, so suction filter devices are essential if this modality is selected for treatment.[57,58]

Electrodesiccation and surgical excision using radiofrequency current may be used for lesions on male external genitalia. These are the same units used to perform loop excision procedures, but shorter shanks and smaller derm loops are substituted. The equipment is less expensive, and the technique is easier to master than laser ablation. For ablation of smaller lesions, the electrosurgical unit (ESU) is set at the coagulation mode. All lesions are merely touched with a 3- to 5-mm ball electrode. The desiccated warts can be wiped away. Any residual tissue can be identified with magnification and then cauterized. Electrodesiccation works best for small lesions. Larger lesions generally require a radiofrequency excision technique.

Radiofrequency excision is best performed under direct colposcopic guidance. The area is anesthetized as discussed previously. The high-frequency ESU is set in *cutting* mode at 15 to 20 watts. As noted, a short-shank dermatologic loop electrode is used to excise the lesion. *The skin on the penis is very thin, and care must be taken to maintain a very superficial excisional plane and to not penetrate too deeply.* Only the smallest lesion should be removed with a single pass. The excision should proceed slowly, layer by layer. Initially, the condylomata may bleed significantly, especially when they are large. However, bleeding stops as all the abnormal tissue is removed. There is enough coagulation, even in pure cutting mode, to stop the minor bleeding. Monsel's solution or aluminum chloride can be used to control any residual bleeding that is not controlled with pressure (Figures 24-12 and 24-13).

Although condylomata may be removed surgically using sharp tissue scissors or by shaving them with a scalpel, the tendency is to go too deep unless the lesions are small.

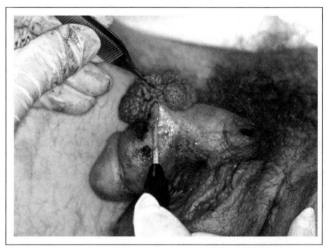

Figure 24-12 Removal of large penile condyloma using radiofrequency surgery. (Courtesy of the National Procedures Institute, 2007.)

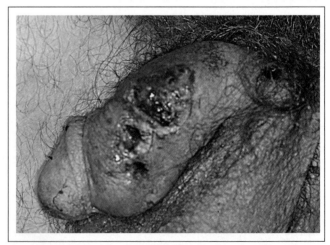

Figure 24-13 Postradiofrequency surgery of large penile condyloma. (Courtesy of the National Procedures Institute, 2007.)

Surgical excision with suture closure is almost never indicated for simple condyloma treatment.

A device called the *infrared coagulator* (Redfield, Montvale, NJ) has received FDA approval for treatment of external lesions. The treatment uses an intense beam of light. The automatic timer controls depth of penetration. The usual setting is 0.75 to 1 second. The unit tip is simply applied to the lesion, and the trigger is pulled. Several applications may be needed to treat an entire lesion if it is large. The treated area immediately turns white and eventually sloughs. Postoperative treatment is the same as for other destructive modalities.

PIN does not always require treatment unless it is severe (PIN 3). When it is treated, any of the previously noted methods may be used, although comparative studies are lacking for outcomes.

Figure 24-14 summarizes options for treatment of lesions of the male genitalia.

POSTOPERATIVE INSTRUCTIONS

Topical anesthetics (e.g., 5% lidocaine ointment) are effective for treatment of postoperative discomfort. A moist healing environment can be obtained with use of over-the-counter antibiotic ointments (e.g., Bacitracin) or petroleum jelly. The treated (denuded) area should be washed three to four times daily with mild soap and water, followed by application of ointment as often as needed to keep the area moist. Ointment also helps prevent clothing from adhering to the tissue. If the patient complains of itching and redness with vesicle formation, a neomycin allergy should be suspected and the patient should be switched to an antibiotic ointment without neomycin.

It is best to schedule a follow-up examination in 2 to 4 weeks to ensure that all lesions have resolved and to treat any lesions that may have appeared in the interim.

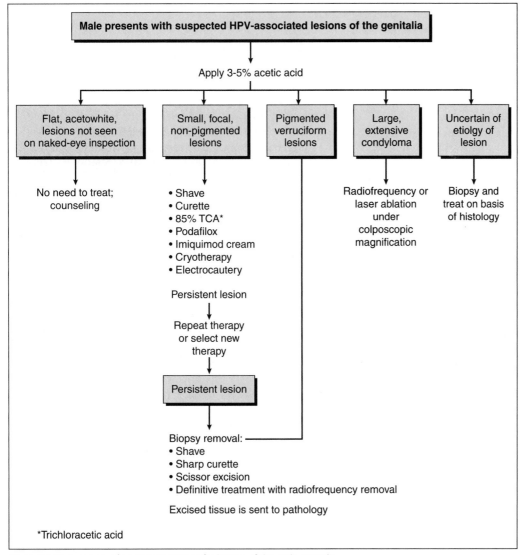

Figure 24-14 Summary of treatment options for lesions of the male genitalia.

COUNSELING

Men should be discouraged from smoking. Smoking increases the risk of penile cancer.[5] Three mechanisms have been postulated: passive smoking effects, agents in tobacco smoke that adhere to the male's fingers and are introduced into vaginal mucus during vaginal and clitoral stimulation using the fingers, and contaminated semen and/or seminal fluid.[57-60]

Monogamy prevents new exposure to other HPV types. Patients infected with non-oncogenic HPV types (HPV 6 or 11) risk exposure to high-risk HPV types (HPV 16 or 18) with each new sexual contact.

It is unknown whether males have the same psychosocial distress as some women with HPV. Asking the patient about anxiety, depression, and other manifestations of distress related to diagnosis and treatment of HPV is advised.

Condom use should be discussed with the patient, but it is important to note that because HPV is a multicentric disease in both men and women, a condom is not fully protective (see previous discussion). However, it should be stressed that condoms will protect against other STIs, including HIV, Chlamydia, and gonorrhea while providing contraceptive benefits.[61] Mutually monogamous partners do not need to continue to use condoms for HPV *protection*.

MANAGEMENT SCENARIOS

Scenario 1

An 18-year-old male presents with five acuminate lesions on the penis that are each 3 to 4 mm. He desires treatment.

Suggested approach: A health and sexual history are obtained. The penis, perineum, and perianal areas are stained with 5% acetic acid. After 5 minutes, the patient is examined with a handheld lens or colposcope at low power. A colposcope may identify smaller lesions that were not seen with the naked eye. A simple method of treating condylomata is to grasp them with pickups and excise them with tissue scissors, being careful to stay in a superficial plane. The penile skin is very thin. Excised specimens are sent to pathology for evaluation. Bleeding is controlled with Monsel's solution, aluminum chloride, or electrocautery. Another approach would be to use cryotherapy or electrocautery with a small ball electrode. Alternatively, one of the topical methods (either patient- or provider-applied) can be used. The patient is generally seen for follow-up in 4 to 6 weeks and re-examined to ensure that all lesions have been removed. He is advised to inform his sexual partner and if female, she should have regular cervical cytology screening.

Scenario 2

A 40-year-old male presents with 25 to 30 condyloma involving the penis and perianal areas. The lesions are 3 to 10 mm each. They have been present for 3 to 5 years. The patient is a smoker.

Suggested approach: An effective method of treating extensive condylomata is to excise them with radiofrequency excision. This technique uses the same equipment as that used to perform a loop excision procedure. Five percent acetic acid is applied to the external genitalia. Two percent lidocaine without epinephrine is used for anesthesia, either to inject the lesions individually (0.52–1 cc) or to use as a dorsal penile block. Additional lidocaine can be placed in a ring block fashion. The frenulum area may need a supplemental injection. The total amount of lidocaine should be no more than 10 cc. Under colposcopic magnification, with a smoke evacuator in place, all lesions are removed using a pure cutting mode. The penile skin is very thin, and use of the colposcope allows controlled removal of the lesion. The loop electrosurgical excision procedure (LEEP) electrodes are not used because they are large and the shafts are long. Short, dermal loops are preferred. Lesions are removed using a *feathering* technique. All lesions should not be removed with a single pass, which often goes too deep. All tissue is sent to pathology for histologic review.

Case 3

A 65-year-old male presents with a lesion under the foreskin. His wife died 20 years previously, and he has had a 2-year relationship with a woman who notices a lesion under the foreskin. He comes in for evaluation. He does not know how long the lesion has been present.

Suggested approach: The foreskin is withdrawn, and a velvety patch of erythematous skin, 10 × 5 mm, is identified on the superior aspect of the penis, just proximal to the corona. The nature of the lesion is uncertain, and a biopsy is indicated. Two percent lidocaine without epinephrine is used for anesthesia (0.5–1 cc). The skin is pinched and a small *snip* biopsy, using tissue scissors, is obtained. The tissue is sent to pathology. Bleeding is controlled with pressure, light ball cautery, aluminum chloride, or ferric subsulfate (Monsel's solution). Pathology returns as erythroplasia of Queyrat (carcinoma *in situ*). A ball cautery could be used to destroy the lesions. These lesions are generally responsive to 5-flurourocil, but treatment may be very uncomfortable, and there are no data to support its use for this indication. Any lesions that fail to resolve must be excised.

Case 4

A 20-year-old male presents with concerns about "white lumps around the rim of his penis." He is concerned about HPV. He has had multiple partners, none of whom have had abnormal Pap smears or condyloma.

Suggested approach: Five percent acetic acid is applied to the external genitalia, and the patient is examined with a handheld lens or colposcope. The only lesions that are identified are at the corona and are small, 2- to 3-mm white papules. They appear *milia-like*. The lesions are believed to be penile pearly papules (PPP), but the patient insists that they be biopsied. After injection of 0.5 to 1 cc of 2%

lidocaine without epinephrine, tissue scissors are used to remove one of the characteristic lesions, which is sent to pathology. Histology confirms PPPs, and the patient is reassured that this is a variant of normal. No treatment is necessary.

REFERENCES

1. von Krogh G. Clinical relevance and evaluation of genitoanal papillomavirus infections in the male. Semin Dermatol 1992;11:229–240.
2. Fine RM. The penile condyloma-cancer connection. Int J Dermatol 1987;26:289.
3. Weiner JS, Liu ET, Walther PJ. Oncogenic human papillomavirus type 16 in association with squamous cell cancer of the male urethra. Cancer Res 1992;52:5018–5023.
4. Noel JC, Vandenbossche M, Peny MO. Verrucous carcinoma of the penis: importance of human papilloma typing for diagnosis and therapeutic decisions. Eur Urol 1992;22:83–85.
5. Malek RS, Goellner JR, Smith T, et al. Human papillomavirus infection and intraepithelial-in-situ, and invasive carcinoma of the penis. Urology 1993;42:159–170.
6. Bosch FX, Castellsague X, Munoz N, et al. Male sexual behavior and human papilloma DNA. J Natl Cancer Inst 1996;88:1060–1067.
7. Munoz N, Castellsague, Bosch FG, et al. Difficulty in elucidating the male role in cervical cancer in Columbia, a high risk area for the disease. J Natl Cancer Inst 1996;88:1068–1075.
8. Boon ME, Susanti I, Tache MJ. Human papillomavirus (HPV): association of male and female genital carcinoma in a Hindu population. Cancer 1989;64:559–565.
9. Brinton LA, Jun-Yao L, Shon-De R, et al. Risk factors for penile cancer: results from a case control study in China. Int J Cancer 1991;47:504–509.
10. Scinicariello F, Rady P, Saltzstein D, et al. Human papillomavirus 16 exhibits a similar integration pattern in primary squamous cell carcinomas of the penis and in its metastases. Cancer 1992;70:2143–2148.
11. Poblet E, Alfaro L, Ferdander-Segoviano P, et al. Human papillomavirus associated with penile squamous cell carcinoma in HIV-positive patients. Am J Surg Path 1999;23:1119–1123.
12. Palefsky JM. Anal cancer and its precursors: an HIV-related disease. Hosp Phys 1993;1:35.
13. Daling JR, Weiss NS, Klopfenstein LL, et al. Correlates of homosexual behavior and the incidence of anal cancer. J Am Med Assoc 1982;247:1988–1990.
14. Xi LF, Critchlow CW, Wheeler CM, et al. Risk of anal carcinoma-in-situ in relation to human papillomavirus type 16 variants. Cancer Res 1998;58:3839–3844.
15. Frisch M, Fenger C, van den Brule AJ, et al. Variants of squamous cell carcinoma: cancer of the anal canal and perianal skin and their relation to human papillomavirus. Cancer Res 1999;59:753–757.
16. Noffsinger A, Witte D, Fenoglio-Preiser CM. The relationship of human papillomaviruses to anorectal neoplasia. Cancer 1992;70:1276–1287.
17. Goldie SJ, Kuntz KM, Weinstein MC. The clinical effectiveness and cost-effectiveness of screening for anal squamous intraepithelial lesions in homosexual and bisexual HIV-positive men. J Am Med Assoc 1999;281:1822–1829.
18. Barasso R, DeBruge J, Croissant O, et al. High prevalence of papilloma-associated penile intraepithelial neoplasia in sexual partners of women with cervical intraepithelial neoplasia. N Engl J Med 1987;317:916–923.
19. Zabbo A, Stein BS. Penile intraepithelial neoplasia in patients examined for exposure to human papillomavirus. J Urol 1993;41:24–26.
20. Schneider A, Sawada E, Gissmanb L, et al. Human papillomavirus in women with a history of abnormal Papanicolaou smears and in their male partners. Obstet Gynecol 1987;69:554–562.
21. Blythe JG, Cheval MJ. Colposcopy of condylomatous men. Missouri Med 1989;86:31–34.
22. Winer RL, Lee SK, Hughes JP, et al. Genital human papilloma virus infection: rates and risk factors in a cohort of female university students. Am J Epidemiol 2003;157:218–226.
23. Marrazzo JM, Kontsky LA, Stine KL, et al. Genital human papillomavirus infection in women who have sex with women. J Infect Dis 1998;178:1604–1609.
24. Krebs HB. Management of human papillomavirus-associated genital lesions in men. Obstet Gynecol 1989;73:312–316.
25. Wikström A, Hedblad MA, Johansson B, et al. The acetic acid test in evaluation of subclinical genital infection: a competence study on penoscopy, histopathology, virology and scanning electron microscopy findings. Genitourinary Med 1992;68:90–99.
26. Pfenninger JL. Androscopy: a technique for examining men for condyloma. J Fam Pract 1989;29:286–288.
27. Sedlacek TV, Cunname M, Carpineilla V. Colposcopy in the diagnosis of penile condyloma. Am J Obstet Gynecol 1986;154:494–496.
28. Epperson WJ. Androscopy for anogenital HPV. J Fam Pract 1991;33:143–146.
29. Epperson WJ. Preventing cervical cancer by treating genital warts in men: why male sex partners need androscopy. Postgrad Med 1990;88:229–236.
30. Newkirk GR, Grannath BD. Teaching colposcopy and androscopy in family practice residencies. J Fam Pract 1990;31:171–178.
31. Patton D, Rodney WM. Androscopy of unproven benefit. J Fam Pract 1991;33:135–136.
32. Strand A, Rylander E, Wilander E, et al. HPV infections in women with squamous intraepithelial neoplasia and/or high risk HPV. Acta Derm Venereol 1995;75:312–316.
33. Rosemberg SK, Greenberg MD, Reid R. Sexually transmitted papillomavirus in men. Obstet Gynecol Clin North Am 1987;14:495–512.
34. Christopher A. Hearing addresses condoms for HPV prevention. J Natl Cancer Inst 2004;96:985.
35. Holmes KK, Levine R, Weaver M. Effectiveness of condoms in preventing sexually transmitted infections. Bull World Health Organ 2004;82:454–461.
36. Zenilman JM, Weisman CS, Rompalo AM, et al. Condom use to prevent incident STD's: the validity of self-reported condom use. Sex Trans Dis 1998;22:15–21.
37. Winer RL, Hughes JP, Feng Q, et al. Condom use and the risk of genital human papillomavirus infection in young women. N Engl J Med 2006;354:2645–2654.
38. Krebs HB, Helmkamp B. Treatment failure of genital condyloma acuminata in women: role of the male sexual partner. Am J Obstet Gynecol 1991;169:337–339.
39. Comite SL, Castadot MJ. Colposcopic evaluation of men with genital warts. J Am Acad Dermatol 1988;18:1274–1278.
40. Krebs HB, Helmkamp B. Does the treatment of genital condyloma in men decrease the treatment failure rate of cervical

dysplasia in the female sexual partner? Obstet Gynecol 1990;76:660–663.

41. Human papillomavirus infections. Morbid Mortal Wkly Rep 1993;42:83.

42. Pfenninger JL Androscopy. In: Pfenninger JL, Fowler GC (eds). Pfenninger and Fowler's Procedures for Primary Care, 2 ed. Mosby, 2003, pp 913–917.

43. Gazzaniga P, Vercillo R, Gradilone AT, et al. Prevalence of papillomavirus, Epstein-Barr virus, cytomegalovirus, and herpes simplex virus type 2 in urinary bladder cancer. J Med Virol 1998;55:262–267.

44. Burmer CG, True LD, Krieger JN. Squamous cell carcinoma of the scrotum associated with human papillomavirus. J Urol 1993;149:374–377.

45. Demeter LM, Stoler MH, Bonnez W, et al. Penile intraepithelial neoplasia: clinical presentation and an analysis of the physical state of human papilloma DNA. J Infect Dis 1993;168:38–46.

46. Habif TP. Pre-malignant and malignant non-melanoma skin tumors and sexually-transmitted viral infections. In: Habif TB (ed). Clinical Dermatology: A Color Guide to Diagnosis and Therapy, ed 3. St Louis: Mosby, 1996, pp 297–345, 649–687.

47. Riva JM, Sedlacek TV, Cunnane MF, et al. Extended carbon dioxide laser vaporization in the treatment of subclinical papillomavirus infections of the lower genital tract. Obstet Gynecol 1989;73:25–30.

48. Richart R. Men and HPV. Prim Care 1995;8:5.

49. Ling MR. Therapy of genital human papillomavirus infections. Part I: indications for the justification of therapy. Int J Dermatol 1992;31:682–686.

50. Kling A. Genital warts therapy. Semin Dermatol 1992;11: 247–255.

51. Maw RD. Treatment of anogenital warts. Dermatol Clin 1998;16:829–834, xv.

52. Beutner KR, Tyring SK, Trofatter KF Jr, et al. Imiquimod, a patient-applied immune-response modifier for treatment of external genital warts. Antimicrob Agents Chemother 1998;42: 789–794.

53. Kraus SJ, Stone KM. Management of genital infections caused by human papillomavirus. Rev Infect Dis 1990;6:S620–S632.

54. Garden JM, O'Banion K, Shelnitz LS, et al. Papillomavirus in the vapor of carbon dioxide laser-treated verrucae. J Am Med Assoc 1988;259:1199–1202.

55. Baggish MS, Poliesz BJ, Joret D, et al. Presence of human immunodeficiency virus DNA in laser smoke. Lasers Surg Med 1991;11:197–203.

56. Tokudome S. Semen of smokers and cervical cancer risk [letter]. J Natl Cancer Inst 1997;89:96–97.

57. Vincent CE, Vincent B, Greiss FC, et al. Some marital-sexual concomitants of carcinoma of the cervix. South Med J 1975; 68:552–558.

58. Brown DC, Pereira L, Garner JB. Cancer of the cervix and the smoking husband. Can Fam Physician 1982;28:499.

59. Whidden P. Cigarette smoking and cervical cancer [letter]. Int J Epidemiol 1994;23:1099–1100.

60. Thomas I, Wright G, Ward B. The effect of condom use on cervical intraepithelial neoplasia grade I (CIN I). Aust N Z J Obstet Gynecol 1990;30:236–239.

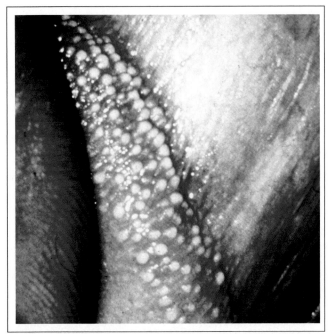

Plate 24-1 PPPs of the corona of the penis. (Courtesy of the National Procedures Institute, 2007.)

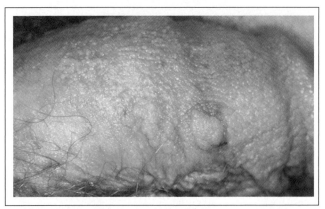

Plate 24-3 Single condyloma of the shaft; also, flat condyloma seen only after the application of 5% acetic acid. (Courtesy of the National Procedures Institute, 2007.)

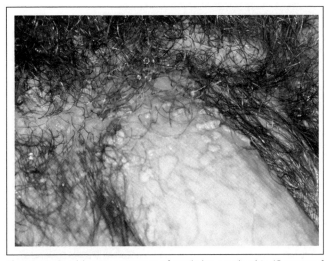

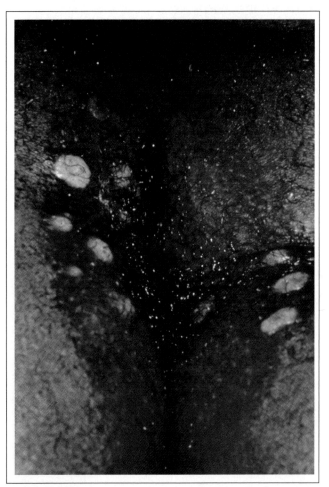

Plate 24-2 Condylomata acuminata of penile base and pubis. (Courtesy of the National Procedures Institute, 2007.)

Plate 24-4 Condyloma latum. (Courtesy of the National Procedures Institute, 2007.)

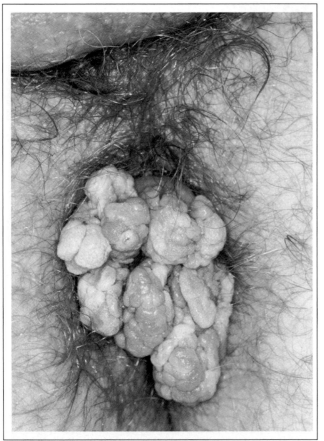

Plate 24-5 Large condylomata of the perianal area. (Courtesy of the National Procedures Institute, 2007.)

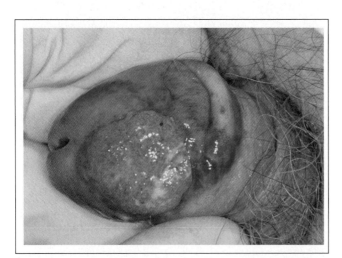

Plate 24-6 Large penile cancer of the glans. (Courtesy of the National Procedures Institute, 2007.)

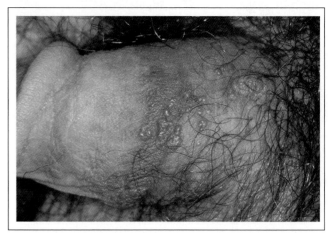

Plate 24-7 Condylomata acuminata of penis. (Courtesy of the National Procedures Institute, 2007.)

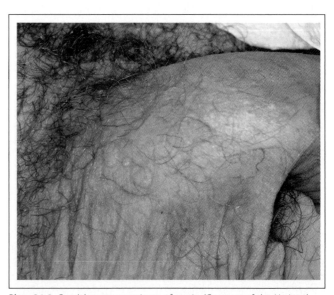

Plate 24-8 Condylomata acuminata of penis. (Courtesy of the National Procedures Institute, 2007.)

CHAPTER 25

Psychosocial Aspects of Colposcopy

Dennis J. Butler • Gregory L. Brotzman

Advances in the detection and treatment of premalignant disease have dramatically reduced the incidence and mortality of cervical cancer. However, this decline has been accompanied by an increase in the recognition of precancerous conditions. With this progress there has been an increased focus on the psychological and emotional reactions of women with abnormal cervical cytology and those referred for colposcopy. *It is now very evident that screening, diagnostic procedures, and treatment may be the cause of a variety of complicated psychological reactions.*

Furthermore, patients' reactions have been found to play a determining role in their adherence to follow-up protocols. In some settings, as many as 45% of women with abnormal cervical cytology do not return for colposcopy or surveillance as recommended.[1,2] Because cervical cancer can be prevented with appropriate monitoring and treatment of precancerous conditions, it is essential to identify and overcome barriers to obtaining medical care.

When informed of an abnormal Papanicalaou (Pap) result, patients experience a heightened sense of vulnerability, uncertainty, fear, and anxiety.[3] It is the clinician's responsibility to reduce a patient's anxiety. However, many patients are not adequately counseled about abnormal cytology and the specific steps involved in diagnostic testing and follow-up. Well-designed patient information material can defuse anxiety and also increase patient participation in follow-up. A comprehensive approach is essential because barriers to compliance are multifactorial and include psychological, educational, logistical, and medical care components.

This chapter reviews the nature and types of reactions that women have to being told that they have an abnormal Pap test and examines preparation for colposcopy. At each step of the process, anticipatory and strategic interventions are identified and evaluated for appropriateness for those women who are at risk for psychological distress. A longitudinal approach is encouraged and emphasizes prevention of dysfunctional reactions to abnormal cytology, preparation for colposcopy, and ongoing care.

ABNORMAL CERVICAL CYTOLOGY

Annual Pap testing is routine for most women, and thus an abnormal result can have a profound psychological impact. There is well-established evidence of a range of emotional, psychological, behavioral, and social disruptions in the lives of women and their families following an abnormal Pap result. From these reports have come recommendations that physicians should anticipate such reactions and develop strategies for enhancing patient follow-up, methods for patient education, and suggestions for reassurance and support. Healthcare professionals can clearly play a role in modifying the psychological impact that abnormal cervical cytology has on patients and their partners.

When a woman learns that she has an abnormal Pap test, she experiences anxiety and a heightened state of apprehension, which has cognitive, emotional, and behavioral components.[3,4] At its most basic level, anxiety is a feeling of increased vulnerability and a sense of loss of control. It serves to alert the individual to a threat and mobilize coping skills. A limited amount of anxiety is appropriate and healthy if it motivates an individual to develop a plan of action. Excessive anxiety and intrusive worrying are associated with such reactions as denial, avoidance, and indecisiveness, which may interfere with compliance.

Two types of anxiety predominate in stressful or threatening medical situations. *Outcome anxiety* refers to patients' apprehension about their medical condition and its potential consequences. *Procedure anxiety* refers to patients' distress about the medical tests and procedures they expect to experience. *Outcome anxiety tends to surface with the abnormal finding, and procedure anxiety commonly increases as the date of the procedure approaches.*

Women with abnormal cervical cytology experience significantly higher anxiety when compared with controls.[3] In some cases, their anxiety has been found to be higher than patients awaiting breast biopsy results and similar in severity to women following an abnormal serum screening for fetal anomalies.[5,6] Patients awaiting colposcopy were also found to have significantly higher anxiety than nonreferred (surveillance) patients.[4,7] Although levels of anxiety are heightened and significant, typically they do not reach the criteria for psychiatric illness.[8]

The routine nature of cervical cytologic screening may actually serve to intensify anxiety when an abnormal result occurs. Patients expect a normal result, and an abnormal finding causes an alteration in their self-perception, making "patients" of people who are asymptomatic and feel well.[9] The disclosure of abnormal cytology can precipitate reactions of depersonalization ("This isn't happening to me!") marked by disbelief and mild to moderate dissociative reactions.

The most common outcome fears that women experience with abnormal cervical cytology include the fear of having cancer, particularly cervical cancer.[10–12] A second fear is that an abnormal cytology is an indication of infertility. A third fear is that a loss of sexual response or functioning will occur.

Although the latter fears can be anticipated, other sensitive concerns are more difficult to elicit. Feelings of guilt may stem from a belief that the abnormal result is punishment for sexual activity or indiscretions.[13] Other women believe they have somehow infected sexual partners or, indirectly, family members.[14] Patients have also attributed abnormal cytology to chance, early sexual activity, use of oral contraceptive pills, pregnancy, and previous infections.[8]

In-depth interviews with women who were told of an abnormal Pap test have uncovered a deeper psychological impact. These women report an experience described as a feeling of "bodily betrayal."[15] This can be understood as a disturbance in the patient's image of self that results in a reduction in her confidence to confront the demands of the abnormal findings. Self-descriptions include viewing oneself as less attractive, tarnished, unclean, or let down by one's body.[8,13] As part of this disruption of self-image, women also report a diminished view of their sexual attractiveness. The feeling of bodily betrayal forces many women, for the first time, to confront their own mortality.

Initial reactions to an abnormal Pap result can be difficult to identify because they are suppressed by the shock of an unexpected result, because they develop over time, and because logistical issues and information sharing are emphasized. Symptomatic reactions may be more accessible on direct inquiry and include sleep disturbance, irritability, depressed affect, crying episodes, outbursts of anger, weight change, loss of interest in sexual activity, and disruptions in sexual relationships.[10,11] Women interviewed about their reactions typically used such affective terms as *worried, nervous, fearful, upset, shocked, panicked, horrified,* or *feeling alone.* Symptomatic reactions are prevalent with as many as 25% of women reporting impairment in daily activities, 50% reporting impairment in sexual interest, and 40% reporting disruption in sleep patterns.[10] One fifth of patients with abnormal results report distressing levels of anxiety prior to their colposcopy.

Another reason that reactions can be difficult to identify is because women may be reluctant to disclose the extent of their anxiety.[16] Disclosure can be inhibited by women's reactions to how they have been told of the abnormal result.[17] Women who perceive that the physician is impersonal will disclose less. Thus, one should not assume that a nonanxious response is adaptive.

The intensity of a woman's reactions cannot always be viewed as a direct response to the news of an abnormal result. Women may have underlying factors including psychiatric difficulties or disrupted relationships that may intensify their reactions.[8] Concurrent stressors such as work, family, other health problems, school responsibilities, financial difficulties or limited social support may also complicate the reaction to abnormal cytology. *Abnormal cytology has also been found to have a reciprocal effect in that the distress of the abnormal Pap result reactivates or intensifies concurrent stressors.*[3,11]

The impact of an abnormal Pap test can have persistent effects. Three months after being told of an abnormal Pap test, some women continued to report elevated levels of anxiety, fear of cancer, and impairment in mood, activity, sexual interest, and sleep patterns.[10]

INTERVENTIONS

The physician's primary task with the woman who has an abnormal Pap test is to acknowledge her distress and encourage appropriate follow-up. *Noncompliance with follow-up is a critical concern and is found among all groups of patients but is highest among women who are young, unmarried, poorly educated, or of lower socioeconomic status.*[18] Unfortunately, those at greatest risk for cervical disease are not only the least likely to be screened, but also less likely to adhere to recommended diagnostic procedures when an abnormality is detected.[2] *Patient involvement in care is associated with improved adherence, greater satisfaction with providers, better understanding of medical details, improved coping, and improved quality of life. Noncompliance may create a self-defeating cycle in which failure to comply sustains uncertainty and distress, which in turn contributes to delay in follow-up.*

Because Pap tests are usually normal, physicians and patients often have a false sense of security prior to the examination.[16] It may be helpful to provide anticipatory guidance through foreshadowing in which the woman is alerted that results may be abnormal but that effective interventions are available.[8] Furthermore, it is also important to inform women that abnormal cytology infrequently implies cancer and that most women are managed with surveillance or low-impact interventions. Identifying support personnel within the clinician's office can also be a source of reassurance in the event of an unexpected result. Forewarning can reduce the initial reactions of shock, disbelief, and the feeling of impending doom that occur when a woman first learns her cytology is abnormal.

Outcome and procedure anxiety can be reduced by providing information, education, support, and reassurance. To alleviate anxiety it is useful to focus on the objective features of the threat, such as the risk factors, and the reasons for further diagnostic steps or treatment options. Although it is not productive to focus exclusively on emotional responses, it is important to elicit the woman's reaction and be supportive in acknowledging her distress.[2]

Information provided to patients should highlight areas known to impede compliance. These include fear of cancer, fear of losing sexual or reproductive functioning, and aversion to medical procedures. Written patient education material has been found to be cost-effective, reduce anxiety, and encourage positive attitudes.[19] This effect even extends to low-effort interventions. For example, women receiving an informational booklet by mail reported less anxiety than those not receiving this information.[17] However, on a cautionary note, providing information may increase knowledge but not reduce anxiety. Providing information best reduces anxiety if it fosters a sense of control over the outcome. Considerations in developing patient information material about abnormal Pap tests include the amount of information, ease of reading, extent of focus on procedures, and extent to which the disease process is highlighted. Brief, simple information may be most effective in reducing anxiety.[6]

When deciding what information to provide patients, three questions should be considered: How much does the patient know, how much would she like to know, and how much does she want to be involved?[20] Some women prefer avoidance and distraction as a means of coping with stressful situations. Thus *providing a patient with written material is not a guarantee that she will read it or understand it or*

that it will serve to reassure her.[21] *In some cases, it might be counterproductive.*[22]

Preparatory information is most beneficial when a woman's preference for information is matched with the amount and specificity of the information she receives. Women who would like to be more informed tend to ask more questions, and women who request written information tend to be more involved in their care.[23] Those women who ask more questions report higher levels of confidence in their care after the examination. However, educational level and social status may also affect the balance of the physician-patient interaction. Less-educated women tend to ask fewer questions and be less assertive during visits in which their Pap results are discussed.[23]

Women may have difficulty understanding the information they receive if healthcare professionals fail to make their recommendations clearly or if they use technical, unfamiliar, or vague terms. *Even terms such as "colposcopy" and "precancerous" have been misunderstood or misinterpreted by patients. For example, patients may interpret "precancerous" as meaning they have an early form of cancer and will eventually die of their disease.*[2] Other research has discovered that patients are confused by procedures and believe that they have had a colposcopy when the speculum was inserted for a normal pelvic examination or that they had a colposcopy when the Pap test was done.[24] Thus, although patients should be encouraged to ask questions, this may be insufficient to assure that they understand key information. *It is helpful if the clinician clearly indicates that abnormal cytology is not a confirmation of cancer but rather is a finding that requires further investigation.*

The success of interventions that provide information about cervical cancer has been documented primarily with higher socioeconomic groups. More intensive specialized efforts are necessary for groups at high risk for noncompliance. Studies of nonadhering groups have found that barriers to follow-up extend beyond a lack of information about results and procedures. These additional barriers include fatalism and hopelessness about cancer, forgetfulness, transportation difficulties, childcare needs, time constraints, conflicting health beliefs, and cultural differences.[2] Many women at high risk for noncompliance have had multiple impersonal or dissatisfying experiences with the healthcare system and have turned to self-care.

Another strategy that has proven successful in modifying poor compliance has been structured telephone counseling.[25] Low-income minority women who had missed a scheduled initial colposcopy appointment received a telephone contact that addressed informational, psychological, and logistical barriers to keeping appointments. *A 15-minute contact was highly effective in addressing the barriers and improved adherence to follow-up. A telephone counseling intervention with high-risk groups is more effective than a telephone confirmation, which is in turn better than standard reminders.*[25,26]

The self-reported tendency to forget appointments is an especially powerful predictor of noncompliance.[25,27] Research suggests that providing telephone reminders to "forgetful" patients can reduce rates of nonadherence. The clinician can ask patients directly whether they tend to be forgetful or whether they can predict their likelihood of compliance. Once patients have identified impediments to follow-up, problem-solving strategies can be individually tailored. For example, once the impediment of transportation difficulty was identified by a group of patients, providing transportation assistance was the most successful intervention for improving attendance at appointments.[27]

Social support also plays a role in managing the distressing emotions that arise when a patient is told that a cervical cytology is abnormal.[12] Support can be of four types: emotional, instrumental (resources), informational, or offering advice. For many medical conditions, patients turn to their reference groups for support, but in studies of women with abnormal Pap results, family and partners are not universally viewed as resources.[4] Elements that inhibit seeking support include the absence of a close partner, stigma, embarrassment discussing anatomy, fear of sexual rejection, and the belief that male partners are disinterested, uninformed, or unable to understand. Failure to inform partners has been reported by more than one fourth of patients. However, after being informed, partners report they experienced increased worry, sought further information, and encouraged their partner to schedule the colposcopy. *Clinicians should encourage women with abnormal cytology to consider disclosure to trusted partners, friends, or family.*

COLPOSCOPY

Although public service educational efforts have improved awareness of the need for annual cervical cytology, women remain less informed about colposcopy. When women's sources of information about colposcopy were examined, it was found that although friends and family were a source of information about cervical cytology, they knew far less about colposcopy.[29] Most women reported that the limited information they had about colposcopy came exclusively from physicians or nurses during brief office encounters. Thus they attend appointments with many unanswered questions.

Individual interviews reveal that patients referred for colposcopy experience four major reactions. Patients had a general sense of something wrong with their health; they were apprehensive about the procedure; they experienced persistent uncertainty about the meaning of an abnormal cytology; and they were confused about the process of referral.[28] In studies of minority women, one fourth had no idea what a colposcopy was, and more than half did not know what having an abnormal Pap test meant or what could be found by colposcopy.[24,29]

Additional investigations suggest that informational deficits are further complicated by the woman's lack of understanding of her basic anatomy. Many women referred for colposcopy do not know the location of the cervix or the site of the Pap testing.[24] Many were unaware that more than

one biopsy might be taken, that an examination of the vulva might be involved, or that the colposcope itself did not enter the vagina.

Patients have expressed uncertainty about what will happen during the procedure and are concerned about pain or discomfort. They subsequently report feeling worried about the loss of sexual functioning or reproductive ability as a result of the procedure.[25] Their questions relate to the actual steps of the examination, the length of the exam, and any pain that may be involved.[28] They also ask questions about the use of the colposcope.

Although colposcopy has not been found to be a significantly painful experience, it may involve mild to moderate discomfort and transient pain. Nearly 50% of women who underwent colposcopy report having been tense and having experienced a fair amount of physical discomfort.[30] However, few studies have systematically examined the issue of pain. In a study of adolescents, they were observed to exhibit three to five behavior expressions of pain during the colposcopy.[31] Self-rated pain scores were found in another study to be significantly lowered with a nonsteroidal anti-inflammatory medication, but all subjects reported tolerating the procedure well.[32]

Long waiting time for the colposcopic examination may also increase anxiety and reduce compliance.[3,33] In one longitudinal study, one fourth of patients were reassured by the long wait, believing that it indicated they did not have a serious problem. However, another fourth expressed impatience and anger at delays in follow-up. Almost 1 year after colposcopy, one third of patients expressed dissatisfaction with the waiting time they had experienced. The clinic involved in the study subsequently reduced wait times for colposcopy to 2 weeks following referral.[8] *In general, scheduling an appointment within 1 month is recommended to foster compliance.* Appointments immediately after an abnormal Pap are likely to be helpful and increase patient satisfaction, but longer waits allow intervening variables to interfere with follow-up.

The completion of the colposcopic examination has been found to be effective in reducing the woman's anxiety.[4] However, some caution is warranted. Improvements in mood might be attributed to relief upon completion of a stressful medical procedure. Research indicates that as many as one fifth of patients remain highly anxious after colposcopy and that others experience heightened levels of anger, distressing thoughts, and avoidance.[34]

INTERVENTION

When information about colposcopy is provided, anxiety tends to decline and compliance improves. However, the timing of information sharing is important. Providing patient education at the colposcopy appointment can be time consuming and ineffective. There is much information to be shared, and patients are known to have a multitude of concerns. Thus anticipatory education and guidance is recommended.

In one study, most women preferred to be told details about colposcopy at the time they were told that they had an abnormal Pap test.[24] Another third of patients indicated they would prefer to receive educational materials and information after the results were discussed but before the procedure was performed. *When very anxious patients were told about colposcopy when their appointment was first scheduled, fewer than 10% were anxious at the time of the procedure.*[35]

The source of information about colposcopy is also relevant. For some women, the annual Pap test is done by the primary care practitioner, but an abnormal result requires referral to another specialist. Under such circumstances, women often prefer to receive colposcopy information from their primary care practitioner.[24]

Not all information about colposcopy is most effective when provided in advance. *Procedural* information is useful to answer a woman's questions about the length, timing, and technical aspects of colposcopy. Such information is most effective when provided in advance because it allows the patient to assess the situation and formulate questions.[36]

At the time of the exam, *sensory* and *behavioral* information should be emphasized. Sensory information orients the patient to the physical sensations that accompany the colposcopy procedure—what is seen, heard, touched, tasted, or smelled.[36] Behavioral information is advice about how patients can make themselves more comfortable or reduce discomfort during the procedure. Sensory and behavioral information should follow procedural information and are optimally effective when shared at the time of the colposcopy. The importance of orienting women to the sensory experience of colposcopy has been supported by extensive interviews. Women experiencing colposcopy for the first time lack an objective physical orientation to the physician's activities.

The experiences of women who have had colposcopic examination have been explored immediately after the procedure. Particular attention has been devoted to their views on how to improve the experience. They reflected little on the procedure but emphasized the need to modify interactional components. *These women expressed a strong desire to speak more with their physician about their concerns*[4,24] *and would have liked the physician to be more supportive and provide more individualized care. Furthermore, patients believed they would have benefited if more understandable terms had been used.* Finally, they wished that the results of the colposcopy had been reported personally rather than by mail or a phone message.

Because it is often difficult and logistically complicated to address the woman's reaction to an abnormal Pap test and colposcopy, clinicians can consider using a patient self-report inventory. The Psychosocial Effects of Abnormal Pap Smears Questionnaire (PEAPS-Q) consists of 14 items that focus on four areas of distress: reaction to the procedure, beliefs or feelings about the significance of the abnormal cytology and alterations in self-perception, worry about infertility, and effect on sexual relationships.[37] This instrument can provide a nonthreatening way to address sensitive concerns, and the clinician can target appropriate counseling and patient education.[30] Because the PEAPS-Q measures reactions after the colposcopy, the responses can be used for debriefing persistent anxiety, concerns, or misinformation.

Most attention about the psychosocial aspects of the abnormal Pap test and colposcopy has been devoted to patient variables (knowledge, anxiety, and compliance), physician–patient relationships, or environmental influences. From a systems perspective, two other considerations emerge. The first involves having a proactive, formalized tracking system for practice management. The second highlights the value of a collaborative, multidisciplinary approach to the patient.

Although clinicians recognize the importance of early intervention and scheduled surveillance, in a busy, multiple-physician environment, many variables interfere with follow-up. *Thus developing a formalized care algorithm and designing a systematic response is fundamental.* By identifying the flow of care and including multiple professionals from the clinic, "critical checkpoints" can be created to facilitate the assessment of the patient's progress.[38] Because of the complexity of the process, it may be necessary to develop a computerized tracking system that reminds women to return and prompts practitioners to respond with specific information and actions at each visit. It has been suggested that published noncompliance rates for colposcopy may actually be misleading because of poor tracking systems. Women may follow up at a better rate than reported but not within the practitioner's recommendations.[39]

The need to educate, reassure, counsel, and support the colposcopy patient begins at the time of the Pap test and continues through the colposcopy results (and subsequent treatment if necessary). Because of the time and effort involved, an individual clinician cannot address all dimensions of care. *The inclusion of a specialized nurse, patient educator, and/or counselor has proven effective in improving patient satisfaction and addressing patient concerns.* When such personnel is available, they are increasingly used, and nonscheduled contact with the physician decreases, patients' anxiety decreases, and patients' adherence to physician recommendations improves.[40]

The use of specific anxiety-reducing techniques such as progressive muscle relaxation or visual imaging has been considered for especially distressed patients. There is an absence of any systematic efforts to determine whether such techniques would be cost-effective in reducing colposcopy patients' anxiety. The use of structured cognitive-behavioral approach has been examined with equivocal results.[21] Although no significant differences were found for typically anxious patients, cognitive-behavioral training may have helped the most distressed patients.

A summary of goals for patient management is listed in Table 25-1.

Table 25-1 Goals of Patient Management to Reduce Anxiety and Increase Compliance

1. Provide accurate information (or correct misinformation) about abnormal cervical cytology.
2. Anticipate and address patient fears and concerns (e.g., cancer, infertility, loss of sexual functioning).
3. Reassure patients and decrease negative expectations.
4. Stress the importance of follow-up and problem-solve factors that contribute to noncompliance.
5. Develop a multidisciplinary approach to provide patient support, education, and clinical interventions.

REFERENCES

1. Lane DS. Compliance with referrals from a cancer-screening project. J Fam Pract 1983;17:811–817.
2. Miller S, Mishel W, O'Leary A, et al. From human papillomavirus (HPV) to cervical cancer: psychosocial processes in infection, detection and control. Ann Behav Med 1996;18:219–228.
3. Nugent LS, Tamlyn-Leaman K, Isa N. Anxiety and the colposcopy experience. Clin Nurs Res 1993;2:267–277.
4. Bell S, Porter M, Kitchner H, et al. Psychological response to cervical screening. Prev Med 1995;24:610–616.
5. Scott DW. Anxiety, critical thinking and information processing during and after breast biopsy. Nurs Res 1983;32:24–28.
6. Marteau TM, Kidd J, Cuddleford L. Reducing anxiety in women referred for colposcopy using an information booklet. Brit J Health Psych 1996;1:181–189.
7. Jones MH, Singer A, Jenkins D: The mildly abnormal cervical smear: patient anxiety and choice of management. J Royal Soc Med 1996;89:257–260.
8. Gath DH, Hallam N, Mynors-Wallis L, et al. Emotional reactions in women attending a UK colposcopy clinic. J Epidem Comm Health 1995;49:79–83.
9. Posner T. Ethical issues and the individual woman in cancer screening programmes. J Advances Health Nurs Care 1993;2:55–69.
10. Lerman C, Miller S, Scarborough R, et al. Adverse psychological consequences of positive cytologic cervical screening. Am J Obst Gyn 1991;165:658–662.
11. Beresford J, Gervaize P. The emotional impact of abnormal Pap smears on patients' referral for colposcopy. Colp Gynecol Laser Surg 1986;2:83–87.
12. Lauver R, Baggot A, Kruse K. Women's experiences in coping with abnormal Papanicolaou results and follow up colposcopy. J Obstet Gynecol Neonat Nurs 1999;28:283–290.
13. Lehr S, Lee M. The psychosocial and sexual trauma of a genital HPV infection. Nurs Pract Forum 1990;1:25–30.
14. McDonald TW, Neutens JJ, Fischer LM, et al. Impact of cervical intraepithelial neoplasia diagnosis and treatment on self-esteem and body image. Gynecol Oncol 1989;34:345–349.
15. Rajoram S, Hill J, Rave C, et al. A biographical disruption: the case of an abnormal Pap smear. Health Care Women Int 1997;18:521–531.
16. Somerset M, Peters TJ. Intervening to reduce anxiety for women with mild dyskaryosis: do we know what works and why? J Adv Nurs 1998;28:563–570.
17. Wilkinson C, Jones JM, McBride J. Anxiety caused by abnormal results of cervical smear tests: a controlled trial. Br Med J 1990;300:440.
18. Michielutte R, Disecker RA, Young LD, et al. Noncompliance in screening follow up among family planning clinic patients with cervical dysplasia. Prev Med 1985;14:248–258.
19. Paskett ED, White E, Carter WB, et al. Improving follow-up after an abnormal Pap smear: a randomized controlled trial. Prev Med 1990;19:630–641.
20. Buckman R. How to Break the Bad News. Baltimore: Johns Hopkins University Press, 1992.
21. Richardson PH, Doherty I, Wolfe CD, et al. Evaluation of cognitive-behavioral counseling for the distress associated with an abnormal cervical smear result. Br J Health Psych 1997;2:327–338.
22. Miller S, Roussi P, Altman D, et al. Effects of coping style on psychological reactions of low income minority women to colposcopy. J Reprod Med 1994;9:711–718.
23. Barsevick AM, Johnson JE. Preference for information and involvement, information seeking and emotional responses of women undergoing colposcopy. Res Nurs Health 1990;13:1–7.
24. Nugent LS, Tamlyn-Leaman K: The colposcopy experience: what do women know? J Adv Nurs 1992;17:514–520.
25. Miller, SM, Siejak, KK, Schroeder CM, et al. Enhancing adherence following abnormal Pap smears among low-income minority women: a preventive telephone counseling strategy. J Nat Cancer Inst 1997;89:703–708.
26. Lerman C, Hanjani P, Caputo C, et al. Telephone counseling improves adherence to colposcopy among lower-income minority women. J Clin Oncol 1992;10:330–333.
27. Marcus AC, Crave LA, Kaplan CP, et al. Improving adherence to screening follow-up among women with abnormal Pap smears: results of a large clinic-based trial of three intervention strategies. Med Care 1992;30:216–230.
28. Tomaino-Brunner C, Freda MC, Runowicz CD. "I hope I don't have cancer": colposcopy and minority women. Oncol Nurs Forum 1996;23:39–44.
29. Massad LS, Meyer P, Hobbs J. Knowledge of cervical cancer screening among women attending urban colposcopy clinics. Cancer Detect Prev 1997;21:103–109.
30. Stinnet BA. Use of the Psychosocial Effects of Abnormal Pap Smears Questionnaire (PEAPS-Q) in a community hospital colposcopy clinic. J Lower Genital Tract Dis 2000;4:34–39.
31. Rickert VI, Kozlowski KJ, Warren AM. Adolescents and colposcopy: the use of different procedures to reduce anxiety. Am J Obstet Gynecol 1994;170:504–508.
32. Rodney WM, Huff M, Euans D, et al. Colposcopy in family practice: pilot studies of pain prophylaxis and patient volume. Fam Prac Res J 1992;12:91–98.
33. Jones MH, Singer A, Jenkins D. The mildly abnormal cervical smear: patient anxiety and choice of management. J Royal Soc Med 1996;89:257–260.
34. Palmer AG, Tucker S, Warren R, et al. Understanding women's response to treatment for cervical intraepithelia neoplasia. Brit J Clin Psych 1993;32:101–112.
35. Boag FC, Dillon AM, Catalan J, et al. Assessment of psychiatric morbidity in patients in a colposcopy clinic situated in a genitourinary clinic. Genitourinary Med 1991;67:481–484.
36. Barsevick AM, Lauver D. Women's informational needs about colposcopy. Image 1990;22:23–26.

37. Bennetts A, Irwig L, Oldenburg B, et al. PEAPS-Q: a questionnaire to measure the psychosocial effects of having an abnormal Pap smear. J Clin Epidemiol 1995;48:1235–1243.

38. Block B, Branham RA. Efforts to improve the follow-up of patients with abnormal Papanicolaou test results. J Am Bd Fam Prac 1998;11:1–11.

39. Patterson T, Roworth M, Hill M. An investigation into the default rate at the Fife clinic: implications for target setting. J Publ Health Med 1995;17:65–69.

40. Baxter K, Peters TJ, Somerset M, et al. Anxiety among women with mild dyskaryosis: costs of an educational intervention. Fam Prac 1999;16:353–359.

CHAPTER 26

Practical Therapeutic Options for Treatment of Cervical Intraepithelial Neoplasia

Mark Spitzer • Gregory L. Brotzman • Barbara S. Apgar

KEY POINTS

▪ The loop electrosurgical excision procedure (LEEP) excises the transformation zone (TZ) with high-frequency (radiofrequency) current using a thin electrode.

▪ Cutting during LEEP requires very high and continuous current density so that the water in the cell rapidly boils and the cell explodes. To accomplish this, the electrode must not come into direct contact with the tissue.

▪ The size and shape of the loop used should be tailored to the size and extent of the TZ and its extension into the endocervical canal.

▪ Complications of LEEP include intraoperative and postoperative bleeding or infection. An unsatisfactory colposcopy occurs in 1.3% to 9% of women after LEEP, and cervical stenosis occurs in 1.3% to 3.85% of treated women.

▪ LEEP appears to approximately double the risk that a woman will subsequently have preterm delivery, a low-birth-weight infant, or premature rupture of membranes, regardless of the size of the excised specimen.

▪ The CO_2 laser produces a monochromatic beam of light in the infrared portion of the spectrum that is coherent and collimated. At its focal point, the energy produced by the laser beam is sufficient to instantaneously boil the intracellular water of the tissue.

▪ In well-selected patients who are candidates for ablative therapy, cryotherapy can effectively treat all grades of CIN.

▪ Cryotherapy involves the cooling of tissue, usually with nitrous oxide, until cryonecrosis has occurred. Freezing of the tissue followed by thawing leads to formation of intracellular ice crystals, expansion of intracellular material, and rupture of the cells with subsequent denaturation of cell proteins.

▪ To ensure an adequate freeze, the ice ball formation should be no less than 5 mm beyond the edge of the cryoprobe.

▪ Cryotherapy may be accompanied by cramping of varying degrees. Most patients will experience a profuse, watery discharge for 2 to 3 weeks after the procedure. Cervical stenosis as a result of the procedure is rare.

▪ Cold-knife conization (CKC) is usually performed when large specimens are needed or when evaluation of the histology is critical and any thermal damage is not acceptable. Such instances include cases of suspected microinvasive carcinoma or adenocarcinoma *in situ*.

▪ Complications of CKC include intraoperative and postoperative hemorrhage, cervical stenosis, and increased pregnancy wastage.

LOOP ELECTROSURGICAL EXCISION

The loop electrosurgical excision procedure (LEEP), also known as electrosurgical loop excision and large loop excision of the transformation zone, has become one of the most common ways to treat cervical intraepithelial neoplasia (CIN), both in the United States and in the rest of the world. Modern electrosurgical units (ESUs) incorporate many advances that allow the surgeon to excise large specimens with a minimal amount of thermal damage and with a minimal risk of bleeding and other complications. Because it is cheaper, faster, and easier to learn and perform, LEEP has replaced laser surgery as the principal method for treating high-grade CIN.

LEEP was first developed in England as a substitute for ablative treatments of the cervix.[1] It was indicated in women who met the criteria for satisfactory colposcopy and therefore were candidates for ablative treatments of the cervix.[2,3] The ease with which LEEP can be done and the fact that it is easily done under local anesthesia with few short-term complications make it an ideal outpatient procedure.[2-4] Early proponents of LEEP recognized that removal of the entire transformation zone (TZ) was theoretically less subject to false-negative results than colposcopy, which might be subject to a misdirected biopsy. In fact, early reports indicated that 1% to 2% of women undergoing LEEP were found to have microinvasive or invasive cancer where none was suspected before the procedure.[2-5] This result, combined with the ease of the procedure, the high patient acceptability, and the low morbidity rate, fostered initial enthusiasm for using a "see and treat" approach rather than colposcopy for all women with abnormal Papanicolaou (Pap) smears.[2,3,6] In this approach, women with abnormal Pap smears were evaluated with LEEP rather than with colposcopy and directed biopsy. Unfortunately, early reports of this approach showed that many women had either very minor abnormalities on their LEEP specimens or only negative metaplastic or inflammatory changes.[7,8] In the United States today, most clinicians use LEEP only after first confirming the histologic grade of disease with a colposcopically directed biopsy.[4,7,9] In the United Kingdom, LEEP is reserved for women whose smears show a high-grade squamous intraepithelial lesion (HSIL) or who have a significant colposcopic lesion extending into the endocervical canal.

Electrosurgical Physics

Modern ESUs must be distinguished from older Bovie units that treated cervical disease by heating and cauterizing the tissue. ESUs apply an alternating current to tissue. Common household current alternates at 60 Hz. Stimulation of nerve and muscle by an alternating current (termed *faradic effects*) occur maximally at frequencies between 10 and 100 Hz. These faradic effects cause muscular tetany and may result in electrocution. However, at frequencies above 2500 Hz, these effects gradually diminish, and above 300 kHz, they are essentially absent. This is why *modern ESUs operate at a frequency between 500 kHz and 4 million Hz and are known as* radiofrequency generators.

All electrical current flows in a closed circuit, and the electrical current always seeks to return to its source. Older ESUs transmitted electricity directly from an electrical outlet and returned it to that outlet (return to ground). Such units placed the patient at risk for alternative pathway burns when the electricity flowing from the ESU through the patient found an alternative path to ground through a conductive substance that inadvertently became grounded (such as a dangling piece of jewelry or an electrocardiogram lead). The electrical current could become focused in that area, causing a burn. *In modern ESUs, passing the main power through a transformer isolates it. In such isolated units, "grounding" the patient does not close the electrical circuit, and no alternative pathway exists through which electricity can flow, eliminating the risk of alternative pathway burns. Only ESUs with such isolated circuitry should be used.*

To properly use electrosurgery, it is important to understand the types of electrosurgical effects one is likely to see. *Desiccation occurs when the electrode is in direct contact with the tissue.* The temperature within the cells rises slowly to less than 100° C. Water evaporates from the cells, and cellular proteins coagulate. Hemostasis results from the drying of blood and the contraction of small blood vessels.

Cutting occurs when the temperature within the cells rises quickly to more than 100° C. The water in the cells rapidly boils, and the cells explode. This requires very high and continuous current density, meaning that the current produced by the ESU must be focused in a very small area. This occurs principally when the electrode is not in physical contact with the tissue and the electric current is traversing the gap between the electrode and the tissue (traveling in an *arc*). LEEP is ideally started with the electrode not in contact with the tissue. *As the tissue is vaporized, steam from the exploding cells forms a steam envelope around the loop. The steam envelope prevents contact between the electrode and the tissue and, combined with ionization of the steam in the electric field, facilitates formation of an arc. Moving the loop too quickly collapses the steam envelope and places the electrode* in direct contact with the tissue. This reduces the power density, and the electrosurgical effect reverts to desiccation rather than cutting. The loop stops cutting, and thermal tissue damage occurs. The observed effect is that the loop drags through the tissue and bends. Proper technique requires that the loop be moved slowly and continuously through the tissue being cut.

The final electrosurgical effect is *spray coagulation*. In this form of coagulation, the electrode does not make contact with the tissue, similar to electrosurgical cutting. *But because the current is interrupted rather than continuous, the steam envelope dissipates, resulting in protein coagulation, hemostasis, and destruction of lesional tissue. Tissue that has been subjected to spray coagulation cannot be used for histopathologic evaluation.*

During LEEP, the ESU is used in a monopolar arrangement. This means that the electricity passes from the electrosurgical loop through the body, back to the grounding pad or dispersive electrode, and then back to the ESU. Reducing the distance that the electricity needs to travel through the patient reduces the resistance encountered and minimizes the amount of electrical current needed to create the desired effects. Therefore the dispersive pad should be positioned as close as possible to the surgical site. The ideal site to place the dispersive pad during LEEP is on the upper thigh.

The amount of electricity flowing during LEEP is the same at the loop electrode and at the dispersive pad. *However, because the surface area at the dispersive pad is much larger, the power density (PD) is lower, and no electrosurgical effects occur at the dispersive pad.* Previous-generation dispersive pads that become partially detached pose a risk of electrosurgical burns at that area. Modern ESUs do not operate if the dispersive pad is partially detached.

Equipment

The equipment required for LEEP is listed in Table 26-1. *One should ensure that the ESU is a newer one with isolated circuitry and that the dispersive pad is of the type that prevents current from flowing if it is not properly applied.* These are important safety precautions that prevent unintended burns. The electrosurgical loop is made of a thin, flexible wire connected to an insulated traverse bar. The loop is fixed into a pencil-type holder. Current is activated either by pressing a button on the holder or by depressing a foot pedal. A thin wire allows a higher PD than does a thicker wire, and it produces less thermal damage to the tissue. Although, intuitively, a thicker and more rigid wire might be more desirable to prevent bending of the wire as it passes through the tissue, in fact the wire should not be making contact with the tissue at all. If the loop is seen to bend, it indicates that the operator is pushing the loop through the tissue too rapidly, causing the steam envelope to collapse and desiccating rather than cutting the tissue. Thicker loops also cause more thermal damage to the tissue. The insulated traverse bar prevents thermal damage to the surface epithelium as it is traversed by the loop. Loops are available in various sizes so that the size of the loop can be individualized to the width and depth of the lesion and the TZ. The traverse bar also limits the depth of excision.

Table 26-1 Equipment Needed for Loop Electrosurgical Excision

Electrosurgical generator

Patient grounding (dispersive) pad

Various sizes and shapes of loop electrodes

Ball electrodes (3- and 5-mm sizes)

Insulated electrode handle

Nonconductive speculum with smoke-evacuator port

Nonconductive vaginal sidewall retractor

Smoke evacuator and filter system

Colposcope

3–5% acetic acid or vinegar

Aqueous Lugol's solution (half strength)

Large cotton swabs

Local anesthetic with vasopressin (in the ratio of 10 units of vasopressin in 30 mL of 1% lidocaine)

Dental-type syringe with 27-gauge needles, 1.5 inches in length

Monsel's paste or gel

Specimen bottles with 10% neutral-buffered formalin

12-inch needle holder

2–0 resorbable suture material

The ball electrode used for cautery hemostasis also comes in varying sizes; usually 3 and 5 mm in diameter. The larger the electrode, the lower the PD. The electrode should be chosen on the basis of the desired effect.

The use of a nonconductive, rather than a metal, speculum prevents transmission of current from the electrode to the unanesthetized vagina. It is important to realize that although contact with a metal speculum will cause a brief shock to the patient, the large surface area of the speculum will likely disperse the current and prevent any burns. Even brief shocks are undesirable, however, because they may cause the patient to jump or move during the excision. The nonconductive speculum includes a smoke-evaluator port. Plastic tubing is placed in the port and then attached to the smoke evacuator unit. The evacuator unit removes the smoke generated in the vagina as the loop excision is performed. Without smoke evacuation, the operator cannot visualize the cervix during the excision.

Technique

As with all surgical procedures for CIN, LEEP is contraindicated in women with active cervical, vaginal, or pelvic infections and in women with known, frankly invasive cervical cancer. It should be used only with caution in women who are pregnant[10] or who have a known bleeding disorder. After informed consent is obtained, the patient is placed in the dorsal lithotomy position, and a nonconductive, coated speculum (or plastic speculum) with smoke evacuation capability is placed into the vagina. Ideally, a vaginal

sidewall retractor will help protect the vaginal sidewall from inadvertent contact with the electrosurgical loop. However, if the vaginal walls are sufficiently distant from the cervix, a sidewall retractor may not be necessary. Three percent to 5% acetic acid is then applied to the cervix, and colposcopy is used to delineate the limits of the lesion. Because the acetic acid effect may be obscured by the injection of a local anesthetic, some have advocated painting the cervix with Lugol's solution to delineate the limits of the lesion before LEEP.

Once the lesion is visualized, an appropriately sized loop is chosen. *The size of the loop chosen should depend on the lateral extent of the TZ and how far the lesion extends into the endocervical canal.* Ideally, the entire TZ should be removed in one piece. However, when the TZ is very large and extends onto the portio of the cervix, it may not be possible to do so without unnecessarily removing too much cervical stroma. In such cases, the central portion of the TZ can be removed with a single sweep, and the remaining anterior and posterior segments of the TZ can be removed with a second, shallower sweep. If the colposcopist can confidently exclude invasion in the peripheral portions of the TZ, these areas can be desiccated or spray coagulated using the ball electrode after removal of the central conization specimen.

The dispersive pad is attached to the patient's upper thigh and to the ESU, and smoke evacuator tubing is attached to the speculum and smoke evacuator. As much as 10 mL of local anesthetic (in a ratio of 10 units of vasopressin in 30 mL of 1% lidocaine) is injected circumferentially into the cervix using a fine needle (27 gauge or finer). The injection should be superficial (only a few millimeters) and should cause the injection site to blanch (Figure 26-1).

The power setting needed to perform LEEP varies with the size of the loop chosen, the placement of the dispersive electrode, and the technique used. Furthermore, the settings on many ESUs (especially older ones) do not provide accurate representation of the unit's power output during a procedure. In general, the lowest power setting should be used that will allow the clinician to easily perform the procedure.

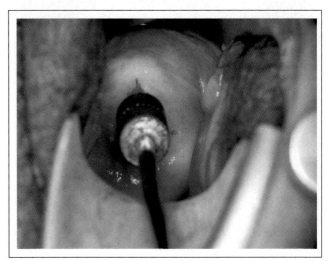

Figure 26-1 Injection of local anesthetic before cervical LEEP or laser surgery.

Lower power settings minimize thermal effects to the tissue, making the pathology specimen easier to interpret, and also reduce the discomfort experienced by the patient.

The procedure is always done under direct colposcopic guidance. The choice of which direction to pass the loop relates to the size and shape of the TZ, the position of the cervix, the amount of room in the vagina, and the laxity of the vaginal walls. The loop should be passed in the direction that makes the procedure easiest. The specimen can then be removed by one of two techniques. One technique begins by placing the tip of the loop approximately 3 to 5 mm beyond the peripheral margin of the TZ and not quite in contact with the cervical tissue (Figure 26-2). After the power is activated, electrical sparks can be seen arcing at the tip of the loop. The loop is then slowly plunged into the cervical stroma to the desired depth. When the colposcopy is satisfactory, the LEEP specimen needs to be 5 to 8 mm in depth. When the lesion or the TZ extends into the endocervical canal, or when the endocervical curettage (ECC) is positive, a deeper LEEP conization should be performed (discussed later). The loop is then brought underneath the TZ (Figure 26-3) and pulled out 3 to 5 mm beyond the peripheral margin of the TZ on the opposite side. The second possible technique begins by laying the loop over the TZ so that it encompasses the lesion, bending the loop slightly in the process. The power is then turned on. After a few seconds, the loop cuts into the cervix. When the wire straightens out, the loop is then brought under the remainder of the TZ and out theopposite side. Although this technique is a little easier, the fact that the loop initially makes contact with the cervix causes it to desiccate the tissue and causes more thermal damage at the ectocervical margin.

In cases where the TZ is not fully visualized, the lesion extends into the endocervical canal, or the ECC result is positive, a cone biopsy is indicated. LEEP can be used as a substitute.[4,11,12] In this case, a larger (deeper) loop may be

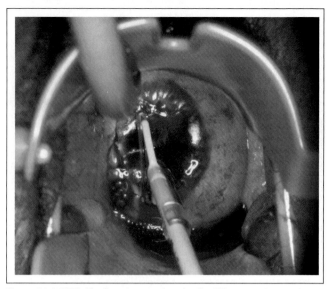

Figure 26-3 LEEP: The loop is passed under the TZ.

used. Alternatively, a shallow, superficial specimen can be obtained, followed by excision of a smaller endocervical specimen. *This so-called top hat technique has the advantage of removing less stroma than does a large LEEP conization. However, the small endocervical specimen frequently suffers from extensive thermal damage and may be uninterpretable histologically.*

Another approach to electrosurgical conization is the use of a device called a *Fisher cone* rather than a wire loop. In the Fisher cone, a fine wire is passed between the insulated stem and the insulated base of the device. The device comes in several sizes, and the angle that the wire makes with the central stem, coupled with the depth to which the device is pushed into the cervix, dictates the depth and width of the cone. When using the Fisher cone, one must take great care to ensure that the correct cone size is chosen. If not, the specimen may be too deep or insufficiently wide to remove the entire TZ. The procedure for electrosurgical conization using the Fisher cone is as follows: After the power is turned on, the wire is plunged into the cervix to its desired depth. The Fisher cone is rotated 360 degrees, using the central stem as a guide to follow the inner aspect of the endocervical canal. One disadvantage of the Fisher cone is that when the shape of the cervix or the TZ is irregular, the Fisher cone may remove too much or not enough tissue. Also, if the procedure must be momentarily interrupted because it is difficult to complete the rotation in one motion, restarting the current while the wire is within the cervical stroma may result in additional thermal injury to the specimen.

Once the cone specimen has been removed with a forceps (Figure 26-4), the defect is carefully cauterized using the ball electrode. *Most of the bleeding is usually found along the ectocervical edge.* For additional hemostasis, thickened Monsel's paste or gel may be applied to the base of the defect.

When fine wire loops are used, the cone specimen exhibits little thermal damage.[13-15] The cure rate for women

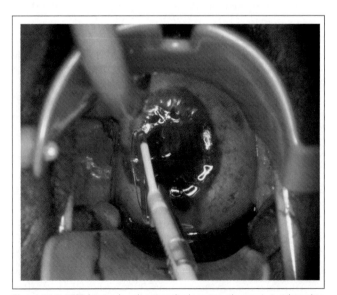

Figure 26-2 LEEP begins by plunging the loop into the cervix just lateral to the TZ.

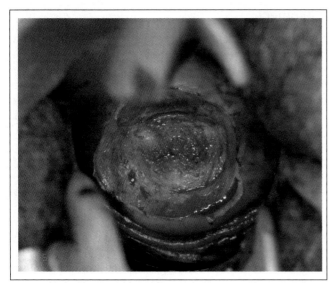

Figure 26-4 Appearance of the cone bed after the LEEP specimen has been removed.

treated with LEEP is comparable to that for women treated with laser or cold-knife conization (CKC) and depends on whether the conization margins are positive or negative. If the margins are negative, a cure rate of approximately 95% can be expected.[1–4,6,16,17] With positive endocervical margins, the cure rate is approximately 70%.[4]

Complications

After LEEP, the patient can expect a heavy, brown, and sometimes malodorous discharge for as long as 2 to 3 weeks.[3,18,19] *Immediate complications occur in 1% to 2% of cases and include heavy vaginal bleeding and infection.*[2–4,6,16,17] A higher rate of hemorrhagic complications occurs when greater amounts of cervical tissue are removed.[3,20,21] Because hemostasis is usually more tenuous immediately after a LEEP, the patient should avoid any heavy lifting or strenuous activity for at least 2 weeks after the procedure and should avoid inserting anything into the vagina for 4 weeks. Because the procedure removes a portion of the endocervical canal, blood flow during the first menses after the procedure may be much heavier than usual. To avoid alarm on the part of the patient, the procedure should be scheduled for immediately after menses, allowing maximal healing before the next menses, and the patient should be alerted to the possibility of heavy bleeding. Bleeding that comes at the time of the expected period should be managed expectantly. Heavy bleeding not associated with menses (heavier than the patient's normal menstrual flow) may need to be treated. If the patient is not hemorrhaging, she should reduce her degree of physical activity. If the bleeding persists, the patient should be examined, and any bleeding sites may be treated with electrocautery or with thickened Monsel's solution. *Clots adherent to the base of the crater should not be removed. They likely represent a vessel that was the source of the bleeding and has now clotted. Removing the clot will only cause the bleeding to resume.*

Postprocedure infection may present as malodorous discharge.[22] However, because discharge is very common in all women undergoing this procedure, distinguishing between a normal discharge and an infection may be difficult. The first indication of cervical infection may be delayed bleeding or delayed healing. Later complications include delayed bleeding and cervical stenosis. An unsatisfactory colposcopy occurs in 1.3% to 9% of women after LEEP, and cervical stenosis occurs in 1.3% to 3.8%.[3,6,16,18] An extreme example of cervical stenosis can be found in postmenopausal women undergoing LEEP, in women undergoing a second LEEP, or in those for whom the LEEP excision is very deep.[23] Cervical stenosis is avoided by having endocervical cells that are stimulated by estrogen. In each of these cases, a necessary element is missing. In postmenopausal women not taking hormone replacement therapy, the endocervical cells are not stimulated because of the hypoestrogenic state. Women undergoing deep conization or repeat conization are at risk for removal of all of their endocervix, leaving nothing to be stimulated by estrogen.[23] In both cases, these women are at risk for cervical os obliteration. When some endocervix remains, stenosis might be prevented by daily application of vaginal estrogen for as long as 1 month after surgery.[23] Little can be done to prevent cervical stenosis when most or all of the endocervical tissue has been removed. Earlier studies suggested that the fertility of women is probably unaffected after a single LEEP.[24–27] However, recent studies have highlighted the potential negative impact of LEEP on subsequent pregnancies. *LEEP appears to approximately double the risk that a woman will subsequently have preterm delivery, a low-birth-weight infant, or premature rupture of membranes, regardless of the size of the excised specimen.*[28,29] Large or repetitive LEEPs may further increase the risk of infertility related to cervical factors, such as cervical stenosis or poor-quality or scanty cervical mucus.

CARBON DIOXIDE LASER

Throughout the 1980s, the carbon dioxide (CO_2) laser became an increasingly more popular modality for treatment of cervical disease. Until the advent of LEEP, the CO_2 laser represented the most versatile and effective tool available for the treatment of CIN. It offered the advantages of a high cure rate,[30,31] the ability to treat almost any extent and grade of disease, the ability to vaporize or excise tissue as needed, excellent healing, and a low complication rate.[32,33] The major disadvantages of the CO_2 laser were the cost of equipment and the need for more extensive physician training. These disadvantages led to diminished use of the CO_2 laser once LEEP became available. Today, *most clinicians reserve CO_2 laser for specific cases in which its versatility offers advantages over LEEP.*

The term *laser* is an acronym for *l*ight *a*mplification by *s*timulated *e*mission of *r*adiation. The CO_2 laser produces a monochromatic beam of light in the infrared portion of the spectrum that is coherent (all waves are exactly in phase with one another) and collimated (all rays are parallel to one another). This allows the beam to be focused through the use of a series of lenses and mirrors. At its focal point, the energy produced by the laser beam is sufficient to instantaneously boil the intracellular water of any tissue with which it comes into contact. The tissue is thus vaporized, producing a crater at the point of contact.

Laser Physics

The amount of energy applied to the tissue is a product of the relationship of two factors. One factor is the energy output of the laser, measured in watts (W). The other factor is the size of the laser spot, measured in square centimeters (cm²). The PD is the unit used to measure the energy that the laser applies to a given area of tissue. The PD is calculated with the formula $PD = 100 \times W/cm^2$. At low PD, the tissue is heated more slowly, and heat is conducted to adjacent tissue, resulting in thermal injury. The amount of heat conducted to the adjacent tissue is directly related to the amount of time that the laser is applied to the tissue. Because a laser used at a lower PD needs more time to achieve its desired effect, it also allows more time for the heat to be conducted to the adjacent tissue and for that tissue to be damaged by the heat. In tissue that has been irreversibly damaged by the heat but not vaporized by the laser, the appearance of cell death is delayed. However, the heat generated by the laser at lower PD also has advantages. It helps achieve hemostasis by coagulating blood and tissue proteins and contracting and sclerosing smaller vessels. The use of a lower PD also allows the operator greater control over the depth of vaporization.

When tissue is subjected to high PD, the tissue will instantaneously vaporize, allowing little time for heat to be conducted to adjacent tissue and minimizing the zone of thermal injury. However, at higher PD, the laser vaporizes tissue very rapidly, forcing the operator to keep the beam in constant rapid motion to avoid the inadvertent creation of deep craters. *The use of lower PD allows the operator greater control over the depth of vaporization. The challenge to the clinician is to use the laser at the highest possible PD that will still allow control of the effects of the beam. Clinicians with greater experience and skill are able to use higher PD and to achieve better and more predictable results.*

Three zones of tissue injury are described when tissue is subjected to laser vaporization. In the innermost zone of the vaporization crater, the tissue has been vaporized. In the next layer, the tissue has been heated and subjected to lethal thermal injury but not vaporized. This tissue will eventually slough. It is this zone that is of greatest concern to the clinician because the extent of devitalized tissue is not apparent at the time of surgery and becomes apparent only later. In the most peripheral zone, the tissue has suffered nonlethal thermal injury. Although the extent of damage is not immediately apparent at the time of surgery, this tissue will recover. The main challenge of CO_2 laser surgery is to minimize the zone of lethal thermal injury and, to some extent, the zone of nonlethal thermal injury, while maintaining control of the depth of laser vaporization.

Equipment

Today, most CO_2 lasers are completely self-contained portable units that may be used in the hospital or office. The size and price of the machine usually relate to the amount of power it is able to generate, but most lower genital tract procedures can be done with machines generating between 20 and 40 W. Because the wavelength of the beam is 10.6 μm (in the invisible infrared portion of the electromagnetic spectrum), CO_2 lasers must have an additional aiming beam. This is usually a second, very-low-power, helium-neon aiming laser beam. The beams are produced by the lasers in the base cabinet and are transferred via a series of mirrors and lenses through an articulated arm to the colposcope. A micromanipulator is attached to the colposcope and allows the clinician to view the laser beam through the colposcope and to control it via a joystick. *When treating lower genital tract lesions with the CO_2 laser, colposcopic magnification and guidance and a micromanipulator must always be used. It is inappropriate to use the laser as a handheld device in this application because this approach deprives the clinician of the control necessary to obtain optimal results.*

One important feature of the micromanipulator is its ability to vary the spot size of the laser. The clinician is able to raise the PD by narrowing the spot size and to lower the PD by using a larger spot size. This ability allows the clinician to easily balance the extent of thermal injury, the speed at which the tissue is being vaporized, and his or her degree of control by using the visible effect on the tissue as a guide.

The equipment required for a laser surgical procedure is listed in Table 26-2. Because of the smoke generated by laser procedures, they should always be done in a well-ventilated room, using a high-efficiency smoke evacuation and filtration device. Before vaporizing tissue, the laser must first vaporize any liquid covering the tissue, so moist gauze pads may be used to protect the area surrounding the operative field from inadvertent laser injury. However, because all laser surgery in this area is done under direct colposcopic guidance, many experienced laser surgeons do not find this precaution necessary. Because the laser beam will be reflected by any shiny surface, laser instruments (speculums, retractors, and manipulators) should all be blackened and nonreflective. For manipulating the cervix, a manipulator with a short, right-angle hook is most effective. Curved hooks are more difficult to use.

Technique

The CO_2 laser can be used as either a vaporization tool or a cutting tool. For a vaporization tool, larger spot sizes are used. The laser is usually set at a high-power setting, and the spot size used is the largest one that will still allow a good balance among tissue vaporization, thermal injury, and control of the laser. In the cutting mode, the spot size is reduced to its narrowest diameter, allowing use of very high PD, even though the overall power output by the laser may be somewhat lower. *At such high PD, tissue vaporization is very rapid, and there is little thermal injury but also little*

Table 26-2 Equipment Needed for CO_2 Laser Surgery

CO_2 laser
Micromanipulator with variable spot size
Blackened nonreflective speculum with smoke-evacuator port
Blackened nonreflective vaginal sidewall retractor
Smoke evacuator and filter system
Right-angle skin hook
Colposcope
3–5% acetic acid or vinegar
Aqueous Lugol's solution (half strength)
Large cotton swabs
Local anesthetic with vasopressin (in the ratio of 10 units of vasopressin in 30 mL of 1% lidocaine)
Dental-type syringe with 27-gauge needles, 1.5 inches in length
Monsel's paste or gel
Specimen bottles with 10% neutral-buffered formalin
12-inch needle holder
2–0 resorbable suture material

CO_2, Carbon dioxide.

hemostatic effect. Control is often achieved by operating the laser in short bursts, manipulating the tissue, and then operating the laser again. Newer and more expensive lasers may have a super-pulse or ultra-pulse mode. In this mode, the laser generates very-high-power output for brief millisecond bursts, followed by a millisecond period of rest. The high power outage allows for vaporization and cutting of tissue with minimal thermal injury, whereas the resting allows the small amount of heat generated to dissipate and gives the operator greater control over the beam.

Three techniques are commonly used to treat cervical disease with the laser. When the TZ and the lesion are fully visualized, they may be vaporized, usually to a depth of 7 to 10 mm. *When the TZ is not fully visualized or the disease extends into the endocervical canal, a laser conization is done, using the laser to cut a cone-shaped specimen to be submitted for histologic evaluation.* The width and depth of the cone are tailored to the degree and extent of disease. When the disease extends well onto the portio of the cervix *and* into the endocervical canal, a combination conization is the ideal technique. The central portion of the TZ is excised to an appropriate depth as a CO_2 laser conization while the peripheral portion of the TZ, which usually contains lower-grade disease, is vaporized. This approach preserves cervical tissue and minimizes both long-term and short-term complications.

Most laser procedures can be done using a local anesthetic, and experienced laser surgeons can perform these procedures in the office setting. Only in rare instances, when the patient is extremely uncooperative or when the anatomy necessitates extreme amounts of manipulation, is it necessary to do such procedures with the patient under general anesthesia. Some clinicians premedicate the patient with ibuprofen before the procedure; however, this is not absolutely necessary.

As with all surgical procedures for CIN, laser surgery is contraindicated in women with active cervical, vaginal, or pelvic infections and in women with known, frankly invasive cervical cancer. It should also be used with caution in women who are pregnant or who have a known bleeding disorder, because blood, just like any other liquid, will interfere with the clinician's ability to achieve the desired tissue effect with the laser. When bleeding is encountered, the blood dissipates the laser energy, preventing it from reaching its intended target. *Because the fluid must be vaporized by the laser before it can sclerose the bleeding vessel, it is somewhat difficult to control brisk bleeding with the laser.* To control such bleeding, all excess blood is removed while a cotton-tipped applicator is used to control the bleeding by direct tamponade of the bleeding vessel. The laser is then used at the lower PD settings to vaporize and coagulate the tissue around the bleeding vessel. The cotton-tipped applicator is slowly rolled away as the laser beam is applied to the tissue and the underlying vessel. When the bleeding is brisk and difficult to temporarily control with focal tamponade, completion of the procedure with the CO_2 laser becomes increasingly difficult.

Laser Procedure

After informed consent is obtained, the patient is placed in the dorsal lithotomy position, and a black, nonreflective speculum with smoke evacuation capability is placed into the vagina. Diluted acetic acid is applied to the cervix, and colposcopy is used to delineate the limits of the lesion. Because the acetic acid effect may be obscured by the injection of local anesthetic, some have advocated painting the cervix with Lugol's solution to delineate the limits of the lesion. After injecting the local anesthetic (in a ratio of 10 units of vasopressin in 30 mL of 1% lidocaine), the laser is used at low PD to outline the areas to be vaporized or excised (Figure 26-5). Beginners may find it helpful to do this by tracing a series of dots using short bursts of the laser and then connecting the dots. More experienced laser surgeons will simply outline this area initially.

Vaporization Technique

The spot size is set at the largest spot that will allow the laser to generate between 500 and 1000 W/cm^2 and still permit the laser surgeon control to vaporize only the areas desired. Ideally, this can be estimated by observing the effects of the laser on the tissue. *When vaporized at an appropriate PD, the tissue in the crater should be mostly white, with small, well-dispersed flecks of black char* (Figure 26-6). The more black char that is seen, the lower the PD and the greater the thermal damage to the tissue. A complete absence of char means that the PD is very high, and the operator may find it difficult to control the laser or may have difficulty achieving hemostasis.

Every laser surgeon develops her or his own method for controlling the effects of the laser. Some use small, slow, overlapping, circular motions of the beam, whereas others

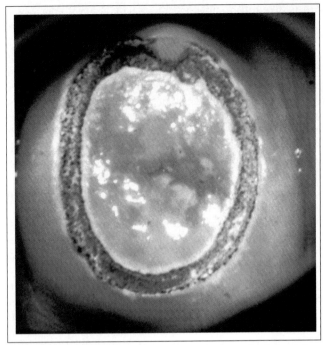

Figure 26-5 Circumference of a laser vaporization (or conization) as it is delineated by the laser. (Image courtesy of V. Cecil Wright, MD.)

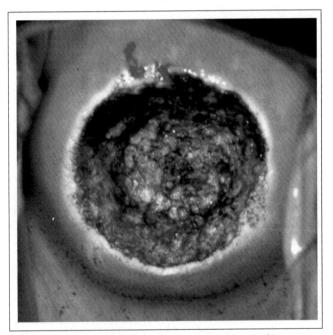

Figure 26-6 Appearance of the cone bed after completion of laser vaporization. (Image courtesy of V. Cecil Wright, MD.)

use rapid, back-and-forth oscillations of the beam. However it is achieved, the desired result is to avoid leaving the beam in any one spot for an extended period of time because this will create a deep crater in the tissue, and any bleeding at the base of this hole will be very difficult to control. The TZ is vaporized until a barrel-shaped defect that is 7 to 10 mm deep is achieved. A rod-shaped measuring device is used to measure the depth. A laser surgeon

may vaporize the stroma immediately surrounding the endocervix to a shallow depth. This will cause the endocervical mucosa to evert *(buttoning)*. The laser surgeon may then continue to vaporize 2 to 3 mm more of the endocervix *(clipping)*. This allows the laser surgeon to exercise some degree of control as to where the squamocolumnar junction (SCJ) will ultimately be located. The laser surgeon can locate the SCJ farther out onto the ectocervix by clipping less of the endocervix or locate it more in the endocervical canal by clipping more. After the vaporization is complete, excess char is gently swabbed out of the crater with large cotton swabs soaked in diluted acetic acid.

Excisional Conization Technique

After the peripheral margin of the cone is outlined with the CO_2 laser, the laser is set at 800 to 1200 W/cm^2 with the smallest possible spot size. The cervix is incised with the laser along the margin of the cone, to a depth of 3 to 5 mm. In narrower and deeper cones, this incision may need to be deeper. Wider and shallower cones may need a shallower incision. Traction is applied to the cut edge of the cone in one direction using a right-angle hook, and the laser beam is directed at the inner margin of the base of the incision (Figure 26-7). This procedure is repeated as traction is applied to the cervical cone sequentially in all directions, gradually undercutting the cone specimen. In an effort to minimize thermal damage to the endocervical portion of the cone, some authors have advocated making the last cut at the endocervical margin with a scalpel or scissors. Others, however, have found it acceptable to cut this margin with the laser at high power.[34]

Some authors follow excision of the cone specimen with ECC or an endocervical biopsy of the canal beyond the

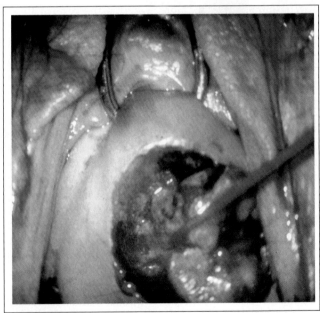

Figure 26-7 Laser excisional conization. The hook is retracting the cone specimen laterally so that the laser can excise it. (Image courtesy of V. Cecil Wright, MD.)

cone specimen. However, this practice is not shared by all. Creation of an endocervical button and clipping of the endocervical tissue may be done as described in the section on laser vaporization.

Combination Laser Cone Biopsy

In instances where the TZ or cervical lesion extends deep into the canal and out onto the portio, some have advocated doing a combination excision/vaporization cone biopsy. This procedure uses aspects of both procedures described previously. The central portion of the TZ is excised as a laser excision cone biopsy, and the outer portion of the lesion or TZ is vaporized as a laser vaporization cone. This minimizes the amount of tissue lost in the procedure (Figure 26-8).

Complications

The immediate postoperative problems seen with laser surgery of the cervix are the same as those seen with any other operative procedures and include bleeding and infection. *The rate of bleeding with laser surgery is less than that with CKC*[34-36] *and comparable to that expected with LEEP.*

As with LEEP, after laser surgery the patient can expect a heavy, brown, and sometimes malodorous discharge for as long as 2 to 3 weeks. Immediate complications occur in 1% to 2% of cases and include heavy vaginal bleeding and infection. As with the instructions for immediately after a LEEP, the patient should avoid any heavy lifting or strenuous activity for at least 2 weeks after the procedure and

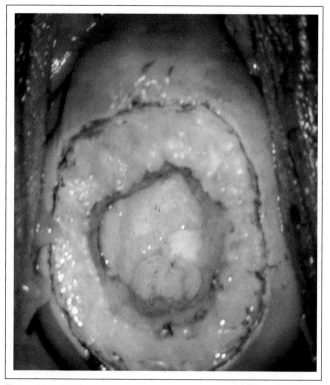

Figure 26-8 Combination laser conization. The laser has vaporized the outer aspect of the TZ. The inner cone specimen will be excised. (Image courtesy of V. Cecil Wright, MD.)

should avoid inserting anything into the vagina for 4 weeks. Blood flow during the first menses after the procedure may be much heavier than normal. Ideally, the procedure should be scheduled for immediately after menses, allowing maximal healing before the next menses, and the patient should be alerted to the possibility of heavy bleeding. At first, any bleeding other than hemorrhage should be managed expectantly. The patient should reduce her degree of physical activity, and if the bleeding continues the patient should be examined; any bleeding sites may be treated with Monsel's paste or gel. Clots adherent to the base of the crater *should not* be removed. They likely represent a vessel that was the source of the bleeding and is now clotted. Removing the clot will only cause the bleeding to resume.

Postprocedure infection may present as a malodorous discharge. However, because discharge is very common in all women undergoing this procedure, distinguishing a normal discharge from an infection may be difficult. Later complications include delayed bleeding and cervical stenosis. *Postmenopausal women or women undergoing a second procedure are at risk of cervical stenosis.*[37] *This may be prevented by treating the women with vaginal estrogen cream.*[23] Just like the experience with LEEP, earlier studies indicated that the fertility of women is probably unaffected following a single laser procedure.[38,39] However, *there is no reason to believe that the fertility-related complications seen in women undergoing LEEP procedures in later studies would not also be seen women undergoing laser procedures.* However, because of the recent popularity of LEEP procedures and unpopularity of laser, there have not been many recent studies that evaluated laser with the same sophistication as recent studies on LEEP. Also, large or repetitive laser procedures may increase the risk of infertility related to cervical factors, such as cervical stenosis or poor-quality or scanty cervical mucus.[39]

CRYOTHERAPY

Even in the midst of newer technologies such as laser and LEEP for the treatment of CIN, cryotherapy remains an effective therapeutic option for treatment of CIN in many patients. Cryotherapy has been used for more than half a century and has a proven efficacy and safety record.[40-45] *In well-selected patients who fit the criteria for ablative therapy, cryotherapy can effectively treat all grades of CIN.* The critical point in the effective application of cryotherapy for treatment of CIN is complete understanding of its limitations. Only patients in whom a high rate of cure can be expected should be treated with cryotherapy, whereas others should be treated with alternative modalities such as LEEP and laser surgery.

Cryotherapy Physics

Cryotherapy involves the cooling of tissue (usually with nitrous oxide) until cryonecrosis has occurred. Freezing of the tissue followed by thawing leads to formation of intracellular ice crystals, expansion of intracellular material, and rupture of the cells with subsequent denaturation of cell proteins. During cryotherapy, freezing of tissue results after formation of an ice ball. When nitrous oxide is used, the temperature at the tip of the cryoprobe is between −65° and −85°C. Cell death occurs at −20°C. At the margin of the ice ball, the temperature is 0°C. *The lethal zone is under the probe at the center of the ice ball and extends to a point 2 mm proximal to the margin of the ice ball.* Distal from that point to the margin of the ice ball is a recovery zone where the temperature of the ice ball is between 0° and −20°C. The extent of the lateral spread of the ice ball also gives a good approximation of the depth of the freeze. An ice ball that forms 7 mm lateral to the probe can be expected to have frozen the tissue about 7 mm deep to the probe. However, because the freeze is nonlethal in the last 2 mm, the freeze cannot be assumed to have treated disease any deeper than 5 mm.

Patient Selection

Histologic evaluations of cervical tissue have shown that the mean depth to which cervical glandular crypts are involved with dysplasia is 1.24 mm. This means that most of the time, when there is extension of dysplasia into the cervical glandular crypts, the disease will be within the depth that can be effectively treated with cryotherapy. However, some dysplasia involves deeper glandular crypts. *Destruction to a depth of 7 mm should eradicate involved crypts in more than 99% of cases.* It is for this reason that most authorities recommend treatment of dysplasia be at least 7 mm deep to maximize the cure rate. Cryotherapy does not reliably treat tissue to that depth. Although cryotherapy is usually effective in the management of CIN, because it usually destroys to a depth of 5 mm as well as 5 mm lateral to the edge of the cryoprobe,[46,47] others have demonstrated that the cure rate for high-grade disease may be lower. In one study in which tissue temperatures during cryotherapy were measured,[48] it was found that use of a small, flat probe could not eradicate disease located deep within glandular crypts. Because crypt involvement is a characteristic of high-grade lesions such as CIN 3, the study's author advocated that such cases be managed with excision rather than cryotherapy.

The location of lesional tissue may also play a role in the effectiveness of cryotherapy. Lesions at the 3- and 9-o'clock positions on the cervix have an increased blood supply from the cervical branches of the uterine artery. The blood flowing through the area warms the tissue and makes it slightly more resistant to reaching the critical lethal temperature with freezing. This reduces the cure rate.[47] Finally, *a large lesion (>two quadrants), a large cervix (>3–3.5 cm), and extension of disease into the endocervical canal all result in a reduced cure rate with cryotherapy.* It is not the grade of the lesion that determines effectiveness of therapy, but rather the size of the lesion being treated.[40,41,43] It has been demonstrated that if disease in the endocervical canal is treated with cryotherapy, the failure rate is higher.[41,50] In each case, the higher failure rate is related to the inability of the probe to freeze all the diseased tissue down to the critical lethal temperature.

Equipment

The equipment required for cryotherapy is listed in Table 26-3. Several types of cryosurgical units are available, with the basic components consisting of a tank of nitrous oxide with a pressure gauge, a handle, and a probe to apply to the cervix. Ferris and Ho reviewed the various cryotherapy units available in 1992.[51] The choice of a cryoprobe to be used depends on the size of the lesion and the morphology of the TZ. *Use of a flat cryoprobe or one with a small central nipple diminishes the possibility of cervical stenosis (Figure 26-9).* This type of probe will also be less likely to cause the SCJ to recess into the endocervical canal, which results in an unsatisfactory colposcopy on follow-up examination.[52–55] Large probes should be avoided on cervices with a portio diameter of less than 3 to 3.5 cm. It is important to use a large nitrous oxide tank with a pressure gauge and at least 20 pounds of pressure. This will allow for a faster and more

Table 26-3 Equipment Needed for Cryosurgery

Cryogun
Large nitrous oxide tank with a pressure gauge and at least 20 psi of pressure in the tank
Various sizes and shapes of cryotips
Water-soluble lubricating gel
Vaginal speculum
Colposcope
3% to 5% acetic acid or vinegar
Vaginal wall retractors
Disinfectant for cryoprobes

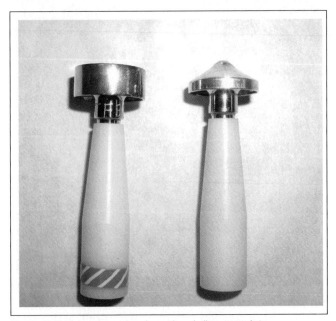

Figure 26-9 Flat probe and probe with a shallow central tip.

effective freeze. With smaller tanks, the pressure may drop below the critical level in the middle of the procedure, making it impossible to achieve an adequately sized ice ball. It is also important to have several cryoprobe tips available to choose from, including an assortment of shapes and sizes. This will allow the clinician to choose the appropriate size and maximize the chances of cure.

Technique

The best time to perform cryosurgery is 1 week after the start of the patient's menses. This ensures that the patient is not pregnant and allows the cervix to heal before the next menses. When cryosurgery is performed immediately before menses, the cervix may swell and block the menstrual outflow, causing cramping. If it is possible that the patient is pregnant, a pregnancy test should be performed before the procedure.

The patient is placed in the dorsal lithotomy position, and an intravaginal speculum is inserted. If the vaginal sidewalls prevent adequate visualization of the cervix, or if they are lax and overlap the cervix, a vaginal sidewall retractor should be used. This prevents inadvertent freezing of the vagina. Colposcopy is performed to confirm the absence of invasive disease. The nitrous oxide tank is activated, and the clinician should check the pressure gauge to confirm that the pressure in the tank is sufficient (at least 20 pounds with the indicator in the green zone) before starting the procedure. If the pressure is inadequate, the treatment will not be successful. A properly sized and shaped cryoprobe is selected, placed on the cryogun, and screwed tightly in place. An improperly secured probe tip can become a projectile when it is subjected to high pressure once the probe is activated. The gun is activated, and the O-ring on the stem is checked. If gas escapes around the contact area between the probe and the stem of the cryogun, the O-ring should be replaced.

The cryogun with the probe attached is inserted into the vagina and applied to the TZ to check whether the size of probe is adequate. *The probe should cover the TZ but not touch the vaginal sidewalls.* When treating a very large TZ, overlapping treatments may be needed. After the correct size of probe is determined, the cryogun is removed from the vagina, and a thin layer of lubricating gel is applied to the cryoprobe to create a sufficient seal with the cervix. The cryogun is placed on the cervix again and is activated to allow gas to flow into the unit. The patient should be warned that she will hear a pop and hiss as the cryogun is activated. The freeze should continue until at least a 7- to 10-mm ice ball is present outside the probe. Time is not as critical as formation of the ice ball because each cervix requires a different time to create the 7- to 10-mm ice ball formation. If the nitrous oxide tank has sufficient pressure at the start of the procedure, a sufficient freeze should be achieved in 3 to 5 minutes, with the time being somewhat less for the second freeze. Freezing for more than 5 minutes does not appreciably increase the size of the ice ball or improve outcome.[49] However, it is important to recognize that the total ice ball lateral spread of freeze of 7 to 10 mm is necessary to ensure a freeze depth of 5 mm.

Although this size of ice ball is ideal, the ice ball should be no less than 5 mm beyond the edge of the cryoprobe to ensure an adequate freeze. The less the lateral spread of the ice ball, the less the depth of the treatment (Figures 26-10 and 26-11).

After the ice ball is sufficiently formed, the cryogun is deactivated, and the cervix is allowed to thaw for approximately 4 to 5 minutes. During thawing, the central zone under the probe tip becomes soft. It is important not to remove the probe tip from the cervix until it is defrosted. Pulling the probe off the cervix before it is defrosted produces pain and bleeding. Although the question of whether a single freeze or a double freeze is more effective is controversial, in general, a freeze-thaw-freeze regimen is recommended.[49,56] If a freeze-thaw-freeze regimen is selected, the cryoprobe is again placed on the cervix, and another freeze is performed. This freeze should also be sufficiently long for a 7-mm ice ball to form. A 10-mm ice ball is ideal but is

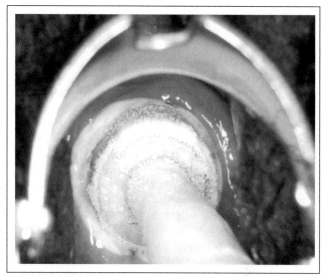

Figure 26-10 Probe applied to the cervical TZ. The ice ball can be seen forming peripheral to the edge of the probe.

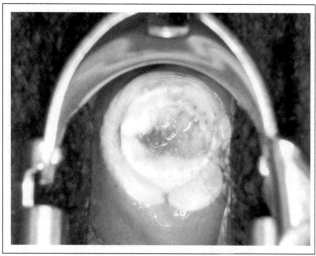

Figure 26-11 Appearance of the cervix after the cryoprobe is removed.

rarely achieved. Once the cervix has thawed, the cryoprobe is removed from the vagina.

On the day of the procedure, the tissue demonstrates erythema and hyperemia. Within the next 24 to 48 hours, bullae or vesicles form with associated edema. The tissue then sloughs. The eschar corresponds to the depth of the freeze. Cervices heal by granulation and re-epithelialization. *Re-epithelialization is complete in 47% of patients 6 weeks post-treatment and in all patients by 3 months*[57] (Figure 26-12).

Side Effects and Complications of Treatment

Cryotherapy of the cervix is usually accompanied by pain and cramping of varying degrees.[58] These cramps are produced by release of prostaglandins and are relieved by non-steroidal anti-inflammatory agents. Some advocate the use of local anesthesia at the time of cryotherapy to reduce pain associated with the procedure. About 3% of patients experience cramps severe enough to warrant stronger drugs. About 20% of patients experience flushing and lightheadedness; therefore patients should rise slowly from the examination table after the procedure. *Patients will experience a profuse, watery discharge for 2 to 3 weeks after the cryotherapy.*[57] Some clinicians believe the discharge may be decreased by the use of Amino-Cerv twice daily for 14 days. Removal of the eschar 2 days after the procedure does not significantly reduce the amount of discharge.[59] Cryotherapy is contraindicated in pregnancy; if there is a suspicion for cancer; if there is a discrepancy among the colposcopy, cytology, and histology results; or if an active cervical, vaginal, or pelvic infection exists.

Some individuals advocate that adolescents be tested for gonorrhea and chlamydia within 2 weeks of therapy.[53] Cervical stenosis sufficient to prevent passage of the cytobrush is rare. To minimize the risk of cervical stenosis, the external os should be probed at each follow-up visit. Serious complications related to cryotherapy are rare.[44] Possible complications include vasovagal episodes, infection, mucometria, infection, and bleeding. *There is no evidence that cryotherapy*

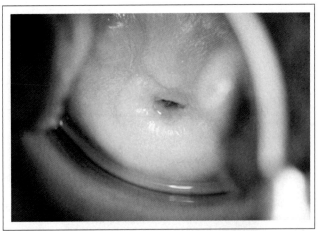

Figure 26-12 Appearance of cervix 3 months after cryotherapy. Note the hypertrophic appearance of the cervix and the paleness, especially near the os. This represents posttreatment stromal fibrosis.

has any adverse impact on fertility or pregnancy outcome,[60] *but these studies are contemporary with or precede studies on laser and LEEP that also showed no efect on fertility and pregnancy, so it may be inappropriate to conclude that cryotherapy is safer based on this comparison.*

COLD-KNIFE CONIZATION

For many years, and even before the popularity of colposcopy, CKC was the standard treatment for treating CIN when uterine conservation was the desired outcome. In more recent years, the ease with which laser conization and LEEP conization may be done, the fact that these procedures can be performed in outpatient settings, and their reduced morbidity relative to CKC have combined to create a trend whereby these newer procedures frequently replace CKC. Many practitioners have limited the use of CKC to situations in which very large conizations are needed or in which evaluation of the histology is critical and the risk of even a small possibility of cautery artifact at the margins cannot be tolerated. Such instances include cases in which invasive or microinvasive carcinoma is suspected and cases of adenocarcinoma *in situ* of the cervix. However, even with these indications, some believe that, in the hands of an experienced practitioner, laser conization or electrosurgical loop conization can provide an adequate specimen with respect to size and histologic quality.

Although some have suggested that CKC can be done with local anesthesia, *the risk of intraoperative bleeding and the need for surgical assistance (retraction) mean that this procedure is almost always done in the operating room.*

Technique

The patient is placed in the dorsal lithotomy position, and a speculum is inserted into the vagina, exposing the cervix. The TZ and the lesion are then delineated. If a colposcope is available, the procedure is done under direct colposcopic guidance, but if one is not available, the cervix is painted with Lugol's iodine to identify the limits of the TZ and the limits of the lesion.

A variety of techniques have been used in an attempt to limit blood loss during CKC. The most popular of these involves laterally placed hemostatic sutures at the proximal portion of the cervix to ligate the descending cervical branches of the uterine artery (Figure 26-13). Another approach is to inject a vasopressor agent directly into the substance of the cervix in a manner similar to that used in laser and LEEP conization. Many clinicians use both techniques. A circumferential incision is then made at the periphery of the TZ as delineated by colposcopy or Lugol's staining. The incision need not be circular and can follow the border of the TZ and lesion. The incision is then continued deeper, gradually tapering toward the endocervical canal until the specimen is removed (Figure 26-14). The size and shape of the specimen and the extent of the taper are all determined by the location and extent of disease. Grasping the cone specimen

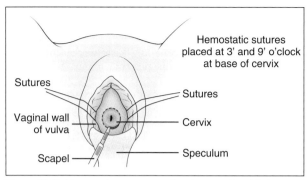

Figure 26-13 Hemostatic sutures are placed at 3 and 9 o'clock.

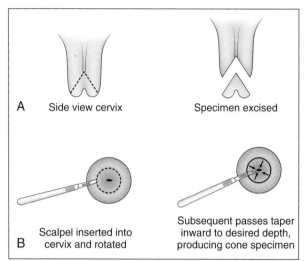

Figure 26-14 Demonstration of CKC.

with a tissue forceps facilitates traction and manipulation of the specimen. However, because this may cause trauma that will denude the cervical epithelium and make it impossible to adequately evaluate the cone histologically, some surgeons place traction sutures into the cone specimen at the start of the procedure and use these sutures to manipulate the specimen. Some of these sutures can be left in place at the conclusion of the procedure to help the pathologist identify the 12-o'clock position on the specimen.

After removal of the specimen, a variety of techniques can be used to achieve hemostasis of the cone bed. The traditional Sturmdorf suture is a vertical mattress suture that folds the remaining ectocervical epithelium into the conization bed and tamponades the bleeding vessels. Although effective at achieving hemostasis, this technique distorts the cervical anatomy and makes it very difficult to adequately visualize the TZ in the future. As a result, most authorities now advocate that bleeding in the conization bed be controlled by electrocautery, simple sutures, or even Monsel's paste, rather than by Sturmdorf sutures.

Complications

CKC has the highest complication rate of any of the treatments for CIN. Short- and long-term complications include primary and secondary hemorrhage, infection, cervical stenosis, and

increased pregnancy wastage. The incidence of significant bleeding after CKC is between 5% and 10%.[61] Should bleeding develop, it is important to evaluate the patient under ideal conditions. This involves visualization of the cervix to identify any bleeding site and treatment of the bleeding point with cautery or simple suturing. Generalized oozing can be treated with Monsel's paste or gel. In rare cases, a tight pack should be inserted into the vagina and the patient observed in the hospital for 24 hours. Despite significant bleeding, blood transfusion is rarely necessary.

Cervical stenosis occurs in 2% to 3% of patients who undergo CKC[61] although this is a relatively rare problem. It is more common that the entire TZ cannot be visualized after CKC, and this may represent a problem in follow-up.

The cause of infertility and pregnancy wastage after CKC is controversial[62–64]; however, *in all likelihood, the incidence of infertility and pregnancy wastage after CKC is directly related to the size of the cone itself.*[65] The larger the cone, the greater the incidence of infertility and preterm labor.

REFERENCES

1. Prendiville W, Cullimore J, Norman S. Large loop excision of the transformation zone (LLETZ). A new method of management for women with cervical intraepithelial neoplasia. Br J Obstet Gynaecol 1989;96:1054–1060.
2. Bigrigg MA, Codling BW, Pearson P, et al. Colposcopic diagnosis and treatment of cervical dysplasia at a single clinic visit: experience of low-voltage diathermy loop in 1000 patients. Lancet 1990;336:229–231.
3. Luesley DM, Cullimore J, Redman CWE, et al. Loop diathermy excision of the cervical transformation zone in patients with abnormal cervical smears. Br Med J 1990;300:1690–1693.
4. Spitzer M, Chernys AE, Seltzer VL. The use of large-loop excision of the transformation zone in an inner-city population. Obstet Gynecol 1993;82:731–735.
5. Gunasekera C, Phipps JH, Lewis BV. Large loop excision of the transformation zone (LLETZ) compared to carbon dioxide laser in the treatment of CIN: a superior mode of treatment. Br J Obstet Gynaecol 1990;97:995–998.
6. Hallam NF, West J, Harper C, et al. Large loop excision of the transformation zone (LLETZ) as an alternative to both local ablative and cone biopsy treatment: a series of 1000 patients. J Gynecol Surg 1993;9:77–82.
7. Alvarez RD, Helm CW, Edwards RP, et al. Prospective randomized trial of LLETZ versus laser ablation in patients with cervical intraepithelial neoplasia. Gynecol Oncol 1994;52:175–179.
8. Bigrigg MA, Codling BW, Pearson P, Read MD, Swingler GR. Colposcopic diagnosis and treatment of cervical dysplasia at a single clinic visit. Experience of low-voltage diathermy loop in 1000 patients. Lancet 1990;336:229–31.
9. Wright TC, Richart RM, Ferenczy AF: Electrosurgery for HPV-Related Lesions of the Anogenital Tract. New York: Arthur Vision, 1992.
10. Robinson WR, Webb S, Tirpack J, et al. Management of cervical intraepithelial neoplasia during pregnancy with loop excision. Gynecol Oncol 1997;64:153–155.
11. Oyesanya O, Amerasinghe C, Manning EAD. A comparison between loop diathermy conization and cold-knife conization

for management of cervical dysplasia associated with unsatisfactory colposcopy. Gynecol Oncol 1993;50:84–88.

12. Mor-Yosef S, Lopes A, Pearson S, et al. Loop diathermy cone biopsy. Obstet Gynecol 1990;775:884–886.

13. Baggish MS, Barash F, Noel Y, et al. Comparison of the thermal injury zones in loop electrical and laser cervical excisional conization. Am J Obstet Gynecol 1992;166:545–548.

14. Wright TC Jr, Richart RM, Ferenczy A, et al. Comparison of specimens removed by CO_2 laser conization and loop electrosurgical excision procedures. Obstet Gynecol 1992;79: 147–153.

15. Turner RJ, Cohen RA, Voet RL, et al. Analysis of tissue margins of cone biopsy specimens obtained with "cold-knife", CO_2 and Nd: YAG lasers and a radio frequency surgical unit. J Reprod Med 1992;37:607–610.

16. Wright TC Jr, Gagnon S, Richart RM, et al. Treatment of cervical intraepithelial neoplasia using the loop electrosurgical excision procedure. Obstet Gynecol 1992;79:173–178.

17. Keijser KG, Kenemans P, van der Zanden PH, et al. Diathermy loop excision in the management of cervical intraepithelial neoplasia: diagnosis and treatment in one procedure. Am J Obstet Gynecol 1992;166:1281–1287.

18. Murdoch JB, Grimshaw RN, Monaghan JM. Loop diathermy excision of the abnormal cervical transformation zone. Int J Gynecol Cancer 1991;1:105–133.

19. Lopes A, Pearson SE, Mor-Yosef S, et al. Is it time for a reconsideration of the criteria for cone biopsy? Br J Obstet Gynaecol 1989;96:1345–1347.

20. Doyle M, Warwick A, Redman C, et al. Does application of Monsel's solution after loop diathermy excision of the transformation zone reduce post-operative discharge? Results of a prospective randomized controlled trial. Br J Obstet Gynaecol 1992;99:1023–1024.

21. Whiteley PF, Olah KS. Treatment of cervical intraepithelial neoplasia: experience with the low-voltage diathermy loop. Am J Obstet Gynecol 1990;162:1272–1277.

22. Cullimore J. Management of complication from LLETZ. In: Prendiville W (ed). Large Loop Excision of the Transformation Zone: A Practical Guide to LLETZ. London: Chapman and Hall Medical, 1993, pp 88–91.

23. Spitzer M. Vaginal estrogen administration to prevent cervical os obliteration following cervical conization in women with amenorrhea. J Lower Genital Tract Dis 1997;1:53–56.

24. Cruickshank ME, Flannelly G, Campbell DM, et al. Fertility and pregnancy outcome following large loop excision of the cervical transformation zone. Br J Obstet Gynaecol 1995;102: 467–470.

25. Bigrigg A, Haffenden DK, Sheehan AL, et al. Efficacy and safety of large-loop excision of the transformation zone. Lancet 1994;343:32–34.

26. Blomfield PI, Buxton J, Dunn J, et al. Pregnancy outcome after large loop excision of the cervical transformation zone. Am J Obstet Gynecol 1993;169:620–624.

27. Haffenden DK, Bigrigg A, Codling BW, et al. Pregnancy following large loop excision of the transformation zone. Br J Obstet Gynaecol 1993;100:1059–1060.

28. Samson SL, Bentley JR, Fahey TJ, et al. The effect of loop electrosurgical excision procedure on future pregnancy outcome. Obstet Gynecol 2005;105:325–332.

29. Kyrgiou M, Koliopoulos G, Martin-Hirsch P, et al. Obstetric outcomes after conservative treatment for intraepithelial or early invasive cervical lesions: systematic review and meta-analysis. Lancet 2006;367:489–498.

30. Anderson MC. Treatment of cervical intraepithelial neoplasia with the carbon dioxide laser. Report of 543 patients. Obstet Gynecol 1982;59:720–725.

31. Wright VC, Davies E, Riopelle MA. Laser surgery for cervical intraepithelial neoplasia: principles and results. Am J Obstet Gynecol 1983;145:181–184.

32. Baggish MS. Laser management of cervical intraepithelial neoplasia. Clin Obstet Gynecol 1983;26:980–995.

33. Baggish MS. Complications associated with carbon dioxide laser surgery in gynecology. Am J Obstet Gynecol 1981;139:568–574.

34. Baggish MS, Dorsey JH, Adelson M. A ten-year experience treating cervical intraepithelial neoplasia with the CO_2. Am J Obstet Gynecol 1989;161:60–68.

35. Larsson G, Alm P, Grundsell H. Laser conization versus cold knife conization. Surg Gynecol Obstet 1982;154:59–61.

36. Fenton DW, Soutter WP, Sharp F, et al. A comparison of knife and CO_2 excisional biopsies. In: Sharp F, Jordan JA (eds). Gynecological Laser Surgery. New York: Perinatology Press, 1986, pp 77–84.

37. Spitzer M, Krumholz BA, Seltzer VL. Cervical os obliteration after laser surgery in patients with amenorrhea. Obstet Gynecol 1990;76:97–100.

38. Spitzer M, Herman J, Krumholz BA, et al. The fertility of women after cervical laser surgery. Obstet Gynecol 1995;86: 504–508.

39. Spitzer M. Fertility and pregnancy outcome after treatment of cervical intraepithelial neoplasia. J Lower Genital Tract Dis 1998;2:225–230.

40. Richart RM, Townsend DE, Crisp W, et al. An analysis of "long term" follow-up results in patients with cervical intraepithelial neoplasia treated with cryosurgery. Am J Obstet Gynecol 1980;137:823–826.

41. Arof H, Gerbie M, Smeltzer J. Cryosurgical treatment of cervical intraepithelial neoplasia: four-year experience. Am J Obstet Gynecol 1984;150:865–869.

42. Einerth Y. Cryosurgical treatment of CIN III. A long term study. Acta Obstet Gynecol Scan 1988;67:627–630.

43. Mitchell MF, Tortolero-Luna G, Cook E, et al. A randomized clinical trial of cryotherapy, laser vaporization, and loop electrosurgical excision for treatment of squamous intraepithelial lesions of the cervix. Obstet Gynecol 1998;92:737–744.

44. Nuovo J, Melnikow J, Willan A, et al. Treatment outcomes for squamous intraepithelial lesions. Int J Gynacol Obstet 2000;68:25–33.

45. Martin-Hirsch PL, Paraskevaidis E, Kitchener H. Surgery for cervical intraepithelial neoplasia. Cochrane Database of Systematic Reviews [computer file]. (2):CD001318, 2000.

46. Anderson M, Hartley R. Cervical crypt involvement by intraepithelial neoplasia. Obstet Gynecol 1980;55:546–550.

47. Boonstra H, Aalders J, Koudstaal J, et al. Minimum extension and appropriate topographic position of tissue destruction for treatment of cervical intraepithelial neoplasia. Obstet Gynecol 1990;75:227–231.

48. Ferris DG. Lethal tissue temperature during cervical cryotherapy with a small flat cryoprobe. J Fam Pract 1994;38:153–156.

49. Boonstra H, Koudstaal J, Oosterhuis J, et al. Analysis of cryolesions in the uterine cervix: application techniques, extensions and failures. Obstet Gynecol 1990;75:232–239.

50. Ferenczy A. Comparison of cryo and carbon dioxide laser therapy for cervical intraepithelial neoplasia. Obstet Gynecol 1985;66:793–798.

51. Ferris D, Ho J. Cryosurgical equipment: a critical review. J Fam Pract 1992;35:185–193.

52. Draeby-Kristiansen J, Garsaae M, Bruun M, et al. Ten years after cryosurgical treatment of cervical intraepithelial neoplasia. Am J Obstet Gynecol 1991;165:43–45.

53. Hillard P, Biro F, Wildey L. Complications of cervical cryotherapy in adolescents. J Reprod Med 1991;36:711–716.

54. Berget A, Andreasson B, Bock J. Laser and cryosurgery for intraepithelial neoplasia. A randomized trial with long-term follow-up. Acta Obstet Gynecol 1991;70:231–235.

55. Stienstra KA, Brewer BE, Franklin LA. A comparison of flat and shallow conical tips for cervical cryotherapy. J Am Board Fam Pract 1999;12:360–366.

56. Bryson S, Lenehan P, Lickrish G. The treatment of grade 3 cervical intraepithelial neoplasia with cryotherapy: an 11-year experience. Am J Obstet Gynecol 1985;151:201–206.

57. Townsend D, Richart R. Cryotherapy and carbon dioxide laser management of cervical intraepithelial neoplasia: a controlled comparison. Obstet Gynecol 1983;61:75–78.

58. Harper DM. Pain and cramping associated with cryosurgery. J Fam Pract 1994;39:551–557.

59. Harper DM, Mayeaux EJ Jr, Daaleman TP, et al. The natural history of cervical cryosurgical healing. The minimal effect of debridement of the cervical eschar. J Fam Pract 2000;49:694–700.

60. Montz FJ. Impact of therapy for cervical intraepithelial neoplasia on fertility. Am J Obstet Gynecol 1996;175:1129–1136.

61. Jones HW 3rd. Cone biopsy and hysterectomy in the management of cervical intraepithelial neoplasia. Clin Obstet Gynecol 1995;9:221–236.

62. Weber T, Obel EB. Pregnancy complications following conization of the uterine cervix. Acta Obstet Gynecol Scand 1979;58:347–351.

63. Bjerre B, Eliasson G, Linell F, et al. Conization as only treatment of carcinoma in situ of the uterine cervix. Am J Obstet Gynecol 1976;125:143–152.

64. Jones JM, Sweetnam P, Hibbard BM. The outcome of pregnancy after cone biopsy of the cervix: a case controlled study. Br J Obstet Gynecol 1979;86:913–916.

65. Leiman G, Harrison NA, Rubin A. Pregnancy following conization of the cervix: complications related to cone size. Am J Obstet Gynecol 1980;136:14–18.

CHAPTER 27

Colposcopy: Pitfalls and Tricks of the Trade

Mark Spitzer

The modern detection and prevention of cervical cancer is both an art and a science. The discrete steps including screening tests, diagnostic evaluation, and confirmatory biopsies have evolved over time based on scientific evidence and practitioner experience. Some expert colposcopists have tried to create objective scientific systems that would allow less-experienced practitioners to replicate the pattern recognition skills they have achieved through years of experience. This approach, called *colposcopic grading*, has become widely accepted in colposcopy as both a teaching and a clinical tool. One of these grading systems is the Reid Colposcopic Index.

Another approach to improving the care of all women has been the development of evidence-based guidelines, the purpose of which is to help guide clinicians toward the best practices in clinical care. Guidelines have been developed for cervical screening and the evaluation, treatment, and follow-up of women with abnormal screening tests and cervical biopsies. By carefully following these guidelines, clinicians avail themselves of the careful scientific analysis of the data used in the development of the guidelines. However, in the final analysis, the art of colposcopy and the scientific management of women with abnormal cervical screening tests and biopsy results are heavily dependent on the experience of the clinician. Clinicians with greater experience are able to use "tricks of the trade" developed over time to detect disease inaccessible to the novice practitioner and avoid errors that would potentially be made by their less-experienced colleagues.

FAILURE TO FOLLOW GUIDELINES

Some of the most common errors include the following: failure to identify significant disease and even cancer, failure to follow established guidelines such as the American Society for Colposcopy and Cervical Pathology (ASCCP) Consensus Guidelines for the Management of Women with Cervical Cytological and Histological Abnormalities, and *failure to follow up known abnormalities* (women with abnormalities who do not come for the initial or follow-up evaluations because they were never instructed to do so or were instructed but did not follow up). *Another major error that results in the failure to prevent cervical cancer is the failure to screen using established screening protocols.* Half of all women with cervical cancer in the United States had never been screened prior to their diagnosis, and another 10% had inadequate screening. *Overaggressive screening, management, and follow-up might also result in unfortunate consequences such as overtreatment, psychological consequences, and unnecessary costs.* All of these errors, their consequences, and strategies to avoid them are reviewed in the respective chapters that discuss these diseases. They will not be discussed in this chapter. Tips for the proper application of various therapeutic modalities such as cryotherapy and the loop electrosurgical excision procedure (LEEP) are reviewed in detail in Chapter 26 and will not be reviewed here.

The goal of this chapter is to try to convey to the reader some of the tricks of the trade and lessons that I have learned over many years of practice. Many of these tips have been mentioned and reviewed elsewhere in this book; others will only be mentioned here. It is my hope that the reader will be able to use my experience to avoid the need to learn from their own mistakes.

TIPS FOR CERVICAL SCREENING

Bleeding is one of the most common problems encountered when using an endocervical brush to do a Papanicolaou (Pap) test. The problem is greater when colposcopy is planned at that visit because persistent bleeding may interfere with the colposcopic examination. In my experience, bleeding sometimes results *when the cervix is deviated away from an axial position toward the direction of one of the vaginal fornices. If the clinician inserts the cytobrush in the axial plane, he or she will drill the brush into the cervical stroma, causing bleeding* (Figure 27-1, *A*). The solution is to *correct the orientation of the cervix by pushing a Pap spatula or tongue*

depressor into the opposite vaginal fornix to straighten the axis of the cervix and allow the brush cytology to be done atraumatically (Figure 27-1, *B*).

Another common mistake when doing a Pap test is twirling the endocervical brush in the endocervical canal. *Endocervical brush cytology is properly performed by turning the brush only 90 to 180 degrees in the canal.* This will minimize endocervical trauma and bleeding.

When I began using liquid-based cytology (using the *broom* collection device), I noticed that I was getting more than the usual number of reports with the absent endocervical cells. I began using a broom and an endocervical brush to obtain the smear and never had that problem again.

When I began screening women over the age of 30 with Pap plus human papillomavirus (HPV) testing, out of convenience, I sent only the liquid-based cytology specimen and asked the laboratory to run the HPV test from the residual fluid of the liquid-based cytology. Unfortunately, I found that 5% to 10% of my reports returned with insufficient fluid to run the HPV test. To understand the underlying reason, one needs to review the mechanics of liquid-based cytology (see Chapter 4.3). After receiving a specimen, the lab processes it in the following manner: The fluid, mixed with the collected cells, is passed through a filter. When enough of the pores in the filter are blocked by cells, the filtration is stopped, and the residual fluid remains for ancillary testing. If the fluid is hypocellular, more of the fluid/cell mixture is needed to create the smear, leaving less for HPV testing. My solution was to *use a separate brush collection device and transport medium (provided by the manufacturer) for the HPV test.* This assures that I will always get the HPV test report.

However, this approach sometimes creates a confusing problem. Consider the following situation: A woman older than age 30 is screened with a Pap plus HPV using liquid-based cytology for the Pap and separate specimen for the HPV test. The HPV test is negative, but the Pap is reported as atypical squamous cells of undetermined significance

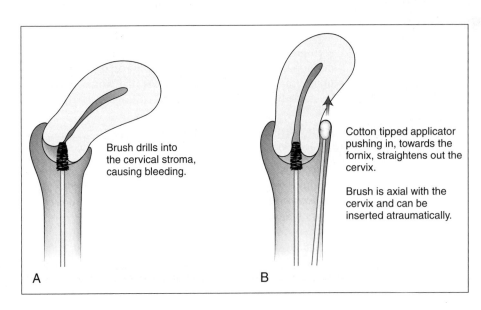

A, Brush drills into the cervical stroma, causing bleeding.

B, Cotton tipped applicator pushing in, towards the fornix, straightens out the cervix.

Brush is axial with the cervix and can be inserted atraumatically.

Figure 27-1 **A,** The cervix is deviated away from an axial position towards the direction of one of the vaginal fornices. If the clinician inserts the cytobrush in the axial plane, he or she will drill the brush into the cervical stroma, causing bleeding. **B,** The orientation of the cervix is corrected by pushing a Pap spatula or tongue depressor into the opposite vaginal fornix, straightening the axis of the cervix and allowing the brush cytology to be done atraumatically.

(ASC-US). The lab does reflex HPV testing on the residual fluid, and the result is positive. Now there are two HPV results: one positive and one negative. It is impossible to say whether this represents a false-positive result, a false-negative result, or a borderline HPV level where either a positive or a negative report are within the margin of error of the test. On a practical level, the patient should be managed according to the positive result, but the best approach is to avoid the problem by *asking the lab not to do reflex HPV testing when a separate specimen is sent for HPV testing.*

PREPARATION FOR COLPOSCOPY

The first and seemingly simplest step in performing colposcopy is the insertion of a vaginal speculum. Here, too, helpful hints are available. Choose the largest speculum that can be comfortably inserted. For most sexually active, premenopausal women, this will be a medium Graves speculum. In multiparous woman, a large speculum may be appropriate. Occasionally, in grand multiparous women or in pregnant women, vaginal laxity can cause the vaginal walls to prolapse through the vaginal speculum blades, blocking the view of the cervix. In such cases, it has been suggested that a condom or a finger of a latex glove with the tip cut off can be slid over the speculum before insertion. This maneuver will prevent the vaginal walls from prolapsing through the sides of the speculum and blocking your view. Those clinicians who have tried to do this know that this is almost impossible to perform with a large speculum

and still open the speculum properly. I prefer to use a lateral vaginal side wall retractor, similar to one used during LEEP procedures. However, even here, tricks of the trade exist. When inserting a vaginal side wall retractor, the pillars of the vaginal speculum limit the extent to which the retractor can be opened (Figure 27-2, *A*). *Using a speculum with pillars that are offset (a fish-mouth speculum) will allow you to take maximal advantage of the vaginal side wall retractor* (Figure 27-2, *B*).

Another obstacle is getting the cervix positioned between the blades of the vaginal speculum. This is especially a problem in obese women, in whom the tips of the speculum blades may not quite reach the vaginal vault. Here *it is helpful to have a longer (not wider) vaginal speculum.* Another approach is to *visualize the cervix just beyond the tips of the vaginal speculum and then have the patient cough strongly.* This will cause the cervix to descend. Once the cervix is between the blades of the speculum, it will usually stay there for the duration of the examination.

In women with vaginal laxity, it may be necessary to hold the speculum in place during the entire colposcopic examination to keep it from slipping out of position. It may also be necessary to manually hold the speculum in place if the cervix is very short (flush with the vaginal vault) or is markedly deviated (anteriorly, posteriorly, or laterally). Such colposcopic examinations are technically very difficult because they require at least three hands (one for the speculum, one for the biopsy forceps, and one to adjust the colposcope). Inexperienced colposcopists may be best advised to refer such patients to more "acrobatic" (experienced) colposcopists.

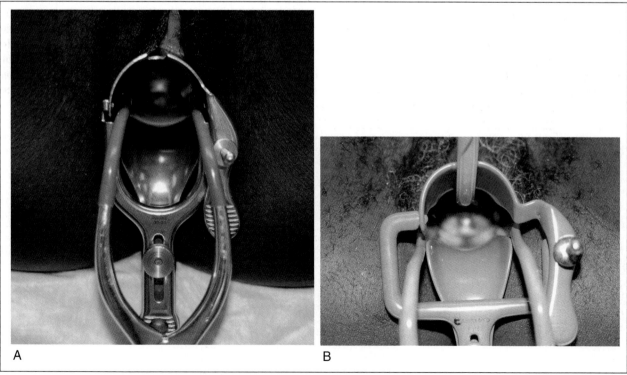

A

B

Figure 27-2 **A,** When inserting a vaginal side wall retractor, the pillars of the vaginal speculum prevent the retractor from being fully opened. **B,** Using a speculum with pillars that are offset will allow the clinician to take maximal advantage of the vaginal side wall retractor and obtain a better view of the cervix.

Colposcopy is best performed with a metal speculum rather than a plastic one. Metal speculums come in a greater variety of sizes and are more finely adjustable to the needs of the individual patient and colposcopic examination. Most metal speculums have two adjustment screws: one on the base that creates a greater opening at the introitus, and another that separates the blades, with the greatest separation at the vaginal vault. *When positioning a vaginal speculum for colposcopy, one should open the speculum a little at the introitus and a lot at the vaginal vault.* This is because opening the blades as much as possible opens and everts the cervix, improving visualization, and also increases the likelihood of a satisfactory colposcopic examination (Figure 27-3, *A*, *B*). Also, the amount of discomfort experienced by the patient is related more to the opening of the speculum at the introitus than at the vaginal vault.

COLPOSCOPIC EXAM

After inserting the vaginal speculum, properly visualizing the cervix, and noting any overt cervical or vaginal lesions, the next step in colposcopy is the application of dilute acetic acid. I find 5% acetic acid works best. This is plain vinegar that can be easily and cheaply obtained in a grocery store. Most brand names have 5% acidity. Some store brands have 4% acidity.

The dilute acetic acid can be applied to the cervix in a variety of ways; however, *the most important common denominator is that it is applied very liberally.* Spray bottles work well, but I prefer to use one or more well-soaked cotton balls placed on the cervix using a sponge forceps and left in place for at least 30 seconds. Gauze 2 × 2 pads do not retain as much acetic acid and can be abrasive to the cervix, so I avoid them. Some colposcopists use proctoswabs (scopettes) to apply acetic acid to the cervix. Although I do not use them because I find that they do not hold as much acetic acid as cotton balls, I have some useful tips for those

who use them. First, cut the swab to a useful length, *most proctoswabs are too long to be used for colposcopy unless they are cut shorter.* Also, *twirl the tip of the proctoswab back and forth in the acetic acid before use. This will loosen the cotton fibers and allow the swab to absorb much more liquid than just letting it sit in the acetic acid for a short period of time.*

One of the most common errors among novice colposcopists is impatience. At first, colposcopy seems quite easy: insert the speculum, apply dilute acetic acid, focus the colposcope, identify and biopsy white lesions. Initially, the most difficult aspect of the procedure is mastering the hand-eye coordination of focusing and taking biopsies. But I noticed that as novice colposcopists improve their hand-eye coordination, the examination takes less time and their ability to identify significant colposcopic lesions diminishes. This is because significant lesions often take time to develop (and also tend to fade more slowly). A clinician who is in a hurry will miss these lesions.

Other changes also occur with time. As acetowhite epithelium with mosaic and punctations begin to fade, the vasoconstrictive effect of acetic acid diminishes and even metaplastic vessels may appear coarse (Figure 27-4). In these cases, the hint that the lesion is not really a high-grade lesion is that it fades very quickly. *Acetowhite change in true high-grade lesions tends to persist for a long time without the need to repeatedly reapply dilute acetic acid.*

One of the biggest obstacles to adequate colposcopy is an obstructed view caused by blood, mucus, vaginal discharge, or even excessive acetic acid. In the presence of cervicitis or a large ectropion, merely dragging the tip of the speculum blades against the cervix while the speculum is being opened may be enough to cause this fragile tissue to bleed. Also, collecting a specimen for cytology or HPV testing using an endocervical brush might cause bleeding, especially when the brush is misdirected (see earlier discussion). *When such bleeding is encountered, the best solution is to apply pressure directly on the bleeding point for a long time (1–2 minutes). I find that a cotton ball soaked in dilute acetic acid works best.* A dry cotton ball leaves cotton fibers stuck to the cervix, and the acetic acid effect wears off

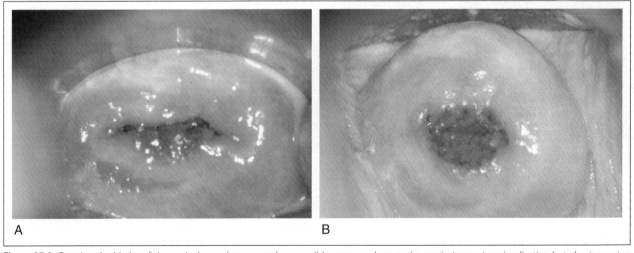

A B

Figure 27-3 Opening the blades of the vaginal speculum as much as possible opens and everts the cervix, improving visualization but also increasing the likelihood of a satisfactory colposcopic examination. **A,** Blades closed; **B,** blades opened.

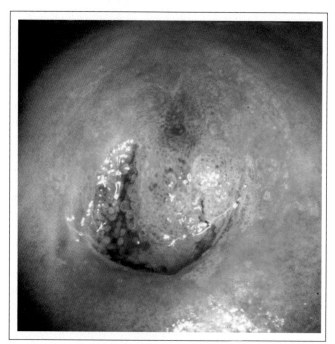

Figure 27-4 Metaplastic epithelium after the acetic acid effect has partially worn off. Punctations appear coarse.

in the interim. The use of acetic acid has the benefit of maintaining the acetic acid effect. Acetic acid also has a vasoconstrictive effect that is helpful in stopping the bleeding. The only place that I find a dry cotton-tipped applicator helpful is in the endocervical canal, which is usually already quite moist.

Troublesome cervical mucus may present in two ways: thick, tenacious mucus; and thin, watery mucus. During the luteal phase of the menstrual cycle and especially during pregnancy, thick, tenacious cervical mucus may be encountered. *The best approach to removing it is to gently twirl a cytobrush within the mucus, snag it, and then pull it off* (Figure 27-5). This may have to be repeated several times with a fresh cytobrush each time. It is important not to traumatize the

endocervix with the cytobrush in the process because doing so may cause bleeding that compounds the problem. The brush rarely needs to be inserted all the way into the canal as during a Pap test. *Another approach to viewing the endocervical canal when encountering thick mucus is to push the mucus farther into the canal, beyond the epithelium you are trying to evaluate.* Leave the applicator in place until you are finished evaluating the endocervical canal; otherwise the mucus will slide right back into your view (Figure 27-6).

The problem with clear mucus is not with the technique used to remove it (it is removed using the same techniques as with thick mucus). Rather, it is the mistaken belief by many colposcopists that because the mucus is so crystal clear, it is easy to see through and to evaluate the underlying epithelium without removing the mucus. This is simply not true. *Clear mucus obscures the visualization of the underlying epithelium just as much as thick mucus, making it impossible to identify any underlying atypical epithelium or evaluate the squamocolumnar junction (SCJ)* (Figure 27-7).

Another common mistake is to misidentify the SCJ when there is a small amount of blood in the endocervical canal. With this appearance, colposcopists may think they are seeing the SCJ when they are really seeing a squamo-blood junction. In order to properly evaluate such patients, the blood must be removed with a dry cotton-tipped applicator and the cervix re-evaluated (Figure 27-8).

Finally, what should be done if the SCJ is not fully visualized? If the canal is narrow, often nothing can be done to improve visualization. But if the canal is somewhat patulous, manipulation may allow visualization of all 360 degrees of the SCJ. The first step would be to open the tips of the speculum blades as much as possible. As mentioned previously, this tends to evert the cervix. The next approach would be to separate the cervix into quadrants and attempt to view each quadrant of the SCJ independently. *Rather than using a cotton-tipped applicator to manipulate or pry open the cervix at the os (this traumatizes the cervix and may cause bleeding or detach dysplastic epithelium), a cotton-tipped applicator should*

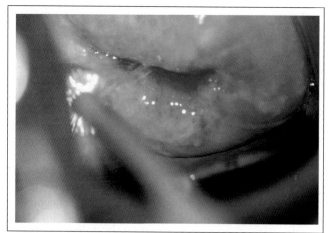

Figure 27-5 Use of a cytobrush to remove cervical mucus. (From Wright VC, Riopelle MA: Gynecologic CO$_2$ Laser Surgery—A Practical Handbook for Lower Genital Disease, 2nd ed. Figure 45, page 64. Houston: Biomedical Communications, 1991).

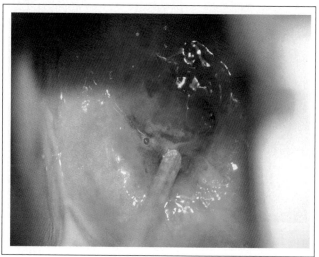

Figure 27-6 Use of a cotton-tipped applicator to push mucus farther into the canal beyond the epithelium being evaluated. (Courtesy of V. Cecil Wright).

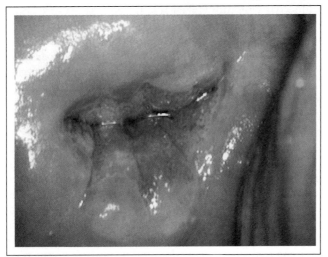

Figure 27-7 Clear mucus obscures the visualization of the underlying epithelium just as much as thick mucus, making it impossible to identify any underlying atypical epithelium or evaluate the SCJ. (From Wright VC, Riopelle MA: Gynecologic CO^2 Laser Surgery—A Practical Handbook for Lower Genital Disease, 2nd edition. Figure 70, page 77. Houseton: Biomedical Communications, 1991).

be inserted into the vaginal fornix and pushed inward to cause the cervix to deviate anteriorly or posteriorly. This allows easier visualization of the SCJ (Figure 27-9).

One approach that I do not use to aid in visualization of the SCJ is the use of an endocervical speculum. When used, this instrument may traumatize the endocervical canal and cause bleeding. Even in the best of circumstances, the blades of the endocervical speculum distort the endocervical epithelium, making it difficult to assess.

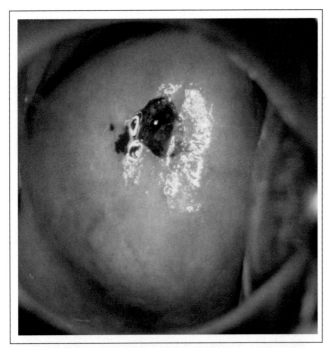

Figure 27-8 Squamo-blood junction. Blood obscures visualization of the SCJ. (From Wright VC, Riopelle MA: Gynecologic CO^2 Laser Surgery—A Practical Handbook for Lower Genital Disease, 2nd edition. Figure 21–24, page 21–19. Houston: Biomedical Communications, 1991).

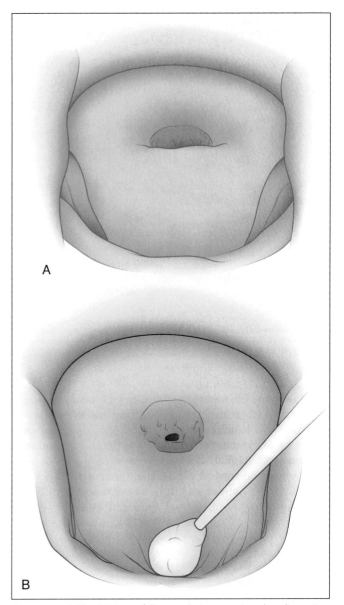

A

B

Figure 27-9 A, The SCJ is not fully seen. B, A cotton-tipped applicator is inserted into the posterior and pushed inward to cause the cervix to deviate posteriorly. This allows for easier visualization of the SCJ.

Before the advent of LEEP and before the implementation of the new 2006 management guidelines, full visualization of the SCJ (transformation zone [TZ]) had greater importance. Treatment often consisted of cervical ablation when the TZ was fully visualized and cold-knife conization when it was not. The difference in morbidity between these two procedures justified extraordinary efforts to visualize the TZ. Today laser ablation has fallen out of favor, and cryotherapy is inappropriate when disease extends into the endocervical canal (even if the SCJ is visualized with an endocervical speculum). Treatment of low-grade CIN is usually not indicated, and most high-grade CIN is treated by LEEP regardless of whether the TZ is fully visualized or not. Thus my practice is to make every attempt to visualize the SCJ, but I do not use an endocervical speculum.

If I cannot see the SCJ without it, I consider the colposcopy unsatisfactory and manage the patient appropriately.

DISCREPANCY BETWEEN CYTOLOGY AND COLPOSCOPY

One of the more difficult patients to manage is the older woman with vaginal atrophy and an abnormal Pap test. Colposcopy shows no atypical epithelium. Although disease in these women is often found in the endocervical canal, it is important to consider the possibility that the dysplastic epithelium is very thin (due to atrophy) and consequently is not presenting with significant acetowhitening. In such instances, *a 2- or 3-week course of nightly vaginal estrogen therapy will thicken the cervicovaginal epithelium and enhance the appearance of dysplastic epithelium that would not otherwise be seen.*

Another common cause of discrepancy between cytology findings and disease seen on the cervix is the presence of disease in the vagina. *Many colposcopists focus so intently on the cervix that they miss disease in the vaginal fornices or even behind the blades of the vaginal speculum* (Figure 27-10, *A* and *B*). My approach is to screen for disease in the vagina while I am applying dilute acetic acid to the cervix by moving the cervix from side to side and up and down, using the ring forceps holding the acetic acid-soaked cotton ball. After evaluating the cervix, if I am unable to identify the source of the abnormal Pap test, I will evaluate the vagina more thoroughly before assuming that the disease cannot be visualized or that the abnormal cytology is falsely positive.

One final attempt to identify previously unseen vaginal lesions is with the use of Lugol's solution. I reserve this as the last step because Lugol's solution will obscure the visualization of all colposcopic features (other than iodine positivity or negativity). Also, it is important to recognize that many benign conditions may cause the epithelium to reject iodine, including atrophy, glandular or metaplastic epithelium, and erosive conditions such as trauma or vaginitis.

SELECTION OF A BIOPSY SITE

Selecting a biopsy site is probably the most difficult colposcopic skill to learn. It requires correlation of the colposcopic appearance with the cervical biopsy result. However, because these results are separated over time, unless the colposcopist can reproducibly describe the colposcopic appearance of the cervix and refer back to it when the biopsy results are available, correlation is difficult to do. One way to effectively correlate colposcopy and pathology is to take colpophotographs and compare them with pathology results. However, colpophotography is also difficult to do well. The best available tool to obtain quality colposcopic images is cervicography, which is not widely available today. Most colposcopists develop their colposcopic correlation skills through mentorship with a more experienced colleague or through long clinical experience.

But using clinical experience or colposcopic grading to select a single worst lesion to biopsy is probably the biggest mistake a novice colposcopist can make. Novice colposcopists have not mastered colposcopic indices sufficiently to reliably and reproducibly apply them without error. But even for experienced colposcopists, grading is too inexact to be relied upon exclusively to identify the location of the highest-grade lesion. Rather, *it is more important to take*

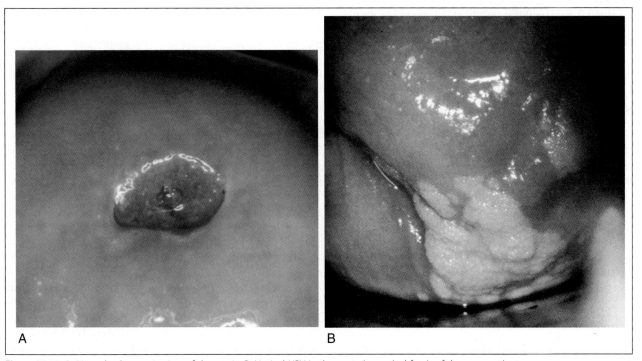

Figure 27-10 A, Normal colposcopic view of the cervix. **B,** Vaginal HPV in the posterior vaginal fornix of the same patient.

multiple biopsies representative of the various epithelial abnormalities identified colposcopically. Biopsies on the posterior aspect of the cervix should be taken first, so that any bleeding will not obscure visualization of subsequent biopsy sites.

ENDOCERVICAL CURETTAGE

A common mistake is the failure to do an endocervical curettage (ECC) when evaluating a previously treated patient. On colposcopy, the clinician may be able to evaluate what they believe to be 360 degrees of the SCJ. The colposcopy is believed to be satisfactory and the ECC optional. However, *in a previously treated patient the colposcopic principle that there is no such thing as a skip lesion is no longer valid.* Once the TZ is disrupted by cervical therapy, islands of metaplastic or lesional tissue may be left behind the newly formed SCJ. The colposcopy appears satisfactory, and yet there may be disease in the endocervical canal. *Whenever there is an abnormal Pap smear in a previously treated patient, ECC is mandatory.*

One controversy that has never been resolved is the timing of an ECC relative to the timing of other cervical biopsies. Two schools of thought exist. One advocates that a cervical biopsy may disrupt epithelium that would result in contamination of a subsequent ECC; therefore the ECC should be done first. The other school says that if the ECC were done first, it would cause bleeding that would obscure visualization and proper placement of subsequent biopsies. In the final analysis, neither argument is dominant and *the order in which an ECC is done is entirely arbitrary.*

Another controversy is how to obtain an ECC. There are two prevalent methods: One involves the use of an endocervical curette, and the other involves the use of an endocervical brush (the same one that is used to obtain endocervical cytology but rotated many more times in order to obtain endocervical tissue, not just exfoliated cells). The specimen is submitted in formalin, rather than in an alcohol-based preservative. The endocervical brush technique is more sensitive, but the endocervical curette is more specific. My approach is to take advantage of the benefits of both techniques. I perform a sharp curettage using an endocervical curette and then collect the specimen by rotating the endocervical brush many times in the endocervical canal to collect the entire specimen that may be trapped in the cervical mucus.

Getting the ECC specimen off the brush and into the formalin is challenging. One approach is to place the brush on a piece of Telfa, fold the Telfa over the cytobrush, and milk off the cellular material using the thumbnail. The Telfa can then be dropped into a formalin container. After collecting the specimen, I prefer to cut off the tip of the brush (or snap it off), put it in formalin, and let the pathologist extract the tissue. Asking the pathologist which method is preferred may answer the question.

HOW TO TAKE A BIOPSY

The goal of a cervical biopsy is to obtain a representative sample of the epithelial lesion while causing the least morbidity (usually bleeding) and discomfort for the patient. Because bleeding and discomfort are usually related to the size of the biopsy, *small biopsies are usually not only sufficient but in many ways better than larger ones, as long as they are representative.* Remember that unless cancer is suspected, little is gained by removing a large amount of cervical stroma. As long as the biopsy samples are just below the basement membrane, removing additional stroma (deeper biopsy) is not beneficial and adds morbidity. Another common mistake is the speed at which the jaws of the biopsy forceps are closed when taking the biopsy. There is apparently a natural instinct among novice colposcopists to snap the jaws quickly (take the biopsy before the patient realizes what is happening). This startles the patient and actually hurts more. In my experience, *if a sharp biopsy forceps is closed very gradually, the patient experiences less pain, and many patients do not even realize that the biopsy was done.* Another approach that minimizes discomfort is to ask the patient to cough when the biopsy is taken. When the colposcopist uses proper instrumentation and proper technique, the use of local or topical anesthesia at the time of colposcopy, or systemic analgesics or anxiolytics prior to colposcopy, is actually counterproductive because it tells the patient that this procedure will hurt a lot (the patient thinks "Otherwise, why would the colposcopist feel the need to give me anesthesia or analgesic or premedicate me with a tranquilizer?"). Rather the colposcopist needs to use proper technique and express confidently to the patient that the biopsy causes only a minor pinch and there is no reason to worry. A clinician who learns how to do painless colposcopic biopsies will often win the patient's confidence for life.

In order to do a small biopsy, many clinicians gravitate towards using smaller biopsy forceps (mini Tischler). I believe this is a mistake. *Small biopsy forceps will often slip off the intended biopsy site, resulting in no biopsy at all, a misdirected biopsy,* or (even worse) scraping a superficial layer of cells off the cervix, enough to damage the epithelium such that a repeat biopsy from that site will be difficult to interpret or *result in a biopsy that is uninterpretable.* The better alternative is to take a small biopsy with a regular biopsy forceps. This allows better control of both the biopsy size and the location.

When using a regular biopsy forceps, it is important to understand that it is not necessary to fill the forceps jaws in their entirety. This just causes unnecessary pain, bleeding, and difficulty in taking the biopsy. The situation is analogous to taking a bite of a sandwich. It is appropriate to take a small bite. In order to do this, you do not need a small mouth; you just need to partially fill a normal-sized mouth. Also, it would be inappropriate to stuff as much of the sandwich as possible into your mouth and then bite.

The technique for taking a biopsy should also be reviewed in a systematic fashion because proper technique will increase the likelihood of a successful biopsy. Most biopsy forceps have a rigid straight jaw and an angled, slightly shorter jaw that slips into the rigid jaw to detach the tissue when the forceps is closed (Figure 27-11). The cervical typography is uneven. Viewed from the introitus, the epithelium in the endocervical canal and the vaginal

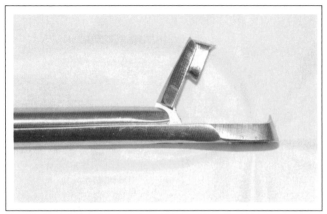

Figure 27-11 Biopsy forceps with a rigid straight jaw and an angled, slightly shorter jaw that slips into the rigid jaw to detach the tissue when the forceps is closed.

fornices are deeper and rise to the tip of the cervix. *When properly positioning the biopsy forceps to perform a biopsy, the jaws of the biopsy forceps should be centered over the lesion with the straight, rigid part of the forceps oriented to the deeper part of the cervix and the angled part of the forceps closer to the crown (apex) of the cervix* (Figure 27-12, *A* and *B*). The jaws of the forceps should be partially rather than completely opened. This approach will require the handle of the forceps be held "upside down" when the lesion is on the *endocervical canal side* of the *posterior lip* or the *vaginal portio side* of the *anterior lip* of the cervix. Depending on the location of the lesion, this will also require that the handle of the forceps be angled to properly center the lesion within the jaws of the forceps (Figure 27-13).

The technique is similar when taking a *vaginal biopsy*, but there is a propensity of the forceps to slip off the biopsy site. This is especially problematic when the epithelium is atrophic and flat, giving the forceps nothing to grip. The solution is either to *loosen the blades of the vaginal speculum,*

releasing the taughtness of the vagina, or *to tent the vaginal epithelium with a hook* (Figure 27-14).

CARE AND MAINTENANCE OF COLPOSCOPIC INSTRUMENTS

In conversations with Steven J. Sullivan, an innovator and developer of many of our modern colposcopy instruments, I learned much about the care of colposcopic instruments. In his experience, *lubrication is the one procedure that will extend the functional life of virtually all instruments with movable parts.* Sterilizing instruments in an autoclave saps vital lubricating oils from the instruments and can cause them to be stiff, close improperly or incompletely, or lock up and not move at all. Forcing the instrument to move without first lubricating it may damage it. The medical assistant who cares for your instruments should review and follow the manufacturer's instruction on lubrication, especially when instruments begin to stiffen or malfunction.

Biopsy forceps should always be kept *sharp*. This minimizes pain and avoids crush artifact when taking a biopsy. However, it is important to realize that biopsy forceps actually use a modified scissor cut, not a knife cut. Biopsy forceps cut by forcing the tissue between two pieces of metal that are very closely aligned. Neither of the jaws is *knife sharp*, nor do they use the sharpness of their edge to cut the tissue. *When a biopsy forceps is dull, it is often actually misaligned, and sharpening it to a knife edge removes metal and actually damages the forceps, making it harder to repair.* A manifestation of a misaligned biopsy forceps is incompletely detached tissue or a *"hanging chad"* biopsy. Having the biopsy forceps *sharpened* by someone unfamiliar with the function of these expensive instruments may damage them beyond repair. Malfunctioning instruments are best returned to the manufacturer for repair.

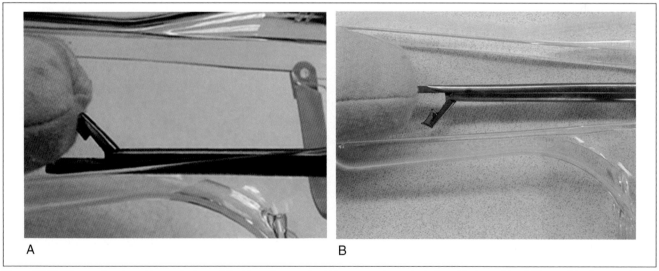

A   B

Figure 27-12 When performing a biopsy, the jaws of the biopsy forceps should be centered over the lesion with the straight, rigid part of the forceps oriented to the deeper part of the cervix and the angled part of the forceps closer to the crown (apex) of the cervix. **A,** Proper position on the posterior portio of the cervix. **B,** Proper position on the posterior endocervical canal side of the cervix.

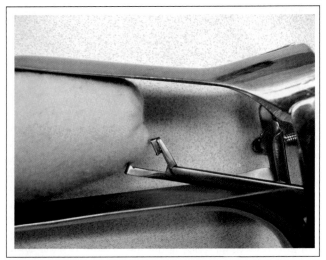

Figure 27-13 When performing a biopsy, the biopsy forceps may need to be angled to properly center the lesion within the jaws of the forceps. A biopsy of the periphery of the anterior lip of the cervix is demonstrated here.

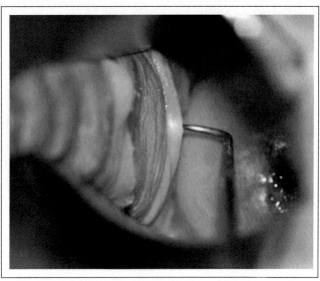

Figure 27-14 Use of a hook to tent the vaginal epithelium to take a biopsy.

Autoclaving instruments that have not first been properly cleaned may bake blood, tissue, or surgical residue on the instrument and interfere with proper function. Certain caustic or corrosive solutions may also damage instruments. Refer to package inserts for the appropriate solutions to use or avoid. Instruments should also be handled gently to avoid physically damaging them. Do not *drop* them or *throw* them into a bucket after use; rather, place them in the bucket gently. Use of a rubber bucket will decrease physical damage.

I hope that the reader found this chapter helpful. I would emphasize that these hints reflect my own experience. The experience of others may have taught them other or different approaches to the colposcopic examination. That is the nature of experience, and there is no substitute for it.

Index